CLINICAL HYPERTENSION

Sixth Edition

Norman M. Kaplan, M.D.

Professor of Medicine
Department of Internal Medicine
University of Texas Southwestern Medical School
Dallas, Texas

WITH A CHAPTER BY

Ellin Lieberman, M.D.

Professor of Pediatrics
University of Southern California
School of Medicine
Los Angeles, California

Editorial Consultant

William W. Neal, M.D.

Staff Physician
Veterans Administration Medical Center
Dallas, Texas

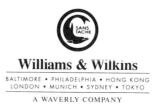

Williams & Wilkins

BALTIMORE • PHILADELPHIA • HONG KONG
LONDON • MUNICH • SYDNEY • TOKYO

A WAVERLY COMPANY

Editor: David C. Retford
Managing Editor: Molly L. Mullen
Copy Editor: John M. Daniel
Designer: Norman W. Och
Illustration Planner: Ray Lowman
Production Coordinator: Barbara J. Felton
Cover Designer: Wilma E. Rosenberger

Copyright © 1994
Williams & Wilkins
428 East Preston Street
Baltimore, Maryland 21202, USA

Accurate indications, adverse reactions, and dosage schedules for drugs are provided in this book, but it is possible that they may change. The reader is urged to review the package information data of the manufacturers of the medications mentioned.

Printed in the United States of America

First Edition 1973
Second Edition 1978
Third Edition 1982
Fourth Edition 1986
Fifth Edition 1990
Chapter reprints are available from the Publisher.

Library of Congress Cataloging-in-Publication Data

Kaplan, Norman M., 1931–
    Clinical hypertension / Norman M. Kaplan: with a chapter by Ellin Lieberman; editorial consultant, William W. Neal.—6th ed.
        p. cm.
    Includes bibliographical references and index.
    ISBN 0-683-04544-X
    1. Hypertension.   I. Lieberman, Ellin.   II. Title.
    [DNLM: 1. Hypertension.   WG 340 K17c 1994]
    RC685.H8K35 1994
    616.1'32—dc20
    DNLM/DLC
    for Library of Congress   93-27557
                                                                        CIP

94 95 96 97 98
1 2 3 4 5 6 7 8 9 10

To those such as:

Goldblatt and Grollman,
Folkow and Pickering,
Braun-Menéndez and Page,
Tobian and Laragh,
Chesley and Freis,
and the many others,

whose work has made it possible for me to
put together what I hope will be a useful book
on clinical hypertension.

Preface to the Sixth Edition

This book represents the distillation of a tremendous volume of literature, filtered through the receptive but, I hope, discriminating awareness of a single author. When I wrote the first edition in 1973, the task was challenging mainly because few had tried a synthesis of what was then known. But—as most who read this book are well aware—in the ensuing 20 years, the task has become much more difficult, mainly because the literature of hypertension has grown so that it is almost beyond the grasp of any one person. I continue to be a single author (with the important exception of the chapter on children written by Dr. Ellin Lieberman) for these two reasons:

- First, a single-authored text should offer more cohesion and completeness and, at the same time, brevity and lack of repetition, in comparison to the usual multi-authored but rarely edited mega-book.

- Second, I have the time, energy, and interest to keep up with the literature, and this book has become the major focus of my professional life. The success of the previous editions and the many compliments received from both clinicians in the field and investigators from the research bench have prompted me to do it again.

The very reason that a single-authored text has become such a rarity explains the need for a new edition fairly often. As with previous editions, almost every page has been revised, using the same goals:

- Give more attention to the common problems. Primary (essential) hypertension takes up almost half of the book.

- Cover every form of hypertension at least briefly, providing references for those seeking more information. Additional coverage is provided to some topics that are unusual but more interesting because new insights about them have become available. An example is glucocorticoid remediable aldosteronism, the genetic basis of which has been uncovered.

- Include the latest data, even if available only in abstract form.

- Provide enough pathophysiology to permit sound clinical judgment.

- Be objective and clearly identify biases. Although my views may counter those of others, I have tried to give reasonable attention to those with whom I disagree.

At the request of readers, the full references are now provided, rather than the abbreviated ones in previous editions. This takes up more space, so to limit the length of the book, some of the original and multiple subsequent sources have been deleted in favor of more recent and inclusive references. Some truly classic references have been kept, but I apoligize to authors whose original contributions have been preempted by references to subsequent work of others.

Once again I am pleased that Dr. Ellin Lieberman, Head of Pediatric Nephrology at the Children's Hospital of Los Angeles, has contributed a chapter on hypertension in children and adolescents. I am particularly indebted to Dr. William Neal for the many hours spent in proofing and organizing the content. I have been fortunate in being in an academic setting wherein such endeavors are nurtured, much to the credit of my former chief, Dr. Donald Seldin, and my current chief, Dr. Daniel Foster. I have been greatly helped by my secretaries, Diana Dubois and Sharon Washington. And lastly, the forbearance of Audrey, my wife, can only be acknowledged by the promise that I will not do it again—at least for another four years.

As with previous editions, I am amazed at the tremendous amount of new information published over the past four years. A considerable amount of significant new information is included in this edition, presented in a manner that I hope enables the reader to grasp its significance and place it in perspective. Once again, I hope that this book will prove both interesting and informative for those who care for the millions of people with hypertension, our most common disease.

Contents

1 Hypertension in the Population at Large

Most people will develop hypertension during their lifetime. As a consequence of the increased awareness of the frequency of hypertension and with the recognition that the progress of hypertension-induced cardiovascular disease can be slowed, if not stopped, by its treatment, the management of hypertension is now the leading indication for both visits to physicians and for the use of prescription drugs in the United States. According to the National Ambulatory Care Survey, there were over 85 million office visits related to hypertension and almost 300 million blood pressure measurements taken in 1991 (Schappert, 1993).

These leading positions are reflected in the data from the surveys of a representative sample of the U.S. population, the National Health and Nutrition Examination Surveys (NHANES), taken over the past 20 years. As seen in Figure 1.1, the percentages of people in the U.S. who are aware of their hypertension, who are receiving treatment, and whose hypertension is controlled have risen progressively. Similar improvements in awareness and control have been reported in other industrialized countries such as Canada (Joffres et al., 1992) and Israel (Green and Peled, 1992).

As impressive as these data are, most hypertension remains poorly controlled, both in industrialized societies (Wilhelmsen and Strasser, 1993) and, even more so, in less developed countries (Elbagir and Ahmed, 1990; Nan et al., 1991). As a result, hypertension-influenced diseases remain the most common causes of morbidity and mortality in developed societies.

Moreover, the main burdens associated with hypertension occur not in the relatively few with severe disease but in the masses of patients with blood pressures that are only minimally elevated (Stamler et al., 1993).

This book will attempt to summarize and analyze the work of thousands of clinicians and investigators worldwide who have advanced our knowledge about the mechanisms behind hypertension and who have provided increasingly effective therapies for its control. Despite their continued efforts, however, hypertension will almost certainly not be conquered because it is one of those diseases that, in the words of a *Lancet* editorialist (Anonymous, 1993), "afflict us from middle age onwards [that] might simply represent 'unfavorable' genes that have accumulated to express themselves in the second half of our lives. This could never be corrected by any evolutionary pressure since such pressures act only on the first half of our lives: once we have reproduced, it does not greatly matter that we grow 'sans teeth, sans eyes, sans taste, sans everything.' "

In this chapter, the overall problems of hypertension for the population at large are considered. I attempt to define the disease, quantify its prevalence and consequences, classify its types, and describe the current status of detection and control. Chapter 2 covers the measurement of the blood pressure and the management of its variability.

CONCEPTUAL DEFINITION OF HYPERTENSION

Although it has been more than 100 years since Mahomed clearly differentiated hyperten-

1

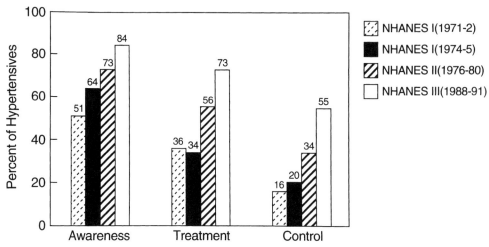

Figure 1.1. Hypertension awareness, treatment, and control (threshold, 160/95). Percentages of the National Health and Nutrition Examination Surveys (NHANES) populations with hypertension (defined as a blood pressure of 160/95 mm Hg or more on one or two examinations) who were aware of the condition, who were receiving treatment, and whose hypertension was controlled. Source: Centers for Disease Control and Prevention, National Center for Health Statistics. (Composed from the Joint National Committee. The fifth report of the Joint National Committee on Detection, Evaluation, and Treatment of High Blood Pressure (JNC V). *Arch Intern Med* 1993;153:154–183.)

sion from Bright's renal disease, authorities still debate the level of blood pressure considered abnormal. Sir George Pickering for many years challenged the wisdom of that debate and decried the search for an arbitrary dividing line between normal and high blood pressure. In 1972 he restated his argument: "There is no dividing line. The relationship between arterial pressure and mortality is quantitative; the higher the pressure, the worse the prognosis." He viewed "arterial pressure as a quantity and the consequence numerically related to the size of that quantity" (Pickering, 1972).

However, as Pickering realized, physicians feel more secure when dealing with precise criteria, even if the criteria are basically arbitrary. To consider a blood pressure of 138/88 mm Hg normal and one of 140/90 high is obviously arbitrary, but medical practice requires that some criteria be used to determine the need for workup and therapy. The criteria should be established on some rational basis that includes the risks of disability and death associated with various levels of blood pressure, as well as the ability to reduce those risks by lowering the blood pressure. As stated by Rose (1980), "The operational definition of hypertension is the level at which the benefits...of action exceed those of inaction."

Even this definition should be broadened because action—that is, making the diagnosis of hypertension at any level of blood pressure—

involves risks and costs as well as benefits, and inaction may provide benefits (Table 1.1). Therefore, in 1983 I proposed that the conceptual definition of hypertension be "that level of blood pressure at which the benefits (minus the risks and costs) of action exceed the risks and costs (minus the benefits) of inaction" (Kaplan, 1983).

Most elements of this conceptual definition are fairly obvious, although some, such as interference with lifestyle and risks from biochemical side effects of therapy, may not be (those will be discussed further in this and later chapters). Let us turn first to the major consequence of inaction, the increased incidence of premature cardiovascular disease, since that is widely considered to be the prime, if not the sole, basis for determining the level of blood pressure which is considered abnormal.

Risks of Inaction: Increased Incidence of Cardiovascular Disease

The risks of elevated blood pressure have been determined from large-scale epidemiologic surveys. MacMahon et al. (1990) performed a meta-analysis of all available major prospective observational studies relating diastolic blood pressure (DBP) level to the incidence of stroke and coronary heart disease (CHD). In the nine studies analyzed, almost 420,000 people were followed up for 6 to 25 years. A total of 599 fatal strokes and 4,260 deaths from CHD were recorded.

Table 1.1   Factors Involved in the Conceptual Definition of Hypertension

	Benefits	Risks and Costs
Action	Reduce risk of cardiovascular disease, debility, and death Decrease monetary costs of catastrophic events	Assume psychological burdens of "the hypertensive patient" Interfere with quality of life Require changes in lifestyle Add risks and side effects from drug therapy Add monetary costs of routine health care
Inaction	Preserve "nonpatient" role Maintain current lifestyle and quality of life Avoid risks and side effects of drug therapy Avoid monetary costs of routine health care	Increase risk of cardiovascular disease, debility, and death Increase monetary costs of catastrophic events

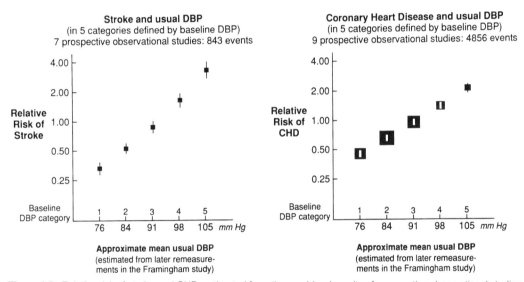

Figure 1.2. Relative risk of stroke and CHD, estimated from the combined results of prospective observational studies for five categories of DBP. (Estimates of the usual DBP in each baseline DBP category are from mean DBP values in the Framingham study recorded 4 years after baseline measurement.) The *solid squares* represent disease risk in each category relative to risk in the whole study population (square size is proportional to the number of events in each DBP category). *Vertical lines* represent 95% confidence intervals for the estimates of relative risk. (Reproduced with permission from MacMahon S, Peto R, Cutler J, et al. Blood pressure, stroke, and coronary heart disease. Part 1, Prolonged differences in blood pressure: prospective observational studies corrected for the regression dilution bias. *Lancet* 1990;335:765–773.)

The overall results demonstrate "direct, continuous and apparently independent associations" with "no evidence of any 'threshold' level of DBP below which lower levels of DBP were not associated with lower risks of stroke and CHD" (Fig. 1.2). In reaching this conclusion, MacMahon et al. considered the common practice in all nine studies to measure DBP only once, which leads to a substantial underestimation of the true association of the usual or long-term average DBP with disease. By applying a correction factor based on three sets of readings recorded over 4 years in the Framingham study to all nine sets of data, MacMahon et al. came up with estimates of risk that are about 60% greater than those previously published using uncorrected data. They estimate that a DBP that is persistently higher by 5.0 mm Hg is associated with at least a 34% increase in stroke risk and at least a 21% increase in CHD risk.

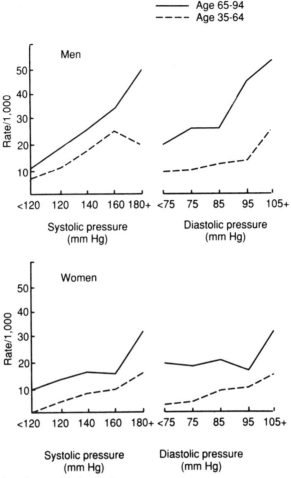

Figure 1.3. Annual rate of cardiovascular disease by age, gender, and level of systolic and diastolic blood pressure based on 30-year follow-up in the Framingham study. (Reproduced with permission from Levy DL, Kannel WB. Cardiovascular risks: new insights from Framingham. *Am Heart J* 1988;116:266–272).

Gender and Risk

Ninety-six percent of the subjects followed up in the nine epidemiologic surveys analyzed by MacMahon et al. (Fig. 1.2) were men. Studies of women have shown that they tolerate hypertension better than men, having lower morbidity and mortality rates from any level of hypertension (Vokonas et al., 1988). Although it takes higher blood pressures to hurt women, when their pressures are high, they *do* suffer. This has been clearly demonstrated in the Framingham study (Fig. 1.3) and in actuarial data (Society of Actuaries, 1979). Nonetheless, the lower rates of cardiovascular disease at all levels of DBP and systolic blood pressure (SBP) among women aged 35 to 64 years and even more strikingly among those aged 65 to 94 years who were followed up for 30 years in the Framingham study suggest that somewhat higher levels of blood pressure could be used to define hypertension among women.

Race and Risk

Blacks tend to have higher levels of blood pressure than non-blacks, and overall mortality rates at all levels are higher among blacks (Neaton et al., 1984). In the Multiple Risk Factor Intervention Trial (MRFIT) which involved more than 23,000 black men and 325,000 white men followed for 10 years, an interesting racial difference was confirmed: the mortality rate of CHD was lower in black men with DBPs above 90 mm Hg than in white men (relative risk, 0.84), but the mortality rate of cerebrovascular disease was higher (relative risk, 2.0) (Neaton et al., 1989).

The greater risk of hypertension among blacks suggests that more attention must be given to even low levels of hypertension among this group, but there seems little reason to use different criteria to diagnose hypertension in blacks than in whites. The special features of hypertension in blacks are discussed in more detail in Chapter 4.

The relative risk of hypertension in both frequency and type of cardiovascular complications differs among other racial groups as well. In particular, the number of deaths due to cardiovascular diseases is lower among Hispanic men in the United States than in non-Hispanic white men despite their higher cardiovascular risk scores (Mitchell et al., 1990) and less adequate control of hypertension than observed among non-Hispanics (Haffner et al., 1993).

Age and Risk: The Elderly

The number of people over age 65 is rapidly increasing and, in less than 50 years, one of every five people in the United States will be older than 65 (Schneider and Guralnik, 1990). Blood pressure, particularly SBP, tends to increase progressively with age (Fig. 1.4) (Row-

land and Roberts, 1982), and elderly people with hypertension have a greater risk of cardiovascular disease (Fig. 1.3). How these risks can be significantly reduced by lowering the blood pressure is covered in Chapter 5, and more about the epidemiology and course of hypertension in this population is provided in Chapter 4.

Isolated Systolic Hypertension. With increasing age, the prevalence of isolated systolic hypertension, defined as a DBP less than 90 mm Hg and a SBP greater than 160 mm Hg, rises progressively and is about 25% in people aged 80 years (Staessen et al., 1990). Over a 30-year interval in the Framingham study, elevations in SBP were more determinate of risk for both strokes and heart attacks than elevations in DBP (Vokonas et al., 1988).

The Old Versus the Very Old. As people advance into their 70s and 80s, hypertension becomes less of a risk factor. In fact, unlike what has been seen in people younger than 65, 3-year mortality rates have been found to be *lower* in those aged 85 to 88 years with blood pressures between 140/70 and 169/99 mm Hg than in those with either higher or lower levels (Heikinheimo

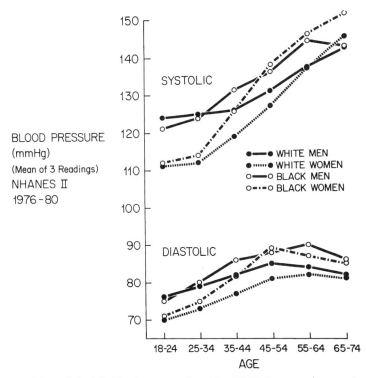

Figure 1.4. Mean systolic and diastolic blood pressures for white and black men and women in various age groups in the 1976–1980 National Health and Nutrition Examination Survey (NHANES II). (Reproduced with permission from Rowland M, Roberts J. Blood pressure levels and hypertension in persons ages 6–74 years. United States, 1976–80. *NCHS Advance Data, No. 84, Vital and Health Statistics of the National Center for Health Statistics.* US Department of Health and Human Services. Washington, DC, Oct 8, 1982.)

et al., 1990). Similar data have been reported in a 10-year follow-up of men aged 80 years or older; all-cause and cardiovascular survival rates were *higher* among those with higher DBP, an observation that could not be explained by multiple biologic or historic factors (Langer et al., 1991).

It may be that people who live to a very old age despite elevated blood pressures are immune to the adverse effects of hypertension or that low blood pressure in the very old is simply a marker of an impending cardiovascular event. Regardless of the explanation, the data suggest that people older than 75 with mildly elevated blood pressures may not require treatment. Nonetheless, hypertension remains a risk for the overall population over the age of 65.

Systolic Versus Diastolic

As noted, isolated systolic hypertension is clearly a marker of cardiovascular disease in the elderly, which is not surprising since such systolic hypertension is in itself a reflection of rigid, atherosclerotic arteries. However, systolic elevations are more determinate of cardiovascular risk than diastolic elevations in all adults, as seen among the 316,000 men followed up for an average of 12 years in the MRFIT (Neaton and Wentworth, 1992) (Fig. 1.5). The high pressures generated during systole place an immediate, direct burden on the heart and vasculature so, logically, all forms of cardiovascular disease occur more frequently with elevated SBP.

Relative Versus Absolute Risk

In most of the data presented to this point, the risks of elevated blood pressure have been presented relative to risks found with lower levels of blood pressure. This way of looking at risk tends to exaggerate its degree. For example, data from the Pooling Project (Pooling Project Research Group, 1978) show a 52% increase in the relative risk for coronary disease over an 8.6-year interval for white men with initial DBP of 80–87 mm Hg, as compared with the risk for those with DBP less than 80 mm Hg (Table 1.2). The 52% increase is derived by taking the rate of major coronary events per 1000 persons in the two groups (100.6 and 66.0, respectively) and dividing the difference (34.6) by the rate of the group with the lower DBP (66.0). This 52% increase in relative risk, then, corresponds to only a 3.5% increase in absolute risk (34.6 per 1000). The importance of this greater risk with higher pressure should not be ignored, but the use of the smaller change in absolute risk rather than the larger change in relative risk seems more appropriate when applying epidemiologic statistics to individual patients.

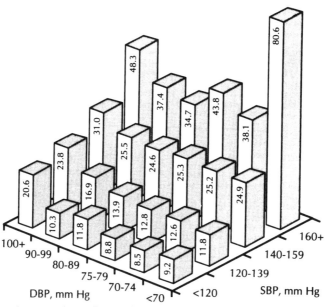

Figure 1.5. Age-adjusted coronary heart disease death rates per 10,000 person-years by level of SBP and DBP for men screened in the Multiple Risk Factor Intervention Trial. (Reproduced with permission from Neaton JD, Wentworth D. Serum cholesterol, blood pressure, cigarette smoking, and death from coronary heart disease. Overall findings and differences by age for 316,099 white men. *Arch Intern Med* 1992;152:56–64.)

Table 1.2.   Risk (8.6-Year) for Major Coronary Events in 7054 White Men

Diastolic BP at Entry[a] (mm Hg)	Major Coronary Events (per 1,000)	Adjusted Rate of Relative Risk	Absolute Excess Risk (per 1,000)
Below 80 (quintiles 1 and 2)	66.0	1.0	–
80–87 (quintile 3)	100.6	1.52	34.6
88–95 (quintile 4)	109.4	1.66	43.4
Above 95 (quintile 5)	143.3	2.17	77.3

Data reprinted with permission of The Pooling Project Research Group. Relationship of blood pressure, serum cholesterol, smoking habit, relative weight, and ECG abnormalities to incidence of major coronary events: final report of the Pooling Project. *J Chronic Dis* 1978;31:201–306. Copyright American Heart Association, Inc.
[a]Blood pressure ranges varied slightly for various 5-year age groups (40–44 years, 45–49, etc.).

Fortunately, data from the Framingham study can be used to assess the actual risk for patients more than 35 years old. As we shall see in Chapter 4, that risk is unevenly distributed and closely related to the number and extent of concomitant risk factors.

For now, the problem seems well defined. For the population at large, risk clearly increases with every increment in blood pressure, and levels of blood pressure that are accompanied by significantly increased risks should be called "high." As Stamler et al. (1993) note: "Among persons aged 35 years or more, most have BP above optimal ($<120/<80$ mm Hg); hence, they are at increased CVD risk, ie, the blood pressure problem involves most of the population, not only the substantial minority with clinical hypertension." However, for individual patients, the absolute risk from slightly elevated blood pressure may be quite small. Therefore, more than just the level of blood pressure should be used to determine risk and, even more importantly, to diagnose a person as hypertensive and begin treatment.

Benefits of Action: Reducing Cardiovascular Disease

Let us now turn to the major benefit listed in Table 1.1 that is involved in a conceptual definition of hypertension, the level at which it is possible to show the benefit of reducing cardiovascular disease by lowering the blood pressure. Inclusion of this factor is predicated on the assumption that it is of no benefit—and, as we shall see, is potentially harmful—to label a person hypertensive if nothing will be done to lower the blood pressure.

Natural Versus Treatment-Induced Blood Pressure

Before proceeding, one caveat is in order. As noted earlier, less cardiovascular disease is seen in people with low blood pressure who are not receiving antihypertensive therapy. However, that fact cannot be used as evidence to support the benefits of therapy because naturally low blood pressure may offer a degree of protection not provided by a similarly low blood pressure resulting from antihypertensive therapy.

The available evidence supports that view: morbidity and mortality rates, particularly those of coronary disease, continue to be higher in patients undergoing antihypertensive drug treatment than in untreated people with similar levels of blood pressure. This has been shown in follow-up studies of multiple populations (Yano et al., 1983; Kannel et al., 1988; Strandberg et al., 1991; Clausen and Jensen, 1992). This issue is discussed in more detail in Chapter 5. For now, let us consider two of these studies. Yano et al. (1983) conducted a 10-year follow-up of 7610 Japanese men in Hawaii aged 45 to 68 years at baseline. Mortality due to cardiovascular diseases overall, coronary heart disease, and stroke was higher in those receiving antihypertensive therapy at baseline than in the untreated men with comparable blood pressures (Fig. 1.6). The authors conclude that "after adjustment of age, blood pressure, and nine other risk factors in multivariate logistic analysis, antihypertensive medication remained significant as a risk factor for CVD, CHD, and stroke."

Using data from the Framingham study, Kannel et al. (1988) reported that the risk of sudden death increased more than twofold over 30 years among people receiving antihypertensive drug treatment. This escalated risk was not accounted for by higher pressure or any other known predisposing factor for sudden death.

These disquieting data should not be taken as evidence against the use of antihypertensive drug therapy. They do not, in any way, deny that protection against cardiovascular complications can be achieved by successful reduction of blood

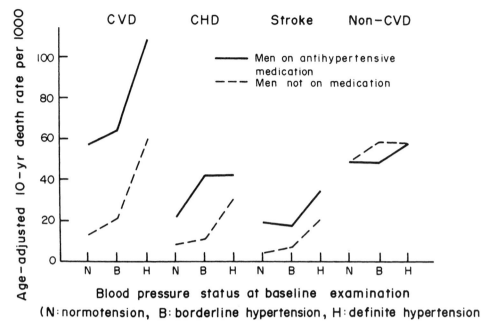

Figure 1.6. Age-adjusted 10-year mortality rates of cardiovascular diseases (CVD), CHD, stroke, and other causes (non-CVD) among men grouped by baseline blood pressure status and use of antihypertensive medication. (Reprinted with permission from Yano K, McGee D, Reed DM. The impact of elevated blood pressure upon 10-year mortality among Japanese men in Hawaii: the Honolulu Heart Program. *J Chronic Dis* 1983;36:569–579. Copyright 1983, Pergamon Press PLC.)

pressure with drugs. They simply indicate that the protection provided may be only partial for one or more reasons, including the following: (*a*) only a partial reduction of blood pressure may be achieved, (*b*) irreversible hypertensive damage may be present, (*c*) other risk factors that accompany hypertension may not be improved, or (*d*) there are dangers inherent to the use of some drugs. Whatever the explanation, these data document a difference between natural and induced levels of blood pressure.

Rationale for Reducing Elevated Blood Pressure

In contrast to the data above, considerable experimental, epidemiologic, and clinical evidence indicates that reducing elevated blood pressure is beneficial. Table 1.3 presents the rationale for lowering elevated blood pressure. The reduction in cardiovascular disease and death (point 5) can be measured to determine the blood pressure level at which a benefit is derived from antihypertensive therapy. That level can be used as part of the operational definition of hypertension.

During the past 25 years, controlled therapeutic trials have included patients with DBP levels

as low as 90 mm Hg. Detailed analyses of these trials are presented in Chapter 5. For now, it is enough to say that there is no question that protection against cardiovascular disease has been documented for reduction of DBP levels that start at or above 100 mm Hg, but there is continued disagreement about whether protection has been shown for those whose DBP starts at or above 90 or even 95 mm Hg. Therefore, expert committees continue to disagree about

Table 1.3. Rationale for the Reduction of Elevated Blood Pressure

1. Morbidity and mortality due to cardiovascular diseases are directly related to the level of blood pressure.
2. Blood pressure rises most in those whose pressures are already high.
3. In humans there is less vascular damage where the blood pressure is lower: beneath a coarctation, beyond a renovascular stenosis, and in the pulmonary circulation.
4. In animal experiments, lowering the blood pressure has been shown to protect the vascular system.
5. Antihypertensive therapy reduces cardiovascular disease and death.

the minimum level of blood pressure that should be treated with drugs.

The differences are highlighted in recent reports of four expert committees. The British Hypertension Society (Sever et al., 1993) and the Canadian Hypertension Society (Haynes et al., 1993) recommend that antihypertensive treatment be started when the DBP is consistently greater than 100 mm Hg for 3 to 4 months. The World Health Organization and the International Society of Hypertension Guidelines Subcommittee (1993) recommend treatment for persons with a DBP greater than 95 mm Hg. The Fifth Joint National Committee on Detection, Evaluation, and Treatment of High Blood Pressure (1993) recommends treatment for those with a persistently elevated DBP greater than 90 mm Hg, "especially in individuals with target organ damage and/or other known risk factors for cardiovascular disease."

When all available data are considered, a DBP of 95 mm Hg seems to be the level at which therapy has been shown to provide protection so that level could be used in the operational definition of hypertension.

Prevention of Progression of Hypertension

Another benefit of action is the prevention of progression of hypertension which should be looked upon as a surrogate for reducing the risk of cardiovascular disease. Evidence of that benefit is strong. Table 1.4 shows the results from five therapeutic trials that followed-up half of the control subjects while they were receiving placebo. Hypertension progressed beyond the threshold level (defined for each trial) in 10–17% of control subjects, but in less than 1% of treated subjects. In three recent large trials of elderly patients, progression of hypertension beyond the predetermined limits for starting

therapy occurred in 9–15% of those on placebo (SHEP Cooperative Research Group, 1991; Dahlöf et al., 1991; MRC Working Party, 1992).

Additional Risks and Costs of Action

The decision to label a person "hypertensive" and begin treatment involves assumption of the role of a patient, changes in lifestyle, possible interference with the quality of life, risks from biochemical side effects of therapy, and financial costs (Table 1.1). As will be emphasized in the next chapter, the diagnosis should not be based on one or only a few readings. In a survey of 6258 adults in two Canadian cities, Birkett et al. (1987) found that 14.3% had been mislabeled as hypertensive and that only 11.4% actually had hypertension. The fact that 85% of U.S. adults had their blood pressure measured in 1985 (Schoenborn, 1988) is then a mixed blessing: blood pressure measurement may identify many who need antihypertensive therapy but may also lead to considerable overdiagnosis and unnecessary treatment.

Assumption of the Role of a Patient

Merely labeling a person "hypertensive" may cause negative effects, as well as enough sympathetic nervous system activity to change hemodynamic measurements (Rostrup et al., 1991). Although some investigators have found no adverse psychological effects related to a person's awareness of having hypertension (Moum et al., 1990), most do (Alderman and Lamport, 1990; Robbins et al., 1990). People who know they are hypertensive may miss work more often because of illness and psychological distress than either normotensive people or those who are unaware of their condition. However, hypertensive people who receive appropriate counseling and comply with therapy usually are

Table 1.4   Progression of Hypertension in Placebo-Controlled Trials of the Treatment of Hypertension

	Veterans Administration (1970)	United States Public Health Service (1977)[a]	Australian (1980)	Oslo[b] (1980)	Medical Research Council (1985)
Number of patients	380	389	3,427	785	17,354
Diastolic blood pressure (mm Hg)					
Initial level	90–114	90–115	95–109	90–109	95–109
Threshold level	125	130	110	110	110
Progression beyond threshold (%)					
Control group	10	12	12	17	11.7
Treatment group	0	0	0.2	0.3	0.9

[a]Smith WM. Treatment of mild hypertension: results of a ten-year intervention trial. *Circ Res* 1977;40(Suppl 1):I–98.
[b]Helgeland A. Treatment of mild hypertension: a five year controlled drug trial. *Am J Med* 1980;69:752.

not absent from work more often and do not have more psychological distress than others (Alderman and Lamport, 1990).

Nonetheless, the consequences of labeling a person hypertensive may be insidious. For example, Johnston et al. (1984) found that the yearly income of 230 hypertensive Canadian steelworkers, 5 years after they were identified, averaged $1093 less than that of a matched group of normotensive workers even though both groups had similar incomes in the year before screening (Johnston et al., 1984).

Changes in Lifestyle and Interferences with Quality of Life

One-third of 3844 patients started on antihypertensive medications for the Hypertension Detection and Follow-up Program experienced side effects; drug treatment was discontinued in about one-third of those patients (Curb et al., 1988). The side effects were recognized by use of detailed surveillance procedures.

In ordinary practice, neither physicians nor patients may be aware of side effects that can impair the patient's quality of life. Jachuck et al. (1982) surveyed 75 consecutive patients from an English group practice who were taking the usual antihypertensive drugs. The patients, their physicians, and their closest relatives were asked a series of questions about the patient's quality of life. Most patients stated that their quality of life had improved or was no different after therapy, and all the physicians stated that the patients had improved. However, 99% of the relatives said that the patients' quality of life was worse after therapy, describing memory loss (33%), irritability (45%), depression (46%), hypochondria (55%), and decreased sexual interest (64%).

This study, although small in scope and uncontrolled, suggests that treatment of hypertension may interfere with a patient's enjoyment of life in ways that neither the patient nor physician is aware of. When objective assessments are used, most patients do not experience any impairments in quality of life (see Chapter 7). Nonetheless, even nonpharmacologic therapies such as a moderate reduction in calories and sodium intake may be perceived as unpleasant.

Risks from Biochemical Side Effects of Therapy

Biochemical risks are less likely to be perceived by the patient than the interferences with lifestyle, but they may actually be more hazardous. These risks are discussed in detail in Chapter 7. For now, only two will be mentioned: hypokalemia develops in about one-third of diuretic-treated patients, and elevations in serum cholesterol or triglyceride level may accompany the use of diuretics or β-blockers.

Overview of Risks and Benefits

We have examined some of the issues involved in determining the level of blood pressure that poses enough risk to mandate the diagnosis of hypertension and to call for therapy, despite the potential risks that appropriate therapy entails. An analysis of issues relating to risk factor intervention by Brett (1984) clearly defines the problem:

Risk factor intervention is usually undertaken in the hope of long-term gain in survival or quality of life. Unfortunately, there are sometimes trade-offs (such as inconvenience, expense, or side effects) and something immediate must be sacrificed. This tension between benefits and liabilities is not necessarily resolved by appealing to statements of medical fact, and it is highlighted by the fact that many persons at risk are asymptomatic. Particularly when proposing drug therapy, the physician cannot make an asymptomatic person feel any better, but might make him feel worse, since most drugs have some incidence of adverse effects. But how should side effects be quantitated on a balance sheet of net drug benefit? If a successful antihypertensive drug causes impotence in a patient, how many months or years of potentially increased survival make the side effect acceptable? There is obviously no dogmatic answer; accordingly, global statements such as "all patients with asymptomatic mild hypertension should be treated" are inappropriate, even if treatment were clearly shown to lower morbidity or mortality rates.

The example of mild hypertension may be developed further. It is widely acknowledged that, with successively higher blood pressure levels, the risk of complications increases gradually rather than abruptly. Therefore, the reasons to intervene should be viewed as gradually more compelling as blood pressure rises, rather than suddenly compelling at a specific level such as 90 mm Hg. Guttmacher et al. (1981) argue persuasively that selection of a cutoff for critically elevated blood pressure reflects a value judgment about the point at which a risk is thought to be serious enough to warrant treatment. Each decision must be individualized, depending on the patient's aversion to risk, perception of the intrusiveness of medical care in his or her life, tolerance for discomfort or untoward drug effects, and other factors. When the medical database contains considerable uncertainty, as it does for mild hypertension, the risk-benefit calculation is even more difficult.

OPERATIONAL DEFINITIONS OF HYPERTENSION

Now that the issues of risk and benefit have been examined, operational definitions of hypertension can be offered.

Fifth Joint National Committee Criteria

The Fifth Joint National Committee on Detection, Evaluation and Treatment of High Blood Pressure (1993) report includes both systolic and diastolic levels in the classification of blood pressure (Table 1.5). The levels used in Table 1.5 are based on at least three sets of readings over several weeks. The minimum average levels of SBP and DBP required for diagnosis are 140 and 90 mm Hg, respectively. Hypertension is then categorized by either systolic or diastolic gradation into one of four stages. If the SBP and DBP correspond to different stages, the highest stage is used.

Systolic Hypertension in the Elderly

In view of the recognized risks of isolated systolic elevations (Fig. 1.5), the Fifth Joint National Committee recommends that, in the presence of a DBP below 90 mm Hg, an SBP

Table 1.5. Classification of Blood Pressure for Adults Aged 18 Years and Older[a]

Category	Systolic	Diastolic
Normal[b]	<130	<85
High normal	130–139	85–89
Hypertension[c]		
Stage 1 (mild)	140–159	90–99
Stage 2 (moderate)	160–179	100–109
Stage 3 (severe)	180–209	110–119
Stage 4 (very severe)	>210	>120

From Joint National Committee. The fifth report of the Joint National Committee on Detection, Evaluation, and Treatment of High Blood Pressure (JNC V). *Arch Intern Med* 1993;153:154–183.

[a]These definitions apply to adults who are not taking antihypertensive drugs and who are not acutely ill. When systolic and diastolic blood pressures fall into different categories, the higher category should be selected to classify the individual's blood pressure status. Isolated systolic hypertension is defined as a systolic blood pressure of 140 mm Hg or more and a diastolic blood pressure of less than 90 mm Hg and staged appropriately.

[b]Optimal blood pressure with respect to cardiovascular risk is less than 120 mm Hg systolic and less than 80 mm Hg diastolic. However, unusually low readings should be evaluated for clinical significance.

[c]Based on the average of two or more readings taken at each of two or more visits after an initial screening.

level of 140 mm Hg or higher be classified as "isolated systolic hypertension." However, most physicians would not consider active drug therapy for patients over age 65 unless the SBP was 160 mm Hg or higher.

Children

For children, the Fifth Joint National Committee uses the definition from the Report of the Second Task Force on Blood Pressure Control in Children which identifies "*significant hypertension* as blood pressure persistently equal to or greater than the 95th percentile for age and *severe hypertension* as blood pressure persistently equal to or greater than the 99th percentile for age." Hypertension in children is covered in Chapter 16.

Operational Definition Based on Risk and Benefit

Considering all the factors shown in Table 1.1, I believe that hypertension in adults, *based on an average of multiple readings*, should be defined as it is in Table 1.5, which is from the Fifth Joint National Committee report.

In using these levels to make the diagnosis, one major caveat should be recognized: the diagnosis of hypertension does not automatically mean that drug treatment should be given to all people with elevated blood pressure levels. Drug treatment should be given to most patients with a DBP above 95 mm Hg, to virtually all with a DBP above 100 mm Hg, and to most with an SBP above 160 mm Hg (see Chapter 5). Moreover, in people susceptible to premature cardiovascular disease because of concomitant risk factors or target organ damage, therapy may be needed for lower levels, even below 140/90 mm Hg.

In addition, many patients whose blood pressure is not high enough to mandate drug therapy may benefit from being diagnosed as hypertensive if, thereby, they are more willing to modify unhealthy lifestyle habits. Such lifestyle modifications may reverse the trend toward progressively higher blood pressure and reduce the level of other cardiovascular risk factors.

More people will obviously be identified as hypertensive with these criteria than would have been with previous criteria that used 160/95 mm Hg as the dividing line. Because this chapter addresses the population at large, let us now consider how use of the lower levels of blood pressure to define hypertension influences the prevalence of the disease and the estimates of overall risk in the population.

PREVALENCE OF HYPERTENSION

The best sources of data for the U.S. population are the National Health and Nutrition Examination Surveys (NHANES). The first survey was performed during 1971–1972 and 1974–1975, the second from 1976 to 1980, and the third during 1988–1991. Each survey examined a large representative sample of the U.S. adult population.

NHANES Surveys

The number of adults in the United States with hypertension, defined in the NHANES surveys as an SBP of 140 mm Hg or higher, a DBP of 90 mm Hg or higher, or a level requiring antihypertensive drug therapy, decreased from about 58 million during 1976–1980 to about 50 million during 1988–1991 (Fig. 1.7). One possible explanation for this decrease in the prevalence of hypertension involves the setting in which the blood pressure measurements were made in these surveys. In NHANES II (1976–1980), blood pressures were measured at special clinics, whereas in NHANES III (1976–1991), they were measured at the subjects' homes and at the clinic several weeks later.

As we examine these data, remember that they are averages of only a few blood pressure readings taken on one or two occasions. A person's blood pressure often remains higher than usual on the first and second examination, so the prevalence of persistent hypertension is probably about one-third lower than indicated by these data. Nonetheless, the data provide an impressive portrayal of how the prevalence of hypertension continues to rise as the population grows older. Although it has been stated that only about 20% of the entire U.S. population has hypertension at any point in time, most people will develop it at some point during their lifetime.

Differences Among Racial Groups

The preceding paragraphs refer to the overall adult population of the United States. However, the prevalence of hypertension varies among different racial groups within the population. Moreover, the prevalence of the disease in non-U.S. populations may differ from that in the U.S. population.

Blacks

Although the complete data from NHANES III are not yet available, those from NHANES II show more blacks than whites in the U.S. have hypertension (Fig. 1.8). Moreover, data from a 10-year follow-up of most of the NHANES I population showed that the incidence of hypertension among black men and women was twice that found among white men and women (Cor-

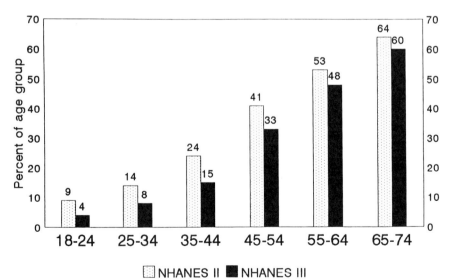

□ NHANES II ■ NHANES III

Figure 1.7. Prevalence of hypertension in US adults according to data from the National Health and Nutrition Examination Surveys conducted during 1976–1980 (NHANES II) and 1988–1991 (NHANES III). Hypertension is defined as mean blood pressure of 140/90 mm Hg or higher based on three readings taken on a single occasion or the use of antihypertensive medications. Source: Center for Disease Control and Prevention, National Center for Health Statistics. (Composed from National High Blood Pressure Education Program Working Group. *Arch Intern Med* 1993;153:186–208.)

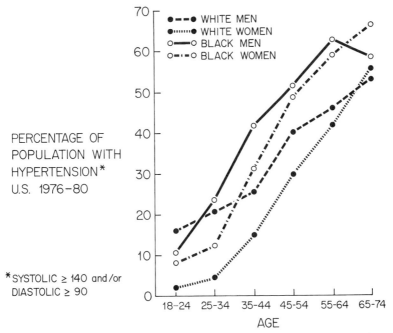

Figure 1.8. Prevalence of hypertension among white and black men and women in the United States according to data from the National Health and Nutrition Examination Survey conducted during 1976–1980 (NHANES II). Hypertension is defined as systolic blood pressure of 140 mm Hg and/or a diastolic blood pressure of 90 mm Hg or higher. (Reproduced with permission from Rowland M, Roberts J. Blood pressure levels and hypertension in persons ages 6–74 years. United States, 1976–80. *NCHS Advance Data, No. 84, Vital and Health Statistics of the National Center for Health Statistics.* US Department of Health and Human Services. Washington, DC, October 8, 1982.)

noni-Huntley et al., 1989). As shown by Neaton et al. (1984), death related to hypertension is more common in black men than in white men. Fortunately, the data from NHANES III show equally good control of hypertension in blacks and the total population in the U.S. Hypertension in blacks is covered in more detail in Chapter 4.

Hispanics

According to data from NHANES II and the Hispanic Health and Nutrition Examination Survey (1982–1984), mean DBP and SBP and the prevalence of hypertension were lower in Mexican-Americans than in Caucasians (Sorel et al., 1991). In an 8-year prospective study, Haffner et al. (1992) found that the incidence of hypertension was similar among 867 Mexican-Americans and 595 non-Hispanic whites in San Antonio, Texas.

Asians

In a survey of Asians and Pacific Islanders living in California, Klatsky and Armstrong (1991) found that the prevalence of hypertension was highest in Filipino and Chinese men born in the U.S., whereas the prevalence in Japanese

and other Asian men was similar to that in Caucasian men.

Native Americans

Hypertension has become considerably more common among Native Americans since about 1950 and is now as common in many Indian tribes as in the surrounding populations (Alpert et al., 1991).

Populations Outside the United States

Many surveys of hypertension in groups throughout the world have been performed, a large number relating blood pressure to dietary sodium intake. Some of the data from those surveys are reviewed in Chapter 3. Most surveys of people in industrialized countries show that the prevalence of hypertension is similar to that in the U.S. white population, whereas most surveys in less developed countries in which the people consume less sodium find a lower prevalence (Green and Peled, 1992; Nan et al., 1991).

Rather marked differences in the prevalence of hypertension among similar populations that cannot be easily explained have also been noted. For example, Shaper et al. (1988) noted a threefold variation among 7735 middle-aged men in 24 towns throughout Great Britain, with higher rates in Northern England and Scotland. Some, but not most, of the variations could be explained by such obvious factors as body weight or alcohol and sodium/potassium intake, leaving most of the variations unexplained (Bruce et al., 1993).

INCIDENCE OF HYPERTENSION

Much less is known about the incidence of newly developed hypertension than about its prevalence. The Framingham study provides one database (Kannel, 1989) and the National Health Epidemiologic Follow-up Study another (Cornoni-Huntley et al., 1989). In the latter study, 14,407 participants in NHANES I (1971–1975) were followed an average of 9.5 years. Unfortunately, blood pressure was measured only once for each participant at the beginning of the study, and only the first of three measured during follow-up was used in the analysis to provide comparability. Therefore, the rates provided by this survey are likely considerably higher than would be found with a more careful assessment based on several readings.

Nonetheless, comparison of the incidence of hypertension (SBP $\geq$ 160 mm Hg; DBP $\geq$ 95 mm Hg) in white men and women shows an approximate 5% increase for each 10-year interval of age at baseline except in the 65–74 year old group (Fig. 1.9). The incidence among blacks was at least twice that among whites. The high incidence in the 55–64 year old and 65–74 year old groups likely represents a considerable proportion of cases of isolated systolic hyperten-

sion because the diagnosis was based on elevations in either SBP or DBP. In the Framingham cohort, of the hypertensive patients more than 65 years old, 60% had isolated systolic hypertension (Kannel, 1990).

CLASSIFICATION OF HYPERTENSION

Hypertension should be categorized on the basis of both severity and cause to facilitate diagnosis and therapy.

Classification by Severity

Level of Blood Pressure

The division of SBP and DBP into grades was recommended by the Fifth Joint National Committee on Detection, Evaluation, and Treatment of High Blood Pressure (Table 1.5) with the hope that the ''mild,'' ''moderate,'' and ''severe'' classifications will no longer be used, particularly since most cardiovascular damage related to hypertension occurs in people with ''mild'' hypertension.

An estimate of the number of people with varying degrees of diastolic hypertension can be made with data from the Hypertension Detection and Follow-up Program (Hypertension Detection and Follow-up Program Cooperative Group, 1977). In this study, 159,000 people aged 30 to 69 years from 14 communities throughout the U.S. were initially examined in their homes (Fig. 1.10). Of all participants with a DBP above 90 mm Hg, 67% had stage 1 hypertension (DBP, 90–99 mm Hg), 22% had stage 2 (DBP, 100–109 mm Hg), and 11% had stage 3 or 4 (DBP, 110 mm Hg or higher). The actual preva-

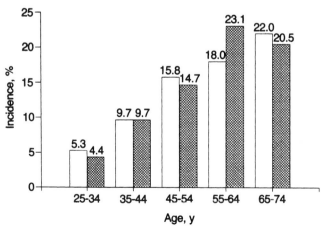

Figure 1.9. Incidence of hypertension in white men (*open bars*) and women (*cross-hatched bars*). Follow-up averaged 9.5 years (National Health Epidemiologic Follow-up Study). (Reproduced with permission from Cornoni-Huntley J, LaCroix AZ, Havlik RJ. *Arch Intern Med* 1989;149:780–788.)

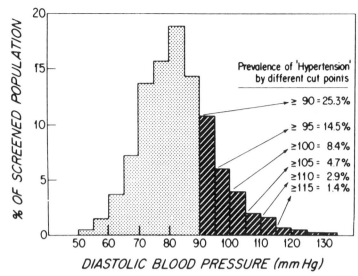

Figure 1.10. Frequency distribution of diastolic blood pressure measured at home screening (158,906 persons aged 30 to 69 years). (From the Hypertension Detection and Follow-up Program Cooperative Group: The hypertension detection and follow-up program: A progress report. *Circ Res* 1977;40(Suppl 1):I-106–I-109. Reprinted with permission of the American Heart Association, Inc.)

lence figures are likely too high because they are based on the second measurements taken on the initial home visit. When the participants were reexamined, their blood pressures were usually lower; 44% of the white men with a DBP of 95 to 104 mm Hg on the first screening had one below 90 mm Hg on the second screening. Nonetheless, the relative distribution of various levels should be correct.

Other Factors

In addition to the level of blood pressure, three other factors are considered to determine the severity of hypertension: (*a*) certain demographic features (e.g., age, sex, and race), (*b*) the extent of vascular damage induced by the high blood pressure, as reflected in target organ involvement, and (*c*) the presence of other risk factors for premature cardiovascular disease. These factors are discussed in more detail in Chapter 4.

Labile Hypertension

Multiple ambulatory readings have been recorded over the full 24 hours, and the marked variability in virtually everyone's blood pressure has become obvious (see Chapter 2). In view of the usual variability of blood pressure, the term "labile" is neither useful nor meaningful.

Borderline Hypertension

The term "borderline" may be used to describe hypertension in which the blood pres-

sure only occasionally rises above 140/90 mm Hg. Persistently elevated blood pressure is more likely to develop in such people than in those with consistently normal readings. However, this progression is by no means certain. In one study of a particularly fit, low-risk group of air cadets with borderline pressures, only 12% developed sustained hypertension over the subsequent 20 years (Madsen and Buch, 1971). Nonetheless, people with borderline pressures tend to have hemodynamic changes indicative of early hypertension and greater degrees of other cardiovascular risk factors, including greater body weight, dyslipidemia, and higher plasma insulin levels (Julius et al., 1990) and should therefore be followed more closely and advised to modify their lifestyle.

Classification by Cause

The list of causes of hypertension (Table 1.6) is quite long; however, the cause of more than 90% of the cases of hypertension is unknown (primary or essential). The proportion of cases secondary to some identifiable mechanism has been debated considerably as more secondary causes have been recognized. Claims that one cause or another is responsible for up to 20% of all cases of hypertension repeatedly appear from investigators who are particularly interested in a certain category of hypertension and therefore see only a highly selected population.

Data from surveys of various populations are available (Table 1.7). Even though the patients

Table 1.6. Types and Causes of Hypertension

Systolic and diastolic hypertension
  Primary, essential, or idiopathic
  Secondary
    Renal
      Renal parenchymal disease
        Acute glomerulonephritis
        Chronic nephritis
        Polycystic disease
        Diabetic nephropathy
        Hydronephrosis
      Renovascular disease
        Renal artery stenosis
        Intrarenal vasculitis
      Renin-producing tumors
      Renoprival
      Primary sodium retention (Liddle's
        syndrome, Gordon's syndrome)
    Endocrine
      Acromegaly
      Hypothyroidism
      Hyperthyroidism
      Hypercalcemia (hyperparathyroidism)
      Adrenal disorders
        Cortical disorders
          Cushing's syndrome
          Primary aldosteronism
          Congenital adrenal hyperplasia
        Medullary tumors
          (pheochromocytoma)
      Extraadrenal chromaffin tumors
      Carcinoids
      Exogenous hormones
        Estrogen
        Glucocorticoids
        Mineralocorticoids
        Sympathomimetics
        Foods containing tyramine and
          monamine oxidase inhibitors
    Coarctation of the aorta
    Pregnancy
    Neurological disorders
      Increased intracranial pressure
        Brain tumor
        Encephalitis
        Respiratory acidosis
      Sleep apnea
      Quadriplegia
      Acute porphyria
      Familial dysautonomia
      Lead poisoning
      Guillain-Barré syndrome
    Acute stress (including surgery)
      Psychogenic hyperventilation
      Hypoglycemia
      Burns
      Pancreatitis
      Alcohol withdrawal
      Sickle cell crisis
      After resuscitation
      After surgery
    Increased intravascular volume
    Alcohol and drug use
Systolic hypertension
  Increased cardiac output
    Aortic valvular insufficiency
    Arteriovenous fistula, patent ductus
    Thyrotoxicosis
    Paget's disease of bone
    Beriberi
    Hyperkinetic circulation
  Rigidity of aorta

Table 1.7. Frequency of Various Diagnoses in Hypertensive Subjects

	Frequency of Diagnosis (%)				
	Gifford (1969)	Berglund et al. (1976)	Rudnick et al. (1977)	Danielson and Dammström (1981)	Sinclair et al. (1987)
No. of patients	4339	689	665	1000	3783
Essential hypertension	89	94	94	95.3	92.1
Chronic renal disease	5	4	5	2.4	5.6
Renovascular disease	4	1	0.2	1.0	0.7
Coarctation of the aorta	1	0.1	0.2	–	–
Primary aldosteronism	0.5	0.1	–	0.1	0.3
Cushing's syndrome	0.2	–	0.2	0.1	0.1
Pheochromocytoma	0.2	–	–	0.2	0.1
Oral contraceptive use	–	(Men only)	0.2	0.8	1.0

in some of these studies were referred specifically to evaluate secondary causes or because they had more severe hypertension (wherein secondary causes are more likely), note that the prevalence of primary (essential) hypertension was 90% or higher.

Perhaps the best data on what could be expected in a medical practice of middle-class whites come from the study by Rudnick et al. (1977), which involved 655 hypertensive patients in a family practice in Hamilton, Ontario, Canada. Each patient had a complete workup, including an intravenous pyelogram. Notice again the rarity of secondary hypertension in this relatively unselected population. The proportion of secondary forms of hypertension does differ in both young and old patients. They are covered in Chapters 4 and 16, respectively.

POPULATION RISK FROM HYPERTENSION

Now that the definition of hypertension and its classification have been provided along with various estimates of its prevalence, the impact of hypertension on the population at large can be considered. As noted, for the individual patient, the higher the level of blood pressure, the greater the risk of morbidity and mortality. However, for the population at large, the greatest burden from hypertension occurs among people with only minimally elevated pressures because there are so many of them. This burden can be seen when the 12-year cardiovascular mortality rates observed with each increment of blood pressure are plotted against the distribution of the various levels of blood pressure among the 350,000 35–57-year-old men screened for MRFIT (Fig. 1.11) (National High Blood Pressure Education Program Working Group, 1993). Although the mortality rates climb progressively, most deaths occur in the much larger proportion of the population with minimally elevated pressures. By multiplying the percentage of men at any given level of blood pressure by the relative risk for that level, it can be seen that more cardiovascular mortality will occur in those with SBP of 110–119 or DBP of 75–79 than among those with SBP of 160+ or DBP of 95–99.

Strategy for the Population

This disproportionate risk for the population at large from relatively mild hypertension bears strongly on the question of how to achieve the greatest reduction in the risks of hypertension.

In the past, most effort has been directed at the group with the highest levels of blood pressure. However, this "high-risk" strategy, as effective as it may be for those affected, does little to reduce total morbidity and mortality if the "low-risk" patients, who make up the largest share of the population at risk, are ignored (Rose, 1985, 1992).

Many more people with mild hypertension are now being treated actively and aggressively with antihypertensive drugs. However, as emphasized by Rose, a more effective strategy would be to lower the blood pressure level of the entire population, as might be accomplished by reduction of sodium intake. Rose estimated that lowering the entire distribution of blood pressure by only 2 to 3 mm Hg by reducing sodium intake would be as effective in reducing the overall risks of hypertension as prescribing current antihypertensive drug therapy for all people with definite hypertension.

This issue is eloquently addressed by Stamler et al. (1993): "A strategy limited solely to efforts for those at very high risk—the main focus to date—fails to realize the opportunity to prevent a sizable proportion of excess deaths attributable to BP level. The high-risk strategy—as useful as it is—has the further serious limitation (if pursued as the *only* strategy) of offering no permanent solution to the BP problem in the population. Its approach involves early detection, evaluation, and care for people *after* they have developed high blood pressure, i.e., it is late and defensive, and above all, it is never-ending, since it does not aim at the *primary prevention* of this major risk factor. In contrast, the broader combined strategy—involving both high-risk and population-wide thrusts—includes in its latter approach safe nutritional-hygienic means for the primary prevention of BP rise with age and high blood pressure. It therefore offers not only a greater potential for saving lives, but also a potential for the final solution of the BP problem."

The broader approach is almost certainly correct on epidemiologic grounds. However, until such mass strategies can be implemented, we are left with the need to better treat those with established hypertension.

DETECTION AND CONTROL OF HYPERTENSION IN THE POPULATION

As seen in Figure 1.1, the percentages of people who are aware of their hypertension, who are receiving treatment, and whose hypertension

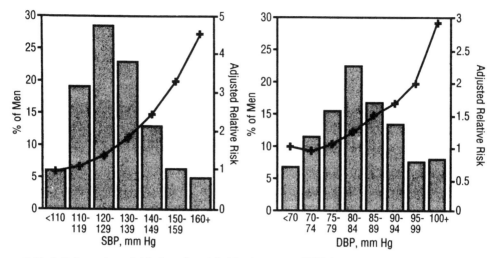

Figure 1.11. *Left.* Percentage distribution of systolic blood pressure (SBP) for men screened for the Multiple Risk Factor Intervention Trial who were aged 35 to 57 years and had no history of myocardial infarction (*n* = 347,978) (*shaded bars*) and corresponding 12-year rates of cardiovascular mortality by SBP level adjusted for age, race, total serum cholesterol level, cigarettes smoked per day, reported use of medication for diabetes mellitus, and imputed household income (using census tract of residence) (*curve with plus signs*). *Right.* Same as at left but for DBP (*n* = 356,222). (Reproduced with permission from National High Blood Pressure Education Program Working Group. *Arch Intern Med* 1993;153:186–208.)

is controlled have risen progressively over the past 20 years. However, if the more appropriate threshold level of 140/90 mm Hg is used, the percentage of people in the U.S. with controlled hypertension as of 1991 was only 43%.

Continued Problems

Whereas the campaign to inform people that hypertension is dangerous and that blood pressure should be measured every year has been successful, the adequate management of the large hypertensive population has proved to be difficult. This difficulty reflects the less than adequate health care provided for the poor in the U.S., a group with a large proportion of blacks in whom the prevalence of hypertension is highest and the largest percentage of uncontrolled disease is present (Shea et al., 1992). The recent cutbacks in Federal funding of health care for the poor have resulted in decreased control of hypertension in that population (Lurie et al., 1986).

The continued difficulties in maintaining adequate follow-up and treatment of the poor are not by any means unique to the United States. Similar problems have been noted in England, where a nationalized health care system should help the poor overcome the economic impediments to adequate blood pressure management (Blane et al., 1990). In less developed countries, even greater problems, including inadequate

funds for medications, continue to impede attempts to control hypertension (Elbagir and Ahmed, 1990).

Proposed Solutions

The major need now is not to educate or screen but to improve adherence to treatment by maintaining contact and encouraging follow-up care (Vallbona and Pavlik, 1992).

Improvements in long-term management can be made both by large-scale approaches and individual providers. Examples of successful large-scale approaches are:

—The North Karelia, Finland, control program that includes intensive community education, hypertension dispensaries run by specially trained nurses, and widespread use of both nondrug and drug therapies (Nissinen et al., 1992);

—Rural control programs such as the one in North Carolina that provides for neighborhood health centers with a community-oriented primary care philosophy (O'Connor et al., 1990);

—Work-site facilities for follow-up care (Foote and Erfurt, 1991); and

—Outpatient hypertension clinics directed by nurses (Schwartz et al., 1990);

Individual providers have found the following techniques to be useful:

—Computers to characterize a patient's cardiovascular risk status, to provide reminders of appointments, and to track patient progress (Degoulet et al., 1990);

—Special nurses or physician's assistants to screen and monitor patients' progress (Robson et al., 1989);

—Home blood pressure monitoring (Soghikian et al., 1992); and

—Community health workers to maintain contact with patients treated in the emergency room (Bone et al., 1989).

Consequences of Improved Control of Hypertension

At least partly as a result of the improved control of hypertension, there has been a steady decrease in the mortality rate of coronary heart disease and an even greater decrease in that of stroke in the U.S. since 1968. The decline in mortality due to these two diseases has been steeper than for noncardiovascular disease (Fig. 1.12). The decrease in hypertension-related mortality has been observed in both men and women, black and white.

Similar decreases in mortality from heart disease have been noted in other countries, such as Finland and Australia, which, like the U.S., have had very high rates (Thom, 1989). On the other hand, in countries such as Poland, Yugoslavia, and Norway, mortality from heart disease has been rising fast, likely because of increased consumption of saturated fat and cigarette smoking.

Contribution of Hypertension Control

The explanation for the reduced mortality rate of cardiovascular disease in the U.S. remains uncertain (Sytkowski et al., 1990). An analysis of the comparative effects of various medical interventions and changes in lifestyle concluded that the latter were responsible for the larger part of the decline in mortality due to coronary disease (Tsevat et al., 1991). Moreover, the prevalence of CHD has continued to increase in the men aged 55 to 64 years over 30-year intervals in the Framingham cohort despite increased treatment of hypertension (D'Agostino et al., 1989).

Stroke is more closely related to hypertension than is coronary heart disease, and the fall in mortality due to stroke would logically be attributable to improved control of hypertension. In the population of Rochester, Minnesota, the incidence of stroke has been found to be closely (inversely) connected to the control of hypertension, more so in women than in men (Garraway and Whisnant, 1987). Analysis of vital statistics for the entire U.S. population, on the other hand, shows no correlation between the decline in mortality due to stroke and improved antihyperten-

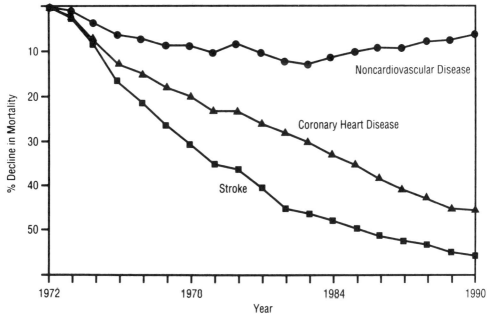

Figure 1.12. Decline in age-adjusted mortality since 1972. Data for 1990 are provisional. Source: National Center for Health Statistics. (Reproduced with permission from the Joint National Committee. The fifth report of the Joint National Committee on Detection, Evaluation, and Treatment of High Blood Pressure (JNC V). *Arch Intern Med* 1993;153:154–183.)

sive therapy (Casper et al., 1992). Moreover, morbidity and mortality from stroke remain considerably higher in treated hypertensives than in normotensive subjects (Lindblad et al., 1993).

Thus, we have to look elsewhere to explain much of the improvement in coronary and cerebrovascular mortality rates which have occurred since 1968. Nonetheless, the increased treatment of hypertension has almost certainly played some role. The evidence that drug therapy for hypertension protects against stroke and heart failure seems strong, although doubts remain about the benefits of therapy for prevention of coronary disease (see Chapter 5). Of particular concern is the continued high occurrence of sudden death, responsible for almost 300,000 deaths per year in the U.S. Although sudden death clearly occurs more frequently among hypertensive patients with left ventricular hypertrophy, its risk was increased an additional twofold among those receiving antihypertensive drug therapy in the Framingham population (Kannel et al., 1988). We obviously have a long way to go, in both the U.S. and elsewhere.

Potential for Prevention

A greater awareness of the causes and accelerators of hypertension may provide insights into the real goal: prevention. Despite more intensive treatment of millions of people with hypertension, we have done little to prevent its onset. The incidence of hypertension in the Framingham population has remained quite stable over 30 years (Kannel et al., 1993).

Increasingly strong evidence documents the ability to delay, if not to prevent, the onset of hypertension (Cutler, 1993). Crucial to that effort is the prevention of obesity since, in the Framingham population, 70% of hypertension in men and 61% in women was directly attributable to excess adiposity (Kannel et al., 1993). Unfortunately, the prevalence of obesity in the United States has risen progressively both in adults and even more disturbingly in children, among whom more obesity-related hypertension has also been noted. We should keep the goal of prevention in mind as we consider the overall problems of hypertension for the individual patient in the ensuing chapters.

References

Alderman MH, Lamport B. Labelling of hypertensives: a review of the data. *J Clin Epidemiol* 1990;43:195–200.

Alpert JS, Goldberg R, Ockene IS, Taylor P. Heart disease in native Americans. *Cardiology* 1991;78:3–12.

Anonymous. Rise and fall of diseases (Editorial). *Lancet* 1993;341:151–152.

Berglund G, Anderson O, Wilhelmsen L. Prevalence of primary and secondary hypertension: studies in a random population sample. *Br Med J* 1976;2:554–556.

Birkett NJ, Evans CE, Haynes RB, et al. Hypertension control in two Canadian communities: evidence for better treatment and overlabelling. *J Hypertens* 1987;4:369–374.

Blane D, Smith GD, Bartley M. Social class differences in years of potential life lost: size, trends, and principal causes. *Br Med J* 1990;301:429–432.

Bone LR, Mamon J, Levine DM, et al. Emergency department detection and follow-up of high blood pressure: use and effectiveness of community health workers. *Am J Emerg Med* 1989;7:16–20.

Brett AS. Ethical issues in risk factor intervention. *Am J Med* 1984;76:557–561.

Bruce NG, Wannamethee G, Shaper AG. Lifestyle factors associated with geographic blood pressure variations among men and women in the UK. *J Hum Hypertens* 1993;7:229–238.

Casper M, Wing S, Strogatz D, Davis CE, Tyroler HA. Antihypertensive treatment and US trends in stroke mortality, 1962 to 1980. *Am J Public Health* 1992;82:1600–1606.

Clausen J, Jensen, G. Blood pressure and mortality: an epidemiological survey with 10 years follow-up. *J Hum Hypertens* 1992;6:53–59.

Cornoni-Huntley J, LaCroix AZ, Havlik RJ. Race and sex differentials in the impact of hypertension in the United States. The National Health and Nutrition Examination Survey I Epidemiologic Follow-up Study. *Arch Intern Med* 1989;149:780–788.

Curb JD, Schneider K, Taylor JO, Maxwell M, Shulman N. Antihypertensive drug side effects in the Hypertension Detection and Follow-up Program. *Hypertension* 1988;11(Suppl II):II-51–II-55.

Cutler JA. Prevention of hypertension. *Curr Opin Nephrol Hypertens* 1993;2:404–414.

D'Agostino RB, Kannel WB, Belanger AJ, Sytkowski PA. Trends in CHD and risk factors at age 55–64 in the Framingham Study. *Int J Epidemiol* 1989;18(Suppl 1):S67–S72.

Dahlöf B, Lindholm LH, Hansson L, Scherstén B, Ekbom T, Wester P-O. Morbidity and mortality in the Swedish Trial in Old Patients with Hypertension (STOP-Hypertension). *Lancet* 1991;338:1281–1285.

Danielson M, Dammström B-G. The prevalence of secondary and curable hypertension. *Acta Med Scand* 1981;209:451–455.

Degoulet P, Chatellier G, Devriès C, Lavril M, Ménard J. Computer-assisted techniques for evaluation and treatment of hypertensive patients. *Am J Hypertens* 1990;3:156–163.

Elbagir M, Ahmed K. Hypertensives who cannot get proper antihypertensive treatment. *J Hum Hypertens* 1990;4:215–216.

Foote A, Erfurt JC. The benefit to cost ratio of work-site blood pressure control programs. *JAMA* 1991;265:1283–1286.

Garraway WM, Whisnant JP. The changing pattern of hypertension and the declining incidence of stroke. *JAMA* 1987;258:214–217.

Gifford RW Jr. Evaluation of the hypertensive patient with emphasis on detecting curable causes. *Milbank Memorial Fund Q* 1969;47:170–186.

Green MS, Peled I. Prevalence and control of hypertension in a large cohort of occupationally-active Israelis examined during 1985–1987: the Cordis Study. *Int J Epidemiol* 1992;21:676–682.

Guidelines Subcommittee of the WHO/ISH Mild Hypertension Liaison Committee. 1993 Guidelines for the Management of mild hypertension. *Hypertension* 1993;22:392–403.

Guttmacher S, Teitelman M, Chapin G, Garbowski G, Schnall P. Ethics and preventive medicine. The case of borderline hypertension. *Hastings Center Rep* 1981;11:12–20.

Haffner SM, Mitchell BD, Valdez RA, Hazuda HP, Morales PA, Stern MP. Eight-year incidence of hypertension in Mexican-Americans and non-Hispanic whites. *Am J Hypertens* 1992;5:147–153.

Haffner SM, Morales PA, Hazuda HP, Stern MP. Level of control of hypertension in Mexican Americans and non-Hispanic whites. *Hypertension* 1993;21:83–88.

Haynes RB, Lacourcière Y, Rabkin SW, et al. Report of the Canadian Hypertension Society Consensus Conference: 2. Diagnosis of hypertension in adults. *Can Med Assoc J* 1993;149:409–418.

Heikinheimo RJ, Haavisto MV, Kaarela RH, Kanto AJ, Koivunen MJ, Rajala SA. Blood pressure in the very old. *J Hypertension* 1990;8:361–367.

Helgeland A. Treatment of mild hypertension: a five year controlled drug trial. *Am J Med* 1980;69:725–732.

Hypertension Detection and Follow-up Program Cooperative Group. The Hypertension Detection and Follow-Up Program. A progress report. *Circ Res* 1977;40(Suppl I):I-106–I-109.

Jachuck SJ, Brierley H, Jachuck S, Willcox PM. The effect of hypotensive drugs on the quality of life. *J Roy Coll Gen Pract* 1982;32:103–105.

Joffres MR, Hamet P, Rabkin SW, Gelskey D, Hogan K, Fodor G. Prevalence, control and awareness of high blood pressure among Canadian adults. *Can Med Assoc J* 1992;146:1997–2005.

Johnston ME, Gibson ES, Terry CW, et al. Effects of labelling on income, work and social function among hypertensive employees. *J Chronic Dis* 1984;37: 417–423.

Joint National Committee on Detection, Evaluation, and Treatment of High Blood Pressure. The fifth report of the Joint National Committee on Detection, Evaluation, and Treatment of High Blood Pressure (JNC V). *Arch Intern Med* 1993;153:154–183.

Julius S, Jamerson K, Mejia A, Krause L, Schork N, Jones K. The association of borderline hypertension with target organ changes and higher coronary risk. Tecumseh Blood Pressure study. *JAMA* 1990;264:354–358.

Kannel WB. Risk factors in hypertension. *J Cardiovasc Pharmacol* 1989;13(Suppl I):S4–S10.

Kannel WB. Hypertension and the risk of cardiovascular disease. In: Laragh JH, Brenner BM, eds. *Hypertension: Pathophysiology, Diagnosis, and Management.* New York: Raven Press, 1990:101–117.

Kannel WB, Cupples LA, D'Agostino RB, Stokes J III. Hypertension, antihypertensive treatment, and sudden coronary death. The Framingham Study. *Hypertension* 1988;11(Suppl II):II-45–II-50.

Kannel WB, Garrison RJ, Dannenberg AL. Secular blood pressure trends in normotensive persons: the Framingham study. *Am Heart J* 1993;125:1154–1158.

Kaplan NM. Hypertension: prevalence, risks, and effect of therapy. *Ann Intern Med* 1983;98:705–709.

Klatsky AL, Armstrong MA. Cardiovascular risk factors among Asian Americans living in northern California. *Am J Public Health* 1991;81:1423–1428.

Langer RD, Ganiats TG, Barrett-Connor E. Factors associated with paradoxical survival at higher blood pressures in the very old. *Am J Epidemiol* 1991;134:29–38.

Levy D, Kannel WB. Cardiovascular risks: new insights from Framingham. *Am Heart J* 1988;116(pt 2):266–272.

Lindblad U, Råstam L, Ranstam J. Stroke morbidity in patients treated for hypertension—the Skaraborg Hypertension Project. *J Intern Med* 1993;233:155–163.

Lurie N, Ward NB, Shapiro MF, Gallego C, Vaghaiwalla R, Brook RH. Termination of Medi-Cal benefits. A follow-up study one year later. *N Engl J Med* 1986;314: 1266–1268.

MacMahon S, Peto R, Cutler J, et al. Blood pressure, stroke, and coronary heart disease. Part 1, Prolonged differences in blood pressure: prospective observational studies corrected for the regression dilution bias. *Lancet* 1990;335:765–774.

Madsen RER, Buch J. Long-term prognosis of transient hypertension in young male adults. *Aerospace Med* 1971;42:752–755.

Mitchell BD, Stern MP, Haffner SM, Hazuda HP, Patterson JK. Risk factors for cardiovascular mortality in Mexican Americans and non-Hispanic whites. San Antonio Heart Study. *Am J Epidemiol* 1990;131: 423–433.

Moum T, Naess S, Srensen T, Tambs K, Holmen J. Hypertension labelling, life events and psychological well-being. *Psychol Med* 1990;20:634–646.

MRC Working Party. Medical Research Council trial of treatment of hypertension in older adults: principal results. *Br Med J* 1992;304:405–412.

Nan L, Tuomilehto J, Dowse G, et al. Prevalence and medical care of hypertension in four ethnic groups in the newly-industrialized nation of Mauritius. *J Hypertens* 1991;9:859–866.

National High Blood Pressure Education Program Working Group. National High Blood Pressure Education Program Working Group report on primary prevention of hypertension. *Arch Intern Med* 1993; 153:186–208.

Neaton JD, Wentworth D. Serum cholesterol, blood pressure, cigarette smoking, and death from coronary heart disease. Overall findings and differences by age for 316,099 white men. *Arch Intern Med* 1992;152: 56–64.

Neaton JD, Kuller LH, Wentworth D, Borhani NO. Total and cardiovascular mortality in relation to cigarette smoking, serum cholesterol concentration, and diastolic blood pressure among black and white males followed up for five years. *Am Heart J* 1984;108(pt 2):759–769

Neaton JD, Wentworth D, Sherwin R, Kittner S, Kuller L, Stamler J. Comparison of 10 year coronary and cerebrovascular disease mortality rates by hypertensive status for black and non-black men screened in the Multiple Risk Factor Intervention Trial (MRFIT) [Abstract]. *Circulation* 1989; 80(Suppl I):II–300.

Nissinen A, Tuomilehto J, Enlund H, Kotte TE. Costs and benefits of community programmes for the control of hypertension. *J Hum Hypertens* 1992;6:473–479.

O'Connor PJ, Wagner EH, Strogatz DS. Hypertension control in a rural community. An assessment of community-oriented primary care. *J Fam Pract* 1990;30:420–424.

Pickering G. Hypertension. Definitions, natural histories and consequences. *Am J Med* 1972;52:570–583.

Pooling Project Research Group. Relationship of blood pressure, serum cholesterol, smoking habit, relative weight and ECG abnormalities to incidence of major coronary events: final report of the Pooling Project. *J Chronic Dis* 1978;31:201–306.

Robbins MA, Elias MF, Schultz NR Jr. The effects of age, blood pressure, and knowledge of hypertensive diagnosis on anxiety and depression. *Exp Aging Res* 1990;16: 199–207.

Robson J, Boomla K, Fitzpatrick S, et al. Using nurses for preventive activities with computer assisted follow up: a randomized controlled trial. *Br Med J* 1989;298: 433–436.

Rose G. Epidemiology. In: Marshall AJ, Barritt DW, eds. *The Hypertensive Patient.* Kent, England: Pitman Medical, 1980:1–21.

Rose G. Sick individuals and sick populations. *Int J Epidemiol* 1985;14:32–38.

Rose G. *The Strategy of Preventive Medicine.* Oxford: Oxford University Press, 1992.

Rostrup M, Mundal MH, Westheim A, Eide I. Awareness of high blood pressure increases arterial plasma catecholamines, platelet noradrenaline and adrenergic responses to mental stress. *J Hypertension* 1991;9:159–166.

Rowland M, Roberts J. Blood pressure levels and hypertension in persons ages 6–74 years. United States, 1976–80. *NCHS Advance Data, No. 84, Vital and Health Statistics of the National Center for Health Statistics.* US Department of Health and Human Services. Washington, DC, October 8, 1982.

Rudnick KV, Sackett DL, Hirst S, Holmes C. Hypertension in a family practice. *Can Med Assoc J* 1977;117:492–497.

Schappert SM. National ambulatory medical survey: 1991 summary. *NCHS Advance Data, No. 230, Vital and Health Statistics of the National Center for Health Statistics.* US Department of Health and Human Services Publication (PHS) 93-1250. Hyattsville, MD, March 29, 1993.

Schneider EL, Guralnik JM. The aging of America. Impact on health care costs. *JAMA* 1990;263:2335–2340.

Schoenborn CA. *NCHS Advance Data, Series 10, No. 163, Vital and Health Statistics of the Center for Disease Control and Prevention.* US Department of Health and Human Services Publication (PHS) 88-1591. Washington, DC, US Government Printing Office, February 1988.

Schwartz LL, Raymer JM, Nash CA, Hanson IA, Muenter DT. Hypertension: role of the nurse-therapist. *Mayo Clin Proc* 1990; 65:67–72.

Sever P, Beevers G, Bulpitt C, Lever A, Ramsay L, Reid J, Swales J. Management guidelines in essential hypertension: report of the second working party of the British Hypertension Society. *Br Med J* 1993;306:983–987.

Shaper AG, Ashby D, Pocock SJ. Blood pressure and hypertension in middle-aged British men. *J Hypertens* 1988;6:367–374.

Shea S, Misra D, Ehrlich MH, Field L, Francis CK. Predisposing factors for severe, uncontrolled hypertension in an inner-city minority population. *N Engl J Med* 1992;327:776–781.

SHEP Cooperative Research Group. Prevention of stroke by antihypertensive drug treatment in older persons with isolated systolic hypertension. Final results of the Systolic Hypertension in the Elderly Program (SHEP). *JAMA* 1991;265: 3255–3264.

Sinclair AM, Isles CG, Brown I, Cameron H, Murray GD, Robertson JWK. Secondary hypertension in a blood pressure clinic. *Arch Intern Med* 1987;147:1289–1293.

Smith WM, for the US Public Health Service Hospitals Cooperative Study Group. Treatment of mild hypertension: results of a ten-year intervention trial. *Circ Res* 1977;40(Suppl I):I-98–I-105.

Society of Actuaries and Association of Life Insurance Medical Directors of America: Blood Pressure Study, 1979 and 1980.

Soghikian K, Casper SM, Fireman BH, Hunkeler EM, Hurley LB, Tekawa IS, Vogt TM. Home blood pressure monitoring. Effect on use of medical services and medical care costs. *Med Care* 1992;30: 855–865.

Sorel JE, Ragland DR, Syme SL. Blood pressure in Mexican Americans, whites, and blacks. The Second National Health and Nutrition Examination Survey and the Hispanic Health and Nutrition Examination Survey. *Am J Epidemiol* 1991;134: 370–378.

Staessen J, Amery A, Fagard R. Isolated systolic hypertension in the elderly. *J Hypertens* 1990;8:393–405.

Stamler J, Stamler R, Neaton JD. Blood pressure, systolic and diastolic, and cardiovascular risks. US population data. *Arch Intern Med* 1993;153:598–615.

Strandberg TE, Salomaa VV, Naukkarinen VA, Vanhanen HT, Sarna SJ, Miettinen TA. Long-term mortality after 5-year multifactorial primary prevention of cardiovascular diseases in middle-aged men. *JAMA* 1991;266:1225–1229.

Sytkowski PA, Kannel WB, D'Agostino RB. Changes in risk factors and the decline in mortality from cardiovascular disease. The Framingham Heart Study. *N Engl J Med* 1990;322:1634–1641.

Thom TJ. International mortality from heart disease: rates and trends. *Int J Epidemiol* 1989;18(Suppl 1):S20–S28.

Tsevat J, Weinstein MC, Williams LW, Tosteson ANA, Goldman L. Expected gains in life expectancy from various coronary heart disease risk factor modifications. *Circulation* 1991;83:1194–1201.

Vallbona C, Pavlik V. Advances in the community control of hypertension: from epidemiology to primary care practice. *J Hypertens* 1992;10(Suppl 7):S51–S57.

Vokonas PS, Kannel WB, Cupples LA. Epidemiology and risk of hypertension in the elderly: the Framingham Study. *J Hypertens* 1988;6(Suppl 1):S3–S9.

Wilhelmsen L, Strasser T, on behalf of the Study Collaborators. WHO-WHL hypertension management audit project. *J Human Hypertens* 1993;7:257–263.

Yano K, McGee D, Reed DM. The impact of elevated blood pressure upon 10-year mortality among Japanese men in Hawaii: the Honolulu Heart Program. *J Chronic Dis* 1983;36:569–579.

2 Measurement of Blood Pressure

Now that some of the major issues about hypertension in the population at large have been addressed, we turn to the evaluation of the individual patient with hypertension. This chapter covers the measurement of the blood pressure (BP), with special attention to the factors that affect its variability.

VARIABILITY OF BLOOD PRESSURE

The variability of the pressure on repeated measurements, both at a single visit and on separate occasions, is much greater than most practitioners realize (Pickering, 1993). Considering the degree of variability found between single measurements made on different occasions, Perry and Miller (1992) concluded: "Perhaps only one-third to two-thirds of people whose measured diastolic pressures exceed 95 mm Hg actually have average pressures that high. . . . In a general population, single measurements of diastolic pressure exceed 95 mm Hg in approximately equal numbers of normotensive, borderline and hypertensive patients; moreover, one-third of those who are usually in the hypertensive range are not identified."

The adverse consequences of not recognizing and dealing with this variability are obvious: individual patients may be falsely labeled "hypertensive" or "normotensive." If falsely labeled as normotensive, needed therapy may be denied. If falsely labeled hypertensive, the label itself may provoke ill effects, as noted in Chapter 1, and unneeded therapy will likely be given with the potential for a lifelong commitment to what is often expensive and bothersome and occasionally hazardous.

Considerable variability has been noted even with the same well-trained observer using a calibrated sphygmomanometer under controlled cir-

cumstances (Watson et al., 1987) (Fig. 2.1). In this study of 32 patients, 12 sets of duplicate readings were obtained over a 3-month interval. Two major findings are shown: initial readings tend to be higher and considerable variability may be seen between the readings at each visit. Watson et al. found that the chance of a 5 mm Hg or greater difference being noted between the average stable BP and that recorded at visit 4 was 50% for the systolic BP (SBP) and 32% for the diastolic BP (DBP).

By Bayesian analysis, the predictive value of the average of two DBP readings above 90 for the presence of "true" DBP above 90 is only 52% (Schechter and Adler, 1988). If the average of eight readings is above 90, the sensitivity or positive predictive value goes up, but only to 73%.

Sources of Variation

As delineated by Rose et al. (1964), BP readings are often variable, because of factors working within the patient ("biological" variation) or problems involving the observer ("measurement" variation).

Measurement Variations

Some of the errors in measurement related to the measurer are listed in Table 2.1. These errors are more common than most realize and regular, frequent retraining of personnel is needed to prevent them (Bruce et al., 1988).

Biological Variations

Biological variations in BP may be either random or systematic. Random variations are uncontrollable but can be reduced simply by repeating the measurement as many times as needed. Systematic variations are introduced by

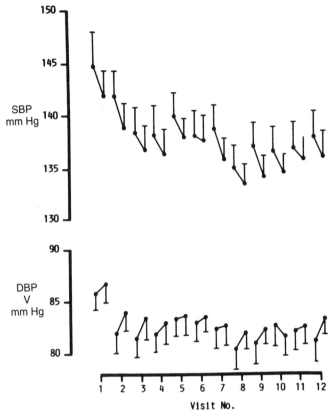

Figure 2.1. Mean values (±SEM) of the first and second readings of systolic blood pressure (*SBP*) and phase V diastolic blood pressure (*DBP*) recorded on 12 visits of 32 patients. (Reproduced with permission from Watson RDS, Lumb R, Young MA, et al. Variation in cuff blood pressure in untreated outpatients with mild hypertension—implications for initiating antihypertensive treatment. *J Hypertens* 1987;5:207–211.)

Table 2.1. Sources of Error in Blood Pressure Measurement

Inappropriate equipment
  Sphygmomanometer with small bladder
  Inaccurate aneroid manometer
Inaccurate reading
  Incorrect position of bladder (not centered
    over brachial artery)
  Use of the wrong values
    Missed auscultatory gap
    Confusion over use of muffling (phase IV)
      for diastolic blood pressure
  Variations due to arrhythmias
  Incorrect positioning of arm (not at level of
    heart)
  Unsupported arm or torso
  Too-slow bladder inflation
  Too-rapid bladder deflation
Observer bias due to digit preference

something affecting the patient and, if recognized, are controllable; however, if not recognized, they cannot be reduced by multiple readings. An example of a systematic variation is that related to environmental temperature: a fall in maximal daily temperatures of 12°C was associated with a rise of 5–10 mm Hg in mean daytime DBP among 22 mildly hypertensive subjects (Giaconi et al., 1989). This difference would not be reduced by repeating the measurements at any given time but if recognized could be taken into account.

The degree of random variation in BP is most apparent with continuous intraarterial measurements (Bevan et al., 1969) (Fig. 2.2). Obviously, considerable differences in readings can be seen at different times of the day. Beyond these, between-visit variations in BP can be substantial. After the first three visits, the standard deviation of the difference in BP from one visit to another in the 32 subjects studied by Watson et al. was 10.4 mm Hg for SBP and 7.0 mm Hg for DBP.

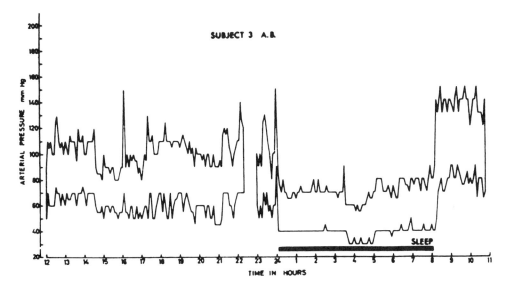

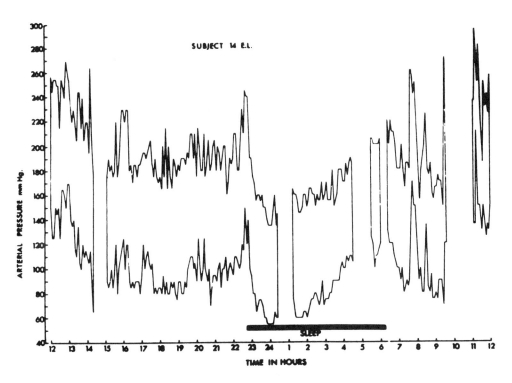

Figure 2.2. Systolic and diastolic blood pressure recorded at 5-minute intervals in a normotensive (*top*) and hypertensive (*bottom*) subject with an intraarterial device. The high pressures in the normotensive subject at 1600 and 2400 are due to a painful stimulus and coitus, respectively. (Reproduced with permission from Bevan AT, Honour AJ, Stott FH. Direct arterial pressure recording in unrestricted man. *Clin Sci* 1969;36:329–344. Copyright 1969, The Biochemical Society, London.)

Types of Variability

As delineated by Conway (1986), variability in BP can be usefully looked at in three ways: short-term, daytime, and diurnal. *Short-term* variability at rest is affected by respiration and heart rate which are under the influence of the autonomic nervous system. *Daytime* variability is mainly determined by the degree of mental and physical activity and is modified by baroreflexes that operate through adjustments in heart rate and peripheral resistance. *Diurnal* variability is substantial, with an average fall in pressure of 20% during sleep, and is partly induced by increased baroreflex sensitivity that decreases sympathetic nervous activity.

The overriding influence of activity on diurnal variations was nicely demonstrated in a study of 461 untreated hypertensive patients whose BP was recorded with a portable noninvasive device every 15 minutes during the day and every 30 minutes at night over a 24-hour interval (Clark et al., 1987). In addition, five readings were taken in the clinic before and another five after the 24-hour recording. When the mean DBP readings for each of the 24 hours were plotted against each patient's mean clinic BP, considerable variations were noted, with lowest pressures during the night and highest near midday (Fig. 2.3, *left*). The patients recorded in a diary where their BP was taken, e.g., at home, work, or other location, and what they were doing at the time, with 15 choices of activity.

When the effects of the various combinations of location and activity on the BP were analyzed, variable effects relative to the BP recorded while relaxing were seen (Table 2.2). When the estimated effects of the various combinations of location and activity were then subtracted from the individual readings obtained throughout the

Table 2.2. Average Changes in Blood Pressure Associated with Commonly Occurring Activities Related to Blood Pressure while Relaxing

Activity	Systolic Blood Pressure	Diastolic Blood Pressure
Meetings	+20.2	+15.0
Work	+16.0	+13.0
Transportation	+14.0	+9.2
Walking	+12.0	+5.5
Dressing	+11.5	+9.7
Chores	+10.7	+6.7
Telephone	+9.5	+7.2
Eating	+8.8	+9.6
Talking	+6.7	+6.7
Desk work	+5.9	+5.3
Reading	+1.9	+2.2
Business (at home)	+1.6	+3.2
Television	+0.3	+1.1
Relaxing	0	0
Sleeping	−10.0	−7.6

Data adapted from Clark LA, Denby L, Pregibon D, et al. A quantitative analysis of the effects of activity and time of day on the diurnal variations of blood pressure. *J Chronic Dis* 1987;40:671–679, copyright 1987. Pergamon Press PLC. Reprinted with permission.

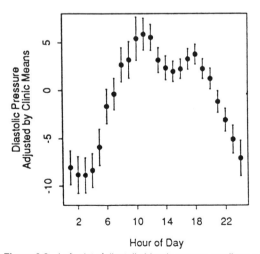 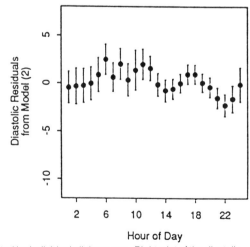

Figure 2.3. *Left*, plot of diastolic blood pressure readings adjusted by individual clinic means. *Right*, plot of the diastolic blood pressure hourly mean residuals after adjustments for various activities by a time-of-day model. The hourly means (*solid circles*) ±2 SEM (*vertical lines*) are plotted versus the corresponding time of day. (Reproduced with permission from Clark LA, Denby L, Pregibon D, et al. A quantitative analysis of the effects of activity and time of day on the diurnal variations of blood pressure. *J Chronic Dis* 1987;40;671–679. Copyright 1987, Pergamon Press PLC.)

24-hour period, very little residual effect related to the time of day was found (Fig. 2.3, *right*). The authors concluded that "there is no important circadian rhythm of BP which is independent of activity."

Blood Pressure During Sleep and on Awakening

Normal Pattern. The usual fall in BP at night is the result of sleep and inactivity rather than the time of day. If people stay awake at night, the pressure falls very little; if they sleep during the day, the pressure falls as expected (Sundberg et al., 1988). The slight rise in BP before awakening and the greater rise after ambulation largely reflect increases in sympathetic nervous activity (Panza et al., 1991; Somers et al., 1993). In a study of 399 randomly selected people, Staessen et al. (1992) found that the degree of fall during sleep follows a normal distribution, averaging 16 ± 9 mm Hg for SBP and 14 ± 7 mm Hg for DBP. Therefore, characterizing patients as "dippers" and "non-dippers" is misleading.

Consequences. The usual fall in pressure during sleep may cause harm by inducing myocardial ischemia in patients with long-standing hypertension who have hypertrophied ventricles or coronary artery disease and therefore impaired coronary vasodilator reserve (Floras, 1988). This fall in perfusion pressure may be particularly ominous when the patient has been inadvertently overtreated with antihypertensive drugs.

On the other hand, the usual abrupt rise in BP after arising in the early morning (Khoury et al., 1992) or in midafternoon after a siesta (Mulcahy et al., 1993) may precipitate serious cardiovascular complications; there is a significantly increased incidence of sudden death (Willich et al., 1992), stroke (Sloan et al., 1992), and myocardial infarction (Fig. 2.4) (Goldberg et al., 1990) in the first few hours after awakening.

Attention must then be directed at ascertaining the degree of the early morning rise in pressure and dampening it with appropriate antihypertensive therapy. This issue is addressed further in Chapter 7, but the proven value of inhibiting both platelet aggregation with aspirin (Ridker et al., 1990) and the degree of rise in BP (Woods et al., 1992) on the incidence of myocardial ischemia in the early morning deserves recognition.

As we shall see, the absence of the usual fall in BP during sleep is also a problem, reflecting,

and likely inducing, additional cardiovascular damage.

Stress of the Measurement

In addition to the changes in BP that occur during sleep and on awakening that are related to sympathetic activation, the actual measurement of the BP may invoke a stress reaction, a reaction that is only transient in most patients but persistent in some. The stress reaction may be partially related to the environment but is mostly related to the measurer.

The Environment. Most patients have a progressive and often dramatic fall in BP after admission to a hospital which may be related to both regression toward the mean and a reduction in anxiety (Nishimura et al., 1987). As will be described more fully later in this chapter, home readings are usually lower than office or clinic readings and are much closer to the average BP recorded by noninvasive ambulatory monitors (Hall et al., 1990).

The Measurer. Figure 2.5 demonstrates that the presence of a physician usually causes a rise in BP that is sometimes very impressive (Mancia et al., 1987b). The data in Figure 2.5 were obtained from patients who underwent a 24-hour intraarterial Oxford recording after 5–7 days in the hospital. When the intraarterial readings were stable, the BP was measured in the noncatheterized arm by both a male physician and a female nurse, half of the time by the physician first, the other half by the nurse first. The patients had not met the personnel but had been told that they would be coming. When the physician took the first readings, the pressures rose an average of 22/14 mm Hg, and as much as 74 mm Hg systolic. Similar rises were seen during three subsequent visits. The rises seen when the nurses took the first set of readings were about half as great as those noted by the physician, and the BP usually returned to near the baseline when measured again after 5 and 10 minutes. The rises were not related to patient age, gender, overall BP variability, or BP levels.

These findings are in keeping with a large amount of data indicating a marked tendency in most patients for BP to fall after repeated measurements regardless of the time interval between readings. They strongly suggest that nurses and not physicians should measure the BP and that at least three sets of readings should be taken before the patient is labeled hypertensive and the need for treatment is determined.

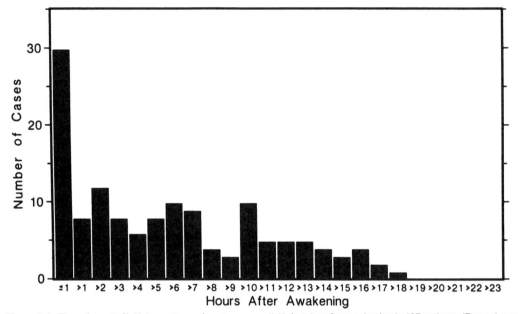

Figure 2.4. Time of onset of initial symptoms of acute myocardial infarction after awakening in 137 patients. (Reproduced with permission from Goldberg RJ, Brady P, Muller JE, et al. Time of onset of symptoms of acute myocardial infarction. *Am J Cardiol* 1990;66:140–144.)

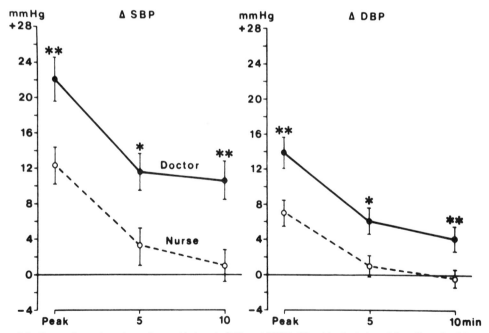

Figure 2.5. Comparison of maximum (or peak) rises in SBP and DBP in 30 subjects during visits with a physician and a nurse. The rises occurring at the 5th and 10th minutes of the visits are shown. Data are expressed as mean ($\pm$SEM) changes from a control value taken 4 minutes before each visit. (Reproduced with permission from Mancia G, Parati G, Pomidossi G, et al. Alerting reaction and rise in blood pressure during measurement by physician and nurse. *Hypertension* 1987;9:209–215. American Heart Association, Inc.)

"White-Coat" Hypertension

Prevalence.   The acute pressor response to the measurement of the blood pressure may persist indefinitely, presumably as a conditioned reflex that increases sympathetic nervous arousal each time the pressure is taken (Pickering, 1992). In a study of 292 patients whose DBP had been repeatedly noted to be between 90 and 104 mm Hg during multiple office visits over an average of 6 years, 21% had persistently normal readings during a 24-hour ambulatory recording taken under usual life conditions (Pickering et al., 1988). The "white-coat" hypertensives were more likely to be younger, nonobese women with a shorter duration of hypertension. White-coat hypertension has been found in about 20% of people diagnosed as hypertensive in routine practice (Hegholm et al., 1992), including elderly patients with predominately systolic hypertension (Cox et al., 1993) and pregnant women (Zuspan and Rayburn, 1991). Moreover, higher office readings are usually noted in those with sustained hypertension as well (Fig. 2.6) (Pickering, 1992). The white-coat effect is responsible for as many as half the cases of "resistant" hypertension which, in fact, is not resistant when the BP is measured outside the office (Mejia et al., 1990a).

Significance.   The definition and prognosis of white-coat hypertension remain in question. Depending on the level chosen as the upper limit of normal for daytime ambulatory blood pressure, the prevalence in a large population of untreated hypertensive patients has been shown to vary from as low as 12.1% to as high as 53.2% (Verdecchia et al., 1992b). Moreover, among 737 young subjects in Tecumseh, Michigan, the 7.1% who had high clinic but normal home readings had early hemodynamic features of persistent hypertension, higher levels of multiple cardiovascular risk factors, including obesity, dyslipidemia, and hyperinsulinemia (Julius et al., 1990), and a higher prevalence of at least one parent with hypertension (Jamerson et al., 1992). Therefore, white-coat hypertensives need counseling to modify unhealthy lifestyles and must remain under observation, much like those with "borderline" hypertension. They should not, however, require antihypertensive therapy, so the need to identify them by out-of-the-office readings is essential.

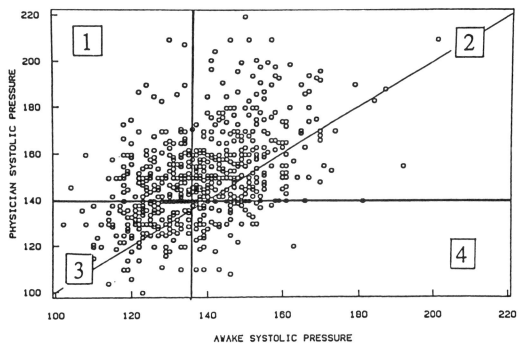

Figure 2.6. Plot of clinic systolic and daytime ambulatory blood pressure in 573 patients. *1*, Patients with white-coat hypertension; *2*, patients with sustained hypertension; *3*, patients with normal blood pressure; *4*, patients whose clinic blood pressure underestimates ambulatory pressure. The majority of patients with sustained hypertension and normal blood pressure had higher clinic pressures than awake ambulatory pressures as shown by the larger number of circles above the line of identity. (Reproduced with permission from Pickering TG. Ambulatory monitoring and the definition of hypertension. *J Hypertens* 1992;10:401–409.)

Other Factors That Affect Variability

Beyond the level of activity and the stresses related to the measurement, a number of other factors affect BP variability, including the sensitivity of baroreflexes and the level of BP, with more variability the higher the pressure (Floras et al., 1988). This latter relationship is probably responsible for the widespread perception that the elderly have more variable BP. When younger and older hypertensives with comparable BP levels were studied, variability was not consistently related to age (Brennan et al., 1986).

It is important to minimize the changes in BP that arise because of variations within the patient. Even little things can have an impact: both SBP and DBP may rise 10 mm Hg with a distended urinary bladder (Fagius and Karhuvaara, 1989) or during relaxed conversation (Silverberg and Rosenfeld, 1980). The pressure rises more when a person talks to someone perceived to be of higher status (Long et al., 1982), which may partly explain why physicians tend to record higher BP readings than their nurses. Interestingly, BP rises in deaf people when they use sign language, suggesting that communication, independent of vocalization, affects the cardiovascular system (Malinow et al., 1986).

Smoking.   Acutely, the surge of nicotine causes a rise in both SBP and DBP that may last for 15 to 30 minutes (Groppelli et al., 1992), likely mediated by release of norepinephrine from adrenergic nerves. Even more prolonged elevations in BP follow use of smokeless tobacco (Hirsch et al., 1992). When their pressures are taken more than 30 minutes after their last cigarette, smokers have generally been found to be no more hypertensive than nonsmokers, and many are often less hypertensive because smokers tend to weigh less than nonsmokers. However, the repeated pressor effects of each cigarette can result in elevated pressures for most of the day in the typical pack-per-day smoker, clearly contributing to the increased risk for cardiovascular diseases noted among smokers.

Caffeine.   Caffeine causes an acute rise in BP and levels of both renin and catecholamines in people who do not normally ingest caffeine-containing beverages. Within a few days, complete tolerance to all of these effects occurs so that the habitual intake of caffeine-containing beverages is unlikely to affect the BP (Shi et al., 1993).

Alcohol.   Acutely, when 0.75 g/kg body weight of ethanol was consumed by a group of young normotensives in 15 minutes so that the blood alcohol level rose quickly to almost 100 mg/dL, a definite rise in BP occurred (Potter et al., 1986). Chronically, alcohol intake beyond 2 ounces/day may induce considerable and persistent rises in BP, so that heavy alcohol intake may be the most common cause of reversible hypertension (see Chapter 3).

OFFICE MEASUREMENT OF BLOOD PRESSURE

Use of the guidelines shown in Table 2.3, adapted from those recommended by the American Heart Association (Frohlich et al., 1988), the British Hypertension Society (Petrie et al., 1986), and the American Society of Hypertension (1992) will prevent most measurement errors. Repeated careful measurements can provide data as reliable as those obtained with ambulatory monitoring (Pearce et al., 1992).

Patient and Arm Position

The patient should be seated comfortably with the arm supported and positioned at the level of the heart (Fig. 2.7). Measurements taken with the arm dependent by the side average 8 mm Hg higher than those taken with the arm supported in a horizontal position at heart level (Mariotti et al., 1987). When sitting upright on a table without support, readings may be as much as 10 mm Hg higher because of the isometric exertion needed to support the body and arm (Cushman et al., 1990).

Differences Between Arms

Initially, the BP should be measured in both arms. Although differences between the two arms are noted only rarely (Gould et al., 1985), if the reading is higher in one arm, that arm should be used for future measurements. Lower pressure in the left arm is seen in patients with subclavian steal caused by reversal of flow down a vertebral artery distal to an obstructed subclavian artery, as noted in 9% of 500 patients with asymptomatic neck bruits (Bornstein and Norris, 1986). On the other hand, BP may be either higher or lower in the paretic arm of a stroke patient (Dewar et al., 1992).

Standing Pressure

Readings should be taken immediately and after standing 2 minutes to check for spontaneous or drug-induced postural changes. In most people, SBP falls and DBP rises a few millimeters of mercury on changing from the supine to

Table 2.3. Guidelines for Measurement of Blood Pressure

Patient conditions
  Posture
    Initially, particularly in patients over age 65, diabetic, or receiving antihypertensive therapy, check for postural changes by taking readings after 5 minutes supine, then immediately and 2 minutes after they stand.
    For routine follow-up, sitting pressures are recommended. The patient should sit quietly with the back supported for 5 minutes and the arm supported at the level of the heart.
  Circumstances
    No caffeine during the hour preceding the reading.
    No smoking during the 15 minutes preceding the reading.
    No exogenous adrenergic stimulants (e.g., phenylephrine in nasal decongestants or eye drops for pupillary dilation).
    A quiet, warm setting.
    Home readings taken under varying circumstances and 24-hour ambulatory recordings may be preferable and more accurate in predicting subsequent cardiovascular disease.
Equipment
  Cuff size: The bladder should encircle and cover two-thirds of the length of the arm; if it does not, place the bladder over the brachial artery. If bladder is too small, high readings may result.
  Manometer: Aneroid gauges should be calibrated every 6 months against a mercury manometer.
  For infants, use ultrasound equipment (e.g., the Doppler method).
Technique
  Number of readings
    On each occasion, take at least two readings, separated by as much time as is practical. If readings vary by more than 5 mm Hg, take additional readings until two are close.
    For diagnosis, obtain three sets of readings at least 1 week apart.
    Initially, take pressure in both arms; if the pressures differ, use the arm with the higher pressure.
    If the arm pressure is elevated, take pressure in one leg, particularly in patients younger than 30.
  Performance
    Inflate the bladder quickly to a pressure 20 mm Hg above the systolic pressure, as recognized by disappearance of the radial pulse.
    Deflate the bladder 3 mm Hg every second.
    Record the Korotkoff phase V (disappearance), except in children, in whom use of phase IV (muffling) may be preferable.
    If the Korotkoff sounds are weak, have the patient raise the arm, open and close the hand 5–10 times, and then inflate the bladder quickly.
Recordings
  Note the pressure, patient position, the arm, cuff size: e.g., 140/90, seated, right arm, large adult cuff.

---

the standing position. In the elderly, significant postural falls of 20 mm Hg or more in SBP are more common, occurring in about 10% of ambulatory people over age 65 and even more frequently in those with systolic hypertension (Lipsitz et al., 1985) (see Chapter 4). Standing pressures should routinely be taken in the elderly to recognize postural falls, particularly before institution of antihypertensive therapy.

Leg Pressure

If the arm reading is elevated, particularly in a patient under age 30, the BP should be taken in one leg to rule out coarctation. The technique for measuring BP in the leg is described in the next section.

The Sphygmomanometer

Cuff Size. The width of the cuff should be equal to about two-thirds of the distance from the axilla to the antecubital space; a 15-cm-wide cuff is adequate for most adults. The bladder within the cuff should be long enough to encircle at least 80% of the arm (Fig. 2.8) (Petrie et al., 1986). Erroneously high readings may occur with use of a cuff that is either too narrow or too short (Croft and Cruickshank, 1990).

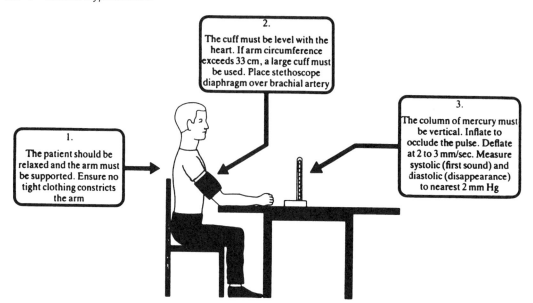

Figure 2.7. Technique of blood pressure measurement recommended by the British Hypertension Society. (Reproduced with permission from British Hypertension Society. *J Hypertens* 1985;3:293.)

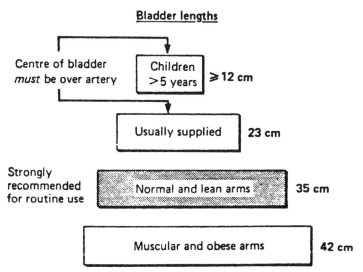

Figure 2.8. Recommendations for the size of blood pressure cuff bladder lengths. (Reproduced with permission from Petrie JC, O'Brien ET, Littler WA, de Swiet M. Recommendations on blood pressure measurement. *Br Med J* 1986;293:611–615.)

Most sphygmomanometers sold in the United States have a cuff with a bladder that is 12 cm wide and 23 cm long, which is too short for patients with an arm circumference greater than 33 cm, whether fat or muscular. The best cuff to use for most adults is the "obese" cuff with a 15 × 33–35 cm bladder; for those with arm circumference greater than 41 cm, the thigh cuff, with a 18 × 36–42 cm bladder, should be used. "Cuff hypertension" can be avoided with use of the recently described tricuff which contains three rubber balloons of different sizes which automatically selects the appropriate size in relation to the arm circumference (Stolt et al., 1993).

Cuff Position.   If the bladder within the cuff does not completely encircle the arm, particular care should be taken to ensure that it is placed over the brachial artery. The lower edge of the cuff should be about 2.5 cm above the antecubital space. In extremely obese people, a more accurate reading may be obtained by placing the cuff on the forearm and listening over the radial artery.

Manometer. Three types of manometers are in use, aneroid, mercury, and a number of electronic devices for out-of-office semiautomatic recordings, as reviewed in Consumer Reports (Anonymous, 1992). Aneroid manometers are frequently inaccurate (Bailey et al., 1991), so they should be checked every few months by connecting a bladder to both the aneroid and a mercury manometer with a Y-tube. With mercury manometers, the reservoir should be full, the meniscus should read zero when no pressure is applied, and the column should move freely when pressure is applied. The filter and vent to the mercury column should be cleaned yearly.

Random-zero manometers have been used to reduce observer bias, but they underestimate the BP (O'Brien et al., 1990a).

New Devices. Beyond the various automatic devices that depend upon compression of the brachial artery, two devices measure the pressure in the fingers, Finapress in one finger (Bos et al., 1992a), Portapres in two (Imholz et al., 1993). If used carefully, these devices can provide noninvasive, continuous 24-hour ambulatory readings as reliably as and more conveniently than other equipment. Another cuffless device that works on the basis of pulse wave velocity, Pulse Time, has been claimed to be reasonably accurate (Carruthers and Taggart, 1988).

Technique for Measuring Blood Pressure

As noted in Table 2.3, care should be taken to raise the pressure in the bladder about 20 mm Hg above the systolic level, as indicated by disappearance of the radial pulse, because patients may have an auscultatory gap, a temporary disappearance of the sound after it first appears. The measurement may be repeated after as little as 15 seconds without significantly affecting accuracy. The cuff should be deflated at a rate of 2–4 mm Hg/second; a slower rate will cause falsely higher readings (Bos et al., 1992b).

Disappearance of the sound (phase V) is a more reliable and reproducible end-point than muffling (phase IV) and is closer to the true intraarterial DBP (Hense et al., 1986). In some patients with a hyperkinetic circulation (e.g., anemia), the sounds do not disappear, and the muffled sound is heard well below the expected

DBP, sometimes near zero. This can also be caused by pressing the stethescope too firmly against the artery. If arrhythmias are present, additional readings may be required to estimate the average SBP and DBP (Sykes et al., 1990).

"Pseudohypertension"

In some elderly patients with very rigid, calcified arteries, the bladder may not be able to collapse the brachial artery, giving rise to falsely high readings or "pseudohypertension" (Spence et al., 1980). The possibility of pseudohypertension should be suspected in elderly people whose vessels feel rigid, who have little vascular damage in the retina or elsewhere despite seemingly high BP readings, and who suffer inordinate postural symptoms despite cautious therapy. An indication of pseudohypertension may be obtained by Osler's maneuver; that is, the radial pulse remains palpable after the pressure in the balloon has occluded the brachial artery, as evidenced by disappearance of the Korotkoff sounds (Messerli et al., 1985). Osler's maneuver has little utility for identifying the few patients with pseudohypertension because of marked intra- and interobserver disagreement (Oliner et al., 1993). If one is suspicious, an automatic oscillometric recorder or finger BP measurement should settle the issue (Zweifler and Shahab, 1993), but a direct intraarterial reading may be needed.

Ways to Amplify the Sounds

The loudness and sharpness of the Korotkoff sounds depend in part on the pressure differential between the arteries in the forearm and those beneath the bladder. To increase the differential and thereby increase the loudness of the sounds, either decrease the amount of blood or increase the capacity of the vascular bed in the forearm. The amount of blood can be decreased by rapid inflation of the bladder, shortening the time when venous outflow is prevented but arterial inflow continues, or by raising the arm for a few seconds to drain venous blood before inflating the bladder. The vascular bed capacity can be increased by inducing vasodilation through muscular exercise, specifically by having the patient open and close the hand 10 times before inflating the bladder. Do not stop between the systolic and diastolic readings; reinflate and start all over again. The vessels will have been partially refilled and the sounds thereby altered.

Taking the Pressure in the Thigh

A large (thigh) cuff should be used to avoid factitiously elevated readings. With the patient lying prone, the leg bent and cradled by the observer, listen with the stethoscope for the Korotkoff sounds in the popliteal fossa. This should be done as part of the initial workup of every hypertensive and with special care in those under age 30 in whom coarctation is more common. Normally, the SBP is higher, the DBP a little lower at the knee than in the arm because of the contour of the pulse wave (Hugue et al., 1988).

Taking Blood Pressure in Children (see Chapter 16)

If the child is calm, the same technique used with adults should be followed; however, smaller, narrower cuffs must be used. As in adults, the bladder should encircle the upper arm (Gómez-Marín et al., 1992), and the fifth Korotkoff phase is more reliable than the fourth (Uhari et al., 1991). If the child is disturbed, the best procedure may be simply to determine the SBP by palpating the radial pulse as the cuff is deflated. In infants, ultrasound techniques are much easier to use (Laaser and Labarthe, 1986).

Blood Pressure During Exercise

The SBP typically rises significantly during isotonic exercise, and both SBP and DBP rise during isometric exercise. A failure of the SBP to rise is indicative of high risk for cardiovascular death (Morrow et al., 1993). Care should be taken in measuring indirect BP during isotonic exercise because the reading may underestimate the true intraarterial change (Kaijser, 1987). More reliable readings have been obtained with Paramed, a device that has differential sensors and a microprocessor to eliminate noise (Ogasawara et al., 1989). The SBP may rise above 195 mm Hg during isotonic exercise, and such a response may indicate the development of soon-to-be persistent hypertension (see Chapter 4).

Recording of Findings

Regardless of which method is used to measure BP, notation should be made of the conditions so that others can compare the findings or interpret them properly. This is particularly critical in scientific reports; yet, most articles about hypertension in prestigious medical journals fail to do so (Roche et al., 1990).

Importance of Office Blood Pressures

Even if all the causes of measurement and biologic variations are recognized and as much care as possible is taken to follow the guidelines listed in Table 2.3, routine office measurements of blood pressure by sphygmomanometry will continue to show considerable variability. However, before discounting even single casual BP readings, recall that almost all the data on the risks of hypertension described in Chapter 1 are based on only one or a few readings taken in large groups of people. There is no denying that such data have epidemiologic value, but a few casual office readings are usually not enough to determine the status of an individual patient. Two actions will minimize variability. First, take at least two readings at every visit, as many as needed to obtain a stable level, with less than 5 mm Hg difference; second, take at least three sets of readings, preferably weeks apart, unless the initial value is so high (e.g., above 180/120) that immediate therapy is needed.

The closer the initial and subsequent readings are to 140/90 mm Hg, the more repeated readings are needed to be able to determine the patient's status (Perry and Miller, 1992). Although multiple carefully taken office readings may be as reliable as those taken by ambulatory monitors (Pearce et al., 1992; Reeves et al., 1992), out-of-office readings do provide additional data, both to confirm the diagnosis and, more importantly, to document the adequacy of therapy. For those with white-coat hypertension, out-of-office readings are essential (Veerman and van Montfrans, 1993); for almost all hypertensives, they will improve management.

HOME AND AMBULATORY MEASUREMENTS

From the preceding, it is clear that pressures recorded in the hospital or office are often affected by both acute and chronic stress reactions and conditioned reflexes that tend to accentuate variability and raise the BP, giving rise to significant white-coat hypertension. Two techniques, home measurements and ambulatory blood pressure monitoring (ABPM), minimize these problems. I believe they will become standard practices in the clinical management of hypertension, as well as mandated practices in the evaluation of new antihypertensive agents. For now, however, the limited amount of long-term follow-up data based upon these techniques and the practical limitations upon their use (Appel and Stason, 1993) have prompted the American College of Physicians (1993) to make these recommendations: ''Available evidence does not warrant widespread dissemination or routine use of automated ambulatory blood pressure measurement at this time. . . . Self-measured blood pressure devices are increasingly being used by patients, and this practice should be encouraged. However, it should also be clear that there has not been sufficient formal evaluation of this method to warrant managing patients solely using blood pressure readings obtained with self-monitoring blood pressure devices. On the other hand, when used as adjunct to physicians' and nonphysicians' office-based measurements, self-measured blood pressures are an invaluable source of information for the management of hypertension.''

Home Measurements

The ''invaluable source of information'' provided by home BP measurements can be of great value for the clinical management of many patients (Julius, 1991) (Table 2.4). Except for the additional information provided by measurements taken during sleep and the inability of a few patients to measure their own BP, self-recorded home measurements give almost all of the information provided by 24-hour ABPM (Stewart and Padfield, 1992). The average BP levels obtained by multiple home readings and those recorded by an ambulatory monitor while the patient is awake are quite close. The self-recorded levels are almost always higher than the full 24-hour ambulatory average because the latter reading includes the pressures taken during sleep, which are almost always lower. Both the home and ambulatory readings are usually quite comparable, reproducible, and considerably lower than office readings (James et al., 1988) (Table 2.5).

In the following sections, the multiple uses for self-recorded measurements are reviewed, and some information about the currently available equipment and guidelines for its use is provided.

Diagnosis

As perhaps first clearly recognized by Ayman and Goldshine in 1940, home recordings are generally lower than office readings and much closer to the levels noted by ''basal'' recordings obtained after prolonged bed rest or ABPM. Home recordings overcome much of the error caused by the acute and persistent pressor-stress response that is responsible for most white-coat hypertension (Hall et al., 1990). The data in Table 2.6 document the significantly lower average of the 32 home readings per patient taken during the 2 weeks between the first and second clinic visits in 268 patients with a BP above 160/95 on three consecutive occasions, twice in the general practitioner's office before the first clinic reading. The home readings were lower in 80% of the patients, by more than 20/10 mm Hg in 40%, so that therapy was deemed unnecessary in 38% of untreated patients and reducible in 16% of treated patients. The accuracy of the home readings taken with the electronic devices is evident by the identical readings taken with that device and the mercury sphygmomanometer at the second clinic visit.

The upper limits of normal for home readings, based on the mean ± 2 standard deviations of 608 healthy young adults, were 142/92 for men and 131/85 for women (Mejia et al., 1990b).

Table 2.4.   Indications for Home Blood Pressure Monitoring

For diagnosis
    To recognize initial, short-term elevations in blood pressure
    To identify persistent white-coat hypertension
    To determine usual blood pressure levels in patients with borderline hypertension
For prognosis
    Inadequate data available except for the relation of hypertension to left ventricular hypertrophy
For therapy
    To monitor response to therapy
        To ensure adequate blood pressure control during awake hours
        To evaluate effects of increasing or decreasing amounts of therapy
        To ascertain whether poor office blood pressure response to increasing treatment represents overtreatment or true resistance
        To identify periods of poor control when office readings are normal but target organ damage progresses
        To identify relation of blood pressure levels to presumed side effects of therapy
        To involve patient and improve adherence

Table 2.5. Average Blood Pressures (BP) in Hypertensive Subjects as Determined by Three Methods of Measurement Compared Over 2 Weeks[a]

Measurement	Ambulatory BP (Awake and Asleep) (mm Hg)	Home BP (mm Hg)	Clinic BP (mm Hg)
Systolic			
Initial	134 ± 11	140 ± 14	158 ± 23[b]
Second	132 ± 12	143 ± 13	152 ± 20
Diastolic			
Initial	85 ± 10	86 ± 12	93 ± 11
Second	86 ± 10	87 ± 12	91 ± 10

Reproduced with permission from James GD, Pickering TG, Yee LS, et al. The reproducibility of average ambulatory, home, and clinic pressures. *Hypertension* 1988;11:545–549. American Heart Association, Inc.
[a]Values are average ± SD.
[b]$p < 0.05$, significantly different from second reading.

Table 2.6. Blood Pressure Recorded at Home Between Clinic Visits

Patient Group	First Clinic Reading (Mercury Manometer)		Home Series (Electronic Device)		Second Clinic Reading			
					Electronic Device		Mercury Manometer	
	SBP	DBP	SBP	DBP	SBP	DBP	SBP	DBP
Untreated $n = 114$	174	103	148	90	165	95	164	97
Treated $n = 154$	177	104	147	87	163	95	164	95

Data from Hall CL, Higgs CMB, Notarianni L. Home blood pressure recording in mild hypertension: value of distinguishing sustained from clinic hypertension and effect on diagnosis and treatment. *J Hum Hypertens* 1990;4:501–507.

Prognosis

There are no data documenting the validity of self-recorded home measurements for ascertainment of long-term prognosis, but they do correlate better with left ventricular hypertrophy than do office readings (Kleinert et al., 1984). Presumably, they will prove to be equal to ABPM.

Therapy

Home recording will be increasingly used to monitor the short- and long-term response to therapy (Table 2.4). Rather than depend on occasional office visits, with their propensity to make the level of hypertension appear to be worse than it is during usual life circumstances, patients should be encouraged to monitor their hypertension with a home device. Perhaps the greatest benefit will be the avoidance of inadvertent overtreatment, a particular need in the elderly (Raccaud et al., 1992).

A striking example of the potential for overtreatment by use of only office readings was reported by Waeber et al. (1987). Although they compared office readings with those obtained by ABPM, it was likely that the values reported by ABPM would be close to those of home recordings because the investigators used only the daytime values. In this study, 17 of 34 hypertensives with office DBP readings above 95 mm Hg despite antihypertensive therapy were noted to have average daytime ambulatory readings below 90 mm Hg. They were given additional treatment on the basis of their office readings; as a result, some ended up with considerably lower BPs than desired (Fig. 2.9).

Equipment

Although mercury and aneroid manometers can be used, semi-automatic electronic devices are only a little more expensive, equally accurate, and much easier to use. Some electronic models are self-inflating, thereby eliminating the potential of transiently high systolic readings from the muscular activity of inflating the cuff (Veerman et al., 1990) but they are double the cost of those that must be inflated manually. Some use a microphone to detect Korotkoff sounds, others are oscillometric devices that do not require as accurate placement of the cuff. The oscillometric devices tend to give less accurate systolic but more accurate diastolic readings (Imai et al., 1989).

Patients with diastolic pressure at beginning ⩽ 90 mmHg
n = 17

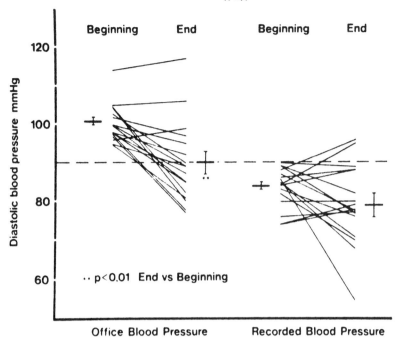

Figure 2.9. Office and ambulatory (recorded) diastolic BP at beginning and end of study in 17 patients with ambulatory diastolic blood pressure of 90 mm Hg or lower at beginning despite office readings above 95 mm Hg. (Reproduced with permission from Waeber B, Scherrer U, Petrillo A, et al. Are some hypertensive patients overtreated? A prospective study of ambulatory blood pressure recording. *Lancet* 1987;2:732–734).

The May 1992 Consumer Reports (Anonymous, 1992) rates 15 electronic models that are available in the U.S. for consistency, accuracy, and ease of use. Among the self-inflating devices, the ratings, in order of estimated quality are: Omron HEM-704C, Sunbeam 7650, Lumiscope 1081, Marshall 91, and Omron HEM-713C. Devices that require manual inflation are rated as follows: Sunbeam 7621, AND UA-701, Sunmark 144, Omron HEM-413C, Walgreens 80WA, Marshall 80, and Lumiscope 1065. Some of these devices can be fitted with an oversized cuff for people with obese or muscular arms, including the Lumiscope 1001, the Marshall 91, and the AND UA-701. The four electronic finger models tested are all rated "not acceptable."

Technique

All the instructions concerning posture, circumstances surrounding the measurement, etc. that are needed for office readings (Table 2.3) need to be followed with home readings, and patients should always be given instructions to supplement those provided with the device. The accuracy of the device and the procedure used by the patient (or person taking the home readings) should be checked by a simultaneous measurement on the other arm in the office with a mercury manometer. These points should be made to the patient:

—Do not be concerned by fluctuations of 5, 10, or even 20 mm Hg, but do inform the physician's office if the pressures are going up progressively over a period of a week or longer.
—If the home readings are being taken to determine the average blood pressure for diagnostic purposes, the readings should be made at different times, e.g., when the patient is either relaxed or stressed, anytime throughout the day or evening.
—If the readings are being taken to determine the adequacy of antihypertensive therapy, the readings should be taken at the same time of day, preferably in the early morning soon after arising from bed, to ensure 24-hour control with the regimen being prescribed. Readings should occasionally be taken repeatedly throughout the interval of a dose of therapy

to ascertain both the peak effect and the duration of effect.

To monitor patients' home readings, the Instromedic Baro-Graf QD device stores and transmits readings over the phone (James et al., 1990).

Stationary Automated Recording

Stationary machines for automated measurements of blood pressure are often found in public places. They substitute human error with the technical errors to which all complex equipment is subject, coupled with the need for maintenance. An evaluation of 10 Vita-Stat machines, the most widely used device in the United States, found them to be less accurate than routine sphygmomanometry and concluded that they are "an unsatisfactory tool for community-based self-measurement of blood pressure" (Salaita et al., 1990).

Ambulatory Monitoring

Noninvasive ABPM is being advocated for additional reasons beyond those for home recordings, mainly for more immediate ascertainment of the usual level of blood pressure and for recognition of the prognostic and therapeutic importance of BP during sleep. More complete coverage of ABPM is provided by Pickering (1991).

The first ABPM, the Remler device, had to be inflated by the patient (Hinman et al., 1962). Although readings could not be obtained during sleep, the use of this device by Sokolow, Perloff and their coworkers provided most of the pertinent information that is known today, even after 30 years of additional work by hundreds of investigators. They showed the value of ABPM in establishing the diagnosis (Perloff and Sokolow, 1978), the prognosis (Sokolow et al., 1966; Perloff et al., 1983), and the need for therapy (Sokolow et al., 1973). Although the clinical application of ABPM has been markedly restrained in the U.S. because most third-party payers will not pay for it, the procedure is now more widely recommended and used. The 1993 report of the Fifth Joint National Committee (1993) states that ABPM "is not necessary for the routine diagnosis and management of most patients," but lists a number of situations in which it would be useful (Table 2.7). In addition, ABPM has been shown to be cost-effective when used appropriately (Krakoff, 1993).

Certain potential problems should be recognized: ABPM may cause mechanical trauma

Table 2.7. Situations in Which Automated Noninvasive Ambulatory Blood Pressure Monitoring Devices May Be Useful

Office or white-coat hypertension
  (blood pressure repeatedly elevated in
    office setting but repeatedly normal out of
    office)
Evaluation of drug resistance
Evaluation of nocturnal blood pressure
  changes
Episodic hypertension
Hypotensive symptoms associated with
  antihypertensive medications or autonomic
  dysfunction
Carotid sinus syncope and pacemaker
  syndromes[a]

The fifth report of the Joint National Committee on Detection, Evaluation, and Treatment of High Blood Pressure (JNC V). *Arch Intern Med* 1993;153:154–183.
[a]Along with electrocardiographic monitoring. (Reproduced with permission from the Joint National Committee on Detection, Evaluation, and Treatment of High Blood Pressure (JNC-V).

(Bottini et al., 1991); the data may show moderate variability on repeated measurements (Reeves and Myers, 1993); unrestricted activity will cause artifactual readings (West et al., 1991); and, as we shall see, the equipment may be unreliable.

Equipment

The noninvasive 24-hour ABPM systems now available use a standard arm cuff that is inflated at predetermined intervals, usually every 15–30 minutes during the day and every 30–45 minutes during the night, by a small pump that is carried on a shoulder strap or attached to the belt. The BP is ascertained either by auscultation through a small microphone placed under the cuff over the brachial artery or by oscillometry which recognizes small changes in air pressure within the inflated cuff, records the SBP and mean BPs, and calculates the DBP. Some of the units using auscultation remove artifactual sounds by accepting only sounds accompanied by an R-wave recorded from a simultaneous electrocardiogram.

The individual BPs measured throughout the 24 hours are stored in the unit worn by the patient and later read by a computer that prints all of the readings (Fig. 2.10) along with the mean ± standard deviations for whatever intervals are desired.

As more of these expensive devices are being marketed, the British Hypertension Society has established a protocol for their evaluation

(O'Brien et al., 1990b) that is even more stringent than the criteria of the United States Association for the Advancement of Medical Instrumentation (AAMI) (White et al., 1993). In evaluations of six currently available models, two (CH-Druck/Pressure Scan ERKA and Profilomat) received an excellent rating, two (Spacelabs 90207, Novacor DIASYS 200) were rated acceptable, and two others (DelMar Avionics Pressurometer IV and Takeda TM-2420) failed (O'Brien et al., 1991, 1992a, 1992b).

Interpretation of ABPM Data

Effects of Activity.
Patients should keep a diary of activities during the 24 hours because of the often marked associated changes in BP (see Table 2.2). A computer-assisted diary (Van Egeren and Madarasmi, 1988) or an electronic activity monitor worn on the dominant wrist (Gretler et al., 1993) may document activity more accurately. To prevent the marked changes induced by activity and position, it may be necessary to limit these factors to ensure more diagnostic accuracy (Pieper et al., 1993).

Summarizing the Data.
Although investigators continue to debate the best way to interpret the data, the best way for clinical use is to simply take the mean of all values (Coats et al., 1991). Most use the average value of all readings obtained throughout the 24 hours. Recognizing that readings during sleep are normally considerably lower than daytime readings, making the 24-hour average lower than the daytime average, there is increasing use of the mean of all daytime (awake) and nighttime (sleep) readings, a procedure that seems sensible and appropriate (Scientific Committee, 1990; Staessen et al., 1994). Therefore, the average daytime value more closely approximates that found by multiple office or home readings, and the nighttime readings receive the attention they deserve. Since virtually all normotensive people have occasional high readings and virtually all fixed hypertensive patients have some normal readings, some advocate use of the "load," i.e., the percentage of ambulatory pressures higher than 140 systolic or 90 diastolic, to diagnose hypertension (Zachariah and Sumner, 1993) and to ascertain the response to therapy (White, 1991).

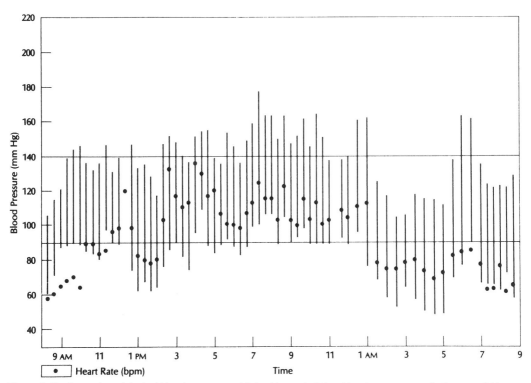

Figure 2.10. Computer printout of blood pressures obtained by ambulatory blood pressure monitoring over 24 hours beginning at 9 am in a 50-year-old man with hypertension receiving no therapy. The patient slept from midnight until 6 am. *Solid circles,* heart rate. (Reproduced with permission from Zachariah PK, Sheps SG, Smith RL. Defining the roles of home and ambulatory monitoring. *Diagnosis* 1988;10:39–50.)

To overcome some of the methodological problems of dealing with literally hundreds of readings, some advocate the use of shorter periods of ABPM (Chanudet et al., 1992). However, others find that the average reading over a few hours may not provide a precise estimate of the daytime or entire 24-hour average (Mancia et al., 1993).

Diagnostic Use

As noted earlier, the definitions of normal and high BP levels obtained by routine sphygmomanometry are arbitrary and still not universally agreed upon. Since ABPM has been performed on many fewer people and since long-term follow-up is not yet available to establish the prognostic meaning of different levels, the definition of normal by ABPM remains uncertain. However, a meta-analysis of data from 23 studies including 3476 normal subjects (Staessen et al., 1991) provides these mean ± 2 standard deviations for the upper limits of normal:

—139/87 for the entire 24 hours (Fig. 2.11)
—146/91 for the daytime
—127/79 for the nighttime

O'Brien et al. (1993) recommend rounding out these data so that the upper limits of normal are 140/90 for the 24-hour period, 150/90 for daytime, and 130/80 for nighttime.

A further expansion of this data base encompasses 4577 normotensives (clinic BP below 140/90), 1324 patients with systolic hypertension (clinic BP 160 mm Hg or higher), and 1310 with diastolic hypertension (clinic BP 95 or higher) (Staessen et al., 1994). The mean ± 2 standard deviations (95th percentile) of the 24-hour levels in the normotensives was 133/82 mm Hg. Of the patients with systolic hypertension, 24% had a 24-hour systolic ambulatory BP below the 95th percentile of normotensives; of those with diastolic hypertension, 30% were below the 95th percentile. These data suggest that as many as 30% of all "clinic hypertensives" will have normal ABPM readings, thereby classifying them as white-coat hypertensives.

The Decision to Treat. Beyond the issue of what is a normal or high BP by ABPM is the larger one: Should ABPM data be used to decide upon the need to treat individual patients? For now, the consensus seems to favor continued use of repeated office readings over ABPM levels (American College of Physicians, 1993). Certainly, disagreements between the two are common. Among 108 patients, the WHO/ISH criteria were used to determine the need for institution of therapy; when criteria based on ABPM were applied to the same patients, the determina-

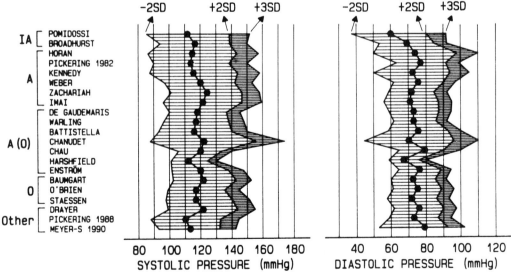

Figure 2.11. Systolic and diastolic blood pressure over 24 hours in various studies. For each study the mean ±2 and ±3 standard deviations are presented. The following abbreviations indicate the technique for recording BP: *A*, auscultatory; *A(O)*, auscultatory with oscillometric backup; *IA*, intraarterial; *O*, oscillometric. Each name refers to a different series of normotensive subjects. (Reproduced with permission from Staessen JA, Fagard RH, Lijnen PJ, et al. Mean and range of the ambulatory pressure in normotensive subjects from a meta-analysis of 23 studies. *Am J Cardiol* 1991;67:723–727.)

tions were the same in 77 patients, but disagreed in 31 (Chatellier et al., 1992). For now, I believe that people with high office readings who are found to be normotensive by either home readings or ABPM, i.e., those with white-coat hypertension, should not be labeled as hypertensive or treated with antihypertensive drugs unless significant hypertensive target organ damage is present. This issue is covered in more detail in Chapter 5.

Prognostic Use

Target Organ Damage. Ambulatory pressures predict the risk for target organ damage and cardiovascular events better than casual or office readings. Most of the data about target organ damage are cross-sectional and show that the extent of left ventricular hypertrophy by echocardiography is more closely correlated with 24-hour ambulatory pressure than casual pressure (Verdecchia and Porcellati, 1993; Cox et al., 1993). This close correlation with ambulatory pressure has also been shown for other indices of target organ damage, including changes in the optic fundi (Palatini et al., 1992) and in renal function (Omboni et al. 1992).

Prognosis. The prognostic value of ABPM is supported by Perloff et al. (1983, 1991) who examined 1076 patients both with multiple office BPs on three visits and with ambulatory readings taken every 30 minutes while the patients were awake over a 1- to 2-day period. The average of the office readings for all patients was 161/101, whereas the ambulatory readings averaged 146/92. In 78% of the patients, the ambulatory readings were lower than the office readings. The patients were followed for as long as 16 years, with the mean duration being 5 years. Life table analyses of their massive set of data showed a significantly greater cumulative 10-year incidence of both fatal and nonfatal cardiovascular events among patients with higher ambulatory BP than those with lower ambulatory BP as compared with their office BP readings (Fig. 2.12).

Blood Pressure During Sleep

BPs recorded during sleep are almost always considerably lower than those recorded while the patient is awake. The failure of BP to fall by 10% or more during sleep has been associated with a number of increased cardiovascular risks, including:

—A first major cardiovascular event over the next 1 to 5 years (Verdecchia et al., 1992a);

—Cerebrovascular damage visualized by MRI (Shimada et al., 1992); and

—Left ventricular hypertrophy (Palatini et al., 1992).

Associations. Moreover, groups of patients known to have higher degrees of overall cardiovascular risk with any given level of daytime blood pressure have been found not to have a normal fall in pressure during sleep. These include:

—Diabetics, either normotensive or hypertensive (Fogari et al., 1993), particularly in the presence of proteinuria (Lurbe et al., 1993). This may reflect diabetic neuropathy (Gambardella et al., 1993);

—American, but not South African, blacks (Fumo et al., 1992);

—Women with preeclampsia (Rath et al., 1990); and

—Patients with chronic renal failure (Baumgart et al., 1991).

A similar lack of the normal fall in BP during sleep has been observed in some patients with various secondary forms of hypertension, including renovascular disease, glucocorticoid and mineralocorticoid excess, and pheochromocytoma (Padfield and Stewart, 1991). This may be related to persistent sympathetic activation or to poorer quality of sleep in patients who are ill.

Therapeutic Response

ABPM has shown that some drugs thought to have a duration of action long enough to allow for once-a-day dosing may turn out not to (Neutel et al., 1990), whereas other drugs thought to be relatively shorter acting may be capable of sustained once-a-day effectiveness (Mancia et al., 1987a). ABPM can be particularly helpful in assessing an individual patient's apparent resistance to increased therapy (Pickering, 1988). As noted (see Fig. 2.9), some patients who appear to be resistant in the office are found to be responsive at home.

New Drug Evaluation

In addition to the more accurate information ABPM provides about efficacy, there are many reasons why ABPM should be a major part of the evaluation of new drugs. First, drugs may have different effects on office and ambulatory readings. In one study, the response to two β-blockers was equal according to office readings, but with ABPM significant differences in both efficacy and duration of action were noted (Neu-

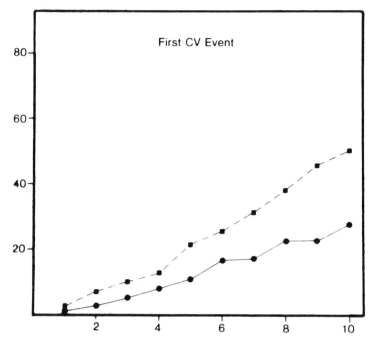

Figure 2.12. Estimated cumulative incidence of cardiovascular morbidity and mortality over 10 years among patients classified according to the difference between their observed ambulatory systolic blood pressure and their office reading. *The dashed line* represents those whose ambulatory SBP was less than 10 mm Hg lower than the office reading; the *solid line* represents those with an ambulatory SBP more than 10 mm Hg lower than the office reading, derived from regression of ambulatory BP on office BP. *CV,* cardiovascular. (Reproduced with permission from Perloff D, Sokolow M, Cowan R. The prognostic value of ambulatory blood pressure. *JAMA* 1983;249:2792–2798. Copyright 1983, American Medical Association.)

tel et al., 1993). Second, to assess the duration of action of a drug, its effect must be measured in ambulatory patients performing their usual activities. In particular, ABPM is the only way to ascertain the efficacy of a drug during the critical early morning hours when the pressure spontaneously rises. Third, by removing the placebo response and improving the accuracy of BP measurements, ABPM will decrease the number of subjects needed to document detectable effects by a factor of four (Coats et al., 1992).

Except for ascertaining the effects of a drug during sleep and before awakening, self-recorded home BP measurements provide the same data as ABPM with a similar level of accuracy at a much lower cost (Mengden et al., 1992). Use of either out-of-office measurement is superior to the traditional use of occasional clinic readings.

CONCLUSION

All in all, ABPM is likely to be more and more widely used, particularly in children (Harshfield et al., 1991) and the elderly (Cox et al., 1993). However, it should not be used promiscuously, because of both its cost and unresolved issues about its proper interpretation. When used appropriately, it may be very cost effective, such as in the detection of white-coat hypertension, thereby saving the financial and other costs of having the diagnosis of hypertension made falsely (Krakoff, 1993). In practice, the appropriate use of ABPM has been shown to have a favorable impact upon the management of patients (Grin et al., 1993).

For now, office sphygmomanometry will continue to be the primary tool for diagnosing and monitoring hypertension. Home readings should be widely used both to confirm the diagnosis and to provide better assurance of appropriate therapy. Ambulatory monitoring should be increasingly used to look for white-coat hypertension, to evaluate apparent resistance to therapy, and to evaluate the adequacy of therapy, particularly during sleep and the early morning hours.

We next turn to the mechanisms responsible for the elevated blood pressure in 95% of those with hypertension, primary (essential) hypertension.

References

American College of Physicians. Automated ambulatory blood pressure and self-measured blood pressure monitoring devices: their role in the diagnosis and management of hypertension. *Ann Intern Med* 1993;118: 889–892.

American Society of Hypertension. Recommendations for routine blood pressure measurement by indirect cuff sphygmomanometry. *Am J Hypertens*1992;5:207–209.

Anonymous. Blood-pressure monitors. *Consumer Reports*, May 1992:295–299.

Appel LJ, Stason WB. Ambulatory blood pressure monitoring and blood pressure self-measurement in the diagnosis and management of hypertension. *Ann Intern Med* 1993;118:867–882.

Ayman D, Goldshine AD. Blood pressure determinations by patients with essential hypertension. I. The difference between clinic and home readings before treatment. *Am J Med Sci* 1940;200:465–474.

Bailey RH, Knaus VL, Bauer JH. Aneroid sphygmomanometers. An assessment of accuracy at a university hospital and clinics. *Arch Intern Med* 1991;151: 1409–1412.

Baumgart P, Walger P, Gemen S, von Eiff M, Raidt H, Rahn KH. Blood pressure elevation during the night in chronic renal failure, hemodialysis and after renal transplantation. *Nephron* 1991;57:293–298.

Bevan AT, Honour AJ, Stott FH. Direct arterial pressure recording in unrestricted man. *Clin Sci* 1969;36:329–344.

Bornstein NM, Norris JW. Subclavian steal: a harmless haemodynamic phenomenon? *Lancet* 1986;2:303–305.

Bos WJW, Imholz BPM, van Goudoever J, Wesseling KH, van Montfrans GA. The reliability of noninvasive continuous finger blood pressure measurement in patients with both hypertension and vascular disease. *Am J Hypertens* 1992a;5:529–535.

Bos WJW, van Goudoever J, van Montfrans GA, Wesseling KH. Influence of short-term blood pressure variability on blood pressure determinations. *Hypertension* 1992b;19:606–609.

Bottini PB, Rhoades RB, Carr AA, Prisant LM. Mechanical trauma and acute neuralgia associated with automated ambulatory blood pressure monitoring. *Am J Hypertens* 1991;4:288.

Brennan M, O'Brien E, O'Malley K. The effect of age on blood pressure and heart rate variability in hypertension. *J Hypertens* 1986;4(Suppl 6):S269–S272.

Bruce NG, Shaper AG, Walker M, Wannamethee G. Observer bias in blood pressure studies. *J Hypertens* 1988;6:375–380.

Carruthers M, Taggart P. Validation of a new, inexpensive, non-invasive miniaturized blood-pressure monitor. *J Ambul Monitor* 1988;1:163–170.

Chanudet X, Chau NP, Lorroque P. Short-term representatives of daytime and night-time ambulatory blood pressures. *J Hypertens* 1992;10:595–600.

Chatellier G, Battaglia C, Pagny J-Y, Plouin P-F, Ménard J. Decision to treat mild hypertension after assessment by ambulatory monitoring and World Health Organization recommendations. *Br Med J* 1992; 305:1062–1066.

Clark LA, Denby L, Pregibon D, et al. A quantitative analysis of the effects of activity and time of day on the diurnal variations of blood pressure. *J Chronic Dis* 1987;40:671–679.

Coats AJS, Clark SJ, Conway J. Analysis of ambulatory blood pressure data. *J Hypertens* 1991;9(Suppl 8):S19–S21.

Coats AJS, Radaelli A, Clark SJ, Conway J, Sleight P. The influence of ambulatory blood pressure monitoring on the design and interpretation of trials in hypertension. *J Hypertens* 1992;10:385–391.

Conway J. Blood pressure and heart rate variability. *J Hypertens* 1986;4:261–263.

Cox JP, Amery A, Clement D, et al. Relationship between blood pressure measured in the clinic and by ambulatory monitoring and left ventricular size as measured by electrocardiogram in elderly patients with isolated systolic hypertension. *J Hypertens* 1993;11:269–276.

Croft PR, Cruickshank JK. Blood pressure measurement in adults: large cuffs for all? *Br Med J* 1990;44:170–173.

Cushman WC, Cooper KM, Horne RA, Meydrech EF. Effect of back support and stethoscope head on seated blood pressure determinations. *Am J Hypertens* 1990;3: 240–241.

Dewar R, Sykes D, Mulkerrin E, Nicklason F, Thomas D, Seymour R. The effect of hemiplegia on blood pressure measurement in the elderly. *Postgrad Med J* 1992;68:888–891.

Fagius J, Karhuvaara S. Sympathetic activity and blood pressure increases with bladder distension in humans. *Hypertension* 1989; 14:511–517.

Floras JS. Antihypertensive treatment, myocardial infarction, and nocturnal myocardial ischaemia. *Lancet* 1988;2:994–996.

Floras JS, Hassan MO, Jones JV, Osikowska BA, Sever PS, Sleight P. Factors influencing blood pressure and heart rate variability in hypertensive humans. *Hypertension* 1988;11:273–281.

Fogari R, Zoppi A, Malamani GD, Lazzari P, Destro M, Corradi L. Ambulatory blood pressure monitoring in normotensive and hypertensive type 2 diabetics: prevalence of impaired diurnal blood pressure patterns. *Am J Hypertens* 1993;6:1–7.

Fredich ED, Grim C, Labarthe DR, Maxwell MH, Perloff D, Weidman WH. Recommendations for human blood pressure determination by sphygmomanometers: report of a special task force appointed by the Steering Committee, American Heart Association. *Hypertension* 1988;11:209A–222A.

Fumo MT, Teeger S, Lang RM, Bednarz J, Sareli P, Murphy MB. Diurnal blood pressure variation and cardiac mass in American blacks and whites and South African blacks. *Am J Hypertens* 1992;5:111–116.

Gambardella S, Frontoni S, Spallone V, et al. Increased left ventricular mass in normotensive diabetic patients with autonomic neuropathy. *Am J Hypertens* 1993; 6:97–102.

Giaconi S, Ghione S, Palombo C, et al. Seasonal influences on blood pressure in high normal to mild hypertensive range. *Hypertension* 1989;14:22–27.

Goldberg RJ, Brady P, Muller JE, et al. Time of onset of symptoms of acute myocardial infarction. *Am J Cardiol* 1990; 66: 140–144.

Gómez-Marín O, Prineas RJ, Råstam L. Cuff bladder width and blood pressure measurement in children and adolescents. *J Hypertens* 1992;10:1235–1241.

Gould BA, Hornung RS, Kieso HA, Altman DG, Raftery EB. Is the blood pressure the same in both arms? *Clin Cardiol* 1985;8:423–426.

Gretler DD, Carlson GF, Montano AV, Murphy MB. Diurnal blood pressure variability and physical activity measured electronically and by diary. *Am J Hypertens* 1993;6:127–133.

Grin JM, McCabe EJ, White WB. Management of hypertension after ambulatory blood pressure monitoring. *Ann Intern Med* 1993;118:833–837.

Groppelli A, Giorgi DMA, Omboni S, Parati G, Mancia G. Persistent blood pressure increase induced by heavy smoking. *J Hypertens* 1992;10:495–499.

Hall CL, Higgs CMB, Notarianni L. Home blood pressure recording in mild hypertension: value of distinguishing sustained from clinic hypertension and effect on diagnosis and treatment. *J Hum Hypertens* 1990;4:501–507.

Harshfield GA, Pulliam DA, Alpert BS, Stapleton FB, Willey ES, Somes GW. Ambulatory blood pressure patterns in children and adolescents: influence of renin-sodium profiles. *Pediatrics* 1991;87:94–100.

Hegholm A, Kristensen KS, Madsen NH, Svendsen TL. White coat hypertension diagnosed by 24-h ambulatory monitoring. *Am J Hypertens* 1992;5:64–70.

Hense H-W, Stieber J, Chambless L. Factors associated with measured differences between fourth and fifth phase diastolic blood pressure. *Int J Epidemiol* 1986; 15:513–518.

Hinman AT, Engel BT, Bickford AF. Portable blood pressure recorder accuracy and preliminary use in evaluating intradaily variations in pressure. *Am Heart J* 1962;63:663–668.

Hirsch J-M, Hedner J, Wernstedt L, Lundberg J, Hedner T. Hemodynamic effects of the use of oral snuff. *Clin Pharmacol Ther* 1992;52:394–401.

Hugue CJ, Safar ME, Aliefierakis MC, Asmar RG, London GM. The ratio between ankle and brachial systolic pressure in patients with sustained uncomplicated essential hypertension. *Clin Sci* 1988;74:179–182.

Imai Y, Abe K, Sasaki S, et al. Clinical evaluation of semiautomatic and automatic devices for home blood pressure measurement: comparison between cuff-oscillometric and microphone methods. *J Hypertens* 1989;7:983–990.

Imholz BPM, Langewouters GJ, van Montfrans GA, et al. Feasibility of ambulatory, continuous 24-hour finger arterial pressure recording. *Hypertension* 1993;21:65–73.

Jamerson KA, Schork N, Julius S. Effect of home blood pressure and gender on estimates of the familial aggregation of blood pressure. The Tecumseh Blood Pressure Study. *Hypertension* 1992;20:314–318.

James GD, Pickering TG, Yee LS, Harshfield GA, Riva S, Laragh JH. The reproducibility of average ambulatory, home, and clinic pressures. *Hypertension* 1988;11:545–549.

James GD, Yee LS, Cates EM, Schlussel YR, Pecker MS, Pickering TG. A validation study of the Instromedix Baro-Graf QD home blood pressure monitor. *Am J Hypertens* 1990;3:717–720.

Joint National Committee on Detection, Evaluation, and Treatment of High Blood Pressure. The fifth report of the Joint National Committee on Detection, Evaluation, and Treatment of High Blood Pressure (JNC V). *Arch Intern Med* 1993;153:154–183.

Julius S. Home blood pressure monitoring: advantages and limitations. *J Hypertens* 1991;9(Suppl 3):S41–S46.

Julius S, Mejia A, Jones K, et al. "White coat" versus "sustained" borderline hypertension in Tecumseh, Michigan. *Hypertension* 1990;16:617–623.

Kaijser L. The indirect method of recording blood pressure during exercise—can the diastolic blood pressure be measured? *Clin Physiol* 1987;7:175–179.

Khoury AF, Sunderajan P, Kaplan NM. The early morning rise in blood pressure is related mainly to ambulation. *Am J Hypertens* 1992;5:339–344.

Kleinert HD, Harshfield GA, Pickering TG, et al. What is the value of home blood pressure measurement in patients with mild hypertension? *Hypertension* 1984;6:574–578.

Krakoff LR. Ambulatory blood pressure monitoring can improve cost-effective management of hypertension. *Am J Hypertens* 1993;6:220S–224S.

Laaser U, Labarthe R. Recommendations for blood pressure measurement in children and adolescents. *Clin Exp Hypertens* 1986;A8:903–911.

Lipsitz LA, Storch HA, Minaker KL, Rowe JW. Intra-individual variability in postural blood pressure in the elderly. *Clin Sci* 1985;69:337–341.

Long JM, Lynch JJ, Machiran NM, Thomas SA, Malinow KL. The effect of status on blood pressure during verbal communication. *J Behav Med* 1982;5:165–172.

Lurbe A, Redón J, Pascual JM, Tacons J, Alvarez V, Batlle DC. Altered blood pressure during sleep in normotensive subjects with type I diabetes. *Hypertension* 1993;21:227–235.

Malinow KL, Lynch JJ, Foreman PJ, Friedmann E, Thomas SA. Blood pressure increases while signing in a deaf population. *Psychosom Med* 1986;48:95–101.

Mancia G, Parati G, Pomidossi G, et al. Evaluation of the antihypertensive effect of once-a-day captopril by 24-hour ambulatory blood pressure monitoring. *J Hypertens* 1987a;5(Suppl 5):S591–S593.

Mancia G, Parati G, Pomidossi G, Grassi G, Casadei R, Zanchetti A. Alerting reaction and rise in blood pressure during measurement by physician and nurse. *Hypertension* 1987b;9:209–215.

Mancia G, Di Rienzo M, Parati G. Ambulatory blood pressure monitoring use in hypertension research and clinical practice. *Hypertension* 1993;21:510–524.

Mariotti G, Alli C, Avanzini F, et al. Arm position as a source of error in blood pressure measurement. *Clin Cardiol* 1987;10:591–593.

Mejia AD, Egan BM, Schork NJ, Zweifler AJ. Artefacts in measurement of blood pressure and lack of target organ involvement in the assessment of patients with treatment-resistant hypertension. *Ann Intern Med* 1990a;112:270–277.

Mejia AD, Julius S, Jones KA, Schork NJ, Kneisley J. The Tecumseh blood pressure study. *Arch Intern Med* 1990b;150:1209–1213.

Mengden T, Binswanger B, Weisser B, Vetter W. An evaluation of self-measured blood pressure in a study with a calcium-channel antagonist versus a β-blocker. *Am J Hypertens* 1992;5:154–160.

Messerli FH, Ventura HO, Amodeo C. Osler's maneuver and pseudohypertension. *N Engl J Med* 1985;312:1548–1551.

Morrow K, Morris CK, Froelicher VF, et al. Prediction of cardiovascular death in men undergoing noninvasive evaluation for coronary artery disease. *Ann Intern Med* 1993;118:689–695.

Mulcahy D, Wright C, Sparrow J, et al. Heart rate and blood pressure consequences of an afternoon SIESTA (*S*nooze-*I*nduced *E*xcitation of *S*ympathetic *T*riggered *A*ctivity). *Am J Cardiol* 1993;71:611–614.

Neutel JM, Schnaper H, Cheng DG, Graettinger WF, Weber MA. Antihypertensive effects of β-blockers administered once daily: 24-hour measurements. *Am Heart J* 1990;120:166–171.

Neutel JM, Smith DHG, Ram CVS, et al. Application of ambulatory blood pressure monitoring in differentiating between antihypertensive agents. *Am J Med* 1993;94:181–187.

Nishimura H, Nishioka A, Kubo S, Suwa M, Kino M, Kawamura K. Multifactorial evaluation of blood pressure fall upon hospitalization in essential hypertensive patients. *Clin Sci* 1987;73:135–141.

O'Brien E, Mee F, Atkins N, O'Malley K. Inaccuracy of the Hawksley random zero sphygmomanometer. *Lancet* 1990a; 336:1465–1468.

O'Brien E, Petrie J, Littler W, et al. The British Hypertension Society protocol for the evaluation of automated and semi-automated blood pressure measuring devices with special reference to ambulatory systems. *J Hypertens* 1990b;8:607–619.

O'Brien E, Mee F, Atkins N, O'Malley K. Accuracy of the Spacelabs 90207, Novacor DIASYS 200, Del Mar Avionics Pressurometer IV and Takeda TM-2420 ambulatory systems according to British and American criteria. *J Hypertens* 1991;9(Suppl 6):S332–S333.

O'Brien E, Mee F, Atkins N, O'Malley K. Accuracy of the CH-Drunk/Pressure San ERKA ambulatory blood pressure measuring system determined by the British Hypertension Society Protocol. *J Hypertens* 1992a;10:1283–1284.

O'Brien E, Mee F, Atkins N, O'Malley K. Accuracy of the Profilomat ambulatory blood pressure measuring system determined by the British Hypertension Society Protocol. *J Hypertens* 1992b;10:1285–1286.

O'Brien E, Atkins N, O'Malley K. Defining normal ambulatory blood pressure from population studies. *Am J Hypertens* 1993;6:201S–206S.

Ogasawara S, Freedman SB, Ram J, Kelly DT. Evaluation of a microprocessor-controlled sphygmomanometer for recording blood pressure during exercise. *Am J Cardiol* 1989;64:806–808.

Oliner CM, Elliott WJ, Gretler ED, Murphy MB. Low predictive value of positive Osler manoeuvre for diagnosing pseudohypertension. *J Hum Hypertens* 1993;7:65–70.

Omboni S, Frattola A, Parati G, Ravogli A, Mancia G. Clinical value of blood pressure measurements: focus on ambulatory blood pressure. *Am J Cardiol* 1992;70:4D–8D.

Padfield PL, Stewart MJ. Ambulatory blood pressure monitoring in secondary hypertension. *J Hypertens* 1991;9(Suppl 8):S69–S71.

Palatini P, Penzo M, Racioppa A, et al. Clinical relevance of nighttime blood pressure and of daytime blood pressure variability. *Arch Intern Med* 1992;152:1855–1860.

Panza JA, Epstein SE, Quyyumi AA. Circadian variation in vascular tone and its relation to α-sympathetic vasoconstrictor activity. *N Engl J Med* 1991;325:986–990.

Pearce KA, Grimm RH Jr, Rao S, et al. Population-derived comparisons of ambulatory and office blood pressures. *Arch Intern Med* 1992;152:750–756.

Perloff D, Sokolow M. The representative blood pressure: usefulness of office, basal, home, and ambulatory readings. *Cardiovasc Med* 1978;June:655–688.

Perloff D, Sokolow M, Cowan R. The prognostic value of ambulatory blood pressure. *JAMA* 1983;249:2792–2798.

Perloff D, Sokolow M, Cowan R. The prognostic value of ambulatory blood pressure monitoring in treated hypertensive patients. *J Hypertens* 1991;9(Suppl 1):S33–S40.

Perry HM Jr, Miller JP. Difficulties in diagnosing hypertension: implications and alternatives. *J Hypertens* 1992;10:887–896.

Petrie JC, O'Brien ET, Littler WA, de Swiet M. Recommendations on blood pressure measurement. *Br Med J* 1986;293:611–615.

Pickering TG. Blood pressure monitoring outside the office for the evaluation of patients with resistant hypertension. *Hypertension* 1988;11:(Suppl II):II-96–II-100.

Pickering TG. *Ambulatory Monitoring and Blood Pressure Variability*. London: Science Press, 1991.

Pickering TG. Ambulatory monitoring and the definition of hypertension. *J Hypertens* 1992;10:401–409.

Pickering TG. Blood pressure variability and ambulatory monitoring. *Curr Opin Nephrol Hypertens* 1993;2:380–385.

Pickering TG, James GD, Boddie C, Harshfield GA, Blank S, Laragh JH. How common is white coat hypertension? *JAMA* 1988;259:225–228.

Pieper C, Warren K, Pickering TG. A comparison of ambulatory blood pressure and heart rate at home and work on work and non-work days. *J Hum Hypertens* 1993; 11:177–183.

Potter JF, Watson RDS, Skan W, Beevers DG. The pressor and metabolic effects of alcohol in normotensive subjects. *Hypertension* 1986;8:625–631.

Raccaud O, Waeber B, Petrillo A, Wiesel P, Hofstetter J-R, Brunner HR. Ambulatory blood pressure monitoring as a means to avoid overtreatment of elderly hypertensive patients. *Gerontology* 1992;38: 99–104.

Rath W, Schrader J, Guhlke U, et al. 24-Hour ambulatory blood pressure measurements in normotensive pregnancy and in pre-eclampsia. *Klin Wochenschr* 1990;68: 768–773.

Reeves RA, Myers MG. Reproducibility of ambulatory blood pressure and assessing treatment withdrawal in hypertension trial. *Am J Hypertens* 1993;6:229S–232S.

Reeves RA, Leenen FHH, Joyner CD. Reproducibility of nurse-measured, exercise and ambulatory blood pressure and echocardiographic left ventricular mass in borderline hypertension. *J Hypertens* 1992;10: 1249–1256.

Ridker PM, Manson JE, Buring JE, Muller JE, Hennekens CH. Circadian variation of acute myocardial infarction and the effect of low-dose aspirin in a randomized trial of physicians. *Circulation* 1990;82:897–902.

Roche V, O'Malley K, O'Brien E. How 'scientific' is blood pressure measurement in leading medical journals? *J Hypertens* 1990;8:1167–1168.

Rose GA, Holland WW, Crowley EA. A sphygmomanometer for epidemiologists. *Lancet* 1964;1:296–300.

Salaita K, Whelton PK, Seidler AJ. A community-based evaluation of the Vita-stat automatic blood pressure recorder. *Am J Hypertens* 1990;3:366–372.

Schechter CB, Adler RS. Bayesian analysis of diastolic blood pressure measurement. *Med Decis Making* 1988;8:182–190.

Scientific Committee. Consensus document on non-invasive ambulatory blood pressure monitoring. *J Hypertens* 1990; 8(Suppl 6):135–140.

Shi J, Benowitz NL, Denaro CP, Sheiner LB. Pharmacokinetic-pharmacodynamic modeling of caffeine: tolerance to pressor effects. *Clin Pharmacol Ther* 1993;53: 6–14.

Shimada K, Kawamoto A, Matsubayashi K, Nishinaga M, Kimura S, Ozawa T. Diurnal blood pressure variations and silent cerebrovascular damage in elderly patients with hypertension. *J Hypertens* 1992;10: 875–878.

Silverberg DS, Rosenfeld JB. The effect of quiet conversation on the blood pressure of hypertensive patients. *Isr J Med Sci* 1980;16:41–43.

Sloan MA, Price TR, Foulkes MA, et al. Circadian rhythmicity of stroke onset. Intracerebral and subarachnoid hemorrhage. *Stroke* 1992;23:1420–1426.

Sokolow M, Werdegar D, Kain HK, Hinman AT. Relationship between level of blood pressure measured casually and by portable recorders and severity of complications in essential hypertension. *Circulation* 1966;34:279–298.

Sokolow M, Perloff D, Cowan R. The value of portably recorded blood pressures in the initiation of treatment of moderate hypertension. *Clin Sci Mol Med* 1973;45: 195s–198s.

Somers VK, Dyken ME, Mark AL, Abboud FM. Sympathetic-nerve activity during sleep in normal subjects. *N Engl J Med* 1993;328:303–307.

Spence JD, Sibbald WJ, Cape RD. Direct, indirect and mean blood pressures in hypertensive patients: the problem of cuff artefact due to arterial wall stiffness, and a partial solution. *Clin Invest Med* 1980; 2:165–173.

Staessen J, Bulpitt CJ, O'Brien E, et al. The diurnal blood pressure profile: a population study. *Am J Hypertens* 1992;5:386–392.

Staessen JA, Fagard RH, Lijnen PJ, Thijs L, Van Hoof R, Amery AK. Mean and range of the ambulatory pressure in normotensive subjects from a meta-analysis of 23 studies. *Am J Cardiol* 1991;67:723–727.

Staessen JA, O'Brien ET, Amery AK, Atkins N, et al. Ambulatory blood pressure in normotensive and hypertensive subjects: results from an international database. *J Hypertens* 1994;12(Suppl 7):S1–S12.

Stewart MJ, Padfield PL. Blood pressure measurement: an epitaph for the mercury sphygmomanometer? *Clin Sci* 1992;83:1–12.

Stolt M, Sjönell G, Åström H, Rössner S, Hansson L. Improved accuracy of indirect blood pressure measurement in patients with obese arms. *Am J Hypertens* 1993; 6:66–71.

Sundberg S, Kohvakka A, Gordin A. Rapid reversal of circadian blood pressure rhythm in shift workers. *J Hypertens* 1988;6:393–396.

Sykes D, Dewar R, Mohanaruban K, et al. Measuring blood pressure in the elderly: does atrial fibrillation increase observer variability? *Br Med J* 1990;300:162–163.

Uhari M, Nuutinen M, Turtinen J, Pokka T. Pulse sounds and measurement of diastolic blood pressure in children. *Lancet* 1991;338:159–161.

Van Egeren LF, Madarasmi S. A computer-assisted diary (CAD) for ambulatory blood pressure monitoring. *Am J Hypertens* 1988;1:179S–185S.

Veerman DP, van Montfrans GA. Nurse-measured or ambulatory blood pressure in routine hypertension care. *J Hypertens* 1993;11:287–292.

Veerman DP, van Montfrans GA, Wieling W. Effects of cuff inflation on self-recorded blood pressure. *Lancet* 1990;335:451–453.

Verdecchia P, Porcellati C. Defining normal ambulatory blood pressure in relation to target organ damage and prognosis. *Am J Hypertens* 1993;6:207S–210S.

Verdecchia P, Schillad G, Boldrini F, et al. Blunted nocturnal fall in blood pressure in hypertensive women with future cardiovascular events [Abstract]. *Circulation* 1992a;86(Suppl I):I–678.

Verdecchia P, Schillaci G, Boldrini F, Zampi I, Porcellati C. Variability between current definitions of 'normal' ambulatory blood pressure: implications in the assessment of white coat hypertension. *Hypertension* 1992b;20:555–562.

Waeber B, Scherrer U, Petrillo A, et al. Are some hypertensive patients overtreated? A prospective study of ambulatory blood pressure recording. *Lancet* 1987;2: 732–734.

Watson RDS, Lumb R, Young MA, Stallard TJ, Davies P, Littler WA. Variation in cuff blood pressure in untreated outpatients with mild hypertension—implications for initiating antihypertensive treatment. *J Hypertens* 1987;5:207–211.

West JNW, Townend JN, Davies P, et al. Effect of unrestricted activity on accuracy of ambulatory blood pressure measurement. *Hypertension* 1991;18:593–597.

White WB. Analysis of ambulatory blood pressure data in antihypertensive drug trials. *J Hypertens* 1991;9(Suppl 1): S27–S32.

White WB, Berson AS, Robbins C, et al. National standard for measurement of resting and ambulatory blood pressures with automated sphygmomanometers. *Hypertension* 1993;21:504–509.

Willich SN, Goldberg RJ, Maclure M, Perriello L, Muller JE. Increased onset of sudden cardiac death in the first three hours after awakening. *Am J Cardiol* 1992;70: 65–68.

Woods KL, Fletcher S, Jagger C. Modification of the circadian rhythm of onset of acute myocardial infarction by long-term antianginal treatment. *Br Heart J* 1992; 68:458–61.

Zachariah PK, Sumner WE III. The clinical utility of blood pressure load in hypertension. *Am J Hypertens* 1993;6:194S–197S.

Zachariah PK, Sheps SG, Smith RL. Defining the roles of home and ambulatory monitoring. *Diagnosis* 1988;10:39–50.

Zuspan FP, Rayburn WF. Blood pressure self-monitoring during pregnancy: practical considerations. *Am J Obstet Gynecol* 1991;164:2–6.

Zweifler AJ, Shahab ST. Pseudohypertension: a new assessment. *J Hypertens* 1993;11:1–6.

3 Primary Hypertension: Pathogenesis

As noted in the previous chapters, as much as 95% of all hypertension is of unknown cause. In the absence of a known cause, there is no obvious name for the disease. "Essential" may be mistakenly interpreted to infer an essential need for higher pressure to push blood through vessels narrowed by age. The term "benign" has been buried along with the millions of unfortunate victims of uncontrolled hypertension. "Idiopathic" seems a bit unwieldy, so I have chosen "primary" simply to distinguish it from all of the remainder, which are "secondary" to known causes.

GENERAL CONSIDERATIONS

The use of the new tools of molecular biology promises to uncover more of the basic mechanisms of primary hypertension than has been possible with the relatively crude observational techniques of the past (Dzau et al., 1993a). In particular, genes that are involved with hypertension will be identified (Morris, 1993).

Nonetheless, the identification of specific genetic linkages and mutations will only point the way to aberrant physiologic pathways, so that the integration of observational data will still be needed. For example, the findings of genetic linkage between the angiotensinogen gene and hypertension (Jeunemaitre et al., 1992b) and the presence of increased levels of plasma angiotensinogen in subjects with higher parental and personal blood pressure (Watt et al., 1992) only support a role for increased synthesis of angiotensinogen in hypertension but do not explain how this translates into elevated blood pressure. We will continue to need to construct reasonable hypotheses from multiple separate pieces of data, hopefully to provide models with broad explanatory powers.

The continued need for such integrated hypotheses is even more obvious given the multifactorial nature of hypertension. As noted by Lifton (1993):

The major advances in genetics and molecular biology of the past decade have lead to the development of powerful techniques for identification of disease-causing genes. Importantly, most successes to date have been with monogenic disorders, *ie*, those in which a single mutation is sufficient to produce the disease trait.

In contrast to such single gene disorders, levels of blood pressure do not generally segregate in families as monogenic traits. Instead, the results of most studies of humans and experimental animal models suggest that variation in blood pressure is due to the combined effects of multiple genes. As a result, different individuals, even within the same family, may be hypertensive due to different combinations of these genetic factors.

Before considering the specific genetic and environmental factors that may be responsible for hypertension, a few generalizations are in order:

—The relevance of data from animal models is highly questionable. Even though 70% of current research on hypertension is being done on rats or other small animals (Carretero et al., 1991), the relevance of such data to the human condition is suspect. For example, linkage of blood pressure to the angiotensin-converting enzyme (ACE) locus has been noted in the spontaneously hypertensive rat (Jacob et al., 1991; Hilbert et al., 1991), but no such linkage has been found in human hypertension (Jeunemaitre et al., 1992a; Harrap et al., 1993; Schmidt et al., 1993). Therefore, whenever possible, this discussion will examine data only from human studies.

—Few analytical techniques are available to measure accurately and repetitively the possibly small changes in various hemodynamic functions that may be involved. Moreover, few investigators or patients have been willing or able to do repetitive studies over the many years it may take for subtle changes to become manifest. Cross-sectional observations may never be able to uncover the sequential changes that could be revealed by longitudinal studies.

—Even when studies are done among adolescent and borderline hypertensives, the beginnings may have already been missed. By the time hypertension is detectable, the initiating factors may be obscured by adaptations invoked by the rising pressure. In the absence of a marker to identify the prehypertensive individual before the blood pressure has risen, we may be viewing the process after the initiating factor(s) is no longer recognizable.

—Although the search for a single underlying abnormality that begins the hemodynamic cascade toward sustained hypertension continues to attract the imagination and energies of numerous investigators, there may be no such single defect. In view of the multiple factors involved in the control of the blood pressure, the concept of a multifaceted mosaic, introduced by Irving Page (1963), may be more appropriate, as unattractive as it may be to those who prefer to believe that for every biologic defect there should be a single specific cause. An editorial some time ago in the *Lancet* (Anonymous, 1977) describes the situation aptly:

Blood pressure is a measurable end product of an exceedingly complex series of factors including those which control blood vessel calibre and responsiveness, those which control fluid volume within and outside the vascular bed, and those which control cardiac output. None of these factors is independent: they interact with each other and respond to changes in blood pressure. It is not easy, therefore, to dissect out cause and effect. Few factors which play a role in cardiovascular control are completely normal in hypertension: indeed, normality would require explanation since it would suggest a lack of responsiveness to increased pressure.

—The search may be misdirected: In looking for the mechanisms of primary hypertension, we may need to separate the disease into many distinct syndromes, each with its own mechanisms. Fifty years ago, almost all hypertension not obviously secondary to intrinsic renal disease was lumped under the term "essential." Since then, coarctation, pheochromocytoma, Cushing's syndrome, renovascular disease, and primary aldosteronism have been identified and a small but insignificant percentage of hypertensive patients put into each category. Additional parts of what is now called primary may be separated into other specific categories. However, as of 1994, no basis for such further division is apparent even though, as we shall see, more and more differences are being identified within the population of patients with primary hypertension. For now, unifying hypotheses seem appropriate, with the recognition that there may be considerable variations in the role of various components at different times and stages and in different people.

Before examining the specific hypotheses that may explain the development of hypertension, the role of genetics will be considered.

ROLE OF GENETICS

Primary hypertension clusters in families. Persons with two or more first-degree relatives with hypertension before age 55 have a 3.8 times greater risk of developing hypertension before age 50 (Williams et al., 1991). However, there are only a few clues as to what specifically may be transmitted genetically.

Genetic Contribution

Estimates of the genetic contribution to the variability of blood pressure vary from 25% in pedigree studies to 65% in twin studies (Williams et al., 1991). Williams et al. estimate that only 7% of the total variance of diastolic pressure is attributable to shared environmental factors so that "most familial aggregation of high blood pressure appears to be due to genes."

Williams et al. are actively studying the genetics of hypertension by examining a variety of traits involved in blood pressure regulation which may be associated with hypertension, i.e., intermediate phenotypes. Although Kurtz and Spence (1993) advise that the relevance of these intermediate phenotypes to the pathogenesis of hypertension is uncertain, Williams et al. (1991) list a number of candidates for gene-environment interaction (Table 3.1). However, Muldoon et al. (1993) find support for only a limited number of these features that are present more frequently in those with a positive family history compared to those with a negative family history, including:

Elevated RBC Na-Li countertransport,
Normodulation of renin-angiotensin in response to changes in sodium uptake,
Left ventricular hypertrophy,
Abnormalities of the peripheral vasculature, and
Greater increases in blood pressure (BP) during exercise.

Mode of Inheritance

Hypertension is "a complex, polygenic, quantitative disease . . . compounded by the late onset of the disease, its unknown penetrance, variable phenotype and the influence of environmental factors" (Morris, 1993). Without marker genes to identify those who are susceptible, and without a link between a genetic alteration and a physiologic dysfunction, the mode of inheritance of primary hypertension cannot be defined clearly. Beyond the presence of hypertension in some forms of congenital adrenal hyperplasia, one small segment of the hypertensive population has been found to have a single mutation with Mendelian autosomal dominant transmission: the syndrome of glucocorticoid-remediable aldosteronism (Lifton et al., 1992) (see Chapter 13).

Search for Markers

Except for these very rare examples of simple Mendelian forms, hypertension is obviously multifactorial. The search for possible biochemical or physiologic markers to identify those people with a genetic predisposition continues in hope of proceeding backward to find DNA markers and thereby prove the existence of major gene-hypertension interactions. A new approach has been taken by Watt et al. (1992). They divided 864 young normotensive adults from 603 families in which both parents had had their pressure measured 8 years previously into four categories or corners (Table 3.2). Those offspring in the highest corner whose parents had higher pressures had four distinguishing characteristics: higher levels of plasma angiotensinogen, cortisol, and 18-OH-corticosteroid, and homozygosity for the glucocorticoid receptor.

The presence of increased plasma angiotensinogen fits nicely with the evidence for genetic linkage between a variant angiotensinogen gene and hypertension found in 379 hypertensive sibling pairs in Salt Lake City and Paris (Jeunemaitre et al., 1992b). Those subjects homozygous for the variant at amino acid 235 had higher

Table 3.1. Candidates for Gene-Environment Interaction

Environmental Factors	Evidence for Genetic Involvement[a]
Sodium and potassium	Na-Li countertransport (H^2)
	Intraerythrocytic sodium (H^2)
	Na pump sites (H^2)
	Urinary kallikrein excretion (H^2)
	Nonmodulation (FHx HBP)
	Intralymphocytic Na (FHx HBP)
	Na sensitivity and haptoglobin phenotype
Calcium	Ionized plasma calcium (FHx HBP)
Exercise	Bicycle exercise diastolic blood pressure (H^2)
	Bicycle diastolic blood pressure and intralymphocytic Na (FHx HBP)
Obesity, fat and calorie intake, insulin resistance	Familial dyslipidemic hypertension
	Type II diabetes
	Fat pattern (H^2)
	Body mass index (H^2)
Stress	Mental arithmetic blood pressure (H^2)

From Williams RR, Hunt SC, Hasstedt SJ, et al. Are there interactions and relations between genetic and environmental factors predisposing to high blood pressure? *Hypertension* 1991;18(Suppl I):I-29–I-37.
[a]Genetic "involvement" means some reported data from genetic heritability (H^2) or family history (FHx) studies link this environmental factor either directly or indirectly to one or more inherited factors. HBP, high blood pressure.

Table 3.2. Offspring Characteristics from the Four Corners Analysis

Offspring Characteristics	Low Parents		High Parents	
	Low Offspring	High Offspring	Low Offspring	High Offspring
Blood pressure	105/56	128/76	110/57	129/75
Angiotensinogen (ng/ml)	1625	1586	1742	2022[a]
Cortisol (μg/100 mL)	11.1	10.4	9.6	14.0[b]
18-OH-Corticosterone (ng/100 mL)	24.2	25.9	17.6	30.2[b]
Glucocorticoid receptor AA	9	19	18	27[c]

From Watt GCM, Harrap SB, Foy CJW, et al. Abnormalities of glucocorticoid metabolism and the renin-angiotensin system: a four-corners approach to the identification of genetic determinants of blood pressure. *J Hypertens* 1992;10:473–482.
[a]$p < 0.01$.
[b]$p < 0.02$.
[c]$p < 0.1$.

plasma levels of angiotensin as well. The variant allele of codon 235 has been found much more frequently in blacks in Birmingham, Alabama (Lifton et al., 1993), but the relevance of the association remains uncertain.

Further support for a possible role of the renin-angiotensin system comes from the creation of a transgenic rat model with overexpression of a mouse renin gene that develops fulminant hypertension, apparently by renin activation of adrenal corticosteroids (Peters et al., 1993). We are then left with a number of provocative clues but little that is certain about the role of heredity in the pathogenesis of hypertension. Certainly, more will soon be known about the genetic determinants of hypertension.

OVERVIEW OF PATHOGENESIS

The pressure required to move blood through the circulatory bed is provided by the pumping action of the heart (cardiac output) and the tone of the arteries (peripheral resistance). Each of these primary determinants of the blood pressure is, in turn, determined by the interaction of the "exceedingly complex series of factors" displayed in part in Figure 3.1.

Hypertension has been ascribed to abnormalities in virtually every one of these factors. Each will be examined, and attempts will be made along the way to integrate them into logical hypotheses. It is unlikely that all of these factors are operative in any given patient, but multiple hypotheses may prove to be correct since the hemodynamic hallmark of primary hypertension, a persistently elevated vascular resistance, may be reached through a number of different paths. Before the final destination, these may converge into either structural thickening of the vessel walls or functional vasoconstriction.

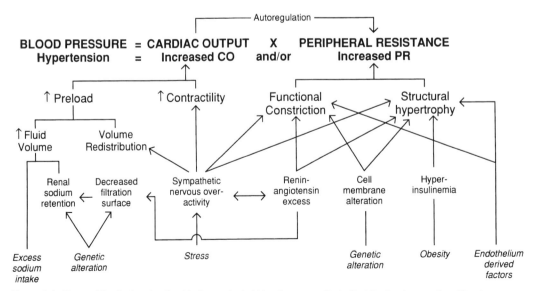

Figure 3.1. Some of the factors involved in the control of blood pressure that affect the basic equation: Blood pressure = cardiac output × peripheral resistance.

Whatever else is involved, heredity must play a role, along with varying contributions of at least three environmental factors for which there is strong support: sodium, stress, and obesity. Each of these environmental factors will be touched upon repeatedly, but just how they interact to induce hypertension remains uncertain, and the interactions are proving to be increasingly complex. For instance, insulin resistance is present even before hypertension develops in those who are genetically predisposed (Allemann et al., 1993); the resultant hyperinsulinemia is associated with sodium sensitivity (Sharma et al., 1993), obesity, and increased sympathetic drive (Modan and Halkin, 1991).

We will follow the outline shown in Figure 3.1, starting on the left side, recognizing that the position of each factor in the outline is not necessarily the order that the hemodynamic cascade follows in the pathogenesis of hypertension. Without knowing what starts the process, we can only lay out a blueprint that can be used by beginning at multiple sites.

CARDIAC OUTPUT

An increased cardiac output has been found in some early, borderline hypertensives, some of whom display a hyperkinetic circulation. If it is responsible for the hypertension, the increase in cardiac output could logically arise in two ways, either from an increase in fluid volume (preload) or from an increase in contractility from neural stimulation of the heart (Fig. 3.1). However, if it is involved in the initiation of hypertension, the increased cardiac output likely does not persist, since the typical hemodynamic finding in established hypertension is an elevated peripheral resistance and normal cardiac output (Julius, 1991).

Hyperkinetic Hypertensives

Numerous investigators have described hypertensives, mostly young, who have definitely high cardiac outputs (Finkielman et al., 1965; Frohlich et al., 1966; Andersson et al., 1989). Using noninvasive echocardiography to study young borderline hypertensives (average age 33), 37 of 99 subjects were found to have increased heart rate, cardiac index, and forearm blood flow caused by an excessive autonomic drive (Julius et al., 1991b).

Most of these features could reflect anxiety over both the knowledge that they were hypertensive (Rostrup et al., 1991) and the invasive procedures used in the studies. When such studies have been repeated within 2 years, cardiac outputs are usually normal (Birkenhäger and de Leeuw, 1984). However, the hypertension in some middle-aged hypertensives may continue to reflect increased cardiac output, as recognized by a high pulse pressure, above 60 mm Hg (Safar, 1989).

Cardiac Hypertrophy

Even if such persistently hyperkinetic patients are relatively rare, echocardiography has made it possible to identify the presence of cardiac hypertrophy in a large portion of early, mild hypertensives, including the normotensive children of hypertensive parents (Koren and Devereux, 1993). Such hypertrophy, described in greater detail in Chapter 4 which deals with the cardiac complications of hypertension, has been generally considered to be a compensatory mechanism to an increased vascular resistance (afterload). However, it could also reflect a primary response to repeated neural stimulation and, thereby, could be an initiating mechanism for hypertension (Julius, 1988a), as well as an ''amplifier'' of cardiac output that reinforces the elevation of BP upstream from the constricted arteriolar bed (Korner et al., 1992).

Increased Neural Stimulation

The increased heart rate and stroke volume found in young hyperkinetic borderline hypertensives have been explained by neurogenic mechanisms that could be both an increased sympathetic and a decreased parasympathetic drive (Julius et al., 1991b). Increased cardiac contractility, rather than an increased preload, has been favored since, as we shall see, intravascular blood volume has been found to be normal or reduced (Tarazi et al., 1983).

Redistribution of Blood Volume

Even without an expanded total volume, blood may be redistributed so that more is in the central or cardiopulmonary component because of greater peripheral vasoconstriction (Fig. 3.1) (London et al., 1978; Schobel et al., 1992). Venous return to the heart would thereby be increased and could mediate an increased cardiac output. However, serious reservations have been expressed, both about the methodology used to measure cardiopulmonary blood volume and the theoretical concept that, if it were increased, it would persist rather than be quickly normalized so that cardiac output would be increased only transiently (Birkenhäger and de Leeuw, 1984).

Increased Fluid Volume

A second mechanism that could induce hypertension by increasing cardiac output would be an increased circulating fluid volume (preload). However, in most studies, patients with established hypertension have a lower blood volume and total exchangeable sodium than do normal subjects (Tarazi et al., 1983; Beretta-Piccoli and Weidmann, 1984).

Relation of Blood Volume to Blood Pressure

However, when the blood pressure was compared with the total blood volume (TBV) in 48 normal subjects and 106 patients with fairly early and mild primary hypertension, an interesting relationship was observed (London et al., 1977b) (Fig. 3.2). A negative correlation was found in the normals but not in the hypertensives, with 80% of the hypertensives being outside the 95% confidence limits of the normal curve. The authors interpret their data to indicate a quantitative disturbance in the pressure-volume relationship in primary hypertension, i.e., a plasma volume that is inappropriately high for the level of blood pressure. Thus, even if absolute values are reduced, a relatively expanded blood volume may be involved in the maintenance of hypertension.

Translocation into Interstitial Space.   One logical explanation for the lower intravascular volume would be the translocation of fluid across the capillary bed into the interstitial space, in keeping with the higher capillary filtration pressure (Williams et al., 1990).

Intracellular Fluid Volume.   Beyond the relative increase in interstitial fluid, there may also be an increase in intracellular fluid volume in established primary hypertension. In one of the few studies that simultaneously measured red blood cell mass, plasma volume, extracellular fluid volume, and total body water in a sizable number of patients with fairly mild hypertension, there was a significant absolute increase of 1.5 liters/m[2] in intracellular fluid among the hypertensives, compared with that of age-matched normotensive controls (Bauer and Brooks, 1979). In a larger population, a significant positive relationship between systolic blood pressure and exchangeable sodium was found in men, but not women, with primary hypertension (Beretta-Piccoli et al., 1984).

This brings us to the final feature about cardiac output. Even if it is involved in the initiation of hypertension, once hypertension is established, cardiac output is usually not increased, but peripheral resistance is elevated.

Autoregulation

A changing pattern of initially high cardiac output giving way to a persistently elevated peripheral resistance has been observed in a few people and many animals with experimental hypertension. When animals with markedly reduced renal tissue are given volume loads, the blood pressure rises initially as a consequence of the high cardiac output, but within a few days, peripheral resistance rises, and cardiac output returns to near the basal level (Guyton, 1992) (Fig. 3.3). The changeover has been interpreted to reflect an intrinsic property of the vascular bed to regulate the flow of blood depending upon the metabolic need of tissues, a process called *autoregulation* described by Borst and Borst-de Geus (1963) and demonstrated experimentally by Guyton and Coleman (1969). With an increased cardiac output, more blood flows through the tissues than is required, and the increased flow delivers extra nutrients or removes additional metabolic products; in response, the vessels constrict, decreasing blood flow and returning the balance of supply and demand to normal. Thereby, peripheral resistance increases and remains high by the rapid induction of structural thickening of the resistance vessels. Autoregulation of tissue blood flow has been documented in conscious dogs where it has been shown to amplify the pressor

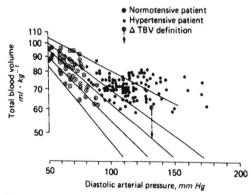

Figure 3.2. Relation between diastolic blood pressure and total blood volume (*TBV*) in 48 normotensive (*open circles*) and 106 hypertensive (*solid circles*) subjects. Only 20% of the hypertensive patients fell within the 95% confidence limits of the normal curve. The "TBV definition" represents the degree of the pressure-volume disturbance. (From London GM, Safer ME, Weiss YA, et al. Volume-dependent parameters in essential hypertension. *Kidney Int* 1977a;11:204–208.)

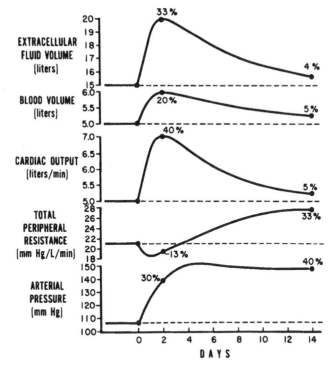

Figure 3.3. Progressive changes in important circulatory system variables during the first weeks of volume-loading hypertension. The initial rise in cardiac output is the basic cause of the hypertension. Subsequently, the autoregulation mechanism returns the cardiac output almost to normal while at the same time causing a secondary increase in total peripheral resistance. (From Guyton AC. Kidneys and fluids in pressure regulation. Small volume but large pressure changes. *Hypertension* 1992;19(Suppl I):I-2–I-8.)

responses to vasoconstrictor agents (Metting et al., 1989).

Similar conversion from initially high cardiac output to later increased peripheral resistance has been shown in some hypertensive people (Julius, 1988a; Lund-Johansen, 1989; Andersson et al., 1989). In Lund-Johansen's study, younger (17–29 year olds) and older (30–39 year olds) mild hypertensives were restudied both at rest and during exercise after 10 and then 20 years without intervening therapy. As the overall blood pressures rose, the cardiac output fell and peripheral resistance increased (Fig. 3.4).

Problems with the Autoregulation Model

The role of autoregulation in the conversion of a high cardiac output to a high peripheral resistance has been questioned for various reasons. These include the finding that patients found to have an increased cardiac output also have an increased oxygen consumption, rather than the lower level that should be seen if there were overperfusion of tissues as entailed in the autoregulation concept (Julius, 1988a).

Julius (1988a) considers autoregulation to be an unlikely explanation for the switch from high cardiac output to increased peripheral resistance and offers another: structural changes that decrease the cardiac responses to nervous and hormonal stimuli but enhance the vascular responses. His proposal states that: "This hemodynamic transition can be explained by a secondary response to elevated blood pressure. The heart becomes less responsive as a result of altered receptor responsiveness and decreased cardiac compliance, whereas the responsiveness of arterioles increases because of vascular hypertrophy, which leads to changes in the wall-to-lumen ratio."

Before discarding the autoregulatory model, we should recognize that it explains the course of hypertension in animals and in people given a volume load, particularly in the presence of reduced renal mass (Fig. 3.3). Admittedly, these experimental and clinical models do not portray the usual picture of primary hypertension. Nonetheless, Ledingham (1989) discounts these objections and defends autoregulation as the "dominant factor" leading to the rise in periph-

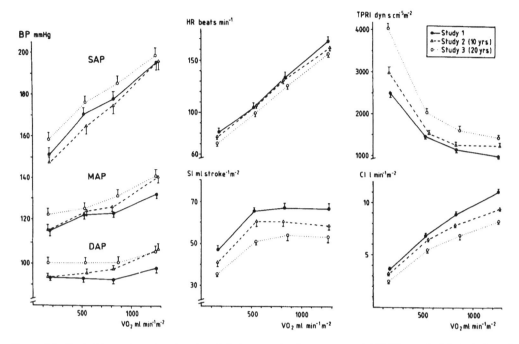

Figure 3.4. Central hemodynamics at rest and during exercise in age group 1 (17–29 years) at first study and at restudy after 10 and 20 years. Mean values: *SAP*, systolic arterial blood pressure; *MAP*, mean arterial blood pressure; *DAP*, diastolic arterial blood pressure; *HR*, heart rate; *SI*, stroke index; *TPRI*, total peripheral resistance index; *CI*, cardiac index; *VO₂*, oxygen consumption. Note the marked increase in TPRI from study I to study III and also the reduction in SI and CI from study I to study III. (From Lund-Johansen P. Central haemodynamics in essential hypertension at rest and during exercise: a 20-year follow-up study. *J Hypertens* 1989;7(Suppl 6):S52–S55.)

eral resistance in hypertension. Moreover, there is additional evidence in favor of volume expansion in the pathogenesis of the disease.

Excess Sodium Intake

Figure 3.1 shows excess sodium intake inducing hypertension by increasing fluid volume and preload, thereby increasing cardiac output. As will become obvious, sodium excess may increase blood pressure in multiple other ways as well, including effects on vascular reactivity (Campese et al., 1993) and contractility (Ashida et al., 1992).

An Overview

After reviewing the available evidence relating sodium intake to hypertension, I conclude that dietary sodium excess is intimately involved in the pathogenesis of primary hypertension. Some reviewing the same evidence do not (Brown et al., 1984), while others accept a role for sodium but question its primacy (Dustan and Kirk, 1989).

The view that excess sodium intake induces hypertension reflects the belief of a large number of investigators, as summarized by Denton in the last 87 pages of his book *The Hunger for Salt* (1982). To quote Denton's nearly final words: "There are good grounds, but by no means a proven case, for suspecting excess salt intake, probably associated with reduced potassium intake, in the aetiology of hypertension in Western-type communities."

My interpretation of these "good grounds" can be summarized as follows. Diets in nonprimitive societies contain many times the daily adult sodium requirement, an amount that is beyond the threshold level needed to induce hypertension (Fig. 3.5). Only part of the population may be susceptible to the deleterious effects of this high sodium intake, presumably because they have an additional renal defect in sodium excretion. As portrayed in Figure 3.5, since almost everyone in nonprimitive societies ingests an excess of sodium beyond the threshold needed to induce hypertension, it may not be possible to show a relationship between sodium intake and blood pressure in these populations. The absence of such a relationship in no way detracts from the possible role of excess dietary sodium in causing hypertension.

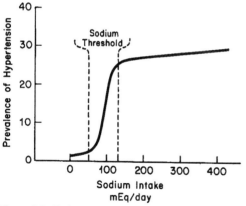

Figure 3.5. Probable association between usual dietary sodium intake and the prevalence of hypertension in large populations. (From Kaplan NM. Dietary salt intake and blood pressure. *JAMA* 1984;251:1429–1430.)

Dietary Sodium:Potassium Ratio

This section relates to sodium excess, but experimental data (Tobian, 1991) and epidemiologic evidence (Khaw and Barrett-Connor, 1988; Geleijnse et al., 1990; He et al., 1991; Bruce et al., 1992) support a close association between hypertension and a high ratio of sodium to potassium intake. A low potassium intake may be as responsible as a high sodium intake (Bulpitt et al., 1986) but, as the following discussion notes, most evidence favors a primary role for sodium excess.

Dietary Chloride

Chloride, and not just sodium, may be involved in the causation of hypertension. In two classic rat models of ''sodium-dependent'' hypertension, hypertension could be induced with sodium chloride but not with sodium bicarbonate or ascorbate (Kurtz and Morris, 1983; Whitescarver et al., 1984). On the other hand, excess chloride without sodium failed to induce hypertension in rats (Whitescarver et al., 1984), so that it may require both sodium and chloride in concert. In people, too, the blood pressure rises more with NaCl than with nonchloride salts of sodium (Boegehold and Kotchen, 1991). The issue is largely academic since chloride is the major anion accompanying sodium in the diet and in body fluids.

Epidemiologic Evidence

The epidemiologic evidence incriminating an excess of sodium includes:

—Primitive, unacculturated people from widely different parts of the world who do not eat sodium have no hypertension, nor does the blood pressure rise with age as it does in all acculturated populations (Page et al., 1981; Carvalho et al., 1989). As an example, the Yanomamo Indians of northern Brazil, who excrete only about 1 mmol of sodium per day, have an average BP of 107/67 among men and 98/62 among women aged 40 to 49 (Oliver et al., 1975).

—The lack of hypertension may be attributable to other differences in lifestyle, but comparisons made in groups living under similar conditions relate the BP most directly to the level of dietary sodium intake (Lowenstein, 1961; Page et al., 1981). Moreover, when unacculturated people, free of hypertension, adopt modern life styles, including increased intake of sodium, their BP rises (Poulter et al., 1990), and hypertension appears (Maddocks, 1967; Poulter et al., 1984).

—In large populations, significant correlations between the level of salt intake and the levels of blood pressure and frequency of hypertension have been found in most (J. Stamler et al., 1989; Law et al., 1991a; Elliott, 1991) but not in all (Smith et al., 1988). Beyond the 28 individual population studies plotted by Elliott (Fig 3.6), the Intersalt study measured 24-hour urine electrolytes and blood pressure in 10,079 men and women aged 20 to 59 in 52 places around the world (Intersalt Cooperative Research Group, 1988). For all 52 centers, there was a positive correlation between sodium excretion and both systolic blood pressure (SBP) and diastolic blood pressure (DBP) but an even more significant association between sodium excretion and the slope of BP with age. In both Elliott's 28 sets of data and Intersalt's 52, few populations were found whose levels of sodium intake were in the 50–100 mmol/day range wherein the threshold for the sodium effect on blood pressure likely resides. However, the virtual absence of either hypertension or a progressive rise in blood pressure with advancing age in those populations wherein average sodium ingestion is less than 50 mmol/day supports the concept of a threshold (Fig. 3.5).

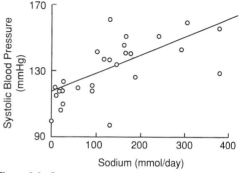

Figure 3.6. Scatterplot showing a cross-population association between mean systolic blood pressure and mean 24-hour sodium excretion for 28 populations; slope = 9.97 mm Hg/100 mmol sodium ($p < 0.001$) (SE, 1.99). (From Elliott P. Observational studies of salt and blood pressure. *Hypertension* 1991;17(Suppl I):I-3–I-8.)

Experimental Evidence

The experimental evidence for a role of sodium excess includes:

—When hypertensives are sodium restricted, their BP falls. As described more fully in Chapter 6, dramatic falls in BP may follow rigid sodium restriction (Kempner, 1948), whereas less rigid restriction to a level of 75–100 mEq/day has been found to lower BP modestly in most studies (Cutler et al., 1991; Law et al., 1991b).

—Although short periods of increased NaCl intake have been shown to raise blood pressure in normotensive subjects (Mascioli et al., 1991), it may never be possible to show conclusively that salt intake causes hypertension in people, but it is fairly easy to do so in genetically predisposed animals (Dahl, 1972; Tobian, 1991). Although long-term intervention studies starting with infants and children to confirm that sodium restriction can prevent hypertension or that sodium excess can cause it in humans are not feasible, a short-term 6-month study on almost 500 newborn infants showed that the half whose sodium intake was reduced by about one-half had a 2.1 mm Hg lower SBP at the end of the 6 months than did the half who were on normal sodium intake (Hofman et al., 1983). Moreover, in randomized controlled studies of hundreds of subjects with high-normal blood pressure, the group who moderately restricted sodium intake for 18 months (Trials of Hypertension Prevention, 1992) to 5 years (R. Stamler et al., 1989) had lower blood pressure and a decreased incidence of hypertension than did the group who did not reduce their sodium intake.

—A high sodium intake may activate a number of pressor mechanisms (Luft and Mann, 1991). These include abnormal vasoconstriction within the renal circulation (Lawton et al., 1988) and enhanced pressor responsiveness to catechols (Campese et al., 1993). High sodium intake raises plasma levels of the Na,K-ATPase inhibitor ouabain (Manunta et al., 1992a) that could lead to an increase of intracellular sodium and calcium.

Parenthetically, cardiovascular damages may be associated with high sodium intake that are not mediated by the effects on sodium on blood pressure. Both in animals (Tobian and Hanlon, 1990) and in humans (Xie et al., 1992; Perry and Beevers, 1992), a high intake of sodium increases the risk of stroke, independent of the effect on blood pressure.

Blood Pressure Sensitivity to Sodium

Since almost everyone in Western countries ingests a high-sodium diet, the fact that only about half will develop hypertension suggests a variable degree of blood pressure sensitivity to sodium, although obviously heredity and interaction with other environmental exposures may be involved (Hamet et al., 1991). Since Luft et al. (1977) and Kawasaki et al. (1978) described varying responses of blood pressure to short periods of low and high sodium intake, numerous protocols have been used to determine "sodium sensitivity" (Sullivan, 1991). Weinberger et al. (1986) defined sodium sensitivity as a 10-mm Hg or greater decrease in mean blood pressure from the level measured after a 4-hour infusion of 2 liters of normal saline compared to the level measured the morning after 1 day of a 10-mmol sodium diet during which three oral doses of furosemide were given at 10 AM, 2 PM, and 6 PM. Using this criterion, they found that 51% of hypertensives but only 26% of normotensives were sodium sensitive (Fig. 3.7).

It is obvious that sodium sensitivity displays a typical bell-shaped distribution with a shift in those who are hypertensive. These investigators observed a further shift with increasing age both in normotensives and even more in hypertensives (Weinberger and Fineberg, 1991) (Fig. 3.8).

A large number of altered responses have been reported in association with sodium sensitivity, as defined in various ways (Table 3.3). Kimura and Brenner (1993) have characterized sodium sensitivity as a reflection of a depressed slope of Guyton's pressure-nutriuresis relationship "caused by or at least strongly associated with elevated glomerular capillary pressure." Of the various features described in sodium-sensitive hypertensive subjects, the most obvious connections are the lower basal levels and the lesser activation of renin-aldosterone with sodium restriction. Thus, in most ways, sodium-sensitive hypertensives appear to be relatively, if not absolutely, volume expanded, with a suppressed, less responsive renin-aldosterone mechanism.

Whatever the mechanism, sodium sensitivity is likely heritable, with close mother-offspring resemblance in blood pressure change with sodium restriction (Miller et al., 1987). A genetic contribution is further supported by an association with haptoglobin 1-1 phenotype (Weinberger et al., 1987).

Recent Changes in Sodium Intake

Those who question the role of dietary sodium excess in the pathogenesis of hypertension should remember that our current high sodium-low potassium intake is a recent phenomenon, beginning only a few hundred years ago and accelerated by modern food processing that adds

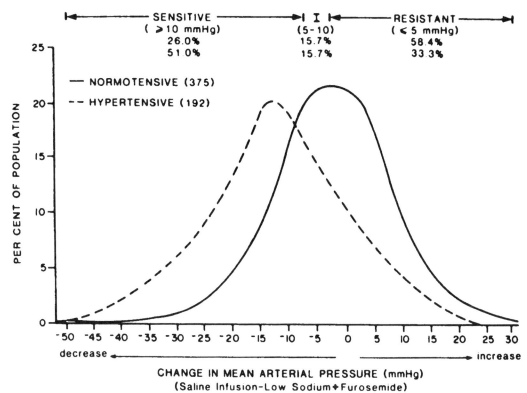

Figure 3.7. Sodium sensitivity and resistance in normal and hypertensive subjects. The lines portray the distribution of blood pressure responses to the maneuvers to assess sodium sensitivity and resistance (saline infusion or a low sodium diet plus furosemide) in normotensive (*solid line*) (*n* = 374) and hypertensive (*dashed line*) (*n* = 192) subjects. The definitions are identified on the top of the figure. The hypertensives are significantly (*p* < 0.001) more sodium sensitive than the normotensives. The distributions are Gaussian. (From Weinberger MH, Miller JZ, Luft FC, Grim CE, Fineberg NS. Definitions and characteristics of sodium sensitivity and blood pressure resistance. *Hypertension* 1986;8(Suppl II):II-127–II-127.)

sodium and removes potassium. Our herbivorous ancestors probably consumed less than 10 mmol of sodium per day, whereas our carnivorous ancestors might have eaten 30 mmol/day (Eaton et al., 1988) (Table 3.4). Human physiology evolved in a low sodium-high potassium environment and we seem ill-equipped to handle the current exposure to high sodium-low potassium.

Our current preference for a high sodium intake likely is an acquired taste, one that may be acquired early in childhood (Beauchamp, 1987). In the typical diet of nonprimitive societies, as little as 15% of total sodium consumption is discretionary, and even less is inherent to the food, with more than three-fourths added in the processing (Mattes and Donnelly, 1991). This increase in sodium intake from processed foods has been so recent that genetic adaptation has not been possible. Since evolutionary changes to preserve Darwinian fitness are not needed if

new environmental factors only produce disability or death after the reproductive years, modern humans may simply not be able to adapt successfully to their high sodium exposure (Trowell, 1980).

RENAL SODIUM RETENTION

With more than enough sodium in the diet and many mechanisms to explain sodium sensitivity, let us consider the hypothesis that patients with primary hypertension are in "a state of continuous correction of a slightly expanded extracellular fluid volume" (de Wardener and MacGregor, 1980). This hypothesis assumes that the excess dietary intake of sodium must be coupled with additional defects, one in the ability of the kidneys to excrete sodium, the other in the handling of sodium within vascular smooth muscle cells. As summarized by de Wardener (1991): "It is proposed that in most forms of hypertension, there is one initiating factor, an

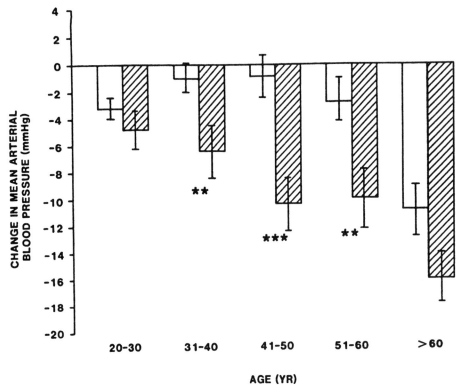

Figure 3.8. This bar graph shows changes in mean arterial pressure in response to maneuvers used to define salt responsivity as a function of age in normotensive (*open bars*) and hypertensive (*hatched bars*) subjects. *Brackets* represent standard deviation of the mean. Significance values between hypertensive and normal subjects are indicated by ** ($p < 0.01$) and *** ($p < 0.001$). (From Weinberger MH, Fineberg NS. Sodium and volume sensitivity of blood pressure. Age and pressure change over time. *Hypertension* 1991;18:67–71.)

abnormal kidney, the functional hypertensinogenic expression of which is a restricted ability to excrete sodium. This sustained restraint on sodium excretion stimulates a sustained activity of volume-controlled mechanisms, including an increase in Na^+,K^+-ATPase inhibitory activity in the plasma and hypothalamus. It is these that raise the blood pressure.''

Functional and Structural Mechanisms

Although a connection between abnormal renal function and hypertension was made by Richard Bright in 1831, the link remained vague until the early 1960s when Guyton (1961) laid out the concept and, soon thereafter, Ledingham and Cohen (1963) in animals and Borst and Borst-de Geus (1963) in a patient independently documented the long-term role of renal excretory function on blood pressure regulation and the presence of expanded fluid volume and cardiac output in the development of hypertension. Guyton and his collaborators have, over the last 30 years, provided an impressive body of experi-

mental and analytical data supporting the central role of renal pressure-natriuresis in the regulation of the normal circulation and its functional resetting in the pathogenesis of hypertension. In addition, reversible renal vasoconstriction has been recognized (Hollenberg et al., 1975) and found even in normotensive young people with hypertensive parents (van Hooft et al., 1991). Beyond these functional changes, Sealey et al. (1988) and Brenner et al. (1988) have proposed that primary structural changes in the kidney could lead to sodium retention and, thereby, to hypertension. Evidence for these various hypotheses will be presented.

Resetting of Pressure-Natriuresis

In normal people, when blood pressure rises, renal excretion of sodium and water increases, shrinking fluid volume and returning the pressure to normal, the phenomenon of *pressure-natriuresis*. On the basis of animal experiments and computer models, Guyton (1992) considers the regulation of body fluid volume by the kid-

Table 3.3. Some of the Reported Associations with Sodium Sensitivity in Hypertension[a]

Finding	Reference
Demographic	
Increasing levels of blood pressure	Weinberger and Fineberg (1991)
Older age	Weinberger and Fineberg (1991)
Black race	Falkner and Kushner (1991)
Positive family history of hypertension	Oshima et al. (1992)
Obesity	Rocchini et al. (1989)
Hormonal	
Insulin resistance and hyperinsulinemia	Sharma et al. (1993)
Low plasma renin-aldosterone levels	Weinberger et al. (1986)
Less activation of renin-aldosterone with sodium restriction	Sullivan (1991)
Higher levels of atrial natriuretic factor	Kohno et al. (1987)
Renal	
Delayed excretion of sodium loads	Luft and Mann (1991)
Increased filtration fraction with sodium loads	Campese et al. (1991)
Increased intraglomerular pressure	Kimura and Brenner (1993)
Nonmodulation of renal and adrenal responses to sodium and angiotensin	Williams and Hollenberg (1991)
Vascular	
Increased forearm vascular resistance	Sullivan (1991)
Increased hypotensive response to calcium blockers	Dichtchekenian et al. (1992)
Sympathetic	
Increased plasma catecholamines	Shimamoto and Shimamoto (1992)
Increased pressor reactivity to norepinephrine	Campese et al. (1993)
Less decrease in plasma catechols with sodium loading	Dimsdale et al. (1990)
Reduced density of β_2-receptors	Kotanko et al. (1992)
Increased urinary excretion of dopa	Gill et al. (1991)
Decreased activation of central dopaminergic system	Hamasaki et al. (1991)
Cellular	
Increased intracellular Ca^{2+} during sodium loading	Alexiewicz et al. (1992)
Increased Na-K cotransport activity	Cacciafesta et al. (1993)
Abnormal intracellular acid-base regulation	Spies et al. (1992)
Increased Na, K-ATPase inhibitor	Iwaoka et al. (1991)

[a]References cited are the most recent; most observations were originally reported prior to those cited.

Table 3.4. Estimated Diet of Late Paleolithic Man Versus That of Contemporary Americans

	Late Paleolithic Diet (Assuming 35% Meat)	Current American Diet
Total dietary energy (%)		
Protein	33	12
Carbohydrate	46	46
Fat	21	42
Polyunsaturated:saturated fat ratio	1.41	0.44
Sodium (mg)	690	3,400
Potassium (mg)	11,000	2,400
K:Na ratio	16:1	0.7:1
Calcium (mg)	1,500–2,000	740

From Eaton SB, Konner M, Shostak M. Stone agers in the fast lane: chronic degenerative diseases in evolutionary perspective. *Am J Med* 1988;84:739–749.

neys to be the dominant mechanism for the long-term control of blood pressure. Therefore, if hypertension develops, he reasons that something must be amiss with this pressure-natriuresis control mechanism.

Experimental Support

The concept is based upon a solid foundation: when arterial pressure is raised, the normal kidney excretes more salt and water, i.e., pressure-natriuresis (Selkurt, 1951). The curve relating arterial pressure to sodium excretion is very steep (Fig. 3.9). A small change in perfusion pressure causes a very large change in the rate of sodium and water excretion, acting as a powerful negative feedback stabilizer of systemic arterial pressure. Under normal conditions, the perfusion pressure is around 100 mm Hg, sodium excretion is about 150 mEq/day, and the two are in a remarkably balanced state. This mechanism is considered to reflect transmission of increased arterial pressure into peritubular capillaries, wherein the increased hydrostatic pressure would reduce sodium reabsorption and increase sodium excretion (Azar et al., 1974). Extracellular fluid (ECF) and plasma volume would presumably shrink enough to lower the blood pressure back to its previous level.

Resetting of Pressure-Natriuresis

In patients with primary hypertension, a rightward resetting of this pressure-sodium excretion curve prevents the return of pressure to normal

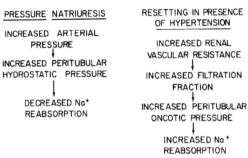

Figure 3.10. Origin of pressure-natriuresis (*left*) and its resetting in the presence of essential hypertension (*right*). (From Brown JJ, Lever AF, Robertson JIS, Schalekamp MA. Renal abnormality of essential hypertension. *Lancet* 1974;2:320–323.)

(Fig. 3.10). The process starts with increased renal vascular resistance, reflecting a preferential constriction of efferent arterioles (Luke, 1993), perhaps by a humoral stimulus with renin-angiotensin being an obvious candidate (Eiskjaer et al., 1992). The release of renin from J-G cells is followed by local generation of angiotensin II (AII) which has immediate access to the efferent arterioles (Romero et al., 1989). The efferent arterioles display heightened reactivity to AII (Ito et al., 1993), and the resultant decrease in renal blood flow increases filtration fraction, the proportion of renal blood flow that is filtered, determined by dividing glomerular filtration rate (GFR) by renal plasma flow (RPF). Numerous studies have shown that in early hypertension, GFR is usually well maintained but RPF is reduced, thereby increasing the filtration fraction (Brod, 1960; London and Safar, 1988). A lower RPF has even been found in the normotensive offspring of hypertensive parents (van Hooft et al., 1991).

As a result of the increased filtration fraction, the peritubular capillary blood, with less sodium and water, will have a higher oncotic pressure, favoring sodium reabsorption. The retained sodium and water overfills the vascular bed, raising blood pressure further. Once a certain level is reached, the higher set pressure-sodium excretion relation comes back into play, returning sodium excretion to balance intake, but at the cost of a persistently elevated blood pressure. This resetting of the renal perfusion pressure-sodium excretion control mechanism has been shown experimentally (Hall et al., 1990) and in patients with two forms of secondary hypertension, primary aldosteronism and renovascular hypertension (Kimura et al., 1987). When the

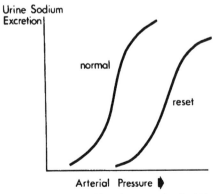

Figure 3.9. Derived renal function curve for the kidneys in people with normal blood pressure and primary hypertension. The resetting of the pressure-natriuresis curve in primary hypertension is shown. (From Guyton AC, Coleman TG, Cowley AW Jr, et al. Arterial pressure regulation. Overriding dominance of the kidneys in long-term regulation and in hypertension. *Am J Med* 1972;52:584–594.)

hypertension was relieved in these patients, the curves shifted leftward, back toward normal.

Inherited Defect in Renal Sodium Excretion

The alteration in renal function responsible for the resetting of the pressure-natriuresis curve may be inherited. Beyond the data noted previously from study of normotensive children of hypertensive parents (van Hooft et al., 1991), most of the evidence comes from rats. Using rats bred to be either sensitive (S) or resistant (R) to the hypertensive action of dietary sodium, Dahl and Heine (1975) showed the primacy of the kidney in the development of hypertension by a series of transplant experiments. These studies show that the blood pressure follows the kidney: When a kidney from a normotensive (R) donor was transplanted to hypertensive (S) host, the blood pressure of the recipient fell to normal (Fig. 3.11). Conversely, when a hypertensive (S) kidney was transplanted into a normotensive (R) host, the blood pressure rose.

Evidence in Humans

The same may be true in people. Curtis et al. (1983) observed long-term remission of hypertension after renal transplantation in six black male patients who likely developed renal failure solely as a consequence of primary hypertension. Since five of these patients had remained hypertensive after removal of their native kidneys, their hypertension was presumably not of renal pressor origin. The most likely explanation for the reversal of hypertension in these patients was the implantation of normal renal tissue that provided control of body fluid volume, something their original kidneys had been unable to manage. Moreover, hypertension develops more frequently in recipients of renal transplants from hypertensive donors than in recipients from normotensive donors (de Wardener, 1990).

As impressive as are both the animal and the human data indicating that resetting of pressure-natriuresis is responsible for the fact that "blood pressure follows the kidney" (Fig. 3.11), other mechanisms may explain abnormal renal sodium retention.

Reduction in Filtration Surface

Brenner et al. (1988) have proposed that hypertension may eventuate from a congenital reduction in the number of nephrons or in the filtration surface area (FSA) per glomerulus, either of which limits the ability to excrete sodium, raising the blood pressure and setting off a vicious cycle whereby systemic hypertension begets glomerular hypertension which begets more systemic hypertension (Fig. 3.12). These investigators point out that as many as 40% of the entire population under age 30 have fewer than the presumably normal number of nephrons (800,000 per kidney) and "speculate that those individuals whose congenital nephron numbers fall in the lower range constitute the population subsets that exhibit enhanced susceptibility to the development of essential hypertension." Similarly, a decrease in filtration surface area, reflected in a decreased glomerular diameter or capillary basement membrane surface area, may be responsible for an increased susceptibility to hypertension even in the presence of a normal nephron number.

Brenner and Anderson (1992) invoke this congenital decrease in filtration surface as a possible explanation for observed differences in suscepti-

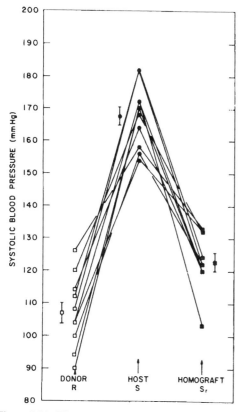

Figure 3.11. Effect of transplanting a "normotensive" kidney from the resistant (*Donor R*) rats to hypertensive sensitive (*Host S*) rats. The resultant blood pressure levels at a median time of 17 weeks after surgery are on the *right*. The mean blood pressure ±SE is indicated for each group. (From Dahl LK, Heine M. Primary role of renal homografts in setting chronic blood pressure and levels in rats. *Circ Res* 1975;36:692–696.)

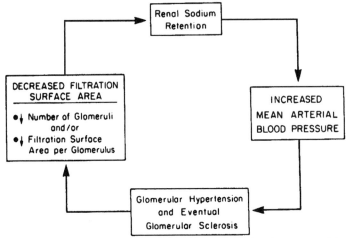

Figure 3.12. Relationship between decreased filtration surface area (*FSA*) and mean arterial pressure. Decreased FSA, due to decreased nephron number and/or FSA per glomerulus, leads to renal sodium retention, and thereby to increased mean arterial pressure. Systemic hypertension in turn promotes glomerular hypertension and eventual sclerosis further decreasing the functioning filtration surface area. (From Brenner BM, Garcia DL, Anderson S. Glomeruli and blood pressure. Less of one, more the other? *Am J Hypertens* 1988;1:335–347.)

bility to hypertension, which characterizes different genetic populations, as well as blacks, women, and older people, all of whom may have smaller kidneys or fewer functioning nephrons. As will be described in Chapter 9, these investigators have developed a similar hypothesis for the progression of renal damage that is commonly observed among diabetics and patients with most forms of acquired kidney disease.

Nephron Heterogeneity

Sealey et al. (1988) have provided another hypothesis for the renal contribution to the pathogenesis of primary hypertension based upon the presence of "a subpopulation of nephrons that is ischemic from either afferent arteriolar vasoconstriction or from an intrinsic narrowing of the lumen. Renin secretion from this subgroup of nephrons is tonically elevated. This increased renin secretion then interferes with the compensatory capacity of intermingled normal nephrons to adaptively excrete sodium and, consequently, perturbs overall blood pressure homeostasis."

This hypothesis is similar to that proposed by Goldblatt who believed that "the primary cause of essential hypertension in man is intrarenal obliterative vascular disease, from any cause, usually arterial and arteriolar sclerosis, or any other condition which brings about the same disturbance of intrarenal hemodynamics" (Goldblatt, 1958). When Goldblatt placed the clamp on the main renal arteries of his dogs, he was trying to explain the pathogenesis of primary

(essential) hypertension rather than what he ended up explaining—the pathogenesis of renovascular hypertension (see Chapter 10). Unable to place minuscule clamps on small arterioles, his experimental concept, nonetheless, is the basis for the more modern model proposed by Sealey et al. (1988) (Table 3.5). The elevated renin from the ischemic population of nephrons, although diluted in the systemic circulation, provides the "normal" renin levels that are usual in patients with primary hypertension, who otherwise would be expected to shut down renin secretion and have low levels. These diluted levels are still high enough to impair sodium excretion in the nonischemic hyperfiltering nephrons but are too low to support efferent tone in the ischemic nephrons, thereby reducing sodium excretion in them as well.

Sealey and associates' concept of nephron heterogeneity differs from Brenner and associates' concept of nephron scarcity but Sealey et al. agree that "a reduction in nephron number related to either age or ischemia could amplify the impaired sodium excretion and promote hypertension" (Sealey et al., 1988).

Sealey et al. expand their model to explain the varying plasma renin levels seen in both normals at different ages and patients with primary hypertension as well as the high renin levels with renovascular hypertension (*RVH*) and the low renin levels with primary aldosteronism (*1° Aldo*) (Fig. 3.13).

Note that even the low-renin form of essential hypertension is shown to involve a few ischemic

Table 3.5. Hypothesis: There Is Nephron Heterogeneity in Essential Hypertension

1. There are ischemic nephrons with impaired sodium excretion intermingled with adapting hyperfiltering hypernatriuretic nephrons.
2. Renin secretion is high from ischemic nephrons and very low from hyperfiltering nephrons.
3. The inappropriate circulating renin-angiotensin level impairs sodium excretion because:
   a. In the adapting hypernatriuretic nephrons
      i. It increases tubular sodium reabsorption.
      ii. It enhances tubuloglomerular feedback-mediated afferent constriction.
   b. As the circulating renin level is diluted by nonparticipation of adapting nephrons, it becomes inadequate to support efferent tone in hypoperfused nephrons.
4. A loss of nephron number with age and from ischemia further impairs sodium excretion.

From Sealey JE, Blumenfeld JD, Bell GM, et al. On the renal basis of essential hypertension: nephron heterogeneity with discordant renin secretion and sodium excretion causing a hypertensive vasoconstriction-volume relation. *J Hypertens* 1988;6:763–777.

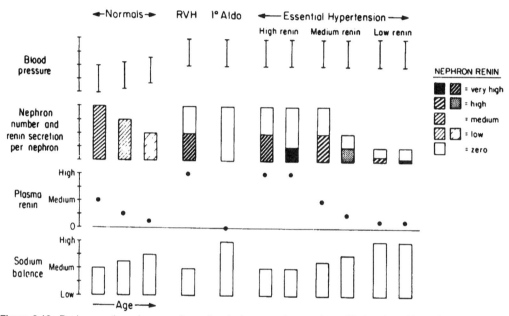

Figure 3.13. Renin secretion, plasma renin, sodium balance, and proportions of ischemic and hyperfiltering nephrons and nephron number in normal subjects with increasing age, in unilateral renovascular hypertension (*RVH*), in primary aldosteronism (*1° Aldo*), and in the three renin subgroups of essential hypertension. Relative values shown are derived from data and a hypothetical model. (From Sealey JE, Blumenfeld JD, Bell GM, et al. On the renal basis for essential hypertension: nephron heterogeneity with discordant renin secretion and sodium excretion causing a hypertensive vasoconstriction-volume relationship. *J Hypertens* 1988;6:763–777.)

nephrons since "*any* renin secretion in the presence of arterial hypertension is abnormal and it works in the same way to impair salt excretion and raise arterial pressure" (Sealey et al., 1988).

This imaginative amplification of Goldblatt's original concept brings us to a consideration of the renin-angiotensin mechanism, skipping for the moment the involvement of the sympathetic nervous system in the pathogenetic scheme for hypertension shown in Figure 3.1.

RENIN-ANGIOTENSIN SYSTEM

As seen in Figure 3.13, plasma renin levels vary within both the normal and hypertensive

populations. Renin may play a critical role in the pathogenesis of most hypertension, a view long espoused by Laragh (1992). Others give it less credit, but all agree that it is involved in cardiovascular homeostasis, perhaps more as a growth factor than as a pressor hormone (Katz, 1992).

Figure 3.14 is a schematic overview of the renin-angiotensin system showing its major components, the regulators of renin release, and the primary effects of AII.

Properties of Renin

Renin was the name given in 1898 by Tigerstedt and Bergman to the pressor material in

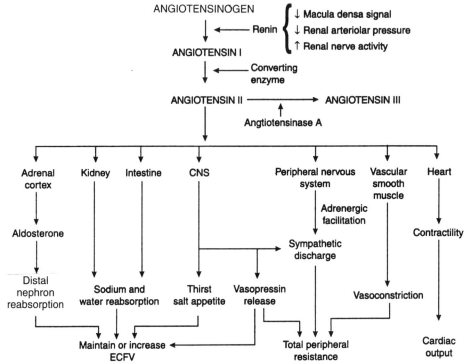

Figure 3.14. Schematic representation of the renin-angiotensin system showing major regulators of renin release, the biochemical cascade leading to AII, and the major effects of AII. *CNS*, central nervous system; *ECFV*, extracellular fluid volume.

extracts of rabbit kidneys (Marks and Maxwell, 1979). In the late 1930s, Page and Helmer and Braun-Menendez et al. showed that the enzyme renin acts upon a protein, angiotensinogen, to release angiotensin (Page, 1975). Renin is stored and secreted from the renal juxtaglomerular (JG) cells located in the wall of the afferent arteriole, which is contiguous with the macula densa portion of the same nephron (Rosivall et al., 1991).

Expression and regulation of the human renin gene and the structure of the enzyme have been elucidated (Griendling et al., 1993). The molecular biology of the renin-angiotensin system has been found to be increasingly more complicated as its intricacies have been revealed.

Forms of Renal Renin

The first product of the translation of renin mRNA is preprorenin, which is processed in the endoplasmic reticulum to a 47-kilodalton (kDa) prorenin. Prorenin may be secreted directly from the JG cell or packaged into immature granules where it is further processed to the active 41-kDa mature (active) renin, which is a glycosylated single-chain polypeptide (Skøtt and Jensen, 1993).

Control of Renal Renin Secretion

The trigger for the secretion of active renin is a *lowering* of cytosolic calcium, which in some manner leads to a fusion of granules that release renin into the cytoplasmic space from which it escapes the cell (Park et al., 1992). The multiple factors that can alter renin secretion include those shown in Figure 3.14, with changes in pressure within the afferent arterioles and sodium concentration in the macula densa likely playing the most important roles. In addition, circulating and intrarenal angiotensin II exerts a direct "short loop" feedback suppression, and other hormones, cytocrines, and neurotransmitters may affect renin release (Skøtt and Jensen, 1993).

Prorenin

Prorenin is the molecular precursor for active renin and is also released from the JG cells. Although it constitutes 80–90% of the renin in human plasma, no physiologic or pathogenic role for prorenin has as yet been established (Osmond et al., 1991). When recombinant human prorenin was infused in large amounts to rhesus monkeys, no effects on cardiovascular or renal functions were noted (Lenz et al., 1991). It does not seem to be converted within the circulation into active renin but such conversion may occur within tissues (Hsueh and Baxter, 1991). Very high concentrations are present in ovarian follicular fluid (Itskovitz et al., 1991), but its possible role in reproduction remains speculative. In addition, high plasma prorenin levels are present in type I diabetics, particularly in those with microvascular complications (Wilson and Luetscher, 1990).

Sealey (1991) has presented an imaginative scheme for an active *vasodilatory* role for prorenin, acting as a balance to the vasoconstrictive effects of renin-angiotensin II. She suggests that "Lack of coordination between the limbs of the greater renin system with a relative excess of renin I [prorenin] would explain the relationship of high prorenin levels to the hyperperfusion injury of diabetes mellitus and the devastating effects of hypertension when it occurs in pregnancy. Conversely, a relative excess of renin II [active renin] would lead to the hypertension and to the ischemic vascular injury of high renin hypertensive disorders." Sealey and co-workers have reported lower plasma prorenin levels in hypertensives than in normotensives (Halimi et al., 1993).

Extrarenal Renin

Low levels of both renin and prorenin are present in the plasma of nephrectomized humans (Opsahl et al., 1993). A number of other tissues have been found to have the various components of the renin-angiotensin system (Paul et al., 1993) and increasing evidence supports their involvement in multiple local and systemic effects (Johnston, 1992) (Table 3.6). In particular, complete renin-angiotensin systems are generated in the brain (Bunnemann et al., 1992), reproductive tract (Samani, 1991) and heart (Dostal and Baker, 1993). Although circulating

AII likely arises from circulating AI, the presence of AII at these various sites may result from its local generation as well.

The issue is not just academic, since the physiologic effects of the system and the actions of various pharmacologic inhibitors upon the system may relate directly to the location of the system.

Functions of Renin

Renin acts as an aspartyl proteinase that catalyzes the hydrolytic release of the decapeptide angiotensin I from its α-globulin substrate, angiotensinogen (Fig. 3.14). Renin itself probably is without effect other than by its activation of angiotensin.

Angiotensinogen

The amount of the renin substrate angiotensinogen in the plasma may vary considerably, and its level may play some role in the overall function of the renin-angiotensin system (Eggena and Barrett, 1992). Estrogens and other stimulators of hepatic microsomal enzyme activity will increase renin substrate levels.

As noted earlier in this chapter, high levels of plasma angiotensinogen have been found in people genetically predisposed to develop hypertension (Watt et al., 1992), and a genetic linkage has been shown between the angiotensinogen gene and hypertension (Jeunemaitre et al., 1992b).

Angiotensin-Converting Enzyme

The two end amino acids histidyl and leucine are removed by a converting enzyme present on the plasma membrane of endothelial cells, forming the 8-amino-acid polypeptide angiotensin II. Conversion occurs throughout the body, particularly in the lung (Erdös, 1990). The endothelial ACE has been found to contain two large homologous domains; the two active sites are

Table 3.6. Functions of Tissue Renin-Angiotensin System

Brain	Neuropeptide processing
	Salt and water balance
Epithelial cells[a]	Ion transport
Reproductive tract	Fertilization
	Peptide processing
Cardiovascular system	Circulatory control
	Cardiovascular structure
Fibroblasts and macrophages	Inflammation and repair

From Johnston CJ. Renin-angiotensin system: a dual tissue and hormonal system for cardiovascular control. *J. Hypertension* 1992;10(Suppl 7):S13–S26.
[a]Epithelial cells include those of the gastrointestinal tract, renal tubule, choroid plexus, eye, and submandibular glands.

inhibited to slightly different degrees by various ACE inhibitors (Wei et al., 1992).

Linkage between the ACE locus and blood pressure has been found in rats but not in humans (Jeunemaitre et al., 1992a). However, a deletion polymorphism in the ACE gene has been found to be associated with the risk for myocardial infarction (MI) (Cambien et al., 1992) and associated with a parental history of fatal MI (Tiret et al., 1993).

AII is inactivated by a series of peptidase enzymes, angiotensinases, which are present in most tissues and in very high concentrations in red blood cells.

Angiotensin Activity

The activity of the final product of this system, AII, is the physiologically important one. This activity reflects complicated interactions.

Angiotensin Receptors

In a manner comparable to that of other peptide hormones, the action of AII is triggered by its interaction with receptors on the plasma membrane of the tissues responsive to the hormone. Two receptors have been cloned, one (AT$_1$) mediating virtually all of the known effects of AII (Timmermans et al., 1992), the other (AT$_2$) apparently involved with cell differentiation and growth (Dzau et al., 1993b).

The binding of circulating AII to its receptors on vascular smooth muscle is impaired during ECF volume depletion as a result of prior occupancy of the receptor sites by increased levels of the hormone (Thurston and Laragh, 1975). Therefore, when ECF volume is shrunken, any given level of AII exerts a lesser response with less vasoconstriction and less of a rise in blood pressure. On the other hand, in adrenal tissue, volume contraction increases both the number of AII receptors and aldosterone synthesis (Hauger et al., 1978). These opposite effects of volume contraction upon the response to AII— a lesser rise in blood pressure, a greater increase in aldosterone synthesis—are physiologically sensible, enabling sodium to be retained without a rise in blood pressure. As we shall see, this modulation of adrenal and vascular responsiveness to angiotensin II with changes in sodium intake has been shown to be altered in 30–50% of patients with primary hypertension who are "nonmodulators" (Williams and Hollenberg, 1991).

Actions of Angiotensin II

As shown in Figure 3.14, AII acts not only on vascular smooth muscle and the adrenal cortex, but also within the heart, kidneys, central nervous system, and adrenergic nerve endings. These actions amplify its volume-retaining and vasoconstrictive effects on the peripheral vascular system. Multiple possible pathogenetic effects of AII are indicated in Figure 3.1 with *arrows* pointing to effects on all four of the primary stimuli to both cardiac output and peripheral resistance.

Vasoconstriction. AII produces sustained rises in blood pressure after binding to vascular AT$_1$ receptors, likely through inhibition of adenylate cyclase mediated through G proteins (Sims et al., 1992). The pressor effect involves facilitation of sympathetic transmission (Hilgers et al., 1993). The greater degree of AII-induced constriction within the renal efferent arterioles than within the afferent arterioles (Denton et al., 1992) is believed to be responsible for the major renal protective effects of ACE inhibitors described in Chapter 7.

Volume. The effects of AII upon adrenal synthesis of aldosterone coupled with its multiple effects on the kidneys (Eiskjaer et al., 1992) place AII as the primary defense against volume depletion and implicate these effects in its hypertensinogenic role.

Hypertrophy. Increasing evidence supports a major role of the renin-angiotensin system in cardiovascular and renal hypertrophy, as noted in the vasculature (Itoh et al., 1993), heart (Dostal and Baker, 1993), and renal mesangium (Anderson et al., 1993). The protective effects of ACE inhibitors on these structures likely reflect an inhibition of this hypertrophy.

Effects of Inhibition of Renin-Angiotensin

There are four sites wherein interruption of the renin-angiotensin system is now feasible (Fig. 3.15). Studies with agents that work at these various sites have provided a great deal of the preceding information about the functions and controls of the renin-angiotensin system. The mechanisms by which agents can act to inhibit the system will be covered in detail in Chapter 7, along with practical considerations about their use to treat hypertension.

Most of the information has come from the use of ACE inhibitors, acting at site 3 in Figure 3.15, which also inhibit the degradation of bradykinin and increase prostaglandins. With the use of specific inhibitors of renin acting at site 2 which do not produce these ancillary effects, no effects on blood pressure or hemodynamics have been noted in sodium-replete, normoten-

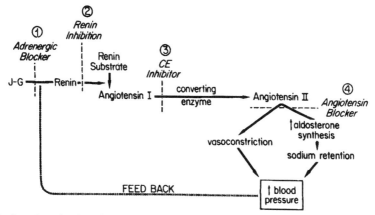

Figure 3.15. The four sites of action of the currently available inhibitors of the renin-angiotensin system.

sive subjects, showing that the renin-angiotensin plays little role under such circumstances (Kiowski et al., 1992). However, when certain perturbations are imposed—volume depletion, sodium restriction, hypotension—the system comes into play and may be essential for survival.

Another global question has been addressed through evidence derived from use of these inhibitors: What role does the renin-angiotensin system play in primary hypertension? This question will be addressed after a brief review of the measurements of these hormones.

Measurements of Plasma Renin

Direct assays of plasma AII have been described (Simon et al., 1992) but are not yet widely available. Currently, it is easier to measure plasma renin activity (PRA) by incubating the patient's plasma containing both angiotensinogen and renin to generate AI which is measured by radioimmunoassay (Sealey, 1991). The amount of AI generated is proportional to the amount of renin present.

Considering all of the factors affecting the level of renin, the agreement noted in the literature is rather surprising: almost all patients with primary aldosteronism have suppressed values; most with renovascular or accelerated-malignant hypertension have elevated levels; and the incidence of suppressed values among patients with primary hypertension is surprisingly similar in different series (Fig. 3.16). Specific information about the use of PRA assays in the evaluation of various secondary forms of hypertension is provided in separate chapters.

The listing in Table 3.7 is not intended to cover every known condition and disease in which a renin assay has been performed, but the more clinically important ones are listed in an attempt to categorize them by mechanism. Some could fit in two or more categories—e.g., upright posture may involve a decreased effective plasma volume, a decreased renal arterial pressure, or catecholamine excess.

Role of Renin-Angiotensin in Primary Hypertension

In keeping with the expected effects of higher perfusion pressure at the JG cell and the high-normal blood volume seen in primary hypertension, suppression of renin release and low levels of PRA are expected. In fact, patients with primary hypertension tend to have lower PRA levels than do age- and sex-matched normotensives (Helmer, 1964; Meade et al., 1983). However, the majority of patients with primary hypertension do not have low, suppressed renin-angiotensin levels, engendering a large amount of clinical research to explain the "inappropriately normal" or even elevated PRA levels seen in most patients (Fig. 3.16). Two logical explanations have been presented: Sealey and associates'

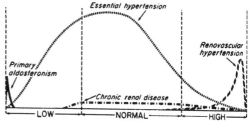

Figure 3.16. Schematic representation of plasma renin activity in various hypertensive diseases. The approximate number of patients with each type of hypertension is indicated along with their proportion of low, normal, or high renin levels. (From Kaplan NM. Renin profiles. The unfulfilled promises. *JAMA* 1977;238:611–613.)

Table 3.7. Clinical Conditions Affecting Renin Levels

Decreased PRA	Increased PRA
Expanded fluid volume	**Shrunken fluid volume**
Salt loads, oral or intravenous	Sodium restriction
Primary salt retention (Liddle's syndrome, Gordon's syndrome)	Fluid losses
Mineralocorticoid excess	Diuretic-induced
Primary aldosteronism	Gastrointestinal losses
Congenital adrenal hyperplasia	Hemorrhage
Cushing's syndrome	Decreased effective plasma volume
11β-Hydroxysteroid dehydrogenase deficiency (licorice)	Upright posture
Deoxycorticosterone (DOC), 18-hydroxy-DOC excess	Cirrhosis with ascites
	Nephrotic syndrome
Sympathetic inhibition	**Decreased renal perfusion pressure**
Autonomic dysfunction	Renovascular hypertension
Therapy with adrenergic neuronal blockers	Accelerated-malignant hypertension
Therapy with β-adrenergic blockers	Chronic renal disease (renin-dependent)
Hyperkalemia	Juxtaglomerular hyperplasia
Decreased renin substrate (?)	**Sympathetic activation**
Androgen therapy	Therapy with direct vasodilators
Decrease of renal tissue	Pheochromocytoma
Hyporeninemic hypoaldosteronism	Stress: hypoglycemia, trauma, exercise
Chronic renal disease (volume-dependent)	Hyperthyroidism
Anephric	Sympathomimetic agents (caffeine)
Increasing age	**Hypokalemia**
Unknown	**Increased renin substrate**
Low renin essential hypertension	Pregnancy
	Estrogen therapy
	Autonomous renin hypersecretion
	Renin-secreting tumors
	Acute damage to juxtaglomerular cells
	Acute glomerulonephritis
	Unknown
	High-renin essential hypertension

(1988) proposal for nephron heterogeneity with a population of ischemic nephrons contributing excess renin described previously in this chapter, and Julius' (1988b) concept of a state of increased sympathetic drive, a concept that will be explored later in this chapter.

Nonmodulation

A third explanation for "normal" renin levels when low levels are to be expected has been proposed by Gordon Williams and Norman Hollenberg on the basis of a series of studies that began in 1970, which indicated that as many as half of normal-renin and high-renin hypertensive patients have a defective feedback regulation of renin-angiotensin within the kidney and the adrenal glands.

Normal Modulation. Normal subjects modulate the responsiveness of their AII target tissues with the level of dietary sodium intake: with sodium restriction, the adrenal secretion of aldosterone is enhanced, whereas vascular responses are reduced; with sodium loading, the adrenal response is suppressed and vascular responses are enhanced, particularly within the renal circulation. With sodium restriction, renal blood flow is reduced, facilitating sodium conservation; with sodium loading, RBF increases, promoting sodium excretion. These changes are mediated mainly by changes in AII, increasing with sodium restriction and decreasing with sodium loading.

Abnormal Modulation. Williams, Hollenberg, and their coworkers have found that about one-half of normal to high renin hypertensives are *nonmodulators*, as characterized by abnormal adrenal and renal responses to AII infusions and salt loads (Williams et al., 1992).

These findings have been attributed to an abnormally regulated and rather fixed level of tissue AII that, in the adrenal tissues, does not increase aldosterone secretion in response to sodium restriction and, in the renal circulation, does not allow renal blood flow to increase with sodium loading. The hypothesis that there is an abnormally regulated fixed local AII concentration in these nonmodulators received support from the correction of both the adrenal and renal defects after suppression of AII by use of converting enzyme inhibitors.

In the overall view of this intriguing set of observations, nonmodulation in the face of relatively high dietary sodium intake could explain the pathogenesis of "sodium-sensitive" hypertension and provide a more targeted, rational therapy for its correction. Part of the nonmodulation profile, a blunted renal blood flow response to sodium loading, has been found in black sodium-sensitive hypertensives (Campese et al., 1991).

Primary Hypertension with Low Renin

We have, then, numerous possible explanations for normal levels of renin in hypertension, the usual finding. Although low renin levels are to be expected in the absence of one or another of the previously described circumstances, a great deal of work has been done to uncover special mechanisms, prognosis, and therapy for hypertensives with low renin.

Mechanism.   The possible mechanisms for low-renin hypertension include volume expansion with or without mineralocorticoid excess as shown in the left side of Table 3.7, but the majority of careful analyses fail to indicate volume expansion (Lebel et al., 1974) or increased levels of mineralocorticoids (Gomez-Sanchez et al., 1985).

Although low renin levels would be expected to be accompanied by low aldosterone levels, plasma aldosterone levels are normal (Griffing et al., 1990). A relatively simple explanation for low renin and normal aldosterone levels is an increased adrenal sensitivity to angiotensin II, as has been demonstrated in some patients (Wisgerhof and Brown, 1978; Griffing et al., 1990). Thus they would need less renin-angiotensin to maintain normal aldosterone levels and volume control.

Prognosis.   A retrospective analysis of the number of strokes and heart attacks over a 7-year interval showed that patients with low renin hypertension had none, whereas 11% of normal-renin and 14% of high-renin patients had experienced one of these cardiovascular complications (Brunner et al., 1972). High renin levels most likely indicate more severe intrarenal vascular damage, so that the higher rate of complications among the high-renin group is not surprising.

However, the data of Brunner et al. posed the possibility of vasculotoxic effects of presumably normal levels of renin.

Although a number of subsequent studies failed to document an improved prognosis in low-renin hypertension (Kaplan, 1975; Birkenhager et al., 1977), Alderman et al. (1991) prospectively tested the prognostic value of the renin-sodium profile in 1717 hypertensive subjects followed for over 8 years while being treated. The incidence of myocardial infarction was 14.7 per 1,000 person-years in the 12% with a high profile, 5.6 in the 56% with a normal profile, and 2.8 in the 32% with a low profile. The incidence of stroke was not correlated with renin status, but the association with heart attack remained significant after adjustment for various possible confounders. In a less direct manner, the increasing evidence of better organ protection with drugs that inhibit the renin-angiotensin system, i.e., ACE inhibitors, has been taken as additional proof of the prognostic value of a lower renin status (Devereux and Laragh, 1992).

Therapy.   In keeping with their presumed but unproven volume excess, patients with low-renin essential hypertension have been found to have a greater fall in blood pressure when given diuretics than do normal-renin patients by some investigators (Vaughan et al., 1973) but not by others (Hunyor et al., 1975; Ferguson et al., 1977; Holland et al., 1979).

If low-renin hypertensive patients do respond better to diuretics, the response does not necessarily indicate a greater volume load. Patients with low renin, by definition, are less responsive to stimuli that increase renin levels, including diuretics, and they therefore experience a lesser rise in PRA with diuretic therapy. Less renin and AII would result in less compensatory vasoconstriction and aldosterone secretion, so that volume depletion would proceed and the blood pressure would fall further in low-renin hypertensive patients given a diuretic.

Overview of Renin-Angiotensin

Although low renin levels are expected in primary hypertension, the presence of normal or high levels in most patients has generated a search for an involvement of such "inappropriate" levels in the pathogenesis of the disease. At least three explanations for higher than expected renin-angiotensin levels have been provided, and it seems likely that this mechanism is abnormally activated in many patients with primary hypertension.

John Laragh and co-workers have long attached a great deal of significance to the various PRA levels found in patients with primary hypertension (Laragh, 1973, 1992). According to this view, the levels of renin can identify the relative contributions of vasoconstriction (peripheral resistance) and body fluid volume expansion to the pathogenesis of hypertension. According to the "bipolar vasoconstriction-volume analysis," arteriolar vasoconstriction by AII is predominantly responsible for the hypertension in patients with high renin, whereas volume expansion is predominantly responsible in those with low renin.

Although actual hemodynamic measurements have not generally confirmed this bipolar relationship with plasma renin levels (Fagard et al., 1977; London et al., 1977b; Julius, 1988b), the problem may be in our dependency, until now, upon their measurements only in plasma rather than from within those tissues where the physiologic and pathologic consequences of renin-angiotensin are occurring. The problem is exemplified in the transgenic rat, which carries an extra load of mouse renin genes and experiences a severe, rapidly lethal form of hypertension (Bachmann et al., 1992). Plasma renin levels are *low*, not high, but—of all places—the adrenal glands show marked overexpression of mouse renin. So, until the entire renin-angiotensin system can be assessed, we have to depend upon measuring its activity in only a single, and perhaps relatively insignificant, site, the circulating blood.

SYMPATHETIC NERVOUS OVERACTIVITY

As shown in Figure 3.1, an excess of renin-angiotensin activity could interact with the sympathetic nervous system (SNS) to mediate most of its effects. On the other hand, stress may activate the SNS directly and SNS overactivity, in turn, may interact with high sodium intake.

The concept has considerable support. Folkow (1989) has concluded that "excitatory psychosocial influences and increased salt intake, which at least partly operate via different genetic elements, are in fact closely intertwined, and are mutually reinforcing as to their actions...to gradually elevate the pressure equilibrium until a state of 'established' hypertension is reached." The evidence, even in a partial listing (Table 3.8), strongly indicates increased SNS activity in early hypertension and, even more impressively, in the still normotensive offspring of

Table 3.8. Evidence for Increased Sympathetic Nervous System Activity in Hypertension

Normotensive offspring of hypertensive parents
Increased heart rate and blood pressure during stress
  Julius et al. *Hypertension* 1991;17(III):12
Increased plasma norepinephrine and total body norepinephrine spillover
  Ferrier et al. *Clin Sci* 1993;84:225
Augmented cardiopulmonary baroreflex restraint
  Rea and Hamdan *Circulation* 1990;82:856
Greater decrease in forearm vascular resistance during stress
  Miller and Ditto *Psychophysiology* 1991;28:103
Increased plasma norepinephrine response to mental stress
  Lenders et al. *J Hypertens* 1989;7:317
Increased plasma norepinephrine response to exercise
  Nielsen et al. *J Hypertens* 1989;7:377
Increased pressor sensitivity to norepinephrine
  Bianchetti et al. *Kidney Int* 1986;29:882
Increased sensitivity of isolated resistance vessels to norepinephrine
  Aalkjaer et al. *Hypertension* 1987;9(Suppl III):III-155
Increased platelet α_2-adrenoreceptor density
  Michel et al. *J Cardiovasc Pharmacol* 1989;13:432
Decreased sodium excretion during stress
  Light et al. *Science* 1983;220:429
Early hypertension
Elevated plasma norepinephrine levels
  Goldstein and Lake *Fed Proc* 1984;43:57
Increased norepinephrine spillover rate
  Esler et al. *Hypertension* 1991;17(Suppl III):29
Increased muscle sympathetic nerve activity
  Anderson et al. *Hypertension* 1989;14:177
Increased heart rate variability
  Guzzetti et al. *J Hypertension* 1991;9:831
Increased α-adrenergic vasoconstriction
  Egan et al. *J Clin Invest* 1987;80:812
Increased vascular reactivity to norepinephrine
  Ziegler et al. *Am J Hypertens* 1991;4:586

hypertensive parents, among whom a large number are likely to develop hypertension.

Before considering further some of the evidence listed in Table 3.8, a brief review of the pertinent physiology of the sympathetic nervous system will be provided.

Normal Physiology

A number of peripheral and central nervous structures are interconnected to provide control over the circulation (Shepherd, 1990). The vasomotor center activates efferent pathways that innervate sympathetic ganglia. From these, an arborizing network of neurons exerts its effects in response to an action potential by release into the synaptic cleft of norepinephrine, which stimulates receptors on target tissues. Sympathetic nerves and their catecholamine secretions induce their effects upon the heart and blood vessels by multiple interactions with both presynaptic and postsynaptic receptors (Langer and Hicks, 1984) (Fig. 3.17).

Role of Epinephrine

A mechanism exists for the translation of intermittent stress into more sustained hypertension. The adrenomedullary secretion of epinephrine may induce far greater and longer effects upon the blood pressure than the relatively short "fight-or-flight" response. After an infusion of epinephrine at levels comparable to those seen during stress, the blood pressure rose and remained elevated for some time thereafter (Blankestijn et al., 1988). Presumably, part of the epinephrine entered the sympathetic nerve endings (5 in Fig. 3.17) and was rereleased into the synaptic cleft as a cotransmitter during subsequent stimulation of the sympathetic nerves. However, in addition, this epinephrine acts upon the presynaptic β2-receptor to facilitate the release of more norepinephrine (7 in Fig. 3.17). Thus, intermittently secreted adrenomedullary epinephrine may invoke a sustained increase in neuronal release of both epinephrine and norepinephrine, in turn causing neurogenic vasoconstriction and a persistent rise in blood pressure (Floras, 1992).

Other Markers

Increased levels of neuropeptide Y, a cotransmitter with norepinephrine in sympathetic neurons supplying arteries and veins, have been reported in hypertensives (Erlinge et al., 1992). In addition, defects in the functions of adenosine (Azevedo and Osswald, 1992) and dopamine (Clark et al., 1992) may be part of the spectrum of SNS involvement in hypertension.

Baroreceptor Dysfunction

Another component of the sympathetic nervous system, the sinoaortic (high pressure) and cardiopulmonary (low pressure) baroreceptors,

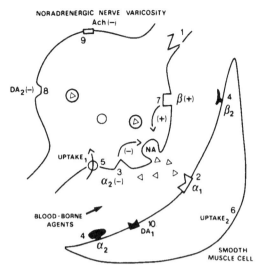

Figure 3.17. Schematic representation of the major receptor types of catecholamines as might be found on the innervation of smooth muscle or cardiac muscle. *1*, electrical stimulation leads to depolarization in the terminal varicosities. The sympathetic varicosity releases noradrenaline (*NA*) into the neuromuscular junction. *2*, the major sympathetic innervation of smooth muscle cells is the α_1-receptor subtype (on cardiac cells it is the β_1-receptor subtype). *3*, noradrenaline released from the varicosity may act on presynaptic α_2-receptors to inhibit the further release of noradrenaline. *4*, α_2-receptors located postjunctionally may be activated by noradrenaline released from the varicosities. α_2-Receptor stimulation mediates contraction; β_2-receptor stimulation leads to dilatation of blood vessels. *5*, the major route of inactivation of noradrenaline is by active neuronal reuptake (*UPTAKE₁*), which may also take up adrenaline. *6*, an extraneuronal uptake mechanism also exists in smooth muscle and cardiac muscle. Both adrenaline and noradrenaline are substrates for this uptake process. *7*, β-receptors are also found on the sympathetic nerve terminals, where their stimulation leads to facilitation of noradrenaline release. These β-receptors (probably β_2-receptor subtype) may be activated by adrenaline. *8*, dopamine (*DA₂*) receptors whose stimulation leads to inhibition of noradrenaline release. *9*, muscarinic cholinergic receptors whose stimulation leads to inhibition of noradrenaline release. *Ach*, acetylcholine. *10*, in certain vascular beds, the smooth muscle possesses dopamine (*DA₁*) receptors that mediate relaxation. (From Langer SZ, Hicks PE. Physiology of the sympathetic nerve ending. *Br J Anaesth* 1984;56:689–700.)

may also be involved. These reflexes, when activated by a rise in blood pressure or central venous pressure, respectively, normally reduce heart rate and lower blood pressure by vagal stimulation and sympathetic inhibition. These reflexes are reset rapidly when hypertension is sustained so that a given increase in BP evokes less decrease in heart rate (Xie et al., 1991).

The lesser sensitivity of the baroreceptors in hypertensive patients is likely the principal determinant of their increased BP variability

(Floras et al., 1988). Beyond rare instances of paroxysmal hypertension in humans with baroreceptor denervation (Aksamit et al., 1987), the effects of the progressive loss of baroreceptor sensitivity as elevated blood pressure persists are uncertain. Shepherd (1990) postulates that the decreased inhibition of the vasomotor center resulting from resetting of the arterial baroreceptors (mechanoreceptors) may be responsible for increased sympathetic outflow and thereby in the perpetuation of hypertension (Fig. 3.18).

Role of Stress

Now that we have seen how repeated stress may lead to sustained hypertension, let us examine the evidence that hypertensives and, even more importantly, those likely to develop hypertension either have more stress or respond differently to stress.

Exposure to Stress

People exposed to repeated psychogenic stresses may develop hypertension more frequently than otherwise similar people not so stressed:

—As an extreme example, the blood pressure remained normal among nuns in a secluded order over a 20-year period whereas it rose with age in women nearby in the outside world (Timio et al., 1988).

—Air traffic controllers, who work under high level psychological stress, annually develop hypertension at a rate 5.6 times greater than do nonprofessional pilots who were initially comparable in physical characteristics (Cobb and Rose, 1973).

—Among healthy employed men, job strain (defined as high psychological demands and low decision latitude on the job) is associated with a 3.1 times greater odds ratio for hypertension, and an increased left ventricular mass index by echo (Schnall et al., 1990).

—Multiple populations living in small, cohesive, protected societies have been found to have low blood pressures that do not rise with aging; those who abandon such an environment and migrate to more urbanized, modern, disorganized societies have higher blood pressures that rise with aging (Salmond et al., 1989; Poulter et al., 1990). Environmental factors such as weight gain and increased sodium intake may be responsible, but there is considerable evidence that social disorganization, as would be expected with migration, is associated with more hypertension (Bland et al., 1991).

—The higher prevalence of hypertension among blacks has been attributed to their increased level of anger and social stresses (Gentry et al., 1982). However, blacks may not be peculiar in this regard: whites in the lower social classes (Tyroler, 1989),

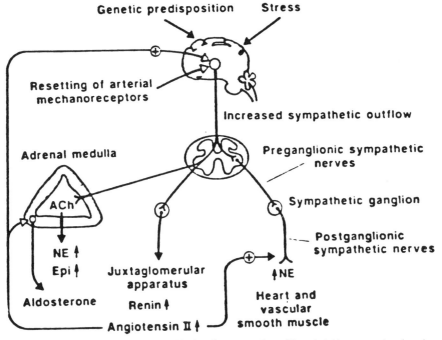

Figure 3.18. Consequence of a genetic predisposition leading to resetting of the arterial baroreceptors (mechanoreceptors) with a resultant increase in sympathetic outflow. This increase could be enhanced further by changes in the cardiovascular centers and an exaggerated cardiovascular response to stress. *ACh*, acetylcholine; *NE*, norepinephrine; *Epi*, epinephrine. (From Shepherd JT. Increased systemic vascular resistance and primary hypertension: the expanding complexity. *J Hypertens* 1990;8(Suppl 7):S15–S27.)

with lower occupational status (Leigh, 1991), or with less formal education (R. Stamler et al., 1992) also have more hypertension and higher mortality associated with it.

Reactivity to Stress

People may become hypertensive not just because they are more stressed but because they respond differently to stress. Greater cardiovascular and sympathetic nervous reactivity to various laboratory stresses has been documented repeatedly in hypertensives and in normotensives at higher risk for developing hypertension (Light et al., 1992; Widgren et al., 1992b). Although the evidence for a different psychological substrate in hypertensive people is impressive, it should be remembered that most of the data are short-term, cross-sectional observations that may not relate to the underlying pathogenesis of hypertension. Julius et al. (1991a) found that hyperreactivity to mental stress was seen more often in the offspring of hypertensive parents but that such hyperreactivity was unrelated to the future development of hypertension. In particular, there is a need to study patients' psychological status before they are aware of their diagnosis since they may display increases in various measures of SNS activity in response to mental stress after becoming aware (Rostrup et al., 1991).

Nonetheless, numerous studies show a greater intensity of anger and hostility, but at the same time a greater suppression of the expression of the anger, among hypertensives (Schneider et al., 1986), patients whose pressure rises over time (Perini et al., 1991), and normotensive offspring of hypertensive parents (Perini et al., 1990). Moreover, hypertensives tend to remain emotionally stressed longer (Melamed, 1987) and to be more disposed to cope actively with stressors (Duijkers et al., 1988).

Despite the rather impressive body of literature supporting higher levels of stress and greater reactivity to that stress, doubts have been raised. Freeman (1990), after reviewing much of this literature, concludes: ''There is no satisfactory evidence that psychosocial stress leads to the elevation of the mean daily blood pressure with its pathogenic connotations.'' Also, Tom Pickering (1990), a major contribution to this literature states: ''The role of mental stress in the development of hypertension remains uncertain. Its effects are likely to depend on an interaction of at least three factors: the nature of the stressor,

its perception by the individual, and the individual's physiological susceptibility.''

Changes with Age

Various indices of sympathetic nervous hyperreactivity are seen exclusively or mainly in younger patients (Ferrier et al., 1993), including higher plasma levels of norepinephrine and norepinephrine spillover. Julius (1990) explains the tendency for previously elevated plasma norepinephrine levels to fall as hypertension becomes established by a negative feedback of the elevated blood pressure per se on the central nervous system. This same explanation is offered for the transition from a high cardiac output to an elevated vascular resistance. In Julius' words: ''This hemodynamic transition is caused by decreased β-adrenergic responsiveness and decreased end-diastolic distention of the heart combined with an increased α-adrenergic responsiveness of the resistance vessels. In parallel, the sympathetic tone decreases in the course of hypertension. This transition in sympathetic tone can be explained by the hypothesis of the 'blood pressure seeking properties of the brain.' The central nervous system 'seeks' to maintain a higher pressure. When vascular overresponsiveness sets in, less sympathetic drive is needed to maintain a neurogenic hypertension.''

Overview of Sympathetic Activity

These various pieces of evidence add up to make a fairly strong case for a role of increased sympathetic nervous system activity in the pathogenesis of hypertension (Wyss, 1993). Catecholamine-induced constriction of renal efferent arterioles has been emphasized previously as a logical way to explain the pressure-natriuresis phenomenon, which is critical to the renal retention of sodium. Moreover, catechols are leading candidates to be both the pressor mechanism that initiates the rise in blood pressure and the trophic mechanism that maintains hypertension via vascular hypertrophy (Fig. 3.1).

Whatever the specific role of SNS activity in the pathogenesis of hypertension, it appears to be involved in the increased cardiovascular morbidity and mortality that afflicts hypertensive patients during the early morning hours. Increased α-sympathetic activity occurs in the early morning, associated with the preawakening increase in REM sleep (Somers et al., 1993) and the assumption of upright posture after overnight recumbency (Cohen and Muller, 1992). The heightened α-sympathetic activity in the early morning is reflected in higher forearm vascular resistance. With the α-blocker, phentolamine, the circadian rhythm is removed; with the direct vasodilator, nitroprusside, the rhythm is preserved but at a lower level (Panza et al., 1991) (Fig. 3.19). As a consequence of the increased SNS activity, blood pressure rises abruptly and markedly and, as detailed in Chapter 2, this rise is at least partly responsible for the increase in sudden death, heart attack, and stroke during the early morning hours.

Increased sympathetic activity is also likely responsible for the increased heart rate present in many hypertensives (Staessen et al., 1991a). In turn, among hypertensives in Framingham, cardiovascular mortality rose progressively with higher heart rate over a 36-year follow-up (Gillman et al., 1993).

PERIPHERAL RESISTANCE

The preceding sections have covered the major elements that could induce hypertension primarily by increasing cardiac output. As noted, both the renin-angiotensin and sympathetic nervous systems may also be directly involved in raising peripheral resistance. We will now consider other factors that may work primarily upon the second part of the equation BP = CO × PR (Fig. 3.1). Most of these can induce both

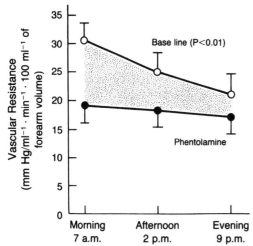

Figure 3.19. Mean vascular resistance at three times of day in 12 healthy subjects. Values shown were obtained at baseline (*open circles*) and after α-sympathetic blockade with the infusion of phentolamine (*solid circles*). The *stippled area* indicates the vascular tone contributed by α-sympathetic vasoconstrictor forces. *P* values refer to the slope of the curve and were obtained by analysis of variance. *Vertical bars* indicate standard errors. (From Panza JA, Epstein SE, Quyyumi AA. Circadian variation in vascular tone and its relation to α-sympathetic vasoconstrictor activity. *N Engl J Med* 1991;325:986–990.)

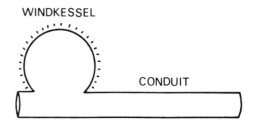

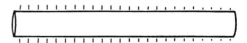

Figure 3.20. The cushioning and conduit functions of the arterial system may be represented (*top*) separately by a Windkessel and distributing tube or (*bottom*) a single distensible tube in which both functions are combined. (From O'Rourke MF, Kelly RP. Wave reflection in the systemic circulation and its implications in ventricular function. *J Hypertens* 1993;11:327–337.)

functional constriction and structural remodeling and hypertrophy. As we shall soon see, the former may be responsible for the latter.

Before proceeding with an overview of the mechanism that raises peripheral resistance, a brief review of some fundamentals should be helpful. In the words of O'Rourke and Brunner (1992): "The arterial system is a complex network of elastic tubes which, at one end, accepts spurts of blood from the left ventricle of the heart, and at its myriad terminations, passes this on in a steady stream into the resistance vessels, which perfuse the organs and tissues of the body. The arterial system acts both as conduit and as cushion, delivering blood with a minimal fall in pressure to peripheral tissues (conduit function) and cushioning pressure fluctuations imposed by intermittent ventricular action (cushioning function). Thus the complex network of tubes can be viewed as a simple system, at least as a first approximation. This simple system is the Windkessel concept, with the distensible Windkessel (cushion) itself linked to peripheral resistance by a rigid conduit" (Fig. 3.20).

As we shall see, hypertension is associated with multiple changes in the properties of different portions of the conduit arteries. However, it is within the smaller resistance arterioles where most of the hemodynamic abnormalities of hypertension occur.

Measurements of Vascular Behavior

In the words of Folkow (1990): "The in vivo hemodynamic behavior of systemic resistance vessels depends not only on 1) their smooth muscle activity and 2) their geometric design, but also on 3) wall distensibility, and 4) the distending pressure. The complex interactions of these four factors, where too often only the first factor is considered . . . should be considered seriously, because the interrelationships . . . are indeed essential for the understanding of the hemodynamics of hypertension.''

Folkow's major conceptual contribution was the recognition that structural changes are responsible for the increased resistance of established hypertension (Fig. 3.21). Because of the increased ratio between wall thickness and lumen diameter, higher wall stress and intraluminal pressure develops when resistance vessels are stimulated.

Whereas total peripheral resistance has usually been measured indirectly by the equation PR = BP/CO (with actual measurements of BP and CO), a number of techniques are being used to assess individual aspects of ''in vivo hemodynamic behavior'' as called for by Folkow. These include measures of *compliance*, the change in vessel diameter for a given change in intravascular pressure, and *wall tension*, the circumferential force in wall per unit vessel length (Mulvany, 1992).

Compliance

More studies of vascular compliance are being reported because it provides a more sensitive, dynamic index of abnormal structure and tone than do static measures of basal caliber. The

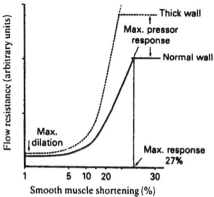

Figure 3.21. Increased vascular reactivity in hypertension explained by structural changes. The differences in flow resistance are calculated in a mathematical model assuming a 30% increased wall thickness being the only difference between hypertensive and normal vessels. (Modified from Folkow B. "Structural factor" in primary and secondary hypertension. *Hypertension* 1990;16:89–101.)

long-time labors of Michel Safar and his co-workers (Safar et al., 1981) are bearing increasing dividends. The field is changing rapidly, but there is basic agreement on these points:

—Compliance overall is decreased in hypertensives due mainly to an intrinsic change in the arterial wall, likely due to increased smooth muscle tone (Yin and Ting, 1992). However, when the impact of the higher pressure per se is accounted for, the difference largely disappears (Roman et al., 1992).

—Measurements of proximal compliance, within the aorta and large arteries, show about a 20% decrease (Weber et al., 1991; McVeigh et al., 1991) most likely due to structural changes.

—Compliance within middle-sized arteries, such as the radial artery, may be increased (Laurent et al., 1993).

—The greatest loss of compliance, as measured with a modified Windkessel model of the circulation, is within the smaller, distal resistance vessels (McVeigh et al., 1991).

Such accurate measures of dynamic vascular function and structure may provide a better way to assess and follow the hemodynamic consequences of hypertension. Evidence is already at hand that pulse pressure, more than mean pressure, acts as the stimulus for alterations of vascular structure, indicating that antihypertensive therapy that most effectively reduces pulse pressure may be most effective in overcoming the small artery damage (Christensen, 1991). As changes in compliance are being recognized even in normotensive subjects with positive family histories of hypertension (Widgren et al., 1992a) and as links between compliance and various humoral factors that can be altered are being found (Neutel et al., 1992), the attention directed to these dynamic measurements almost certainly will continue to escalate. Moreover, as noted in Chapter 4, the travel and reflection of the pressure wave generated by the heart as it traverses the arterial tree clearly is involved in the vascular damage that accompanies hypertension (O'Rourke and Kelly, 1993).

Meanwhile, the underlying role of increased peripheral resistance mediated by vascular remodeling and hypertrophy, however it is measured, must be recognized as a major contributor to the pathogenesis of hypertension.

Role of Vascular Hypertrophy

Regardless of what starts the process, the perpetuation of hypertension clearly depends upon the development of vascular hypertrophy (Folkow, 1990). In studies of small resistance vessels from subcutaneous tissue from hypertensive subjects, an average 29% increase in the media thickness: lumen diameter ratio was found, closely matching the 32% elevation in blood pressure, without any hypersensitivity to vasoconstrictors (Aalkjaer et al., 1987). Although this increase has been attributed mainly to vascular wall growth, increasing evidence supports a greater role for a rearrangement of a normal amount of tissue around a smaller lumen, a process known as *remodeling* (Heagerty et al., 1993) (Fig. 3.22).

Initiating Pressor Mechanism

The search for the pathogenesis of sustained hypertension has increasingly focused on vascular hypertrophy, particularly since multiple vasoactive substances are known to serve as growth or trophic factors for vascular hypertrophy (Dzau et al., 1993a). This knowledge has come, in part, from the study of certain forms of endocrine hypertension, including pheochromocytoma, primary aldosteronism, and renovascular disease. Each of these secondary forms of hypertension is known to arise from the direct effect of a specific pressor hormone. What has now become obvious is that, regardless of the initial hormonal effect, whether it be volume retention as with primary aldosteronism or vasoconstriction as with pheochromocytoma or renovascular disease, maintenance of hypertension derives from vascular hypertrophy that increases peripheral resistance. As summarized by Lever and Harrap (1992): "Most forms of secondary

hypertension have two pressor mechanisms; a primary cause, e.g., renal clip, and a second process, which is slow to develop, capable of maintaining hypertension after removal of the primary cause, and probably self-perpetuating in nature. We suggest that essential hypertension also has two mechanisms, both based upon cardiovascular hypertrophy: 1) a growth-promoting process in children (equivalent to the primary cause in secondary hypertension); and 2) a self-perpetuating mechanism in adults."

Sustaining Hypertrophic Response

Lever and Harrap start with the original proposal of Folkow (Fig. 3.23) wherein hypertension is initiated by a minor overactivity of a specific fast-acting pressor mechanism (Fig. 3.23*A*), e.g., angiotensin II, that raises blood pressure slightly and initiates a positive feedback (*B-C-B*) that induces vascular hypertrophy and maintains the hypertension. The amplification (BCB) is "slowly progressive, ultimately large and probably nonspecific. Thus different forms of chronic hypertension may resemble each other because part of the hypertension in each has the same mechanism" (Lever, 1986). In the second and third proposals, two additional elements are added: *D*, a genetically determined reinforced hypertrophic response, and *E*, the direct contribution of one or more trophic mechanisms for hypertrophy.

This scheme, involving both an immediate pressor action and a slow hypertrophic effect,

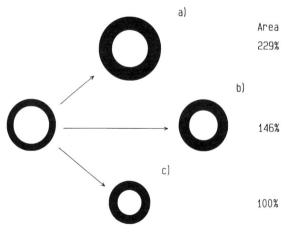

Figure 3.22. Schematic drawing shows different modes of structural change of arteries. Silhouette on the left shows the media cross-section of the control vessel. On the *right* are shown various ways in which the media thickness:lumen diameter ratio can be doubled. In *a*), material has been added to the outer surface. In *b*), material has been added to the inner surface. In *c*), there has been rearrangement of existing material (remodeling), with consequent reduction in lumen diameter. The percentages on the right show the relative cross-sectional areas. (From Heagerty AM, Aalkjaer C, Bund SJ, et al. Small artery structure in hypertension. Dual processes of remodeling and growth. *Hypertension* 1993;21:391–397.)

(a) <u>First hypothesis</u>

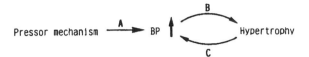

(b) <u>Second and third hypotheses</u>

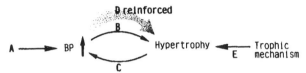

Figure 3.23. Hypotheses for the initiation and maintenance of hypertension: (*a*) Folkow's first proposal that a minor overactivity of a pressor mechanism (*A*) raises blood pressure slightly, initiating positive feedback (*BCB*) and a progressive rise of blood pressure. (*b*) As in (*a*) with two additional signals: *D*, an abnormal or "reinforced" hypertrophic response to pressure, and *E*, increase of a humoral agent causing hypertrophy directly. (From Lever AF, Harrap SB. Essential hypertension: a disorder of growth with origins in childhood? *J Hypertens* 1992;10:101–120.)

may be common to the action of various pressor-growth promoters. In the majority of hypertensive patients, no marked excess of any of the known pressor hormones is identifiable. Nonetheless, a lesser excess of one or more may have been responsible for initiation of the process that is sustained by the positive feedback postulated by Folkow (1990) and the trophic effects emphasized by Lever and Harrap (1992). This sequence encompasses a variety of specific initiating mechanisms that accentuate and maintain the hypertension by a nonspecific feedback-trophic mechanism. In the past few years, two additional factors have been added to this scheme: the major role played by both autocrine and paracrine factors arising from the endothelial cells (Gibbons, 1993) and the apparent involvement of protooncogenes and growth factors (Itoh et al., 1993). Their roles will be discussed later in this chapter.

If this double process is involved in the pathogenesis of primary hypertension, as seems likely, the difficulty in recognizing the initiating, causal factor is easily explained. In the words of Lever (1986):

The primary cause of hypertension will be most apparent in the early stages; in the later stages, the cause will be concealed by an increasing contribution from hypertrophy. . . . A particular form of hypertension may wrongly be judged to have "no known cause" because each mechanism considered is insufficiently abnormal by itself to have produced the hypertension. The cause of essential hypertension may have been considered already but rejected for this reason.

Cell Membrane Alterations

The next potential mechanism shown in Figure 3.1 relates to alterations in the cell membrane that could influence both tone and hypertrophy. Although Swales (1990a) argues that "if disturbances in cell membrane function reflect the causal abnormality in hypertension, they must be related to structural changes in the resistance vessel," most of the reported disturbances primarily affect tone. Nonetheless, as shown by Swales (1990a) (Fig. 3.24), hypotheses incorporating abnormal ionic fluxes across cell membranes can be linked to both tone (contractility) and hypertrophy (growth).

Ion Transport Across Membranes

Figure 3.25 portrays some of the transport systems present in the cell membrane that control the movement of sodium, potassium, calcium, and other ions in order to maintain the marked differences in concentration of these ions on the outside and inside of cells which, in turn, provide the electrochemical gradients needed for various cell functions.

Abnormalities of the physical properties of the membrane and of multiple transport systems have been implicated in the pathogenesis of hypertension. Most of what follows relates to vascular smooth muscle cells but, since such cells are not available for study in humans, surrogates such as red and white blood cells have been used. There are serious reservations about the pertinence of these in vitro measurements to in vivo changes (Swales, 1991), but at least some

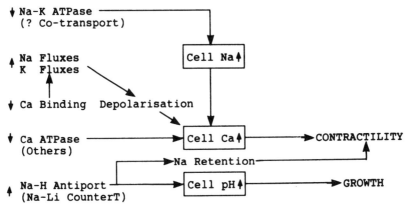

Figure 3.24. Hypotheses linking abnormal ionic fluxes to increased peripheral resistance through increases in cell sodium, calcium, or pH. *CounterT*, countertransport. (From Swales JD. Functional disturbance of the cell membrane in hypertension. *J Hypertens* 1990;8(Suppl 7):S203–S211.)

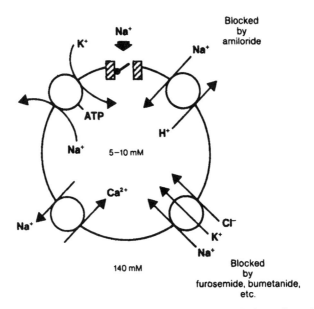

Figure 3.25. Sodium transport systems. Clockwise from the top, these include the sodium channel, Na^+-H^+ antiport exchange, Na-K cotransport, Na^+-Ca^{2+} exchange, and the Na^+-K^+ ATPase pump. (From Lazdunski M. Transmembrane ionic transport system and hypertension. *Am J Med* 1988;84(Suppl 1B):3–9.)

have also been seen in vascular smooth muscle cells of hypertensive rats (Orlov et al., 1992) and humans (Rosskopf et al., 1993). However, the reservations voiced by Swales need to be kept in mind: whereas the intracellular pH of platelets from hypertensives was reported to be more alkaline (Astarie et al., 1992), no such raised pH was found in human resistance arteries (Izzard et al., 1991).

Sodium Transport Abnormalities

Garay (1990) has characterized the abnormalities in sodium transport found in the most widely studied surrogate, red blood cells. He divides them into the following groups.

Stable abnormalities: These precede and are not modified by changes in hypertension and are genetic, found in both hypertensives and in their normotensive offspring (as well as in genetically hypertensive rats). These abnormalities involve two systems—the Na^+-K^+ pump and Na^+, K^+, Cl^- cotransport—that are regulatory, "characterized by a decreased apparent affinity for internal sodium, thus decreasing the ability to rapidly extrude any excess in physiologic cell Na^+ content."

The other three abnormalities—in Na^+, Li^+ countertransport, the sodium channel leak, and in the maximal rate of cotransport—''are characterized by increased maximal rates of cation translocation. They tend to permanently increase cell Na^+ content.''

Compensatory abnormalities: These include increases in the maximal rate of the Na,K pump which compensate for the stable defects, thereby preventing increases in cell Na^+ content.

Acquired abnormalities: This specifically refers to the endogenous natriuretic factor that arises after volume expansion and inhibits the Na,K pump.

With the tremendous amount of research in this area over the past 15 years, it has become obvious that none of these defects is present in all or even the majority of hypertensives, and Swales in particular has questioned their pathogenetic role. He concludes that ''The best unifying hypothesis is that all the reported abnormalities are markers for a disturbance of physicochemical properties of the cell membrane lipids of hypertensive patients'' (Swales, 1990b). He notes that the active transport of sodium is a fundamental property of all cells so that even minor changes in the properties of cell membranes could lead to secondary alterations in Na^+ transport (Swales, 1991).

Intracellular Sodium. The likely wisdom of Swales' view may even apply to the most basic and perhaps most widely accepted abnormality: an increase in intracellular Na^+ content (Table 3.9). This was first shown by Tobian and Binion (1952) in measurements of electrolyte content of renal arteries obtained from hypertensive patients at autopsy. In retrospect, their data also could reflect a small increase in the high Na^+ interstitial fluid (Hilton, 1991), the sodium perhaps bound to the glycosaminoglycans that accumulate in hypertrophied vessels (Simon, 1990).

The majority of studies with red cells that control for confounding factors do *not* show increased sodium content (Simon, 1989). Simon ascribes the in vitro findings to increased membrane permeability to sodium in hypertensives, resulting in more rapid uptake of Na^+ during the preparation of cells for measurement.

Abnormalities in Cell Membrane Permeability

The cell membrane is semipermeable and allows the passive movement of some ions. An increase in the permeability to sodium has been

found to be a generalized characteristic of cell membranes in sodium-dependent forms of hypertension in animals and in man (Furspan and Bohr, 1988). The structure of the cell membrane both in spontaneously hypertensive rats and in patients with primary hypertension is altered (Postnov, 1990), including a reduction in the cholesterol/phospholipid ratio that could be responsible for destabilizing the plasma membrane resulting in an increase in membrane permeability (Ronquist et al., 1992).

The probable involvement of an altered composition of the lipids in the cell membrane in producing the various abnormalities in transport fluxes described in blood cells from hypertensives and their offspring (Table 3.9) is supported by the finding that an elevated level of erythrocyte membrane lipids is accompanied by lower Na^+-Li^+ countertransport, Na^+-K^+ cotransport, and Na^+, K^+-ATPase pump activities (Lijnen et al., 1992). In turn, these same cation transport systems have been correlated with plasma lipid levels (Hajem et al., 1990), offering another possible explanation for the known increased association between dyslipidemias and hypertension (Weder, 1993). Moreover, lovastatin-induced reductions in plasma cholesterol were accompanied by decreases in red blood cell sodium content and Na^+-H^+ exchange (Weder et al., 1991).

Sodium-Lithium Countertransport

Of all the abnormalities of sodium transport with a genetic component listed in Table 3.9, the evidence is most convincing for an increase in the Na^+-Li^+ countertransport system described by Canessa et al. (1980). As reviewed by Rutherford et al. (1992), Na^+-Li^+ countertransport is increased in a portion of patients with several conditions: hypertension, dyslipidemia, pregnancy, and diabetes. Although they recognize the view of some investigators that this may play a direct pathophysiologic role in hypertension, they believe it more reasonable to consider it ''an epiphenomenon resulting from changes in erythrocyte membrane structure and function.'' Regardless, there is evidence obtained by measuring the disposition of oral lithium in red cells for altered Na^+-Li^+ countertransport in vivo in patients with untreated essential hypertension (Brearley et al., 1993).

Sodium-Hydrogen (Proton) Exchange

Increased Na^+-H^+ exchange has been measured in blood cells from both animals and humans with hypertension and found to persist

Table 3.9. Changes in Sodium Calcium Content and Transport in Blood Cells from Hypertensive Patients

Measurement	Defect	Reference
Red blood cells		
Intracellular Na content	Increased	Losse et al., *Klin Wochenschr* 1960;38:393–395
Passive Na influx	Increased	Wessels and Zumkley (1980)
Na efflux (ouabain-resistant)	Increased	Postnov et al., *Pflugers Arch* 1977;371:263–269
Na efflux rate constant	Increased	Fitzgibbon et al. *Clin Sci* 1980;59(Suppl 6):195s–197s
Na efflux (ouabain-sensitive)	Decreased	Walter and Distler, *Hypertension* 1982;4:205–210
Na-K cotransport	Low Na-K flux ratio[a]	Garay and Meyer, *Lancet* 1979;1:349–353
Na-Li countertransport	Increased rate[a]	Canessa et al., *N Engl J Med* 1980;302:722–726
K-Na countertransport	Increased K efflux	Adragna et al., *Clin Sci* 1981;61(Suppl 7):11s–12s
Na-K pump (ouabain-sensitive)	Increased Rb influx[a]	Woods et al., *Br Med J* 1981;282:1186–1188
Na-H exchange	Increased	Canessa et al., *Hypertension* 1991;17:340–348
Calcium binding	Decreased[a]	Postnov et al., *Pflugers Arch* 1977;371:263–269
Calcium pump activity	Decreased	Devynck et al., *Hypertension* 1981;3:397–403
Cell membrane fluidity	Decreased	Orlov et al., *Clin Sci* 1982;63:43–47
White blood cells		
Intracellular Na content	Increased	Edmondson et al. (1975)
Na influx	Increased[a]	Nielsen et al., *Scand J Clin Lab Invest* 1989;49:293–300
Na-K pump (ouabain-sensitive)	Decreased Na$^+$ efflux	Edmondson et al. (1975)
	Increased Na$^+$ efflux	Pedersen et al., *Am J Hypertens* 1990;3:182–187
Membrane permeability	Increased	Forrester and Alleyne, *Br Med J* 1981;283:5–8
Intracellular calcium	Increased	Oshima et al., *Hypertension* 1988;11:703–707
Na-H exchange	Increased	Goldsmith et al. (1991)
Platelets		
Intracellular Na content	Decreased	Tepel et al., *J Hypertens* 1992;10:991–996
Na-H exchange	Increased	Livne et al., *J Hypertens* 1991;9:1013–1019
Intracellular calcium	Increased	Erne et al., *N Engl J Med* 1984;310:1084–1088

[a]Defect also found in normotensive relatives of patients with primary hypertension.

after blood pressure is normalized by antihypertensive therapy (Rosskopf et al., 1993). Such increased exchange, if unopposed, would lead not only to increased intracellular sodium but also to intracellular alkalinization. Such an alkaline intracellular pH has been reported by some (Astarie et al., 1992) but not by others (Goldsmith et al., 1991). If intracellular pH were higher as a result of increased Na$^+$-H$^+$ exchange, this could serve as a stimulus for cell growth, as will be described under Mechanisms for Cell Proliferation.

Acquired Inhibition of the Sodium Pump

In addition to the putative abnormalities in the "stable" or genetic transport systems in Garay's classifications, there is increasingly strong evidence for an acquired inhibition of the sodium pump in many, if not most, forms of hypertension.

The extrusion of sodium within cells is the primary task of the membrane-bound, magnesium-dependent enzyme Na^+,K^+-ATPase, the Na^+ pump. This enzyme catalyzes the breakdown of adenosine triphosphate (ATP) to provide the energy for ionic movements. The activity of the pump is stimulated by an increase of sodium on the inside or of potassium on the outside of the cell membrane and is inhibited by cardiac glycosides such as ouabain. The difference between sodium movement before and after ouabain is taken as the level of pump activity.

Defects in Hypertension. A *decrease* in the activity of the sodium pump, measured as the rate of ouabain-sensitive sodium efflux, has been found in the leukocytes of patients with essential hypertension (Edmundson et al., 1975) and in some of their first-degree relatives (Heagerty et al., 1982). The inhibition of pump activity was later ascribed to an agent circulating in the plasma of hypertensive subjects, since normal cells could be inhibited by incubation in hypertensive subjects' plasma, whereas incubation in the plasma of a normotensive subject had no such effect (Gray et al., 1986).

An Acquired Pump Inhibitor. With volume expansion, partial inhibition of the sodium pump had been seen in experimental animals and attributed to the production of a circulating pump inhibitor (Haddy, 1990). Blaustein (1977) postulated that such a circulating pump inhibitor could induce hypertension by inhibiting the sodium-calcium exchange in vascular tissue. Subsequently de Wardener and MacGregor (1980, 1982) put together the hypothesis that the pump inhibitor was the same as the hypertensinogenic substance postulated by Dahl et al. (1967) to be responsible for the hypertension in their sodium-sensitive rats. The hypothesis (Fig. 3.26) was summarized as follows:

Essential hypertension in man is due to an inherited variability in the ability of the kidney to eliminate sodium. This variability becomes increasingly obvious the greater the sodium intake. The difficulty in eliminating sodium increases the concentration of a circulating sodium transport inhibitor. This substance affects sodium transport across cell membranes. In the kidney, it adjusts urinary sodium excretion so that sodium balance is near that of normal subjects on the same intake of sodium, thus making it difficult to demonstrate an increase in extracellular fluid volume. In the arteriole, it causes a rise in intracellular sodium concentration, which in turn raises the intracellular calcium concentration and thus increases vascular reactivity (de Wardener and MacGregor, 1980).

Nature of the Natriuretic Hormone. The search for a natriuretic substance that appears in plasma after volume expansion, chemically and functionally distinct from the atrial natriuretic peptide, has gone on for over 30 years. Despite experimental evidence for its origin in the hypothalamus (Anner et al., 1990), investigators at the University of Maryland and Upjohn have provided strong evidence that the inhibitor is ouabain (Hamlyn et al., 1991) and that the adrenal cortex may be a major site for its synthesis (Ludens et al., 1992). The evidence for its presence and involvement in volume-expanded forms of hypertension continues to mount (Hamlyn and Manunta, 1992), including the recognition of a patient with an adrenocortical tumor associated with hypertension and elevated plasma ouabain levels, both of which receded after surgical removal (Manunta et al., 1992b).

Abnormal Calcium Handling

In addition to these various possible abnormalities in sodium transport, the red blood cells of both genetically hypertensive rats (Devynck et al., 1982) and patients with essential hypertension (Postnov, 1990) do not bind calcium as avidly nor pump calcium out of cells normally. Since increased concentrations of free calcium found within the cytosol of vascular smooth muscle cells are held responsible for the increased contractility of vessels in hypertension, such defects in calcium binding or extrusion could be central to the development of hypertension (Fig. 3.27).

Decreased Binding. Lesser binding of calcium to the cell membrane has been shown to destabilize the membrane, leading to a more rapid influx of calcium and vascular smooth muscle contraction (Dominiczak and Bohr, 1990).

Decreased Extrusion. Defects have been noted in the two mechanisms involved in removing calcium, the Ca^{2+} pump and Na^+-Ca^{2+} exchange, in addition to the dynamic processes of release and sequestration of free calcium between cytosol and endoplasmic reticulum and mitochondria (Adeoya et al., 1988). Blaustein

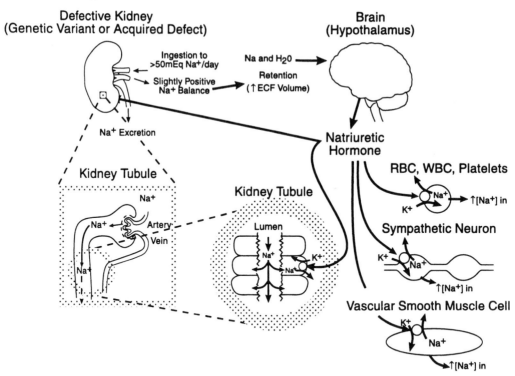

Figure 3.26. Diagram of how an inherited defect in renal sodium excretion may lead to inhibition of sodium transport in erythrocytes (*RBC*), leukocytes (*WBC*), sympathetic neurons, and vascular smooth muscle. These effects appear to be mediated by a circulating natriuretic hormone (*NH*). *ECF*, extracellular fluid. (From Blaustein MP, Hamlyn JM. Role of a natriuretic factor in essential hypertension: an hypothesis. *Ann Intern Med* 1983;98(Part 2):785–792.)

(1988) has shown the importance of Na^+-Ca^{2+} exchange for extrusion of calcium after contractile activation, and his observation has been amply confirmed (Rembold et al., 1992). Blaustein has provided evidence that as little as a 5% increase in intracellular sodium via inhibition of the sodium pump would inhibit Na^+-Ca^{2+} exchange enough to raise intracellular calcium so that the resting tone of vascular smooth muscle would increase by as much as 50%.

A Unifying Hypothesis

By incorporating various abnormalities in sodium and calcium handling described in the previous sections, a unifying hypothesis can be constructed, linking many of the components shown in Figure 3.1. As seen in the bottom portion of Figure 3.28, hypertension could be induced by the direct mediation of increased intracellular calcium by either a primary membrane defect or secondary to increased intracellular sodium arising from a membrane defect. On the other hand, a stronger argument can be fashioned for the top portion of Figure 3.28, despite its increased complexity. The evidence

that a natriuretic hormone arises in the presence of increased vascular volume seems persuasive and the evidence for involvement of the factors shown on the right—high sodium intake, stress, sympathetic nervous, and renin-angiotensin—has been described in the earlier sections of this chapter.

We will now consider additional mechanisms that could induce vascular hypertrophy, some in more direct ways than those previously covered.

VASCULAR HYPERTROPHY

As seen in the top portion of Figure 3.23, vascular hypertrophy may arise secondary to repeated rises in pressure from various pressor agents, with signals from the endothelial cells almost certainly involved in the translation of increased pressure into smooth muscle cell hypertrophy.

On the other hand, as shown on the bottom of Figure 3.23, a number of trophic mechanisms have been recognized that may induce vascular hypertrophy either in concert with an initial pressor stimulus or in a manner independent of a rise in pressure (Lever and Harrap, 1992). Some

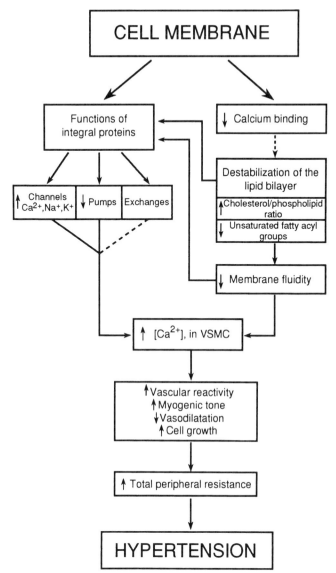

Figure 3.27. Relationship between cell membrane abnormalities and increased total peripheral resistance in hypertension. *Broken lines* indicate mechanisms which are not yet clearly defined. *VSMC*, vascular smooth muscle cells. (From Dominiczak AF, Bohr DF. Cell membrane abnormalities and the regulation of intracellular calcium concentration in hypertension. *Clin Sci* 1990;79:415–423.)

of these are shown in Figure 3.29, and they may be interrelated (Dzau et al., 1993a). Angiotensin II increases protein synthesis in an in vitro preparation of aortic cells by 80% in 24 hours (Berk et al., 1989) and induces protooncogene and growth factor genes within 30 minutes (Naftilan et al., 1989). Experimental evidence exists for involvement of a host of growth factors for smooth muscle cells (Itoh et al., 1993), with at least seven expressed in the aorta of hypertensive rats, including platelet-derived growth factor

(PDGF), insulin-like growth factor (IGF), and transforming growth factor-β (TGF-β) (Sarzani et al., 1989).

Mechanisms of Cellular Proliferation

As seen in Figure 3.30, when a growth factor occupies its membrane receptor, it activates membrane phosphodiesterase which hydrolyzes the phosphatidylinositol biphosphate (*PIP*) that comprises 5 to 15% of the total membrane phospholipid content (Berridge, 1993; Ohanian and

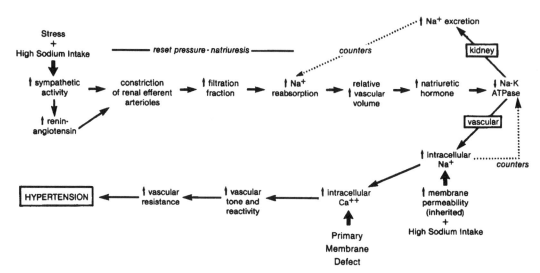

Figure 3.28. Hypothesis for the pathogenesis of primary (essential) hypertension, starting from one of three points, shown as *heavy arrows*. The first, starting on the *top left*, is the combination of stress and high sodium intake, which induces an increase in natriuretic hormone and thereby inhibits sodium transport. The second, at the *bottom right*, invokes an inherited defect in sodium transport to induce an increase in intracellular sodium. The third, at the *bottom middle*, suggests a primary membrane defect that directly leads to increased free intracellular calcium. (From Kaplan NM. Systemic hypertension: mechanisms and diagnosis. In: Braunwald E, ed. *Heart Disease*. Philadelphia: WB Saunders, 1988:817–851.)

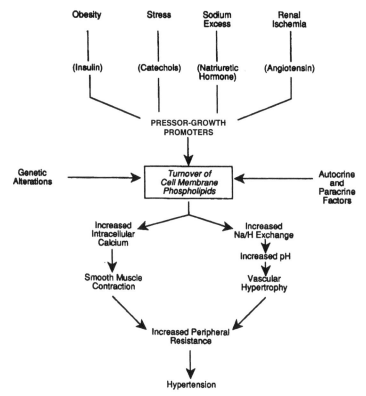

Figure 3.29. Scheme for the induction of hypertension by numerous pressor hormones that act as vascular growth promoters.

Heagerty, 1992). This hydrolysis produces two compounds: the water-soluble inositol triphosphate (IP_3) which is released into the cytosol, and the hydrophobic 1,2-diacylglycerol (DG) which is retained in the membrane. These two compounds have two major, separate functions: IP_3 releases calcium from nonmitochondrial organelles, which, in smooth muscle cells, triggers contraction; DG has a second-messenger role in the cell membrane, activating protein kinase C, which controls the activity of the amiloride-sensitive Na^+-H^+ exchanger. As more sodium enters and hydrogen exits, the cell becomes more alkaline; the increased alkalinity is the cell signal to provoke the nucleus to initiate protein synthesis and division.

The intricacies of this mechanism may be much beyond those schematically shown in Figure 3.30 (Touyz and Schiffrin, 1993). Nonetheless, it is clear that various pressor-trophic factors, including AII both in vitro (Lyall et al., 1992) and in vivo (Simon and Altman, 1992), induce this dual effect. These effects are separable: "The constrictor stimulus is short-term and sufficient to initiate contraction but not proliferation. Cellular growth only occurs when the tissue is stimulated excessively for a long time" (Heagerty et al., 1988).

This process has great explanatory power, as noted by Heagerty et al. (1988): "In a disease such as hypertension where abnormal medial thickening is observed, the process of activation of (the phosphoinositide) system such as by autonomic excess, and the possibility of a genetically inherited abnormal smooth muscle cell reinforcing the stimulus by proliferating more avidly, might hold the key....It is conceivable that an overactive phosphoinositide system could underlie the structural changes in hypertension."

Beyond the effects of pressor-trophic factors, the elevated pressure per se may lead to further structural change. Turbulent flow over cultured vascular smooth muscle cells provoked changes in membrane ion transport that were associated with cell hyperplasia (Rosati and Garay, 1991). The effect of pressure was shown in vivo by inducing coarctation of the aorta in normotensive rats (Ollerenshaw et al., 1988). With the elevated pressures above the coarctation, inositol phosphate accumulated in the aorta and its medial cross-sectional area and thickness increased. Despite the common hormonal milieu, the vessels below the coarctation did not hypertrophy, presumably because their hypertrophic machinery was not turned on by exposure to a higher pressure. Of great significance, the increase in phosphoinositide hydrolysis proximal to the coarctation preceded any significant rise in blood pressure. Thus, hypertrophy appears to have been triggered very early by the stretch induced by the initial load placed upon the aorta and not as a later consequence of high pressure.

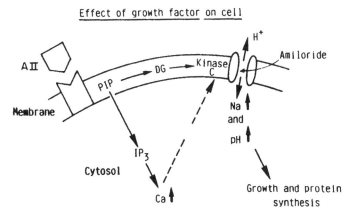

Figure 3.30. Schematic representation of the main events in a signaling system activated by growth factors. For example, angiotensin II occupies a membrane receptor; phosphatidylinositol biphosphate (*PIP*) is hydrolyzed by phosphodiesterase in the membrane; inositol triphosphate (*IP₃*) is released into the cytosol and diacylglycerol (*DG*) in the plane of the membrane. The latter activates protein kinase C linked to an amiloride-sensitive Na^+-H^+ exchanger whose activity increases. Sodium enters the cell down an electrochemical gradient and protons are extruded. The increased intracellular pH that results promotes growth and protein synthesis. (From Lever AF. Slow pressor mechanisms in hypertension: a role for hypertrophy of resistance vessels? *J Hypertens* 1986;4:515–524.)

Microvascular Rarefaction

Along with the changes in larger vessel caliber and thickness, the increased resistance and subsequent elevation of pressure in hypertension may also reflect a permanent closure of capillaries and arterioles, i.e., structural rarefaction of microvessels. Such has been seen in animal models (le Noble et al., 1990) and muscle biopsies from hypertensive patients (Henrich et al., 1988).

ENDOTHELIUM-DERIVED FACTORS

These effects on smooth muscle cell growth and remodeling may be mediated through endothelium-derived factors. Over the last few years, it has become obvious that endothelial cells, rather than serving as a passive covering for the conduit of blood, are constantly producing mediators which communicate with underlying smooth muscle cells. These mediators are produced in response to shear forces, intravascular pressure, circulating hormones, and platelet factors (Lüscher et al., 1993a). The products arising from within the endothelial cells may influence both contraction-relaxation and cell growth (Flavahan, 1992) (Fig. 3.31).

Alterations in the production of these mediators are involved in the induction and persistence of hypertension in both experimental models (Bell, 1993) and humans (Panza et al., 1990, 1993a, 1993b, 1993c). As will be noted, the effects of hypercholesterolemia and the development of atherosclerosis also may relate to these factors.

Endothelium-derived Relaxing Factor

In 1980, Furchgott and Zawadzki reported that an intact endothelium was required for acetylcholine-induced vasodilation, a process that normally "stimulates release of a substance(s) that causes relaxation of the vascular smooth muscle." Seven years later, Palmer et al. (1987) and Ignarro and co-workers (1987) identified the endothelium-derived relaxing factor (EDRF) as the gas nitric oxide (NO). Since then, the biochemistry of NO has been defined and a host of biologic responses attributed to its release (J.S. Stamler et al., 1992). Not the least of these responses is vasodilation, which is intimately involved in the regulation of the blood pressure (Rees et al., 1989) and renal function (Romero and Strick, 1993).

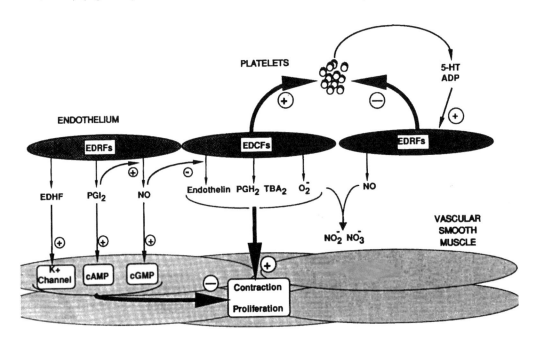

Figure 3.31. Schematic diagram of proposed interactions between endothelial mediators. *PGI$_2$*, prostacyclin; *NO*, nitric oxide; *EDHF*, endothelium-derived hyperpolarizing factor; *PGH$_2$*, prostaglandin H$_2$; *TXA$_2$*, thromboxane A$_2$; *O^{2-}*, superoxide anion; *5-HT*, serotonin; *ADP*, adenosine diphosphate; *EDRFs*, endothelium-derived relaxing factors; *EDCFs*, endothelium-derived contracting factors. (From Flavahan NA. Atherosclerosis or lipoprotein-induced endothelial dysfunction. Potential mechanisms underlying reduction in EDRF/nitric oxide activity. *Circulation* 1992;85:1927–1938.)

Abnormality in Hypertension

Hypertensive patients have a reduced vasodilatory response to various stimuli of endothelium-dependent vascular relaxation (Panza et al., 1993b) that is not restored by effective antihypertensive therapy (Panza et al., 1993c) or by provision of additional substrate for the synthesis of NO (Panza et al., 1993a), suggesting that the NO system is somehow fundamentally altered in primary hypertension. Inhibition of NO synthesis with the inhibitor of nitric oxide synthase, nitro-L-arginine, causes hypertension in animals (Dananberg et al., 1993), a process which may involve elimination of NO-induced neural processes rather than just impairment of release of NO from endothelium (Toda et al., 1993). Local infusions of such NO synthase inhibitors invoke less vasoconstriction in hypertensive patients (Calver et al., 1992). Moreover, hypertensive patients with left ventricular hypertrophy have markedly impaired endothelium-dependent vasodilation of coronary resistance vessels which "may contribute to disordered coronary flow regulation and the ischemic manifestations of hypertensive heart disease" (Treasure et al., 1993).

While NO-donors (nitroprusside, isosorbide) are being widely used in the treatment of hypertension and coronary artery disease, the recognition of the molecular basis for NO synthesis (Nishida et al., 1992) provides even more exciting potential for the prevention and treatment of hypertension and vascular diseases (Corbett et al., 1992).

Relations to Hypercholesterolemia

Hypercholesterolemia, in addition to promoting atherosclerosis, may aggravate hypertension by impairing vasodilation as seen in coronary arteries (Cohen et al., 1988) and forearm resistance vessels (Creager et al., 1990). The effect likely is mediated by inactivation of NO by the lysolecithin component (Mangin et al., 1993) of oxidized lipoprotein (Chin et al., 1992) and can be corrected by L-arginine-induced stimulation of NO production (Drexler et al., 1991).

Other Vasodilatory Substances

In the excitement over NO, the role of other putative relaxing factors shown in Figure 3.31 is seldom mentioned. Prostacyclin (de Nucci et al., 1988) and endothelium-derived hyperpolarizing factor (Flavahan, 1992) may also be involved.

Endothelins

The middle of Figure 3.31 portrays a number of endothelium-derived contracting factors. Of these, endothelin has been increasingly emphasized since its discovery in 1988 (Yanagisawa et al., 1988). Now known to be composed of three distinct peptides, the endothelins have been shown to have a wide range of biologic actions (Simonson and Dunn, 1991) that may involve them in numerous pathologic conditions (Haynes and Webb, 1993).

The role of endothelins in human hypertension remains uncertain (Vanhoutte, 1993). Circulating levels have been reported to be normal or high, the higher values possibly caused by the contribution of vascular damage, heart failure, or renal insufficiency (Lüscher et al., 1993b). There is no doubt that endothelin can raise blood pressure, as demonstrated in a patient with an endothelin-secreting tumor (Yokokawa et al., 1991). The role of endothelin may turn out to be primarily as a promotor of vascular hypertrophy (Chua et al., 1992).

Other Constricting Factors

Prostaglandin H_2 (Ito et al., 1991), superoxide anion (Katusic and Vanhoutte, 1989), and PDGF-B (Kourembanas et al., 1990) are among other possibly important constricting factors.

INSULIN RESISTANCE AND HYPERINSULINEMIA IN HYPERTENSION WITH OR WITHOUT OBESITY

We will now consider the last of the possible pressor-growth promoters shown in Figure 3.29: hyperinsulinemia. This will be examined in the broader context of the associations among hypertension, obesity, diabetes, and dyslipidemias: the insulin resistance syndrome (Kaplan, 1989).

Insulin resistance and consequent hyperinsulinemia are present in as many as half of nonobese patients with primary hypertension and in virtually all patients with two conditions that are commonly accompanied by hypertension: obesity and adult-onset, non-insulin-dependent diabetes mellitus. Over the past few years, an "insulin hypothesis" has evolved, attributing the development of hypertension to the effects of hyperinsulinemia (DeFronzo and Ferrannini, 1991; Reaven, 1991). More recently, counter views have been expressed, some proposing a reverse sequence in which the development of hypertension leads to insulin resistance and hyperinsulinemia (Anderson and Mark, 1993a); others doubting any causal connection (Jarrett, 1992). The associations between hypertension and insulin resistance are well established, but as of now, their meaning is uncertain.

Observations on the Association with Hypertension

Hyperinsulinemia was first reported in nonobese hypertensive patients by Welborn et al. in 1966, reconfirmed by Berglund et al. in 1976 and Singer et al. in 1985, but not widely appreciated until 1987 when Ferrannini et al. reported a 40% decrease in insulin sensitivity in nonobese hypertensives with the more precise and specific euglycemic insulin-clamp technique. Their study documented that the insulin resistance of primary (essential) hypertension involved the peripheral utilization of glucose but not the renal, lipid, or potassium effects of insulin. Reaven and co-workers (Fuh et al., 1987; Shen et al., 1988) simultaneously reported insulin resistance in hypertensives, whether treated or not.

Positive Observations

Since then, a large number of reports have documented hyperinsulinemia in hypertensives, both fasting (Denker and Pollock, 1992) and post-glucose load (Zavaroni et al., 1992). With more sophisticated measures, resistance to peripheral insulin-mediated glucose utilization has been repeatedly found in about half of nonobese hypertensives (Pollare et al., 1990; Rooney et al., 1992). In addition, a decreased clearance of insulin may contribute to the hyperinsulinemia (Salvatore et al., 1992). The data in humans are supported by just as impressive data in rat models of induced hypertension (Reaven, 1991). On the other hand, hypertension per se has been shown not to lead to insulin resistance, both in humans with various forms of secondary hypertension (Sechi et al., 1992; Shamiss et al., 1992) and in rats with genetic forms of hypertension (Frontoni et al., 1992).

Prospective Data.   The most impressive data supporting a causal role for hyperinsulinemia in the pathogenesis of hypertension come not from various cross-sectional studies but from prospective follow-up observations. Among 50-year-old women in Gothenburg followed for 12 years (Lissner et al., 1992) and in 1440 Caucasian and Mexican-American subjects in San Antonio followed for 8 years (Haffner et al., 1992), the presence of high fasting insulin levels

was predictive of the development of hypertension. The relative risk for hypertension for those with plasma insulin levels in the upper 25th percentile was threefold greater in the Swedish study and twofold greater for those in the upper third in the Texas study. Although other abnormalities in body weight and lipids were also more common in those with higher baseline insulin levels, the association of hyperinsulinemia with hypertension remained significant when these possibly confounding features were excluded by multivariate analyses.

These findings are supported by the presence of insulin resistance in younger normotensive offspring of hypertensive parents (Allemann et al., 1993; Ohno et al., 1993) and by the positive cross-sectional relation between plasma insulin levels and blood pressure in children (Florey et al., 1976; Jiang et al., 1993; Srivinasan et al., 1993).

Negative Observations

Despite these impressive positive data, a number of observations do not support a role for insulin resistance in the induction of hypertension. Some ethnic groups apparently do not display the association between hyperinsulinemia/insulin resistance and hypertension repeatedly found in Caucasian subjects, the populations in most of the studies referred to above. Although marked insulin resistance has been found in Pima Indians (Saad et al., 1991) and Mexican-Americans (Ferrannini et al., 1991), they do not have an increased prevalence of hypertension. No differences in plasma insulin levels were found between normotensive and hypertensive Micronesian, Polynesian, and Melanesian Pacific Islanders (Dowse et al., 1993) or blacks on the island of Seychelles (Tappy et al., 1991).

On the other hand, a positive association between insulin and blood pressure has been found among Chinese men and women living in Hong Kong (Woo et al., 1992) and young black men in Philadelphia (Falkner et al., 1990).

The fact that certain ethnic groups may not have the association most likely means that genetic mechanisms and possibly environmental factors must also play a role and that they may override the influence of insulin (Reaven, 1993). Taken together, the data support an important role for insulin resistance and hyperinsulinemia, but it is a role that is influenced strongly by environmental factors, e.g., the presence of obesity, and genetics. Not all who are insulin-resistant are hypertensive, and not all (nonobese) hypertensives are insulin resistant. However, the two go together more than by chance, and there are known mechanisms for their interaction.

Mechanisms for Insulin Resistance

Insulin Resistance with Obesity

Virtually every obese person is insulin resistant, possibly secondary to decreased numbers and impaired functions of insulin receptors (Caro, 1991). Such receptor defects are manifested by decreased insulin-mediated uptake of glucose into skeletal muscle, but the insulin resistance of obesity also reflects a defect in insulin's usual hemodynamic action to increase blood flow through the muscle bed (Laakso et al., 1990). The degree of insulin resistance that accompanies obesity (or type II diabetes) is not increased further by the presence of hypertension, suggesting that the resistance in all three conditions involves the same mechanisms and is maximally induced by obesity (or diabetes) (Bonora et al., 1993).

Beyond the resistance to insulin found with obesity of any form, there is even greater insulin resistance in those whose obesity is predominantly located in the upper body or abdomen (Peiris et al., 1992). This ''android'' pattern of obesity is associated with decreased hepatic extraction of insulin, thereby adding further to the delivery of more insulin to the systemic circulation (Fig. 3.32).

Insulin Resistance in Hypertension without Obesity

As shown in Figure 3.32, the manner by which obesity, particularly when predominantly abdominal, evokes hyperinsulinemia seems easy to explain. The explanation for the insulin resistance found in about half of nonobese hypertensives, however, is not obvious and may involve one or more aspects of insulin's action (Table 3.10). Support exists for virtually each aspect:

—Delivery may be reduced by diminished blood flow as seen acutely with sympathetic activation (Jamerson et al., 1993) or chronically from capillary rarefaction. Moreover, the usual insulin-mediated vasodilatory action that normally increases muscle blood flow is attenuated in patients with hypertension (Baron et al., 1993).

—Transport, shown to be rate limiting for insulin action (Yang et al., 1989), may be reduced.

—The action of insulin within skeletal muscle may be impaired for multiple reasons. Of these, an inherited or acquired predominance of type 2B (white) muscle fibers which are more resistant to the effects of insulin than are type 1 and 2A (red) fibers (James et al., 1985) has been demonstrated (Juhlin-Dannfelt et al., 1979) and shown to be associated with in vivo insulin resistance (Lillioja et al., 1987).

The phospholipids in skeletal muscle of insulin-resistant patients have decreased concentrations of polyunsaturated fatty acids which may modulate the action of insulin (Borkman et al., 1993). Obviously, the number of possible causes for insulin resistance in hypertension is large and expanding; which are responsible remains to be established.

Effects of Hyperinsulinemia on Blood Pressure

Figure 3.32 portrays three ways by which hyperinsulinemia could induce hypertension. Even more have been proposed and have experimental

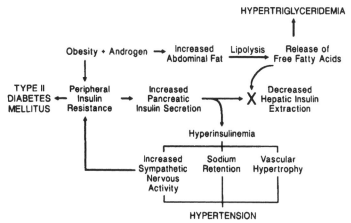

Figure 3.32. Overall scheme for the mechanism by which upper body obesity could promote glucose intolerance, hypertriglyceridemia, and hypertension via hyperinsulinemia.

Table 3.10. Factors That May Induce Insulin Resistance in Hypertension

Aspect	Normal Site of Action	Effect of Hypertension
Insulin delivery	Capillary bed	Vasoconstriction Attenuated vasodilation Capillary rarefaction
Insulin transport	Interstitium	Impaired transport
Insulin action	Muscle fiber	Genetic/acquired increase in type 2B fibers Hormonal interference with insulin effects Decreased glucose transporter protein

support (Donnelly and Connell, 1992) (Table 3.11).

Of these, impaired vasodilation may be particularly important. Insulin acutely acts as a vasodilator, both in experimental models (Hall et al., 1992) and in humans (Anderson and Mark, 1993a, 1993b). The latter investigators have shown that although insulin increases sympathetic noradrenergic activity to skeletal muscle, the effect is normally overridden by the direct vasodilatory effect of insulin (Fig. 3.33, *left*). However, patients with hypertension have a defect in this vasodilatory action, failing to increase muscle blood flow in response to insulin infusions (Baron et al., 1993). In combination with high levels of sympathetic nervous activation such as described earlier in this chapter, the effects of attenuated vasodilation could enable insulin to raise the blood pressure in patients who are obese or hypertensive (Fig. 3.33, *right*).

Thus, there are differences between relatively short-term effects of insulin in normal people and the long-term effects of hyperinsulinemia in patients who are genetically predisposed to express prohypertensive effects. Such differences may also explain the absence of hypertension in patients with rather chronic hyperinsulinemia from insulinomas (O'Brien et al., 1993) or with the polycystic ovary syndrome (Zimmermann et al., 1992).

Additional evidence in favor of a hypertension-inducing effect of hyperinsulinemia is the lowering of blood pressure by the use of agents that increase insulin sensitivity and lower insulin levels, accomplished in humans with the biguanide metformin (Landin et al., 1991), and in animals with glitazones (Pershadsingh et al., 1993). Uncertainty remains over the effect of exogenous insulin in diabetic patients.

In total, the evidence for a pressor effect of hyperinsulinemia seems impressive. Nonetheless, Anderson and Mark (1993a) conclude that ''Despite the recent surge of interest, it is not yet clear whether insulin resistance and hyperinsulinemia promote hypertension or whether these are secondary to abnormal skeletal muscle

Table 3.11. Proposed Mechanisms by Which Insulin Resistance and/or Hyperinsulinemia May Lead to Increased Blood Pressure

1. Enhanced renal sodium and water reabsorption (Gupta et al., 1992)
2. Increased blood pressure sensitivity to dietary salt intake, i.e., salt sensitivity (Sharma et al., 1993)
3. Augmentation of the pressor and aldosterone responses to angiotensin II (Rocchini et al., 1990)
4. Changes in transmembrane electrolyte transport
   Increased intracellular sodium (Barbagallo et al., 1993)
   Decreased Na^+, K^+-ATPase activity (Pontremoli et al., 1991)
   Increased Na^+-H^+ pump activity (Aviv, 1992)
5. Increased intracellular Ca^{2+} accumulation (Aviv, 1992)
6. Stimulation of growth factors, especially in vascular smooth muscle (Bornfeldt et al., 1992)
7. Stimulation of sympathetic nervous activity (Lembo et al., 1992)
8. Reduced synthesis of vasodilatory prostaglandins (Axelrod, 1991)
9. Impaired vasodilation (Baron et al., 1993)
10. Increased secretion of endothelin (Hu et al., 1993)

Modified from Donnelly R, Connell JMC. Insulin resistance: possible role in the aetiology and clinical course of hypertension. *Clin Sci* 1992;83:265–275.

sympathetic and vascular mechanisms in obesity and hypertension.''

Consequences of Insulin Resistance

In addition to hypertension, insulin resistance and consequent hyperinsulinemia are often accompanied by dyslipidemia and glucose intolerance that may lead into type II diabetes. This constellation in nonobese subjects was termed ''syndrome X'' by Reaven (1988) but is best referred to as the ''insulin resistance syndrome,'' particularly since cardiologists have priority for the use of ''syndrome X'' as angina without obvious coronary atherosclerosis.

Obesity, diabetes, and dyslipidemia are each associated with an increased prevalence of hypertension (see Chapter 4). These associations may involve mechanisms in addition to or distinct from insulin resistance, but insulin resistance is common and potentially hazardous, interacting with genetic endowments to contribute to many of the causes for premature cardiovascular diseases that are rampant in industrialized societies (McKeigue et al., 1993). For over 20 years, Stout (1990) has warned of the role of insulin in the pathogenesis of atherosclerosis.

Since hyperinsulinemia precedes the development of overt disease (Haffner et al., 1992), the need for prevention of insulin resistance through diet and exercise is obvious.

OTHER POSSIBLE MECHANISMS

The preceding exposition of the multiple factors shown in Figure 3.1 does not, unfortunately, exhaust the possible mechanisms for primary hypertension. The evidence for those that follow is less impressive or they seem to affect only a portion of the larger hypertensive population.

Natriuretic Peptide Family

The discovery by deBold et al. (1981) of a rapid natriuretic effect of injection of atrial extract led to a tremendous amount of research to define the physiologic role and pathologic place of what was first considered only an atrial natriuretic peptide, but what has now become a family of natriuretic peptides (Nakao et al., 1993). The family includes three additional peptides that share both structure and function with the atrial peptide—brain (Richards et al., 1993), C-type (Koller and Goeddel, 1992), and urodilatin, which has been found only in the urine

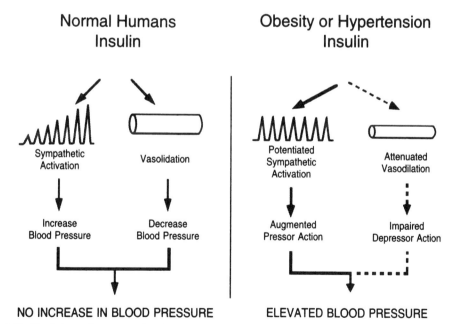

Figure 3.33. The *left panel* represents insulin's actions in normal humans. Although insulin causes marked increases in sympathetic neural outflow which would be expected to increase blood pressure, it also causes vasodilation which would decrease blood pressure. The net effect of these two opposing influences is no change or a slight decrease in blood pressure. There may be an imbalance between the sympathetic and vascular actions of insulin in conditions such as obesity or hypertension. As shown in the *right panel*, insulin may cause potentiated sympathetic activation or attenuated vasodilation. An imbalance between these pressor and depressor actions of insulin may result in elevated blood pressure. (From Anderson EA, Mark AL. Cardiovascular and sympathetic actions of insulin: the insulin hypothesis of hypertension revisited. *Cardiovasc Risk Factors* 1993b;3:159–163.)

(Valentin and Humphreys, 1993). These peptides are entirely unlike the ouabain-like natriuretic factor described earlier.

The natriuretic peptides respond to an increase in intravascular volume, acting primarily upon the kidney to increase sodium excretion, on the vasculature to induce vasodilation, and on the adrenal glands to reduce aldosterone secretion, effects that counter the major effects of the renin-aldosterone mechanism. However, there is no convincing evidence for a role of the natriuretic family in the pathogenesis of hypertension (Tan et al., 1993). Blood levels may be slightly elevated, but to a lesser degree than expected for the expanded intravascular volume described earlier in this chapter (Hollister and Inagami, 1991).

Prostaglandins

Various prostaglandins (PGs) have different sites of origin and different effects on the blood pressure. Platelet-derived thromboxanes promote platelet aggregation, constrict vascular smooth muscle, and may inhibit sodium excretion. Prostacyclin, synthesized within the blood vessel wall, inhibits platelet aggregation, relaxes vascular smooth muscle, and by reducing renal vascular resistance promotes natriuresis. PGE_2 is vasodilatory, and $PGF_{2\alpha}$ is vasoconstrictive. Products of the lipoxygenase pathway of arachidonic acid metabolism may mediate the intracellular actions of pressor hormones by regulation of intracellular calcium movements (Saito et al., 1992).

Prostaglandins and Primary Hypertension

Despite numerous findings suggesting a role for PGs in primary hypertension, the general impression is that PGs probably are not major players in primary hypertension although clearly they are important in circulatory control and thrombosis (Oates et al., 1988). Nonetheless, reduced excretion of prostacyclin metabolites has been found in mild primary hypertension, with impressively negative correlations with the level of elevated pressure (Minuz et al., 1990). As will be noted in Chapter 11, there is stronger evidence for a role for PGs in the pathogenesis of preeclampsia.

Renal Prostaglandins. The kidney synthesizes several different PGs; which of these is physiologically important remains in question since considerable interconversion occurs between them, and most assays, until recently, have been nonspecific. Intrarenal PGs modify the renal response to various vasoconstrictor stimuli, including angiotensin and norepinephrine (Inscho et al., 1990). Thus the major function of intrarenal prostaglandins is to sustain the renal circulation in the face of any situation wherein it is threatened. The inhibition of renal prostaglandins may be responsible for the slight rise in blood pressure and the more impressive inhibition of the action of various antihypertensive agents with the use of nonsteroidal antiinflammatory drugs (Pope et al., 1993).

Medullipin: The Renomedullary Vasodepressor Lipid

After 40 years of persistent work, Muirhead (1991) and coworkers have documented both the existence and the role of a substance secreted from renal medullary cells that appears to function as a counterbalance to the effects of angiotensin II. The renomedullary hormone, called medullipin I, requires activation by the cytochrome P-450-dependent enzyme system of the liver into medullipin II.

The structure of this hormone remains unknown but its existence has been strongly inferred from multiple experiments in animals, wherein a rise in renal perfusion causes arterial pressure to fall. This hypotensive response is dependent upon an intact renal medulla and is not altered by renal denervation or inhibition of renin-angiotensin or autonomic nervous function (Christy et al., 1991). The actions of the renomedullary lipid are not inhibited by blockade of both prostaglandins and kinins, pointing further to its separate status (Muirhead et al., 1992a). Whether it functions under normal circumstances and is involved in various human hypertensive diseases remains to be seen. A patient with persistent hypotension associated with elevated medullipin levels has been described (Muirhead et al., 1992b).

Kallikrein-Kinin System

Kallikrein acts upon the kininogen substrate to release bradykinins (Fig. 3.34). These kinins may be involved in the control of blood flow, electrolyte excretion, and blood pressure (Fitzgibbon et al., 1993). Although much is known about the genetic regulation of kallikrein and kininogen synthesis, very little is known about the functions of the vasoactive product bradykinin. In vitro, bradykinin constricts vascular smooth muscle cells but, at the same time, stimulates the release of vasodilators, likely EDRF (Briner et al., 1993). The availability of specific

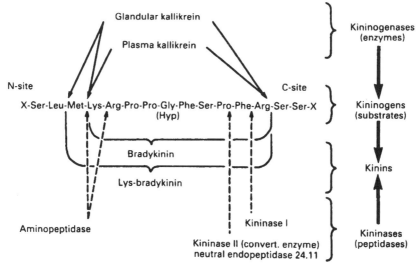

Figure 3.34. Site of kininogen cleavage (*solid arrows*) by the main kininogenases (glandular and plasma kallikrein). Site of kinin cleavage (*broken arrows*) by kininases (kininase I and II, neutral peptidase, and aminopeptidase). (From Carretero OA, Scicli AG. Kinins: paracrine hormone. *Kidney Int* 1988;34(Suppl 26):S-52–S-59.)

bradykinin antagonists is providing a new tool to explore the functions of the system (Plante et al., 1992).

Vasopressin

The antidiuretic hormone vasopressin probably is not involved in the pathogenesis of hypertension, although subtle increases in its secretion may be present (Henneberry et al., 1992).

Other Vasoactive Factors

Beyond those referred to earlier in this chapter, a host of vasoactive peptides and growth factors may be involved in the pathogenesis of hypertension, including platelet-derived, insulin-like, and fibroblast growth factors (Scott-Burden et al., 1992). The evidence for their involvement is unimpressive, as it is for a possible lack of the potent vasodilator calcitonin gene-related peptide (Portaluppi et al., 1992).

Abnormal Steroid Metabolism

Through the years, claims have been made for a number of abnormal patterns of adrenocortical response to stimulation and types of hormones secreted. In reviewing these claims, Connell and Fraser (1991) conclude: ''Many of the studies in which abnormalities have been reported were small and few findings have been confirmed by subsequent investigations.''

More recently, suggestions of subtle abnormalities in glucocorticoid metabolism have been made, in particular the cortisol-cortisone shuttle described in Chapter 14 (Walker et al., 1992) that could lead to increased levels of plasma cortisol as noted by Watt et al. (1992) in their four-corner analysis.

POSSIBLE CONTRIBUTING FACTORS

A number of secondary features may contribute to the role of the primary mechanisms covered earlier in this chapter, for example, the additional burden of sleep apnea on obesity (see Chapter 15). Beyond these primary and secondary mechanisms, a variety of factors may raise the blood pressure in those who are exposed and susceptible to them. Either because they do not impact on the majority who develop hypertension or because they have only a minimal effect, they are considered to be ''contributing'' rather than causal.

Fetal Environment

Beyond genetic influences described at the beginning of this chapter, the development of hypertension may begin in utero: low birth weight, particularly in concert with large placental size, is associated with the subsequent development of hypertension in most surveys (Gennser et al., 1988; Whincup et al., 1992; Law et al., 1993) but not all (Seidman et al., 1991). The inverse relation between systolic BP and birth weight progressively increases with advancing age: at ages 64–71, SBP was decreased by 5.2 mm Hg for every kilogram increase in birth weight (Law et al., 1993).

Explanations for this imprinting include the induction of insulin resistance by fetal undernutrition. Adults whose birth weights were below 6.5 pounds had 10 times the prevalence of the insulin resistance syndrome than those whose birth weights were above 9.5 pounds (Barker et al., 1993). Another intriguing possible explanation for this association is increased exposure of the poorly nourished fetus to maternal glucocorticoids, "the glucocorticoids acting during critical periods of prenatal development, exerting organizational effects or imprint patterns of response that persist throughout life" (Edwards et al., 1993). Fetal protection from the high levels of maternal glucocorticoids is normally provided by placental 11β-hydroxysteroid dehydrogenase (11β-OHSD) which converts the active cortisol to inactive cortisone. In rats, placental 11β-OHSD actively correlated positively with term fetal weight and negatively with placental weight, thereby matching the associations that have been correlated with subsequent hypertension in humans (Benediktsson et al., 1993).

Calcium and Parathyroid Hormone

Beyond the probability that an increased intracellular calcium is involved in the pathogenesis of hypertension as noted earlier in this chapter, there are other aspects of the relationship between calcium and hypertension.

Serum Calcium and Phosphorus

Hypertension is more common in the presence of hypercalcemia and, in most studies with sizeable numbers of patients, there is a direct relationship between total serum calcium and blood pressure (Staessen et al., 1991b). On the other hand, levels of plasma ionized calcium are generally lower in hypertensives (Hvarfner et al., 1990). Some find that the relationship varies with the level of plasma renin activity: inverse in those with low PRA, none with normal PRA, and direct with high PRA (Resnick et al., 1983; Hunt et al., 1991a). In surveys of large populations, low serum phosphorus levels are more common in those with hypertension (Selby et al., 1990; Hunt et al., 1991b).

Dietary Calcium Intake

Despite the evidence that total serum calcium and blood pressure are related in a direct, positive manner, most find lower intake of dietary calcium intake in hypertensives (McCarron et al., 1984; Cutler and Brittain, 1990; Gillman et al., 1992).

Increased Renal Excretion of Calcium

As first noted by McCarron et al. (1980) and confirmed by Strazzullo (1991), hypertensives excrete more calcium both under basal circumstances and during a calcium infusion, and they have a high incidence of kidney stones (Cappuccio et al., 1990). The renal leak could represent a decreased binding of calcium to kidney cells. However, another explanation is the well-described increase in calcium excretion whenever intravascular volume is expanded and sodium excretion is increased (Suki et al., 1968), as seen in patients with volume-expansion forms of hypertension, e.g., primary aldosteronism (Resnick and Laragh, 1985). The simple intake of increased amounts of sodium leads directly to an increase in calcium excretion (Breslau et al., 1982).

Whether or not the development of hypertension is related to excess sodium intake and retention, an increase in urine calcium excretion can be identified even in the normotensive offspring of hypertensive parents (van Hooft et al., 1993).

Increased Levels of Parathyroid Hormone (PTH)

Probably as a homeostatic response to their urinary calcium leak, hypertensives tend to have increased levels of plasma PTH (McCarron et al., 1980; Grobbee et al., 1988). Although not nearly so high as those seen with primary hyperparathyroidism (wherein hypertension is frequent), these elevated PTH levels could exert a pressor effect (Campese, 1989) and be involved in the hypertension of volume-expanded states.

Selective Benefit of Calcium Supplementation

This scenario implies that PTH levels elevated in response to ionized calcium levels that are lowered by hypercalciuria could be responsible for at least some of the hypertension seen in volume-expanded states (Fig. 3.35). This scheme is carried one step further: the provision of additional calcium that would raise plasma calcium (at the price of even more hypercalciuria) would shut off PTH and thereby lower the blood pressure.

The scheme fits clinical practice. As will be noted in Chapter 6, most properly performed clinical studies have shown little or no overall effect of calcium supplementation among unselected hypertensives. However, in patients with low ionized calcium or increased PTH levels, calcium supplements often cause a significant

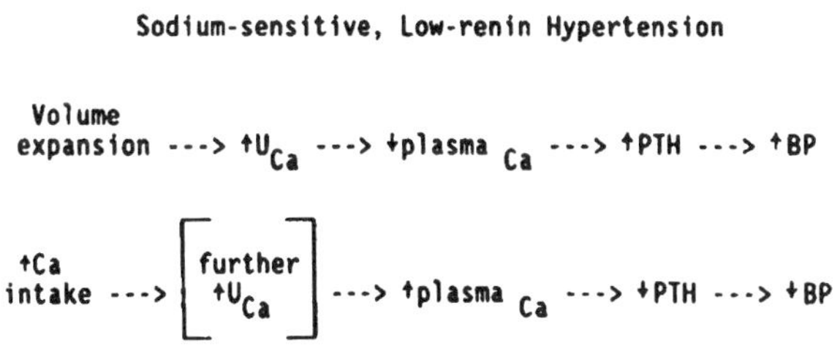

Sodium-sensitive, Low-renin Hypertension

$$\text{Volume expansion} \dashrightarrow \uparrow U_{Ca} \dashrightarrow \downarrow \text{plasma}_{Ca} \dashrightarrow \uparrow PTH \dashrightarrow \uparrow BP$$

$$\uparrow Ca \text{ intake} \dashrightarrow \left[\begin{array}{c} \text{further} \\ \uparrow U_{Ca} \end{array}\right] \dashrightarrow \uparrow \text{plasma}_{Ca} \dashrightarrow \downarrow PTH \dashrightarrow \downarrow BP$$

Figure 3.35. A potential explanation for the involvement of PTH in volume-expanded forms of hypertension and for a hypotensive action of increased dietary calcium intake. U_{Ca}, urinary calcium; *BP*, blood pressure.

fall in blood pressure (Grobbee and Hofman, 1986).

Other Minerals

Potassium Deficiency

As noted earlier in this chapter when the possible role of a high sodium:low potassium ratio was described, there are considerable data suggesting a lack of potassium as being involved in hypertension (Tobian, 1988). These include population surveys showing an inverse relation between dietary potassium intake and blood pressure (Khaw and Barrett-Connor, 1988) particularly in blacks (Veterans Administration Cooperative Study Group, 1987) and extending down to children (Geleijnse et al., 1990). Skeletal muscle potassium is decreased in untreated hypertensives (Ericsson, 1984). As noted in Chapter 6, potassium depletion will raise blood pressure and potassium supplementation may lower the blood pressure. The overall potassium intake of modern people has certainly been reduced below that of our ancestors (Table 3.4), so there are logical reasons to advocate a return to a more ''natural'' higher potassium-lower sodium diet.

Magnesium

Magnesium, beyond its role in activation of many critical enzymes involved in intermediary metabolism and phosphorylation, works as a natural antagonist to many of the actions of calcium (Gilbert D'Angelo et al., 1992). Magnesium deficiency in rats induced significant hypertension associated with marked reductions in the size of the lumen of small vessels (Altura et al., 1984).

In untreated hypertensives, serum and total red blood cell magnesium levels are not low (Kjeldsen et al., 1990). The free magnesium concentration in erythrocytes, measured by the same technique, was low in 17 hypertensives in New York (Resnick et al., 1988) but was normal in 14 hypertensives in England (Woods et al., 1988). The effect of magnesium supplements is covered in Chapter 6.

Lead

In the second National Health and Nutrition Examination Survey (NHANES II) performed from 1976 to 1980, a direct relationship was found between blood lead levels and systolic and diastolic pressures for men and women, white and black, aged 12 to 74 (Harlan et al., 1985). In multiple regression analyses, the relationship was independent of other variables for men, but not for women.

Although no such relation has been noted in Welshmen (Elwood et al., 1988) or Belgians (Dolenc et al., 1993), it has been seen in other groups, including Boston policemen (Weiss et al., 1986) and Danes (Grandjean et al., 1989). In this latter group, the association was largely attributable to alcohol intake, which could either alter lead metabolism or, more likely, provide the source for lead exposure.

Other Trace Metals: Zinc and Cadmium

The same NHANES II data found an inverse relation between serum zinc levels and blood pressure (Harlan et al., 1985). There are considerable data in animals but few in man incriminating a direct relation of blood pressure with cadmium (Staessen et al., 1991b), with the possible exception of patients with renal insufficiency (Geiger et al., 1989). Beyond these, there are no other known significant associations between trace elements and blood pressure (Saltman, 1983). However, textile workers exposed to carbon disulfide had higher diastolic pressures (Egeland et al., 1992).

Caffeine

People not tolerant to caffeine will have a pressor effect from it, but tolerance develops rapidly so that caffeine does not produce a persistent increase in blood pressure (Shi et al., 1993).

Antioxidants

Two cross-sectional surveys have reported an inverse relation between plasma concentrations of ascorbic acid and blood pressure, one from eastern Finland (Salonen et al., 1988), and the other from southern U.S. (Moran et al., 1993).

Alcohol

The possible role of alcohol, in amounts consumed by a large part of the overall population, needs special emphasis. In contrast to its immediate vasodepressor effect (Kojima et al., 1993), chronic consumption, even of small quantities, may raise the blood pressure; in larger quantities, alcohol may be responsible for a significant amount of hypertension.

Nature of the Relationship

The association was reported in 1915 (Lian, 1915), but not until Klatsky et al. (1977) documented it in a large population was alcohol recognized as a pressor substance. The association has been seen in over 40 population studies, some showing a linear relationship throughout the entire range of consumption, others showing a J-shaped relationship (Shaper et al., 1988) (Fig. 3.36), with slightly less hypertension in those who consume fewer than two drinks a day, compared to those who abstain (World Hypertension League, 1991). This J-shaped pattern parallels

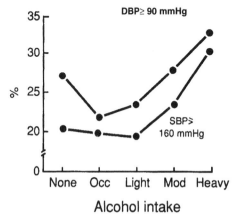

Figure 3.36. Age-adjusted prevalence rates (%) of measured systolic and diastolic hypertension by levels of alcohol intake in drinks: occasional (*Occ*), light (one to two daily), moderate (*Mod*) (three to six daily), and heavy (more than six daily). (From Shaper AG, Wannamethee G, Whincup P. Alcohol and blood pressure in middle-aged British men. *J Hum Hypertens* 1988;2:71–78S.)

the association with total and coronary mortality (Marmot and Brunner, 1991; Klatsky et al., 1992).

Based upon these associations, as much as 10% of hypertension in men can be attributed directly to alcohol excess (MacMahon, 1987). Less hypertension may be seen among those who drink wine rather than beer or spirits (Kimball et al., 1992) and those who drink episodically rather than daily (Russell et al., 1991). Those who quit drinking have pressures similar to those who never drank (Klatsky et al., 1977), and those who are hypertensive while consuming 2 or more ounces of ethanol per day will have a significant fall in pressure if they reduce intake to 1 ounce per day (Ueshima et al., 1993).

Possible Mechanisms

The pressor effects of alcohol may arise from:

—Alterations of cell membranes, allowing more calcium to enter (Vasdev et al., 1991), perhaps by inhibition of sodium transport (Kojima et al., 1993).
—Stimulation of sympathetic nervous activity (Grassi et al., 1989).
—Induction of insulin resistance with subsequent hyperinsulinemia (Shelmet et al., 1988). The lower blood pressures noted among light consumers may be related to lower plasma insulin levels (Mayer et al., 1992).
—Increases in cortisol secretion, leading to a ''pseudo-Cushing's'' appearance in some heavy drinkers (Kirkman and Nelson, 1988).

Physical Inactivity

People who are physically active and fit may develop less hypertension, and those who are hypertensive may lower their blood pressure by regular isotonic exercise (Arroll and Beaglehole, 1992). The prevention of hypertension may be one of the ways exercise protects against the development of cardiovascular disease. Among 14,998 Harvard male alumni followed for 16 to 50 years, those who did not engage in vigorous sports play were at 35% greater risk for developing hypertension, whether or not they had higher blood pressures while in college, a family history of hypertension, or obesity, all of which also increased the risk of hypertension (Paffenbarger et al., 1983). In a similar vein, normotensive people who were at a low level of physical fitness, assessed by maximal treadmill testing, had a 52% greater relative risk for developing hypertension over the next 1 to 12 years when compared with people initially at a high level of physical fitness (Blair et al., 1984).

Temperature and Altitude

For individuals, blood pressure tends to be higher in colder weather (Kunes et al., 1991), but environmental temperature is not an important determinant of population differences in blood pressure (Bruce et al., 1991).

Similarly, ascent to higher altitude may raise the blood pressure (Reeves et al., 1992), but no more hypertension is seen among those who live at higher altitude (Jongbloed and Hofman, 1983).

ASSOCIATIONS WITH HYPERTENSION

In addition to all of these possible mechanisms, surveys of large populations reveal a number of associations with hypertension that are likely not directly causal but are reflective of shared mechanisms (e.g., glaucoma) or of consequences of the hypertension (e.g., hyperuricemia) (Selby et al., 1990; Hunt et al., 1991b).

Hyperuricemia

Hyperuricemia is found in as many as half of untreated hypertensives (Cannon et al., 1966). Whereas this may simply reflect nephrosclerosis and reduced renal function (Messerli et al., 1980), other possible reasons include an increased proximal tubular reabsorption of uric acid in concert with sodium (Cappuccio et al., 1991), an effect of upper body obesity, insulin resistance, and glucose intolerance (Modan et al., 1987), and the contribution of excessive alcohol intake.

Hematologic Findings

Red Cells. Probably related to decreased plasma volume, higher hematocrits are found in hypertensives and the prevalence of hypertension doubles with an increase of 10% in the hematocrit (Cirillo et al., 1992). The other red cell indices are comparable to the hematocrit (Göbel et al., 1991). Such ''pseudopolycythemia'' has long been identified with hypertension and, when associated with obesity and stress, is called Gaisbock's syndrome.

White Cells. Elevated white blood cell counts are predictive of the development of hypertension (Friedman et al., 1990) and are likely related to insulin resistance and hyperinsulinemia (Facchini et al., 1992). In the Framingham population, higher white blood cell counts were associated with increased risk of cardiovascular disease (Kannel et al., 1992).

Platelets. Platelet counts are usually normal, but a number of changes in platelet function have been described (De Clerck, 1986), including an increased aggregatory response, usually reflected by elevated levels of plasma β-thromboglobulin, a platelet-specific protein released when platelets are activated (Islim et al., 1992).

Fibrinogen. Elevated plasma fibrinogen levels are a major risk factor for coronary heart disease (Yarnell et al., 1991) and have been noted, along with increased plasminogen activator inhibitor levels (PAI-1), in hypertensives with insulin resistance (Landin et al., 1990).

Hypofibrinolysis. Decreased fibrinolytic activity, along with higher PAI-1 and lower tissue plasminogen activator activity, has been found in patients with hypertension and hypercholesterolemia (Jansson et al., 1991) and hypertensive premenopausal women (Nordby et al., 1992).

Viscosity. Not surprisingly, in view of the findings noted above, blood viscosity is increased in hypertensives (Smith et al., 1992; Zannad and Stoltz, 1992). As noted years ago (Letcher et al., 1981), but given little attention until recently, increased blood viscosity may play a significant role in raising peripheral resistance, interfering with the microcirculation, and enhancing thrombosis, all increasing the risk for cardiovascular disease (Yarnell et al., 1991).

Sex Hormones

Menopause

A rise in blood pressure is not part of the menopausal syndrome, but women do show a rising incidence of hypertension after menopause, and this is associated with a major increase in cardiovascular risk (Kitler, 1992). A simple explanation for the increased incidence of hypertension after menopause is that the monthly menses keeps fluid volume slightly lower in women before menopause so that the hemodynamic cascade toward hypertension is slowed (Seely, 1976).

Estrogen

Premenopausal women with hypertension usually have a higher heart rate and cardiac output and a lower peripheral resistance than do men with similar degrees of hypertension (Messerli et al., 1987). These differences could reflect higher estrogen levels, which have been found to be even higher in premenopausal hypertensive women than in normotensive subjects (Hughes et al., 1989). In that same study, estrogen levels were also higher in hypertensive than in normotensive men although still well below those in women.

Testosterone

Hypertensive men have also been reported to have lower testosterone levels than do normotensives (Barrett-Connor and Khaw, 1988).

Other Associations

The following have been found to have an increased association with hypertension:

Open-angle glaucoma (Quigley, 1993);
Senile cataracts (Clayton et al., 1980);
Color blindness (Morton, 1975);
Blood group MN (Gleiberman et al., 1984);
Serum IgG levels (Khraibi, 1991);
Aortic stenosis (Beevers et al., 1983);
Pseudoxanthoma elasticum (Parker et al., 1964);
Cancer incidence (Muldoon and Kuller, 1993)
Gastric ulcer and cancer (Sonnenberg, 1988);
Reduced forced vital capacity (Selby et al., 1990);

A number of other diseases wherein hypertension is frequently noted are described in Chapter 15.

CONCLUSION

The preceding coverage may not exhaust the possible mechanisms for primary hypertension, but it at least touches upon all that have received serious attention until now. It should be reemphasized that multiple defects are likely involved and some of the initiating factors may no longer be discernible, having been dampened as hypertension develops. Without a certain genetic marker, it is impossible to know whether a normotensive, even with a strongly positive family history, will definitely develop hypertension so that long-term prospective studies are difficult to design and perform. Nonetheless, attempts are being made to follow the hemodynamic and hormonal changes that accompany the development of hypertension (Julius et al., 1990).

In the absence of certainty about the pathogenesis, it will be difficult to convince many that preventive measures should be undertaken. However, there seems no possible harm and a great deal of potential good to be gained from encouraging moderation in intake of sodium, calories, and alcohol, maintenance of good physical condition, and avoidance of unnecessary stress. As will be described in Chapter 6, the value of these preventive measures has now been demonstrated, and their use should be strongly encouraged (National High Blood Pressure Education Program, 1993).

Now that the possible causes of primary hypertension have been examined, we will turn to the natural history and clinical consequences of the disease. Regardless of cause, its consequences must be dealt with.

References

Aalkjaer C, Heagerty AM, Petersen KK, Swales JD, Mulvany MJ. Evidence of increased media thickness, increased neuronal amine uptake, and depressed excitation-contraction coupling in isolated resistance vessels from essential hypertensives. *Circ Res* 1987;61:181–186.

Adeoya SA, Norman RI, Bing RF. Erythrocyte membrane calcium adenosine 5'-triphosphate activity in the spontaneously hypertensive rat. *Clin Sci* 1988;77: 395–400.

Aksamit TR, Floras JS, Victor RG, Aylward PE. Paroxysmal hypertension due to sinoaortic baroreceptor denervation in humans. *Hypertension* 1987;9:309–314.

Alderman MH, Madhavan S, Ooi WL, Cohen H, Sealey JE, Laragh JH. Association of the renin-sodium profile with the risk of myocardial infarction in patients with hypertension. *N Engl J Med* 1991;324: 1098–1104.

Alexiewicz JM, Gaciong Z, Parise M, Karubian F, Massry SG, Campese VM. Effect of dietary sodium intake on intracellular calcium in lymphocytes of salt-sensitive hypertensive patients. *Am J Hypertens* 1992;5:536–541.

Allemann Y, Horber FF, Colombo M, et al. Insulin sensitivity and body fat distribution in normotensive offspring of hypertensive parents. *Lancet* 1993;341:327–331.

Altura BM, Altura BT, Gebrewold A. Magnesium deficiency and hypertension: correlation between magnesium deficient diets and microcirculatory changes in situ. *Science* 1984;223:1315–1317.

Anderson EA, Mark AL. The vasodilator action of insulin. Implications for the insulin hypothesis of hypertension. *Hypertension* 1993a; 21: 136–141.

Anderson EA, Mark AL. Cardiovascular and sympathetic actions of insulin: the insulin hypothesis of hypertension revisited. *Cardiovasc Risk Factors* 1993b;3: 159–163.

Anderson PW, Do YS, Hsueh WA. Angiotensin II causes mesangial cell hypertrophy. *Hypertension* 1993;21:29–35.

Andersson OK, Beckman-Suurküla M, Sannerstedt R, Magnusson M, Sivertsson R. Does hyperkinetic circulation constitute a pre-hypertensive stage? A 5-year follow-up of haemodynamics in young men with mild blood pressure elevation. *J Intern Med* 1989;226:401–408.

Anner BM, Rey HG, Moosmayer M, Meszoely I, Haupert GT Jr. Hypothalamic Na$^+$-K$^+$-ATPase. *Am J Physiol* 1990;258:F144–F153.

Anonymous. Catecholamines in essential hypertension. *Lancet* 1977;1:1088–1099.

Arroll B, Beaglehole R. Does physical activity lower blood pressure: a critical review of the clinical trials. *J Clin Epidemiol* 1992;45:439–447.

Ashida T, Kawano Y, Yoshimi H, Kuramochi M, Omae T. Effects of dietary salt on sodium-calcium exchange and ATP-drive calcium pump in arterial smooth muscle of Dahl rats. *J Hypertens* 1992;10: 1335–1341.

Astarie C, Le Quan Sang K-H, David-Dufilho M, Devynck M-A. Further investigation of platelet cytosolic alkalinization in essential hypertension. *J Hypertens* 1992;10: 849–854.

Aviv A. The role of cell Ca^{2+}, protein kinase C and the Na$^+$-H$^+$ antiport in the development of hypertension and insulin resistance. *J Am Soc Nephrol* 1992;3: 1049–1063.

Axelrod L. Insulin, prostaglandins, and the pathogenesis of hypertension. *Diabetes* 1991;40:1223–1227.

Azar S, Tobian L, Johnson MA. Glomerular, efferent arteriolar, peritubular capillary, and tubular pressures in hypertension. *Am J Physiol* 1974;227:1045–1050.

Azevedo I, Osswald W. Does adenosine malfunction play a role in hypertension? *Pharmacol Res* 1992;25:227–236.

Bachmann S, Peters J, Engler E, Ganten D, Mullins J. Transgenic rats carrying the mouse renin gene—morphological characterization of a low-renin hypertension model. *Kidney Int* 1992;41:24–36.

Barbagallo M, Gupta RK, Resnick LM. Independent effects of hyperinsulinemia and hyperglycemia on intracellular sodium in normal human red cells. *Am J Hypertens* 1993;6:264–267.

Barker DJP, Hale CN, Fall CHD, Osmond C, Phipps K, Clark PMS. Type 2 (non-insulin-dependent) diabetes mellitus, hypertension and hyperlipidaemia (syndrome X): relation to reduced fetal growth. *Diabetologia* 1993;36:62–67.

Baron AD, Brechtel-Hook G, Johnson A, Hardin D. Skeletal muscle blood flow. A possible link between insulin resistance and blood pressure. *Hypertension* 1993;21:129–135.

Barrett-Connor E, Khaw K-T. Endogenous sex hormones and cardiovascular disease in men. *Circulation* 1988;78:539–545.

Bauer JH, Brooks CS. Volume studies in men with mild to moderate hypertension. *Am J Cardiol* 1979;44:1163–1170.

Beauchamp GK. The human preference for excess salt. *Am Scientist* 1987;75:27–33.

Beevers DG, Sloan PJM, Mackinnon J. Aortic stenosis and systemic hypertension. *Br Med J* 1983;286:1960–1961.

Bell DR. Vascular smooth muscle responses to endothelial autocoids in rats with chronic coarctation hypertension. *J Hypertens* 1993;11:65–75.

Benediktsson R, Lindsay RS, Noble J, Seckl JR, Edwards CR. Glucocorticoid exposure in utero: new model for adult hypertension. *Lancet* 1993;341:339–341.

Beretta-Piccoli C, Weidmann P. Circulatory volume in essential hypertension. *Mineral Electrolyte Metab* 1984;10:292–300.

Beretta-Piccoli C, Weidmann P, Brown JJ, Davies DL, Lever AF, Robertson JIS. Body sodium blood volume state in essential hypertension: abnormal relation of exchangeable sodium to age and blood pressure in male patients. *J Cardiovasc Pharmacol* 1984;6:S134–S142.

Berglund G, Larsson B, Andersson O, et al. Body composition and glucose metabolism in hypertensive middle-aged males. *Acta Med Scand* 1976;200:163–169.

Berk BC, Vekshtein V, Gordon HM, Tsuda T. Angiotensin II-stimulated protein synthesis in cultured vascular smooth muscle cells. *Hypertension* 1989;13:305–314.

Berridge MJ. Inositol trisphosphate and calcium signalling. *Nature* 1993;361: 315–325.

Birkenhäger WH, de Leeuw PW. Cardiac aspects of essential hypertension. *J Hypertens* 1984;2:121–125.

Birkenhäger WH, Kho TL, Schalekamp MADH, Kolsters G, Wester A, de Leeuw PW. Renin levels and cardiovascular morbidity in essential hypertension. *Acta Clin Belg* 1977;32:168–172.

Blair SN, Goodyear NN, Gibbons LW, Cooper KH. Physical fitness and incidence of hypertension in healthy normotensive men and women. *JAMA* 1984;252:487–490.

Bland SH, Krogh V, Winkelstein W, Trevisan M. Social network and blood pressure: a population study. *Psychosom Med* 1991;53:598–607.

Blankestijn PJ, Man in't Veld AJ, Tulen J, et al. Support for adrenaline-hypertension hypothesis: 18 hour pressor effect after 6 hours adrenaline infusion. *Lancet* 1988;2:1386–1389.

Blaustein MP. Sodium ions, calcium ions, blood pressure regulation, and hypertension: a reassessment and a hypothesis. *Am J Physiol* 1977;232:C165–C173.

Blaustein MP. Sodium/calcium exchange and the control of contractility in cardiac muscle and vascular smooth muscle. *J Cardiovasc Pharmacol* 1988; 12(Suppl 5): S56–S68.

Blaustein MP, Hamlyn JM. Role of a natriuretic factor in essential hypertension: an hypothesis. *Ann Intern Med* 1983;98(Part 2):785–792.

Boegehold MA, Kotchen TA. Importance of dietary chloride for salt sensitivity of blood pressure. *Hypertension* 1991;17(Suppl I):I-158–I-161.

Bonora E, Bonadonna RC, Del Prato S, et al. In vivo glucose metabolism in obese and type II diabetic subjects with or without hypertension. *Diabetes* 1993;42:764–772.

Borkman M, Strolien LH, Pan DA, Jenkins AB, Chisholm DJ, Campbell LV. The relation between insulin sensitivity and the fatty-acid composition of skeletal-muscle phospholipids. *N Engl J Med* 1993;328: 238–244.

Bornfeldt KE, Arnqvist HJ, Capron L. In vivo proliferation of rat vascular smooth muscle in relation to diabetes mellitus insulin-like growth factor I and insulin. *Diabetologia* 1992;35:104–108.

Borst JGG, Borst-de Geus A. Hypertension explained by Starling's theory of circulatory homeostasis. *Lancet* 1963;1:677–682.

Brearley CJ, Wood AJ, Aronson JK, Grahame-Smith DG. Evidence for an altered mode of action of the sodium-lithium countertransporter in vivo in patients with untreated essential hypertension. *J Hypertens* 1993;11:147–153.

Brenner BM, Anderson S. The interrelationships among filtration surface area, blood pressure, and chronic renal disease. *J Cardiovasc Pharmacol* 1992;19(Suppl 6): S1–S7.

Brenner BM, Garcia DL, Anderson S. Glomeruli and blood pressure. Less of one, more the other? *Am J Hypertens* 1988;1:335–347.

Breslau NA, McGuire JL, Zerwekh JE, Pak CYC. The role of dietary sodium on renal excretion and intestinal absorption of calcium and on vitamin D metabolism. *J Clin Endocrinol Metab* 1982;55:369–373.

Briner VA, Tsai P, Schrier RW. Bradykinin: potential for vascular constriction in the presence of endothelial injury. *Am J Physiol* 1993;264:F322–F327.

Brod J. Essential hypertension. Haemodynamic observations with a bearing on its pathogenesis. *Lancet* 1960;2:773–778.

Brown JJ, Lever AF, Robertson JIS, Schalekamp MA. Renal abnormality of essential hypertension. *Lancet* 1974;2:320–323.

Brown JJ, Lever AF, Robertson JIS, et al. Salt and hypertension [Letter]. *Lancet* 1984;2:456.

Bruce N, Elford J, Wannamethee G, Shaper AG. The contribution of environmental temperature and humidity to geographic variations in blood pressure. *J Hypertens* 1991;9:851–858.

Bruce NG, Cook DG, Shaper AG, Ratcliffe JG, Thomson AG. Casual urine concentrations of sodium and potassium and geographic blood pressure variations in Great Britain. *J Hum Hypertens* 1992;6: 157–164.

Brunner HR, Laragh JH, Baer L, et al. Essential hypertension: renin and aldosterone, heart attack and stroke. *N Engl J Med* 1972;286:441–449.

Bulpitt CJ, Broughton PMG, Markowe HLJ, et al. The relationship between both sodium and potassium intake and blood pressure in London civil servants. A report from the Whitehall Department of Environment Study. *J Chronic Dis* 1986;39: 211–219.

Bunnemann B, Fuxe K, Ganten D. The brain renin-angiotensin system: localization and general significance. *J Cardiovasc Pharmacol* 1992;19(Suppl 6):S51–S62.

Cacciafesta M, Ferri C, De Angelis C, et al. Is the Na$^+$/K$^+$ cotransport activity a marker of salt sensitivity [Abstract]? *Am J Hypertens* 1993;6:70A.

Calver A, Collier J, Moncada S, Vallance P. Effect of local intra-arterial N^G-monomethyl-L-arginine in patients with hypertension: the nitric oxide dilator mechanism appears abnormal. *J Hypertens* 1992;10: 1025–1031.

Cambien F, Poirier O, Lecerf L, et al. Deletion polymorphism in the gene for angiotensin-converting enzyme is a potent risk factor for myocardial infarction. *Nature* 1992;359:641–643.

Campese VM. Calcium, parathyroid hormone, and blood pressure. *Am J Hypertens* 1989;2:34S–44S.

Campese VM, Parise M, Karubian F, Bigazzi R. Abnormal renal hemodynamics in black salt-sensitive patients with hypertension. *Hypertension* 1991;18:805–812.

Campese VM, Karubian F, Chervu I, Parise M, Sarkies N, Bigazzi R. Pressor reactivity to norepinephrine and angiotensin in salt-sensitive hypertensive patients. *Hypertension* 1993;21:301–307.

Canessa M, Adragna N, Solomon HS, Connolly TM, Tosteson DC. Increased sodium-lithium countertransport in red cells of patients with essential hypertension. *N Engl J Med* 1980;302:772–776.

Cannon PJ, Stason WB, Demartini FE, Sommers SC, Laragh JH. Hyperuricemia in primary and renal hypertension. *N Engl J Med* 1966;275:457–464.

Cappuccio FP, Strazzullo P, Mancini M. Kidney stones and hypertension: population based study of an independent clinical association. *Br Med J* 1990;300: 1234–1236.

Cappuccio FP, Iacone R, Strazzullo P. Serum uric acid and proximal sodium excretion: an independent association in man (the Olivetti study). *J Hypertens* 1991; 9(Suppl 6):S280–S281.

Caro JF. Insulin resistance in obese and nonobese man. *J Clin Endocrinol Metab* 1991;73:691–695.

Carretero OA, Scicli AG. Kinins: paracrine hormone. *Kidney Int* 1988;34(Suppl 26): S-52–S-59.

Carretero OA, Barman SM, Berecek KH, et al. Major pathogenetic factors in hypertension. *Hypertension* 1991;18(Suppl I): I-70–I-73.

Carvalho JJM, Baruzzi RG, Howard PF, et al. Blood pressure in four remote populations in the INTERSALT study. *Hypertension* 1989;14:238–246.

Chin JH, Azhar S, Hoffman BB. Inactivation of endothelial derived relaxing factor by oxidized lipoproteins. *J Clin Invest* 1992;89:10–18.

Christensen KL. Reducing pulse pressure in hypertension may normalize small artery structure. *Hypertension* 1991;18:722–727.

Christy IJ, Woods RL, Courneya CA, Denton KM, Anderson WP. Evidence for a renomedullary vasodepressor system in rabbits and dogs. *Hypertension* 1991;18:325–333.

Chua BHL, Krebs CJ, Chua CC, Diglio CA. Endothelin stimulates protein synthesis in smooth muscle cells. *Am J Physiol* 1992;262:E412–E416.

Cirillo M, Laurenzi M, Trevisan M, Stamler J. Hematocrit, blood pressure, and hypertension. The Gubbio Population Study. *Hypertension* 1992;20:319–326.

Clark BA, Rosa RM, Epstein FH, Young JB, Landsberg L. Altered dopaminergic responses in hypertension. *Hypertension* 1992;19:589–594.

Clayton RM, Cuthbert J, Phillips CI, et al. Analysis of individual cataract patients and their lenses: a progress report. *Exp Eye Res* 1980;31:553–566.

Cobb S, Rose RM. Hypertension, peptic ulcer, and diabetes in air traffic controllers. *JAMA* 1973;224:489–492.

Cohen MC, Muller JE. Onset of acute myocardial infarction—circadian variation and triggers. *Cardiovasc Res* 1992;26: 831–838.

Cohen RA, Zitnay KM, Haudenschild CC, Cunningham LD. Loss of selective endothelial cell vasoactive functions caused by hypercholesterolemia in pig coronary arteries. *Circ Res* 1988;63:903–910.

Connell JMC, Fraser R. Adrenal corticosteroid synthesis and hypertension. *J Hypertens* 1991;9:97–107.

Corbett JA, Tilton RG, Chang K, et al. Aminoguanidine, a novel inhibitor of nitric oxide formation, prevents diabetic vascular dysfunction. *Diabetes* 1992;41:552–556.

Creager MA, Cooke JP, Mendelsohn ME, et al. Impaired vasodilation of forearm resistance vessels in hypercholesterolemic humans. *J Clin Invest* 1990;86:228–234.

Curtis JJ, Luke RG, Dustan HP, et al. Remission of essential hypertension after renal transplantation. *N Engl J Med* 1983;309: 1009–1015.

Cutler JA, Brittain E. Calcium and blood pressure. An epidemiologic perspective. *Am J Hypertens* 1990;3:137S–146S.

Cutler JA, Follmann D, Elliott P, Suh I. An overview of randomized trials of sodium reduction and blood pressure. *Hypertension* 1991;17(Suppl I):I-27–I-33.

Dahl LK. Salt and hypertension. *Am J Clin Nutr* 1972;25:231–244.

Dahl LK, Heine M. Primary role of renal homografts in setting chronic blood pressure and levels in rats. *Circ Res* 1975;36:692–696.

Dahl LK, Knudsen KD, Heine M, Leitl G. Effects of chronic excess salt ingestion. *J Exp Med* 1967;126:687–699.

Dananberg J, Sider RS, Grekin RJ. Sustained hypertension induced by orally administered nitro-L-arginine. *Hypertension* 1993;21:359–363.

deBold AJ, Borenstein HB, Veress AT, Sonnenberg H. A rapid and potent natriuretic response to intravenous injection of atrial myocardial extract in rats. *Life Sci* 1981;28:89–94.

De Clerck F. Blood platelets in human essential hypertension. *Agents Action* 1986;18:563–580.

DeFronzo RA, Ferrannini E. Insulin resistance. A multifaceted syndrome responsible for NIDDM, obesity, hypertension, dyslipidemia, and atherosclerotic cardiovascular disease. *Diabetes Care* 1991;14:173–194.

Denker PS, Pollock VE. Fasting serum insulin levels in essential hypertension. A meta-analysis. *Arch Intern Med* 1992; 152:1649–1651.

Denton D. *The Hunger for Salt*. New York: Springer-Verlag, 1982.

Denton KM, Fennessy PA, Alcorn D, Anderson WP. Morphometric analysis of the actions of angiotensin II on renal arterioles and glomeruli. *Am J Physiol* 1992; 262:F367–F372.

de Nucci G, Gryglewski RJ, Warner TD, Vane JR. Receptor-mediated release of endothelium-derived relaxing factor and prostacyclin from bovine aortic endothelial cells is coupled. *Proc Natl Acad Sci USA* 1988;85:2334–2338.

Devereux RB, Laragh JH. Angiotensin converting enzyme inhibition of renin system activity induces reversal of hypertensive target organ changes. Do these effects predict a reduction in long-term morbidity? *Am J Hypertens* 1992;5:923–926.

Devynck MA, Pernollet MG, Nunez AM, et al. Diffuse structural alterations in cell membranes of spontaneous hypertensive rats. *Proc Natl Acad Sci USA* 1982;79: 5057–5060.

de Wardener HE. The primary role of the kidney and salt intake in the aetiology of essential hypertension: part I. *Clin Sci* 1990;79:193–200.

de Wardener HE. Kidney, salt intake, and Na$^+$,K$^+$-ATPase inhibitors in hypertension. *Hypertension* 1991;17:830–836.

de Wardener HE, MacGregor GA. Dahl's hypothesis that a saluretic substance may be responsible for a sustained rise in arterial pressure: its possible role in essential hypertension. *Kidney Int* 1980;18:1–9.

de Wardener HE, MacGregor GA. The natriuretic hormone and essential hypertension. *Lancet* 1982;1:1450–1454.

Dichtchekenian V, Gisiger S, Quental I, Santos SRC, Marcondes M, Heimann JC. Higher salt consumption, digoxin-like factor, and nifedipine response are associated with salt sensitivity in essential hypertension. *Am J Hypertens* 1992;5:707–712.

Dimsdale JE, Ziegler M, Mills P, Berry C. Prediction of salt sensitivity. *Am J Hypertens* 1990;3:429–435.

Dolenc P, Staessen JA, Lauwerys RR, Amery A, on behalf of the Cadmibel Study Group. Short report: low-level exposure does not increase the blood pressure in the general population. *J Hypertens* 1993;11:589–593.

Dominiczak AF, Bohr DF. Cell membrane abnormalities and the regulation of intracellular calcium concentration in hypertension. *Clin Sci* 1990;79:415–423.

Donnelly R, Connell JMC. Insulin resistance: possible role in the aetiology and clinical course of hypertension. *Clin Sci* 1992;83:265–275.

Dostal DE, Baker EM. Evidence for a role of an intracardiac renin-angiotensin system in normal and failing hearts. *Trends Cardiovasc Med* 1993;3:67–74.

Dowse GK, Collins VR, Alberti GMM, Zimmet PZ, Tuomilehto J, Chitson P, Gareeboo H, for the Mauritius Non-communicable Disease Study Group. Insulin and blood pressure levels are not independently related in Mauritians of Asian Indian, Creole or Chinese origin. *J Hypertens* 1993;11:297–307.

Drexler H, Zeiher AM, Meinzer K, Just H. Correction of endothelial dysfunction in coronary microcirculation of hypercholesterolaemic patients by L-arginine. *Lancet* 1991;338:1546–1550.

Duijkers TJ, Drijver M, Kromhout D, James SA. ''John Henryism'' and blood pressure in a Dutch population. *Psychosom Med* 1988;50:353–359.

Dustan HP, Kirk KA. Corcoran Lecture: the case for or against salt in hypertension. *Hypertension* 1989;13:696–705.

Dzau VJ, Gibbons GH, Cooke JP, Omoigui N. Vascular biology and medicine in the 1990s: scope, concepts, potentials, and perspectives. *Circulation* 1993a;87:705–719.

Dzau VJ, Sasamura H, Hein L. Heterogeneity of angiotensin synthetic pathways and receptor subtypes: physiological and pharmacological implications. *J Hypertens* 1993b;11(Suppl 3):S13–S18.

Eaton SB, Konner M, Shostak M. Stone agers in the fast lane: chronic degenerative diseases in evolutionary perspective. *Am J Med* 1988;84:739–749.

Edmondson RPS, Thomas RD, Hilton PJ, Patrick J. Abnormal leucocyte composition and sodium transport in essential hypertension. *Lancet* 1975;1:1003–1005.

Edwards CRW, Benediktsson R, Lindsay RS, Seckl JR. Dysfunction of placental glucocorticoid barrier: link between fetal environment and adult hypertension? *Lancet* 1993;341:355–357.

Egeland GM, Burkhart GA, Schnorr TM, Hornung RW, Fajen JM, Lee ST. Effects of exposure to carbon disulphide on low density lipoprotein cholesterol concentration and diastolic blood pressure. *Br J Indust Med* 1992;49:287–293.

Eggena P, Barrett JD. Regulation and functional consequences of angiotensinogen gene expression. *J Hypertens* 1992;10: 1307–1311.

Eiskjaer H, Sørensen SS, Danielsen H, Pedersen EB. Glomerular and tubular antinatriuretic actions of low-dose angiotensin II infusion in man. *J Hypertens* 1992; 10: 1033–1040.

Elliott P. Observational studies of salt and blood pressure. *Hypertension* 1991;17(Suppl I):I-3–I-8.

Elwood PC, Yarnell JWG, Oldham PD, et al. Blood pressure and blood lead in surveys in Wales. *Am J Epidemiol* 1988;127: 942–945.

Erdös EG. Angiotensin I converting enzyme and the changes in our concepts through the years. Lewis K. Dahl memorial lecture. *Hypertension* 1990;16:363–370.

Erlinge D, Ekman R, Thulin T, Edvinsson L. Neuropeptide Y-like immunoreactivity and hypertension. *J Hypertens* 1992;10: 1221–1225.

Ericsson F. Potassium in skeletal muscle in untreated primary hypertension and in chronic renal failure, studied by X-ray fluorescence technique. *Acta Med Scand* 1984;215:225–230.

Facchini F, Hollenbeck CB, Chen YN, Chen Y-DI, Reaven GM. Demonstration of a relationship between white blood cell count, insulin resistance, and several risk factors for coronary heart disease in women. *J Intern Med* 1992;232:267–272.

Fagard R, Amery A, Reybrouck T, Lijnen P, Billiet L, Joossens JV. Plasma renin levels and systemic haemodynamics in essential hypertension. *Clin Sci Mol Med* 1977;52:591–597.

Falkner B, Kushner H. Interaction of sodium sensitivity and stress in young adults. *Hypertension* 1991;17(Suppl I):I-162–I-165.

Falkner B, Hulman S, Tannenbaum J, Kushner H. Insulin resistance and blood pressure in young black men. *Hypertension* 1990;16:706–711.

Ferguson RK, Turek DM, Rovner DR. Spironolactone and hydrochlorothiazide in normal-renin and low-renin essential hypertension. *Clin Pharmacol Ther* 1977;21: 62–69.

Ferrannini E, Buzzigoli G, Bonadonna R, et al. Insulin resistance in essential hypertension. *N Engl J Med* 1987;317:350–357.

Ferrannini E, Haffner SM, Stern MP, et al. High blood pressure and insulin resistance: influence of ethnic background. *Eur J Clin Invest* 1991;21:280–287.

Ferrier C, Cox H, Esler M. Elevated total body noradrenaline spillover in normotensive members of hypertensive families. *Clin Sci* 1993;84:225–230.

Finkielman S, Worcel M, Agrest A. Hemodynamic patterns in essential hypertension. *Circulation* 1965;31:356–368.

Fitzgibbon WR, Ploth DW, Margolius HS. Kinins and vasoactive peptides. *Curr Opin Nephrol Hypertens* 1993;2:283–290.

Flavahan NA. Atherosclerosis or lipoprotein-induced endothelial dysfunction. Potential mechanisms underlying reduction in EDRF/nitric oxide activity. *Circulation* 1992;85:1927–1938.

Floras JS. Epinephrine and the genesis of hypertension. *Hypertension* 1992;19: 1–18.

Floras JS, Hassan MO, Jones JV, Osikowska BA, Sever PS, Sleight P. Consequences of impaired arterial baroreflexes in essential hypertension: effects on pressor responses, plasma noradrenaline and blood pressure variability. *J Hypertens* 1988;6:525–535.

Florey CDV, Uppal S, Lowy C. Relation between blood pressure, weight, and plasma sugar and serum insulin levels in schoolchildren aged 9–12 years in Westland, Holland. *Br Med J* 1976;1: 1368–1371.

Folkow B. Sympathetic nervous control of blood pressure. Role in primary hypertension. *Am J Hypertens* 1989;2:103S–111S.

Folkow B. ''Structural factor'' in primary and secondary hypertension. *Hypertension* 1990;16:89–101.

Freeman ZS. Stress and hypertension—a critical review. *Med J Aust* 1990;153: 621–625.

Friedman GD, Selby JV, Quesenberry CP Jr. The leukocyte count: a predictor of hypertension. *J Clin Epidemiol* 1990;43: 907–911.

Frohlich ED, Dustan HP, Page IH. Hyperdynamic beta-adrenergic circulatory state. *Arch Intern Med* 1966;117:614–619.

Frontoni S, Ohman L, Haywood JR, DeFronzo RA, Rossetti L. In vivo insulin action in genetic models of hypertension. *Am J Physiol* 1992;262:E191–E196.

Fuh MM-T, Shieh S-M, Wu D-A, Chen Y-DI, Reaven GM. Abnormalities of carbohydrate and lipid metabolism in patients with hypertension. *Arch Intern Med* 1987;147:1035–1038.

Furchgott RF, Zawadzki JV. The obligatory role of endothelial cells in the relaxation of arterial smooth muscle by acetylcholine. *Nature* 1980;288:373–376.

Furspan PB, Bohr DF. Cell membrane permeability in hypertension. *Clin Physiol Biochem* 1988;6:122–129.

Garay R. Typology of Na^+ transport abnormalities in erythrocytes from essential hypertensive patients. A first step towards the diagnosis and specific treatment of different forms of primary hypertension. *Cardiovasc Drug Ther* 1990;4:373–378.

Geiger H, Bahner U, Anders S, Schaefer RM, Schaller K-H. Cadmium and renal hypertension. *J Hum Hypertens* 1989;3:23–27.

Geleijnse JM, Grobbee DE, Hofman A. Sodium and potassium intake and blood pressure change in childhood. *Br Med J* 1990;300:899–902.

Gennser G, Rymark P, Isberg PE. Low birth weight and risk of high blood pressure in adulthood. *Br Med J* 1988;296: 1498–1500.

Gentry WD, Chesney AP, Gary HE Jr, Hall RP, Harburg E. Habitual anger-coping styles: I. effect on mean blood pressure and risk for essential hypertension. *Psychosom Med* 1982;44:195–202.

Gibbons GH. Autocrine-paracrine factors and vascular remodeling in hypertension. *Curr Opin Nephrol Hypertens* 1993;2:291–298.

Gilbert D'Angelo EK, Singer HA, Rembold CM. Magnesium relaxes arterial smooth muscle by decreasing intracellular Ca^{2+} without changing intracellular Mg^{2+}. *J Clin Invest* 1992;89:1988–1994.

Gill JR Jr, Grossman E, Goldstein DS. High urinary dopa and low urinary dopamine-to-dopa ratio in salt-sensitive hypertension. *Hypertension* 1991;18:614–621.

Gillman MW, Oliveria SA, Moore LL, Ellison RC. Inverse association of dietary calcium with systolic blood pressure in young children. *JAMA* 1992;267: 2340–2343.

Gillman MW, Kannel WB, Belanger A, D'Agostino RB. Influence of heart rate on mortality among persons with hypertension: the Framingham study. *Am Heart J* 1993;125:1148–1154.

Gleiberman L, Gershowitz H, Harburg E, Schork MA. Blood pressure and blood group markers: association with the MN locus. *J Hypertens* 1984;2:337–341.

Göbel BO, Schulte-Göbel A, Weisser B, Glänzer K, Vetter H, Düsing R. Arterial blood pressure. Correlation with erythrocyte count, hematocrit, and hemoglobin concentration. *Am J Hypertens* 1991;4: 14–19.

Goldblatt H. Experimental renal hypertension. Mechanism of production and maintenance. *Circulation* 1958;17:642–647.

Goldsmith DJA, Tribe RM, Poston L, et al. Leucocyte intracellular pH and Na^+-H^+ exchange activity in essential hypertension: an in vitro study under physiological conditions. *J Hypertens* 1991;9:645–653.

Gomez-Sanchez CE, Holland OB, Upcavage R. Urinary free 19-nor-deoxycorticosterone and deoxycorticosterone in human hypertension. *J Clin Endocrinol Metab* 1985;60:234–238.

Grandjean P, Hollnagel H, Hedegaard L, Christensen JM, Larsen S. Blood lead-blood pressure relations: alcohol intake and hemoglobin as confounders. *Am J Epidemiol* 1989;129:732–739.

Grassi GM, Somers VK, Renk WS, Abboud FM, Mark AL. Effects of alcohol intake on blood pressure and sympathetic nerve activity in normotensive humans: a preliminary report. *J Hypertens* 1989;7(Suppl 6):S20–S21.

Gray HH, Hilton PJ, Richardson PJ. Effect of serum from patients with essential hypertension on sodium transport in normal leucocytes. *Clin Sci* 1986;70:583–586.

Griendling KK, Murphy TJ, Alexander RW. Molecular biology of the renin-angiotensin system. *Circulation* 1993;87:1816–1828.

Griffing GT, Wilson TE, Melby JC. Alterations in aldosterone secretion and metabolism in low renin hypertension. *J Clin Endocrinol Metab* 1990;71:1454–1460.

Grobbee DE, Hofman A. Effect of calcium supplementation on diastolic blood pressure in young people with mild hypertension. *Lancet* 1986;2:703–707.

Grobbee DE, Hackeng WHL, Birkenhäger JC, Hofman A. Raised plasma intact parathyroid hormone concentrations in young people with mildly raised blood pressure. *Br Med J* 1988;296:814–816.

Gupta AK, Clark RV, Kirchner KA. Effects of insulin on renal sodium excretion. *Hypertension* 1992;19(Suppl I):I-78–I-82.

Guyton AC. Physiologic regulation of arterial pressure. *Am J Cardiol* 1961;8:401–407.

Guyton AC. Kidneys and fluids in pressure regulation. Small volume but large pressure changes. *Hypertension* 1992;19(Suppl I):I-2–I-8.

Guyton AC, Coleman TG. Quantitative analysis of the pathophysiology of hypertension. *Circ Res* 1969;24(Suppl I):I-1–I-14.

Haddy FJ. Digitalis-like circulating factor in hypertension: potential messenger between salt balance and intracellular sodium. *Cardiovasc Drug Ther* 1990;4:343–349.

Haffner SM, Ferrannini E, Hazuda HP, Stern MP. Clustering of cardiovascular risk factors in confirmed prehypertensive individuals. *Hypertension* 1992;20:38–45.

Hajem S, Moreau T, Hannaert P, et al. Erythrocyte cation transport systems and plasma lipids in a general male population. *J Hypertens* 1990;8:891–896.

Halimi J-M, James G, Cohen H, Alderman M, Laragh JH, Sealey JE. Hypertensives (HT) have lower plasma prorenin (PRO) than normotensives (NT) [Abstract]. *Am J Hypertens* 1993;6:23A.

Hall JE, Mizelle HL, Hildebrandt DA, Brands MW. Abnormal pressure natriuresis. A cause or a consequence of hypertension? *Hypertension* 1990;15:547–559.

Hall JE, Brands MW, Hildebrandt DA, Mizelle HL. Obesity-associated hypertension. Hyperinsulinemia and renal mechanisms. *Hypertension* 1992;19(Suppl I):I-45–I-55.

Hamasaki S-I, Umeda T, Sato T. Salt sensitivity and central dopaminergic activity in patients with essential hypertension. *Am J Hypertens* 1991;4:745–751.

Hamet P, Mongeau E, Lambert J, et al. Interactions among calcium, sodium, and alcohol intake as determinants of blood pressure. *Hypertension* 1991;17(Suppl I):I-150–I-154.

Hamlyn JM, Manunta P. Ouabain, digitalis-like factors and hypertension. *J Hypertens* 1992;10(Suppl 7):S99–S111.

Hamlyn JM, Blaustein MP, Bova S, et al. Identification and characterization of a ouabain-like compound from human plasma. *Proc Natl Acad Sci USA* 1991;88:6259–6263.

Harlan WR, Landis JR, Schmouder RL, Goldstein NG, Harlan LC. Blood lead and blood pressure. Relationship in the adolescent and adult US population. *JAMA* 1985;253:530–534.

Harrap SB, Davidson HR, Connor JM, et al. The angiotensin I converting enzyme gene and predisposition to high blood pressure. *Hypertension* 1993;21:455–460.

Hauger RL, Aguilera G, Catt KJ. Angiotensin II regulates its receptor sites in the adrenal glomerulosa zone. *Nature* 1978;271:176–178.

Haynes WG, Webb DJ. The endothelin family of peptides: local hormones with diverse roles in health and disease? *Clin Sci* 1993;84:485–500.

He J, Tell GS, Tang Y-C, Mo P-S, He G-Q. Relation of electrolytes to blood pressure in men. The Yi people study. *Hypertension* 1991;17:378–385.

Heagerty AM, Milner M, Bing RF, Thurston H, Swales JD. Leucocyte membrane sodium transport in normotensive populations: dissociation of abnormalities of sodium efflux from raised blood pressure. *Lancet* 1982;2:894–896.

Heagerty AM, Izzard AS, Ollerenshaw JD, Bund SJ. Blood vessels and human essential hypertension. *Int J Cardiol* 1988;20:15–28.

Heagerty AM, Aalkjaer C, Bund SJ, Korsgaard N, Mulvany MJ. Small artery structure in hypertension. Dual process of remodeling and growth. *Hypertension* 1993;21:391–397.

Helmer OM. Renin activity in blood from patients with hypertension. *Can Med Assoc J* 1964;90:221–225.

Henneberry HP, Slater JDH, Eisen V, Führ S. Arginine vasopressin response to hypertonicity in hypertension studied by arginine vasopressin assay in unextracted plasma. *J Hypertens* 1992;10:221–228.

Henrich HA, Romen W, Heimgärtner W, Hartung E, Bäumer F. Capillary rarefaction characteristic of the skeletal muscle of hypertensive patients. *Klin Wochenschr* 1988;66:54–60.

Hilbert P, Lindpaintner K, Beckmann JS, et al. Chromosomal mapping of two genetic loci associated with blood-pressure regulation in hereditary hypertensive rats. *Nature* 1991;353:521–529.

Hilgers KF, Veelken R, Rupprecht G, Reeh PW, Luft FC, Mann JFE. Angiotensin II facilitates sympathetic transmission in rat hind limb circulation. *Hypertension* 1993;21:322–328.

Hilton PJ. Na$^+$ transport in hypertension. *Diabetes Care* 1991;14:233–239.

Hofman A, Hazebroek A, Valkenburg HA. A randomized trial of sodium intake and blood pressure in newborn infants. *JAMA* 1983;250:370–373.

Holland OB, Gomez-Sanchez C, Fairchild C, Kaplan NM. Role of renin classification for diuretic treatment of black hypertensive patients. *Arch Intern Med* 1979;139:1365–1370.

Hollenberg NK, Adams DF, Solomon H, et al. Renal vascular tone in essential and secondary hypertension: hemodynamic and angiographic responses to vasodilators. *Medicine* 1975;54:29–41.

Hollister AS, Inagami T. Atrial natriuretic factor and hypertension. A review and metaanalysis. *Am J Hypertens* 1991;4:850–865.

Hsueh WA, Baxter JD. Human prorenin. *Hypertension* 1991;17:469–479.

Hu R-m, Levin ER, Pedram A, Frank HJL. Insulin stimulates production and secretion of endothelin from bovine endothelial cells. *Diabetes* 1993;42:351–358.

Hughes GS, Mathur RS, Margolius HS. Sex steroid hormones are altered in essential hypertension. *J Hypertens* 1989;7:181–187.

Hunt SC, Williams RR, Kuida H. Different plasma ionized calcium correlations with blood pressure in high and low renin normotensive adults in Utah. *Am J Hypertens* 1991a;4:1–8.

Hunt SC, Stephenson SH, Hopkins PN, Williams RR. Predictors of an increased risk of future hypertension in Utah. A screening analysis. *Hypertension* 1991b;17:969–976.

Hunyor SN, Zweifler AJ, Hansson L, Schork MA, Ellis C. Effect of high dose spironolactone and chlorthalidone in essential hypertension: relation to plasma renin activity and plasma volume. *Aust NZ J Med* 1975;5:17–24.

Hvarfner A, Mörlin C, Präntare H, Wide L, Ljunghall S. Calcium metabolic indices, vascular retinopathy, and plasma renin activity in essential hypertension. *Am J Hypertens* 1990;3:906–911.

Ignarro LJ, Buga GM, Wood KS, Byrns RE, Chaudhuri G. Endothelium-derived relaxing factor produced and released from artery and vein is nitric oxide. *Proc Natl Acad Sci USA* 1987;84:9265–9269.

Inscho EW, Carmines PK, Navar LG. Prostaglandin influences on afferent arteriolar responses to vasoconstrictor agonists. *Am J Physiol* 1990;259:157–F163.

Intersalt Cooperative Research Group. Intersalt: an international study of electrolyte excretion and blood pressure. Results for 24 hour urinary sodium and potassium excretion. *Br Med J* 1988;297:319–328.

Islim IF, Beevers DG, Bareford D. The effect of antihypertensive drugs on *in vivo* platelet activity in essential hypertension. *J Hypertens* 1992;10:379–383.

Ito S, Arima S, Ben YL, Juncos LA, Carretero OA. Endothelium-derived relaxing factor/nitric oxide modulates angiotensin II action in the isolated microperfused rabbit afferent but not efferent arteriole. *J Clin Invest* 1993;91:2012–2019.

Ito T, Kato T, Iwama Y, et al. Prostaglandin H$_2$ as an endothelium-derived contracting factor and its interaction with endothelium-derived nitric oxide. *J Hypertens* 1991;9:729–736.

Itoh H, Mukoyama M, Pratt RE, Gibbons GH, Dzau VJ. Multiple autocrine growth factors modulate vascular smooth muscle cell growth response to angiotensin II. *J Clin Invest* 1993;91:2268–2274.

Itskovitz J, Rubattu S, Rosenwaks Z, Liu HC, Sealey JE. Relationship of follicular fluid prorenin to oocyte maturation, steroid levels, and outcome of in vitro fertilization. *J Clin Endocrinol Metab* 1991;72:165–171.

Iwaoka T, Umeda T, Miura F, et al. Renal sodium handling and sodium transport inhibitor in salt-sensitive essential hypertension. *J Hypertens* 1991;9:49–54.

Izzard AS, Cragoe EJ Jr, Heagerty AM. Intracellular pH in human resistance arteries in essential hypertension. *Hypertension* 1991;17:780–786.

Jacob HJ, Lindpaintner K, Lincoln SE, et al. Genetic mapping of a gene causing hypertension in the stroke-prone spontaneously hypertensive rat. *Cell* 1991;67:213–224.

Jamerson KA, Julius S, Gudbrandsson T, Andersson O, Brant DO. Reflex sympathetic activation induces acute insulin resistance in the human forearm. *Hypertension* 1993;21:618–623.

James DE, Jenkins AB, Kraegen EW. Heterogeneity of insulin action in individual muscles in vivo: euglycemic clamp studies in rats. *Am J Physiol* 1985;248:E567–E574.

Jansson J-H, Johansson B, Boman K, Nilsson TK. Hypofibrinolysis in patients with hypertension and elevated cholesterol. *J Intern Med* 1991;229:309–316.

Jarrett RJ. In defense of insulin: a critique of syndrome X. *Lancet* 1992;340:469–471.

Jeunemaitre X, Lifton RP, Hunt SC, Williams WR, Lalouel J-M. Absence of linkage between the angiotensin converting enzyme locus and human essential hypertension. *Nature Genet* 1992a;1:72–75.

Jeunemaitre X, Soubrier F, Kotelevtsev YV, et al. Molecular basis of human hypertension: role of angiotensinogen. *Cell* 1992b;71:169–180.

Jiang X, Srinivasan SR, Bao W, Berenson GS. Association of fasting insulin with blood pressure in young individuals. *Arch Intern Med* 1993;153:323–328.

Johnston CJ. Renin-angiotensin system: a dual tissue and hormonal system for cardiovascular control. *J Hypertens* 1992;10(Suppl 7):S13–S26.

Jongbloed LS, Hofman A. Altitude and blood pressure in children. *J Chronic Dis* 1983;36:397–404.

Juhlin-Dannfelt A, Frisk-Holmberg M, Karlsson J, Tesch P. Central and peripheral circulation in relation to muscle-fibre composition in normo- and hyper-tensive man. *Clin Sci* 1979;56:335–340.

Julius S. Transition from high cardiac output to elevated vascular resistance in hypertension. *Am Heart J* 1988a;116:600–606.

Julius S. Interaction between renin and the autonomic nervous system in hypertension. Am Heart J 1988b;116:611–616.

Julius S. Changing role of the autonomic nervous system in human hypertension. *J Hypertens* 1990;8(Suppl 7):(S59–S65).

Julius S. Clinical implications of pathophysiologic changes in the midlife hypertensive patient. *Am Heart J* 1991;122:886–891.

Julius S, Jamerson K, Mejia A, Krause L, Schork N, Jones K. The association of borderline hypertension with target organ changes and higher coronary risk. *JAMA* 1990;264:354–358.

Julius S, Jones K, Schork N, Johnson E, Krause L, Nazzaro P, Zemva A. Independence of pressure reactivity from pressure levels in Tecumseh, Michigan. *Hypertension* 1991a;17(Suppl I):III-12–III-21.

Julius S, Krause L, Schork NJ, et al. Hyperkinetic borderline hypertension in Tecumseh, Michigan. *J Hypertens* 1991b;9:77–84.

Kannel WB, Anderson K, Wilson PWF. White blood cell count and cardiovascular disease. Insights from the Framingham study. *JAMA* 1992;267:1253–1256.

Kaplan NM. The prognostic implications of plasma renin in essential hypertension. *JAMA* 1975;231:167–170.

Kaplan NM. Renin profiles. The unfulfilled promises. *JAMA* 1977;238:611–613.

Kaplan NM. Dietary salt intake and blood pressure. *JAMA* 1984;251:1429–1430.

Kaplan NM. Systemic hypertension: mechanisms and diagnosis. In: Braunwald E, ed. *Heart Disease*. Philadelphia: WB Saunders, 1988:817–851.

Kaplan NM. The deadly quartet. Upper-body obesity, glucose intolerance, hypertriglyceridemia, and hypertension. *Arch Intern Med* 1989;149:1514–1520.

Katusic ZS, Vanhoutte PM. Superoxide anion is an endothelium-derived contracting factor. *Am J Physiol* 1989;257:H33–H37.

Katz AM. Is angiotensin II a growth factor masquerading as a vasopressor? *Heart Dis Stroke* 1992;1:151–154.

Kawasaki T, Delea CS, Bartter FC, Smith H. The effect of high-sodium and low-sodium intakes on blood pressure and other related variables in human subjects with idiopathic hypertension. *Am J Med* 1978;64:193–198.

Kempner W. Treatment of hypertensive vascular disease with rice diet. *Am J Med* 1948;4:545–577.

Khaw K-T, Barrett-Connor E. The association between blood pressure, age, and dietary sodium and potassium: a population study. *Circulation* 1988;77:53–61.

Khraibi AA. Association between disturbances in the immune system and hypertension. *Am J Hypertens* 1991;4:635–641.

Kimball AW, Friedman LA, Moore RD. Nonlinear modeling of alcohol consumption for analysis of beverage type effects and beverage preference effects. *Am J Epidemiol* 1992;135:1287–1292.

Kimura G, Brenner BM. A method for distinguishing salt-sensitive from non-salt-sensitive forms of human and experimental hypertension. *Curr Opin Nephrol Hypertens* 1993;2:341–349.

Kimura G, Saito F, Kojima S, et al. Renal function curve in patients with secondary forms of hypertension. *Hypertension* 1987;10:11–15.

Kiowski W, Linder L, Kleinbloesem C, van Brummelen P, Bühler FR. Blood pressure control by the renin-angiotensin system in normotensive subjects. Assessment by angiotensin converting enzyme and renin inhibition. *Circulation* 1992;85:1–8.

Kirkman S, Nelson DH. Alcohol-induced pseudo-Cushing's disease: a study of prevalence with review of the literature. *Metabolism* 1988;37:390–394.

Kitler ME. Differences in men and women in coronary artery disease, systemic hypertension and their treatment. *Am J Cardiol* 1992;70:1077–1080.

Kjeldsen SV, Sejersted OM, Frederichsen P, Leren P, Eide IK. Increased erythrocyte magnesium in never treated essential hypertension. *Am J Hypertens* 1990;3:573–575.

Klatsky AL, Friedman GD, Siegelaub AB, Gérard MJ. Alcohol consumption and blood pressure. *N Engl J Med* 1977;296:1194–1200.

Klatsky AL, Armstrong MA, Friedman GD. Alcohol and mortality. *Ann Intern Med* 1992;117:646–654.

Kohno M, Yasunari K, Murakawa K, Kanayama Y, Matsuura T, Takeda T. Effects of high-sodium and low-sodium intake on circulating atrial natriuretic peptides in salt-sensitive patients with systemic hypertension. *Am J Cardiol* 1987;59:1212–1213.

Kojima S, Kawano Y, Abe H, et al. Acute effects of alcohol ingestion on blood pressure and erythrocyte sodium concentration. *J Hypertens* 1993;11:185–190.

Koller KJ, Goeddel DV. Molecular biology of the natriuretic peptides and their receptors. *Circulation* 1992;86:1081–1088.

Koren MJ, Devereux RB. Mechanism, effects, and reversal of left ventricular hypertrophy in hypertension. *Curr Opin Nephrol Hypertens* 1993;2:87–95.

Korner PI, Bobik A, Angus JJ. Are cardiac and vascular "amplifiers" both necessary

for the development of hypertension? *Kidney Int* 1992;41(Suppl 37):S38–S44.

Kotanko P, Höglinger O, Skrabal F. β_2-Adrenoceptor density in fibroblast culture correlates with human NaCl sensitivity. *Am J Physiol* 1992;263:C623–C627.

Kourembanas S, Hannan RL, Faller DV. Oxygen tension regulates the expression of the platelet-derived growth factor-B chain gene in human endothelial cells. *J Clin Invest* 1990;86:670–674.

Kunes J, Tremblay J, Bellavance F, Hamet P. Influence of environmental temperature on the blood pressure of hypertensive patients in Montréal. *Am J Hypertens* 1991;4:422–426.

Kurtz TW, Morris RC Jr. Dietary chloride as a determinant of "sodium-dependent" hypertension. *Science* 1983;222:1139–1141.

Kurtz TW, Spence MA. Genetics of essential hypertension. *Am J Med* 1993;94:77–84.

Laakso M, Edelman SV, Brechtel G, Baron AD. Decreased effect of insulin to stimulate skeletal muscle blood flow in obese men. A novel mechanism for insulin resistance. *J Clin Invest* 1990;85:1844–1852.

Landin K, Tengborn L, Smith U. Elevated fibrinogen and plasminogen activator inhibitor (PAI-1) in hypertension are related to metabolic risk factors for cardiovascular disease. *J Intern Med* 1990;27:273–278.

Landin K, Tengborn L, Smith U. Treating insulin resistance in hypertension with metformin reduces both blood pressure and metabolic risk factors. *J Intern Med* 1991;229:181–187.

Langer SZ, Hicks PE. Physiology of the sympathetic nerve ending. *Br J Anaesth* 1984;56:689–700.

Laragh JH. Vasoconstriction-volume analysis for understanding and treating hypertension: the use of renin and aldosterone profiles. *Am J Med* 1973;55:261–274.

Laragh JH. The renin system and four lines of hypertension research. Nephron heterogencity, the calcium connection, the prorenin vasodilator limb, and plasma renin and heart attack. *Hypertension* 1992;20:267–279.

Laurent S, Hayoz D, Trazzi S, et al. Isobaric compliance of the radial artery is increased in patients with essential hypertension. *J Hypertens* 1993;11:89–98.

Law CM, de Swiet M, Osmond C, et al. Initiation of hypertension in utero and its amplification throughout life. *Br Med J* 1993;306:24–27.

Law MR, Frost CD, Wald NJ. By how much does dietary salt reduction lower blood pressure? I. Analysis of observational data among populations. *Br Med J* 1991a;302:811–815.

Law MR, Frost CD, Wald NJ. III. Analysis of data from trials of salt reduction. *Br Med J* 1991b;302:819–824.

Lawton WJ, Sinkey CA, Fitz AE, Mark AL. Dietary salt produces abnormal renal vasoconstrictor responses to upright posture in borderline hypertensive subjects. *Hypertension* 1988;11:529–536.

Lazdunski M. Transmembrane ionic transport system and hypertension. *Am J Med* 1988;84(Suppl 1B):3–9.

le Noble JLML, Tangelder GJ, Slaaf DW, van Essen H, Reneman RS, Struyker-Boudier HAJ. A functional morphometric study of the cremaster muscle microcirculation in young spontaneously hypertensive rats. *J Hypertens* 1990;8:741–748.

Lebel M, Schalekamp MA, Beevers DG, et al. Sodium and the renin-angiotensin system in essential hypertension and mineralocorticoid excess. *Lancet* 1974;2: 308–310.

Ledingham JM. Autoregulation in hypertension: a review. *J Hypertens* 1989;7(Suppl 4): S97–S104.

Ledingham JM, Cohen RD. The role of the heart in the pathogenesis of renal hypertension. *Lancet* 1963;2:979–981.

Leigh JP. A ranking of occupations based on the blood pressure of incumbents in the National Health and Nutrition Examination Survey I. *J Occup Med* 1991;33: 853–861.

Lembo G, Napoli R, Capaldo B, et al. Abnormal sympathetic overactivity evoked by insulin in the skeletal muscle of patients with essential hypertension. *J Clin Invest* 1992;90:24–29.

Lenz T, Sealey JE, Maack T, et al. Half-life, hemodynamic, renal, and hormonal effects of prorenin in cynomolgus monkeys. *Am J Physiol* 1991;260:R804–R810.

Letcher RL, Chien S, Pickering TG, Sealey JE, Laragh JH. Direct relationship between blood pressure and blood viscosity in normal and hypertensive subjects. *Am J Med* 1981;70:1195–1202.

Lever AF. Slow pressor mechanisms in hypertension: a role for hypertrophy of resistance vessels? *J Hypertens* 1986;4: 515–524.

Lever AF, Harrap SB. Essential hypertension: a disorder of growth with origins in childhood? *J Hypertens* 1992;10:101–120.

Lian C. L'alcoolisme, cause d'hypertension arterielle. *Bull L'Acad Med* 1915;74: 525–528.

Lifton RP. Genetic factors in hypertension. *Curr Opin Nephrol Hypertens* 1993;2:258–264.

Lifton RP, Dluhy RG, Powers M, et al. Hereditary hypertension caused by chimaeric gene duplications and ectopic expression of aldosterone synthase. *Nature Genet* 1992;2:66–74.

Lifton RP, Warnock D, Acton RT, Harman L, Lolouel JM. High prevalence of hypertension-associated angiotensinogen variant T235 in African Americans [Abstract]. *Clin Res* 1993;41:260A.

Light KC, Dolan CA, Davis MR, Sherwood A. Cardiovascular responses to an active coping challenge as predictors of blood pressure patterns 10 to 15 years later. *Psychosom Med* 1992;54:217–230.

Lijnen P, Fagard R, Staessen J, Thijs L, Amery A. Erythrocyte membrane lipids and cationic transport systems in men. *J Hypertens* 1992;10:1205–1211.

Lillioja S, Young AA, Cutler CL, et al. Skeletal muscle capillary density and fiber type are possible determinants of in vivo insulin resistance in man. *J Clin Invest* 1987;80:415–424.

Lissner L, Bengtsson C, Lapidus L, Kristjansson K, Wedel H. Fasting insulin in relation to subsequent blood pressure changes and hypertension in women. *Hypertension* 1992;20:797–801.

London GM, Safar ME. Renal haemodynamics, sodium balance and the capacitance system in essential hypertension. *Clin Sci* 1988;74:449–453.

London GM, Safar ME, Weiss YA, et al.. Volume-dependent parameters in essential hypertension. *Kidney Int* 1977a;11: 204–208.

London GM, Safar ME, Weiss YA, et al. Relationship of plasma renin activity and aldosterone levels with hemodynamic functions in essential hypertension. *Arch Intern Med* 1977b;137:1042–1047.

London GM, Safar ME, Simon AC, Alexandre JM, Levenson JA, Weiss YA. Total effective compliance, cardiac output and fluid volumes in essential hypertension. *Circulation* 1978;57:995–1000.

Lowenstein FW. Blood-pressure in relation to age and sex in the tropics and subtropics. *Lancet* 1961;1:389–392.

Ludens JH, Clark MA, Robinson FG, DuCharme DW. Rat adrenal cortex is a source of a circulating ouabainlike compound. *Hypertension* 1992;19:721–724.

Luft FC, Mann JFE. Sodium and its interrelationships with other pressor systems in hypertension. *Curr Opin Cardiol* 1991;6:697–703.

Luft FC, Grim CE, Higgins JT Jr, Weinberger MH. Differences in response to sodium administration in normotensive white and black subjects. *J Lab Clin Med* 1977;90: 555–562.

Luke RG. Essential hypertension: a renal disease? A review and update of the evidence. *Hypertension* 1993;21:380–390.

Lund-Johansen P. Central haemodynamics in essential hypertension at rest and during exercise: a 20-year follow-up study. *J Hypertens* 1989;7(Suppl 6):S52–S55.

Lüscher TF, Boulanger CM, Yang Z, Noll G, Dohi Y. Interactions between endothelium-derived relaxing and contracting factors in health and cardiovascular disease. *Circulation* 1993a;87(Suppl V):V-36–V-44.

Lüscher TF, Oemar BS, Boulanger CM, Hahn AWA. Molecular and cellular biology of endothelin and its receptors—Part II. *J Hypertens* 1993b;11:121–126.

Lyall F, Dornan ES, McQueen J, Boswell F, Kelly M. Angiotensin II increases proto-oncogene expression and phosphoinositide turnover in vascular smooth muscle cells via the angiotensin II AT_1 receptor. *J Hypertens* 1992;10:1463–1469.

MacMahon S. Alcohol consumption and hypertension. *Hypertension* 1987;9: 111–121.

Maddocks I. Blood pressures in melanesians. *Med J Aust* 1967;1:1123–1126.

Mangin EL Jr, Kugiyama K, Nguy JH, Kerns SA, Henry PD. Effects of lysolipids and oxidatively modified low density lipoprotein on endothelium-dependent relaxation of rabbit aorta. *Circ Res* 1993;72:161–166.

Manunta P, Hamilton BP, Pruce E, Hamlyn JM. High dietary sodium raises plasma levels of ouabain in normal man [Abstract]. *J Hypertens* 1992a;10(Suppl 4):S96.

Manunta P, Evans G, Hamilton BP, Gann D, Resau J, Hamlyn JM. A new syndrome with elevated plasma ouabain and hypertension secondary to an adrenocortical tumor [Abstract]. *J Hypertens* 1992b;10(Suppl 4):S27.

Marks LS, Maxwell MH. Tigerstedt and the discovery of renin. An historical note. *Hypertension* 1979;1:384–398.

Marmot M, Brunner E. Alcohol and cardiovascular disease: the status of the U shaped curve. *Br Med J* 1991;303:565–568.

Mascioli S, Grimm R Jr, Launer C, et al. Sodium chloride raises blood pressure in normotensive subjects. The study of sodium and blood pressure. *Hypertension* 1991;17(Suppl I):I-21–I-26.

Mattes RD, Donnelly D. Relative contributions of dietary sodium sources. *J Am Coll Nutr* 1991;10:383–393.

Mayer EJ, Newman B, Quesenberry CP, King M-C, Friedman GD, Selby JV. Alcohol intake and insulin concentrations in nondiabetic women twins [Abstract]. *Circulation* 1992;85:20.

McCarron DA, Pingree PA, Rubin RJ, Gaucher SM, Molitch M, Krutzik S. Enhanced parathyroid function in essential hypertension: a homeostatic response to a urinary calcium leak. *Hypertension* 1980; 2:162–168.

McCarron DA, Morris CD, Henry HJ, Stanton JL. Blood pressure and nutrient intake in the United States. *Science* 1984;224:1392–1397.

McKeigue PM, Ferrie JE, Pierpoint T, Marmot MG. Association of early-onset coronary heart disease in South Asian men with glucose intolerance and hyperinsulinemia. *Circulation* 1993;87:152–161.

McVeigh GE, Burns DE, Finkelstein SM, et al. Reduced vascular compliance as a marker for essential hypertension. *Am J Hypertens* 1991;4:245–251.

Meade TW, Imeson JD, Gordon D, Peart WS. The epidemiology of plasma renin. *Clin Sci* 1983;64:273–280.

Melamed S. Emotional reactivity and elevated blood pressure. *Psychosom Med* 1987;49:217–225.

Messerli FH, Frohlich ED, Dreslinski R, Suarez DH, Aristimuno GG. Serum uric acid in essential hypertension: an indicator of renal vascular involvement. *Ann Intern Med* 1980;93:817–821.

Messerli FH, Garavaglia GE, Schmieder RE, Sundgaard-Riise K, Nunez BD, Amodeo C. Disparate cardiovascular findings in men and women with essential hypertension. *Ann Intern Med* 1987;107:158–161.

Metting PJ, Stein PM, Stoos BA, Kostrzewski KA, Britton SL. Systemic vascular autoregulation amplifies pressor responses to vasoconstrictor agents. *Am J Physiol* 1989;256:R98–R105.

Miller JZ, Weinberger MH, Christian JC, Daugherty SA. Familial resemblance in the blood pressure response to sodium restriction. *Am J Epidemiol* 1987;126:822–830.

Minuz P, Barrow SE, Cockcroft JR, Ritter JM. Prostacyclin and thromboxane biosynthesis in mild essential hypertension. *Hypertension* 1990;15:469–474.

Modan M, Halkin H. Hyperinsulinemia or increased sympathetic drive as links for obesity and hypertension. *Diabetes Care* 1991;14:470–487.

Modan M, Halkin H, Karasik A, Lusky A. Elevated serum uric acid—a facet of hyperinsulinaemia. *Diabetologia* 1987;30:713–718.

Moran JP, Cohen L, Greene JM, et al. Plasma ascorbic acid concentrations relate inversely to blood pressure in human subjects. *Am J Clin Nutr* 1993;57:213–217.

Morris BJ. Identification of essential hypertension genes. *J Hypertens* 1993;11:115–120.

Morton WE. Hypertension and color blindness in young men. *Arch Intern Med* 1975;135:653–656.

Muirhead EE. The medullipin system of blood pressure control. *Am J Hypertens* 1991;4:556S–568S.

Muirhead EE, Brooks B, Byers LW. Biologic differences between vasodilator prostaglandins and medullipin I. *Am J Med Sci* 1992a;303:86–89.

Muirhead EE, Streeten DHP, Brooks B, Schroeder ET, Byers LW. Persistent hypertension associated with hypermedullipinemia: a new syndrome. *Blood Pressure* 1992b;1:138–148.

Muldoon MF, Kuller LH. Hypertension and cancer. *Br Med J* 1993;306:598–599.

Muldoon MF, Terrell DF, Bunker CH, Manuck SB. Family history studies in hypertension research. Review of the literature. *Am J Hypertens* 1993;6:76–88.

Mulvany MJ. A reduced elastic modulus of vascular wall components in hypertension? *Hypertension* 1992;20:7–9.

Naftilan AJ, Pratt RE, Dzau VJ. Induction of platelet-derived growth factor a-chain and c-myc gene expressions by angiotensin II in cultured rat vascular smooth muscle cells. *J Clin Invest* 1989;83:1419–1424.

Nakao K, Itoh H, Suga S-i, Ogawa Y, Imura H. The natriuretic peptide family. *Curr Opin Nephrol Hypertens* 1993;2:45–50.

National High Blood Pressure Education Program. Working group report on primary prevention of hypertension. *Arch Intern Med* 1993;153:186–208.

Neutel JM, Smith DHG, Graettinger WF, Weber MA. Dependency of arterial compliance on circulating neuroendocrine and metabolic factors in normal subjects. *Am J Cardiol* 1992;69:1340–1344.

Nishida K, Harrison DG, Navas JP, et al. Molecular cloning and characterization of the constitutive bovine aortic endothelial cell nitric oxide synthase. *J Clin Invest* 1992;90:2092–1096.

Nordby G, Haaland A, Os I. Evidence of decreased fibrinolytic activity in hypertensive premenopausal women. *Scand J Clin Lab Invest* 1992;52:275–281.

Oates JA, FitzGerald GA, Branch RA, Jackson EK, Knapp HR, Roberts LJ II. Clinical implications of prostaglandin and thromboxane A_2 formation. *N Engl J Med* 1988;319:761–767.

O'Brien T, Young WF Jr, Palumbo PJ, O'Brien PC. Hypertension and dyslipidemia in patients with insulinoma. *Mayo Clin Proc* 1993;68:141–146.

Ohanian J, Heagerty AM. The phosphoinositide signaling system and hypertension.

Curr Opin Nephrol Hypertens 1992;1:73–82.

Ohno Y, Suzuki H, Yamakawa H, Nakamura M, Otsuka K, Saruta T. Impaired insulin sensitivity in young, lean normotensive offspring of essential hypertensives: possible role of disturbed calcium metabolism. *J Hypertens* 1993;11:421–426.

Oliver WJ, Cohen EL, Neel JV. Blood pressure, sodium intake, and sodium related hormones in the Yanomamo Indians, a "no-salt" culture. *Circulation* 1975;52:146–151.

Ollerenshaw JD, Heagerty AM, West KP, Swales JD. The effects of coarctation hypertension upon vascular inositol phospholipid hydrolysis in Wistar rats. *J Hypertens* 1988;6:733–738.

Opsahl JA, Smith KL, Murray RD, Abraham PA, Katz SA. Renin and renin inhibition in anephric man. *Clin Exp Hypertens* 1993;15:289–306.

Orlov SN, Resink TJ, Bernhardt J, Bühler FR. Na^+-K^+ pump and Na^+-K^+ co-transport in cultured vascular smooth muscle cells from spontaneously hypertensive and normotensive rats: baseline activity and regulation. *J Hypertens* 1992;10:733–740.

O'Rourke MF, Brunner HR. Introduction to arterial compliance and function. *J Hypertens* 1992;10(Suppl 6):S3–S5.

O'Rourke MF, Kelly RP. Wave reflection in the systemic circulation and its implications in ventricular function. *J Hypertens* 1993;11:327–337.

Oshima T, Matsuura H, Ishibashi K, et al. Familial influence upon NaCl sensitivity in patients with essential hypertension. *J Hypertens* 1992;10:1089–1094.

Osmond DH, Sealey JE, McKenzie JK. Activation and function of prorenin: different viewpoints. *Can J Physiol Pharmacol* 1991;69:1308–1314.

Paffenbarger RS Jr, Wing AL, Hyde RT, Jung DL. Physical activity and incidence of hypertension in college alumni. *Am J Epidemiol* 1983;117:245–257.

Page IH. The nature of arterial hypertension. *Arch Intern Med* 1963;111:103–115.

Page IH. The discovery of angiotensin. *Perspect Biol Med* 1975;18:456–462.

Page LB, Vandevert DE, Nader K, Lubin NK, Page JR. Blood pressure of Qash' qai pastoral nomads in Iran in relation to culture, diet, and body form. *Am J Clin Nutr* 1981;34:527–538.

Palmer RMJ, Ferrige AG, Monacada S. Nitric oxide release accounts for the biological activity of endothelium-derived relaxing factor. *Nature* 1987;327:524–526.

Panza JA, Quyyumi AA, Brush JE Jr, Epstein SE. Abnormal endothelium-dependent vascular relaxation in patients with essential hypertension. *N Engl J Med* 1990;323:22–27.

Panza JA, Epstein SE, Quyyumi AA. Circadian variation in vascular tone and its relation to α-sympathetic vasoconstrictor activity. *N Engl J Med* 1991;325:986–990.

Panza JA, Casino PR, Badar DM, Quyyumi AA. Effect of increased availability of endothelium-derived nitric oxide precursor on endothelium-dependent vascular relaxation in normal subjects and in patients

with essential hypertension. *Circulation* 1993a;87:1475–1481.

Panza JA, Casino PR, Kilcoyne CM, Quyyumi AA. Role of endothelium-derived nitric oxide in the abnormal endothelium-dependent vascular relaxation of patients with essential hypertension. *Circulation* 1993b;87:1468–1474.

Panza JA, Quyyumi AA, Callahan TS, Epstein SE. Effect of antihypertensive treatment on endothelium-dependent vascular relaxation in patients with essential hypertension. *J Am Coll Cardiol* 1993c;21:1145–1151.

Park CS, Hong CD, Honeyman TW. Calcium-dependent inhibitory step in control of renin secretion. *Am J Physiol* 1992;262:F793–F798.

Parker JC, Friedman-Kien AE, Levin S, Bartter FC. Pseudoxanthoma elasticum and hypertension. *N Engl J Med* 1964;271:1204–1206.

Paul M, Wagner J, Dzau VJ. Gene expression of the renin-angiotensin system in human tissues. Quantitative analysis by the polymerase chain reaction. *J Clin Invest* 1993;91:2058–2064.

Peiris AN, Stagner JI, Vogel RL, Nakagawa A, Samols E. Body fat distribution and peripheral insulin sensitivity in healthy men: role of insulin pulsatility. *J Clin Endocrinol Metab* 1992;75:290–294.

Perini C, Müller FB, Rauchfleisch U, Battegay R, Hobi V, Bühler FR. Psychosomatic factors in borderline hypertensive subjects and offspring of hypertensive parents. *Hypertension* 1990;16:627–634.

Perini C, Müller FB, Bühler FR. Suppressed aggression accelerates early development of essential hypertension. *J Hypertens* 1991;9:499–503.

Perry IJ, Beevers DG. Salt intake and stroke: a possible direct effect. *J Hum Hypertens* 1992;6:23–25.

Pershadsingh HA, Szollosi J, Benson S, Hyun WC, Feuerstein BG, Kurtz TW. Effects of ciglitazone on blood pressure and intracellular calcium metabolism. *Hypertension* 1993;21:1020–1023.

Peters J, Münter K, Bader M, Hackenthal E, Mullins JJ, Ganten D. Increased adrenal renin in transgenic hypertensive rats, TGR (mREN2)27, and its regulation by cAMP, angiotensin II, and calcium. *J Clin Invest* 1993;91:742–747.

Pickering TG. Does psychological stress contribute to the development of hypertension and coronary heart disease? *Eur J Clin Pharmacol* 1990;39(Suppl 1):S1–S7.

Plante GE, Bissonnette M, Sirois MG, Regoli D, Sirois P. Renal permeability alteration precedes hypertension and involves bradykinin in the spontaneously hypertensive rat. *J Clin Invest* 1992;89:2030–2032.

Pollare T, Lithell H, Berne C. Insulin resistance is a characteristic feature of primary hypertension independent of obesity. *Metabolism* 1990;39:167–174.

Pontremoli R, Zavaroni I, Mazza S, et al. Changes in blood pressure, plasma triglyceride and aldosterone concentration, and red cell cation concentration in patients with hyperinsulinemia. *Am J Hypertens* 1991;4:159–163.

Pope JE, Anderson JJ, Felson DT. A meta-analysis of the effects of nonsteroidal anti-inflammatory drugs on blood pressure. *Arch Intern Med* 1993;153:477–484.

Portaluppi F, Trasforini G, Margutti A, et al. Circadian rhythm of calcitonin-gene related peptide in uncomplicated essential hypertension. *J Hypertens* 1992;10: 1227–1234.

Postnov YV. An approach to the explanation of cell membrane alteration in primary hypertension. *Hypertension* 1990; 15:332–337.

Poulter N, Khaw KT, Hopwood BEC, Mugambi M, Peart WS, Sever PS. Salt and blood pressure in various populations. *J Cardiovasc Pharmacol* 1984; 6: S197–S203.

Poulter N, Khaw KT, Hopwood BEC, Mugambi M, Peart WS, Rose G, Sever PS. The Kenyan Luo migration study: observations on the initiation of a rise in blood pressure. *Br Med J* 1990;300:967–972.

Quigley HA. Open–angle glaucoma. *N Engl J Med* 1993;328:1097–1106.

Reaven GM. Role of insulin resistance in human disease. *Diabetes* 1988; 37: 1595–1607.

Reaven GM. Insulin resistance, hyperinsulinemia, hypertriglyceridemia, and hypertension. Parallels between human disease and rodent models. *Diabetes Care* 1991;14:195–202.

Reaven GM. Treatment of hypertension: focus on prevention of coronary heart disease. *J Clin Endocrinol Metab* 1993; 76:537–540.

Rees DD, Palmer RMJ, Moncada S. Role of endothelium-derived nitric oxide in the regulation of blood pressure. *Proc Natl Acad Sci USA* 1989;86:3375–3378.

Reeves JT, Mazzeo RS, Wolfel EE, Young AJ. Increased arterial pressure after acclimatization to 4300 m: possible role of norepinephrine. *Int J Sports Med* 1992; 13(Suppl 1):S18–S21.

Rembold CM, Richard H, Chen X-L. Na$^+$-Ca^{2+} exchange, myoplasmic Ca^{2+} concentration, and contraction of arterial smooth muscle. *Hypertension* 1992;19:308–313.

Resnick LM, Laragh JH. Calcium metabolism and parathyroid function in primary aldosteronism. *Am J Med* 1985;78: 385–389.

Resnick LM, Laragh JH, Sealey JE, Alderman MH. Divalent cations in essential hypertension. Relations between serum ionized calcium, magnesium, and plasma renin activity. *N Engl J Med* 1983;309: 888–891.

Resnick LM, Gupta RK, Gruenspan H, Laragh JH. Intracellular free magnesium in hypertension: relation to peripheral insulin resistance. *J Hypertens* 1988;6(Suppl 4):S199–S201.

Richards AM, Crozier IG, Holmes SJ, Espiner EA, Yandle TG, Frampton C. Brain natriuretic peptide: a natriuretic and endocrine effects in essential hypertension. *J Hypertens* 1993;11:163–170.

Rocchini AP, Key J, Bondie D, Chico R, Moorehead C, Katch V, Martin M. The effect of weight loss on the sensitivity of blood pressure to sodium in obese adolescents. *N Engl J Med* 1989;321:580–585.

Rocchini AP, Moorehead C, DeRemer S, Goodfriend TL, Ball DL. Hyperinsulinemia and the aldosterone and pressor responses to angiotensin II. *Hypertension* 1990;15:861–866.

Roman MJ, Pini R, Pickering TG, Devereux RB. Non-invasive measurements of arterial compliance in hypertensive compared with normotensive adults. *J Hypertens* 1992;10(Suppl 6):S115–S118.

Romero JC, Strick DM. Nitric oxide and renal function. *Curr Opin Nephrol Hypertens* 1993;2:114–121.

Romero JC, Bentley MD, Textor SC, Knox FG. Alterations in blood pressure by derangement of the mechanisms that regulate sodium excretion. *Mayo Clin Proc* 1989;64:1425–1435.

Ronquist G, Frithz G, Gunnarsson K, Arvidson G. Decreased erythrocyte cholesterol/phospholipid ratio in untreated patients with essential hypertension. *J Intern Med* 1992;232:247–251.

Rooney DP, Neely RDG, Ennis CN, et al. Insulin action and hepatic glucose cycling in essential hypertension. *Metabolism* 1992;41:317–324.

Rosati C, Garay R. Flow-dependent stimulation of sodium and cholesterol uptake and cell growth in cultured vascular smooth muscle. *J Hypertens* 1991;9:1029–1033.

Rosivall L, Rázga Z, Ormos J. Morphological characterization of human juxtaglomerular apparatus. *Kidney Int* 1991;39(Suppl 32):S-9–S-12.

Rosskopf D, Düsing R, Siffert W. Membrane sodium-proton exchange and primary hypertension. *Hypertension* 1993;21: 607–617.

Rostrup M, Mundal HH, Westheim A, Eide I. Awareness of high blood pressure increases arterial plasma catecholamines, platelet noradrenaline and adrenergic responses to mental stress. *J Hypertens* 1991;9:159–166.

Russell M, Cooper ML, Frone MR, Welte JW. Alcohol drinking patterns and blood pressure. *Am J Pub Health* 1991;81: 452–457.

Rutherford PA, Thomas TH, Laker MF, Wilkinson R. Plasma lipids affect maximum velocity not sodium affinity of human sodium-lithium countertransport: distinction from essential hypertension. *Eur J Clin Invest* 1992;22:719–724.

Saad MF, Lillioja S, Nyomba BL, et al. Racial differences in the relation between blood pressure and insulin resistance. *N Engl J Med* 1991;324:733–739.

Safar ME. Pulse pressure in essential hypertension: clinical and therapeutic implications. *J Hypertens* 1989;7:769–776.

Safar ME, Peronneau PP, Levenson JA, Simon AC. Pulsed Doppler: diameter, velocity and flow of the brachial artery in sustained essential hypertension. *Circulation* 1981;63:393–400.

Saito F, Hori MT, Ideguchi Y, Berger M, Golub M, Stern N, Tuck ML. 12-Lipoxygenase products modulate calcium signals in vascular smooth muscle cells. *Hypertension* 1992;20:138–143.

Salmond CE, Prior IAM, Wessen AF. Blood pressure patterns and migration: a 14-year cohort study of adult Tokelauans. *Am J Epidemiol* 1989;130:37–52.

Salonen JT, Salonen R, Ihanainen M, et al. Blood pressure, dietary fats, and antioxidants. *Am J Clin Nutr* 1988;48:1226–1232.

Saltman P. Trace elements and blood pressure. *Ann Intern Med* 1983;98(Part 2): 823–827.

Salvatore T, Cozzolino D, Giunta R, Giugliano D, Torella R, D'Onofrio F. Decreased insulin clearance as a feature of essential hypertension. *J Clin Endocrinol Metab* 1992;74:144–149.

Samani NJ. New developments in renin and hypertension. Tissue generation of angiotensin I and II changes the picture. *Br Med J* 1991;302:981–982.

Sarzani R, Brecher P, Chobanian AV. Growth factor expression in aorta of normotensive and hypertensive rats. *J Clin Invest* 1989;83:1404–1408.

Schmidt S, van Hooft IMS, Grobbee DE, Ganten D, Ritz E. Polymorphism of the angiotensin I converting enzyme gene is apparently not related to high blood pressure: Dutch Hypertension and Offspring Study. *J Hypertens* 1993;11:345–348.

Schnall PL, Pieper C, Schwartz JE, et al. The relationship between "job strain," workplace diastolic blood pressure, and left ventricular mass index. Results of a case-control study. *JAMA* 1990;263:1929–1935.

Schneider RH, Egan BM, Johnson EH, Drobny H, Julius S. Anger and anxiety in borderline hypertension. *Psychosom Med* 1986;48:242–248.

Schobel HP, Schmieder RE, Gatzka C, Messerli FH. Intravascular volume—a determinant of early cardiac adaptation in hypertension [Abstract]? *Circulation* 1992;86(Suppl I):I-65.

Scott-Burden T, Hahn AWA, Bühler FR, Resink TJ. Vasoactive peptides and growth factors in the pathophysiology of hypertension. *J Cardiovasc Pharmacol* 1992; 20(Suppl 1):S55–S64.

Sealey JE. Plasma renin activity and plasma prorenin assays. *Clin Chem* 1991;37: 1811–1819.

Sealey JE, Blumenfeld JD, Bell GM, Pecker MS, Sommers SC, Laragh JH. On the renal basis for essential hypertension: nephron heterogeneity with discordant renin secretion and sodium excretion causing a hypertensive vasoconstriction-volume relationship. *J Hypertens* 1988;6:763–777.

Sechi LA, Melis A, Tedde R. Insulin hypersecretion: a distinctive feature between essential and secondary hypertension. *Metabolism* 1992;41:1261–1266.

Seely S. Possible reasons for the comparatively high resistance of women to heart disease. *Am Heart J* 1976;91:275–280.

Seidman DS, Laor A, Gale R, Stevenson DK, Mashiach S, Danon YL. Birth weight, current body weight, and blood pressure in late adolescence. *Br Med J* 1991;302: 1235–1237.

Selby JV, Friedman GD, Quesenberry CP Jr. Precursors of essential hypertension: pulmonary function, heart rate, uric acid, serum cholesterol, and other serum chemistries. *Am J Epidemiol* 1990;131: 1017–1027.

Selkurt EE. Effect of pulse pressure and mean arterial pressure modification on renal hemodynamics and electrolyte and water excretion. *Circulation* 1951;4:541–551.

Shamiss A, Carroll J, Rosenthal T. Insulin resistance in secondary hypertension. *Am J Hypertens* 1992;5:26–28.

Shaper AG, Wannamethee G, Whincup P. Alcohol and blood pressure in middle-aged British men. *J Hum Hypertens* 1988;2: 71–78.

Sharma AM, Schorr U, Distler A. Insulin resistance in young salt-sensitive normotensive subjects. *Hypertension* 1993; 21:273–279.

Shelmet JJ, Reichard GA, Skutches CL, Hoeldtke RD, Owne OE, Boden G. Ethanol causes acute inhibition of carbohydrate, fat, and protein oxidation and insulin resistance. *J Clin Invest* 1988;81:1137–1145.

Shen D-C, Shieh S-M, Fuh MM-T, Wu D-A, Chen Y-DI, Reaven GM. Resistance to insulin-stimulated glucose uptake in patients with hypertension. *J Clin Endocrinol Metab* 1988;66:580–583.

Shepherd JT. Increased systemic vascular resistance and primary hypertension: the expanding complexity. *J Hypertens* 1990;8(Suppl 7):S15–S27.

Shi J, Benowitz NL, Denaro CP, Sheiner LB. Pharmacokinetic-pharmacodynamic modeling of caffeine: tolerance to pressor effects. *Clin Pharmacol Ther* 1993;53: 6–14.

Shimamoto H, Shimamoto Y. Plasma norepinephrine is a major determinant of hemodynamic alterations with sodium loading. *J Hypertens* 1992;10:855–860.

Simon D, Romestand B, Huang H, et al. Direct simplified, and sensitive assay of angiotensin II in plasma extracts performed with a high-affinity monoclonal antibody. *Clin Chem* 1992;38:1963–1967.

Simon G. Is intracellular sodium increased in hypertension? *Clin Sci* 1989;76:455–461.

Simon G. Increased vascular wall sodium in hypertension: where is it, how does it get there and what does it do there? *Clin Sci* 1990;78:533–540.

Simon G, Altman S. Subpressor angiotensin II is a bifunctional growth factor of vascular muscle in rats. *J Hypertens* 1992;10: 1165–1171.

Simonson MS, Dunn MJ. Endothelins: a family of regulatory peptides. *Hypertension* 1991;17:856–863.

Sims C, Ashby K, Douglas JG. Angiotensin II-induced changes in guanine nucleotide binding and regulatory proteins. *Hypertension* 1992;19:146–152.

Singer P, Gödicke W, Voigt S, Hajdu I, Weiss M. Postprandial hyperinsulinemia in patients with mild essential hypertension. *Hypertension* 1985;7:182–186.

Skøtt O, Jensen BL. Cellular and intrarenal control of renin secretion. *Clin Sci* 1993;84:1–10.

Smith WCS, Crombie IK, Tavendale RT, Gulland SK, Tunstall-Pedoe HD. Urinary electrolyte excretion, alcohol consumption, and blood pressure in the Scottish heart health study. *Br Med J* 1988;297: 329–330.

Smith WCS, Lowe GDO, Lee AJ, Tunstall-Pedoe H. Rheological determinants of blood pressure in a Scottish adult population. *J Hypertens* 1992;10:467–472.

Somers VK, Dyken ME, Mark AL, Abboud FM. Sympathetic-nerve activity during sleep in normal subjects. *N Engl J Med* 1993;328:303–307.

Sonnenberg A. Concordant occurrence of gastric and hypertensive diseases. *Gastroenterology* 1988;95:42–48.

Spies K-P, Wenzlaff V, Sharma AM, Distler A. Effects of dietary salt intake on NA$^+$/H$^+$-antiport activity and intracellular pH in salt-resistant and salt-sensitive normotensive young men [Abstract]. *J Hypertens* 1992;10(Suppl 4):S72.

Srinivasan SR, Bao W, Berenson GS. Coexistence of increased levels of adiposity, insulin, and blood pressure in a young adult cohort with elevated very-low-density lipoprotein cholesterol: the Bogalusa Heart Study. *Metabolism* 1993;42:170–176.

Staessen J, Bulpitt CJ, Thijs L, Fagard R, Joossens JV, Van Hoof R, Amery A. Pulse rate and sodium intake interact to determine blood pressure. A population study. *Am J Hypertens* 1991a;4:107–112.

Staessen J, Sartor F, Roels H, et al. The association between blood pressure, calcium and other divalent cations: a population study. *J Hum Hypertens* 1991b;5:485–494.

Stamler J, Rose G, Stamler R, Elliott P, Dyer A, Marmot M. INTERSALT study findings. Public health and medical care implications. *Hypertension* 1989;14:570–577.

Stamler JS, Singel DJ, Loscalzo J. Biochemistry of nitric oxide and its redox-activated forms. *Science* 1992;258:1898–1902.

Stamler R, Stamler J, Gosch FC, Civinelli J, Fishman J, McKeever P, McDonald A, Dyer AR. Primary prevention of hypertension by nutritional-hygienic means. *JAMA* 1989;262:1801–1807.

Stamler R, Shipley M, Elliott P, Dyer A, Sans S, Stamler J. Higher blood pressure in adults with less education. Some explanations from INTERSALT. *Hypertension* 1992;19:237–241.

Stout RW. Insulin and atheroma. 20-Yr perspective. *Diabetes Care* 1990;13:631–654.

Strazzullo P. The renal calcium leak in primary hypertension: pathophysiological aspects and clinical implications. *Nutr Metab Cardiovasc Dis* 1991;1:98–103.

Suki WN, Schwettmann RS, Rector FC Jr, Seldin DW. Effect of chronic mineralocorticoid administration on calcium excretion in the rat. *Am J Physiol* 1968;215:71–74.

Sullivan JM. Salt sensitivity. Definition, conception, methodology, and long-term issues. *Hypertension* 1991;17(Suppl I): I-61–I-68.

Swales JD. Functional disturbance of the cell membrane in hypertension. *J Hypertens* 1990a;8(Suppl 7):S203–S211.

Swales JD. Membrane transport of ions in hypertension. *Cardiovasc Drug Ther* 1990b;4:367–372.

Swales JD. Is there a cellular abnormality in hypertension? *J Cardiovasc Pharmacol* 1991;18(Suppl 2):S39–S44.

Tan ACITL, Russel FGM, Thien T, Benraad TJ. Atrial natriuretic peptide. An overview of clinical pharmacology and pharmacokinetics. *Clin Pharmacokinet* 1993;24: 28–45.

Tappy L, Bovet P, Jéquier E, Shamlaye C, Darioli R, Burnand B. Relationship of fasting serum insulin concentrations with blood pressure in a representative sample of the adult population of the Seychelles. *Int J Obesity* 1991;15:669–675.

Tarazi RC, Fouad FM, Ferrario CM. Can the heart initiate some forms of hypertension? *Fed Proc* 1983;42:2691–2697.

Thurston H, Laragh JH. Prior receptor occupancy as a determinant of the pressor activity of infused angiotensin II in the rat. *Circ Res* 1975;36:113–117.

Timio M, Verdecchia P, Venanzi S, Gentili S, Ronconi M, Francucci B, Montanari M, Bichisao E. Age and blood pressure changes: a 20-year follow-up study in nuns in a secluded order. *Hypertension* 1988;12:457–461.

Timmermans PBMWM, Chiu AT, Herblin WF, Wong PC, Smith RD. Angiotensin II receptor subtypes. *Am J Hypertens* 1992;5:406–410.

Tiret L, Kee F, Poirier O, et al. Deletion polymorphism in angiotensin-converting enzyme gene associated with parental history of myocardial infarction. *Lancet* 1993;341:991–992.

Tobian L. Potassium and sodium in hypertension. *J Hypertens* 1988;6(Suppl 4): S12–S24.

Tobian L. Salt and hypertension. Lessons from animal models that relate to human hypertension. *Hypertension* 1991; 17(Suppl I):I-52–I-58.

Tobian L, Binion JT. Tissue cations and water in essential hypertension. *Circulation* 1952;5:754–758.

Tobian L, Hanlon S. High sodium chloride diets injure arteries and raise mortality without changing blood pressure. *Hypertension* 1990;15:900–903.

Toda N, Kitamura Y, Okamura T. Neural mechanism of hypertension by nitric oxide synthase inhibitor in dogs. *Hypertension* 1993;21:3–8.

Touyz RM, Schiffrin EL. Signal transduction in hypertension: part II. *Curr Opin Nephrol Hypertens* 1993;2:17–26.

Treasure CB, Klein L, Vita JA, et al. Hypertension and left ventricular hypertrophy are associated with impaired endothelium-mediated relaxation in human coronary resistance vessels. *Circulation* 1993;87: 86–93.

Trowell HC. Salt and hypertension. *Lancet* 1980;2:88.

Trials of Hypertension Prevention Collaborative Research Group. The effects of non-pharmacologic interventions on blood pressure of persons with high normal levels. *JAMA* 1992;267:1213–1220.

Tyroler HA. Socioeconomic status in the epidemiology and treatment of hypertension. *Hypertension* 1989;13(Suppl I):I-94–I-97.

Ueshima H, Mikawa K, Baba S, et al. Effect of reduced alcohol consumption on blood pressure in untreated hypertensive men. *Hypertension* 1993;21:248–252.

Valentin J-P, Humphreys MH. Urodilatin: a paracrine renal natriuretic peptide. *Semin Nephrol* 1993;13:61–70.

van Hooft IMS, Grobbee DE, Derkx FHM, de Leeuw PW, Schalekamp MADH, Hofman A. Renal hemodynamics and the renin-angiotensin-aldosterone system in normotensive subjects with hypertensive and normotensive parents. *N Engl J Med* 1991;324:1305–1311.

van Hooft IMS, Grobbee DE, Frölich M, Pols HAP, Hofman A. Alterations in calcium metabolism in young people at risk for primary hypertension. The Dutch Hypertension and Offspring Study. *Hypertension* 1993;21:267–272.

Vanhoutte PM. Is endothelin involved in the pathogenesis of hypertension? *Hypertension* 1993;21:747–751.

Vasdev S, Sampson CA, Prabhakaran VM. Platelet-free calcium and vascular calcium uptake in ethanol-induced hypertensive rats. *Hypertension* 1991;18:116–122.

Vaughan ED Jr, Laragh JH, Gavras I, et al. Volume factor in low and normal renin essential hypertension. Treatment with either spironolactone or chlorthalidone. *Am J Cardiol* 1973;32:523–532.

Veterans Administration Cooperative Study Group on Antihypertensive Agents. Urinary and serum electrolytes in untreated black and white hypertensives. *J Chronic Dis* 1987;40:839–847.

Walker BR, Connacher AA, Webb DJ, Edwards CRW. Glucocorticoids and blood pressure: a role for the cortisol/cortisone shuttle in the control of vascular tone in man. *Clin Sci* 1992;83:171–178.

Watt GCM, Harrap SB, Foy CJW, et al. Abnormalities of glucocorticoid metabolism and the renin-angiotensin system: a four-corners approach to the identification of genetic determinants of blood pressure. *J Hypertens* 1992;10:473–482.

Weber MA, Smith DHG, Neutel JM, Graettinger WF. Arterial properties of early hypertension. *J Hum Hypertens* 1991;5:417–423.

Weder AB. Is there a metabolic link between increased red blood cell lithium-sodium countertransport and hypertension? *Nutr Metab Cardiovasc Dis* 1993;3:38–45.

Weder AB, Serr C, Torretti BA, Bassett DR, Zweifler AJ. Effects of lovastatin treatment on red blood cell and platelet cation transport. *Hypertension* 1991;17:203–209.

Wei L, Clauser E, Alhenc-Gelas F, Corvol P. The two homologous domains of human angiotensin I-converting enzyme interact differently with competitive inhibitors. *J Biol Chem* 1992;267:13398–13405.

Weinberger MH, Fineberg NS. Sodium and volume sensitivity of blood pressure. Age and pressure change over time. *Hypertension* 1991;18:67–71.

Weinberger MH, Miller JZ, Luft FC, Grim CE, Fineberg NS. Definitions and characteristics of sodium sensitivity and blood pressure resistance. *Hypertension* 1986;8(Suppl II):II-127–II-134.

Weinberger MH, Miller JZ, Fineberg NS, Luft FC, Grim CG, Christian JC. Association of haptoglobin with sodium sensitivity and resistance of blood pressure. *Hypertension* 1987;10:443–446.

Weiss ST, Muñoz A, Stein A, Sparrow D, Speizer FE. The relationship of blood led to blood pressure in a longitudinal study of working men. *Am J Epidemiol* 1986;123:800–808.

Welborn TA, Breckenridge A, Rubinstein AH, Dollery CT, Fraser TR. Serum-insulin in essential hypertension and in peripheral vascular disease. *Lancet* 1966;1:1336–1337.

Wessels F, Zumkley H. Sodium metabolism of RBC in hypertensive patients. In: Losse H, Zumkley H, eds. *Intracellular Electrolytes and Arterial Hypertension*. Stuttgart: Georg Thieme Verlag, 1980:59–68.

Whincup PH, Cook DG, Papacosta O. Do maternal and intrauterine factors influence blood pressure in childhood? *Arch Dis Child* 1992;67:1423–1429.

Whitescarver SA, Ott CE, Jackson BA, Guthrie GP Jr, Kotchen TA. Salt-sensitive hypertension: contribution of chloride. *Science* 1984;223:1430–1432.

Widgren BR, Berglund G, Wikstrand J, Andersson OK. Reduced venous compliance in normotensive men with positive family histories of hypertension. *J Hypertens* 1992a;10:459–465.

Widgren BR, Wikstrand J, Berglund G, Andersson OK. Increased response to physical and mental stress in men with hypertensive parents. *Hypertension* 1992b;20:606–611.

Williams GH, Hollenberg NK. Non-modulating hypertension. A subset of sodium-sensitive hypertension. *Hypertension* 1991;17(Suppl I):I-81–I-85.

Williams GH, Dluhy RG, Lifton RP, et al. Non-modulation as an intermediate phenotype in essential hypertension. *Hypertension* 1992;20:788–796.

Williams RR, Hunt SC, Hasstedt SJ, et al. Are there interactions and relations between genetic and environmental factors predisposing to high blood pressure? *Hypertension* 1991;18(Suppl I):I-29–I-37.

Williams SA, Boolell M, MacGregor GA, Smaje LH, Wasserman SM, Tooke JE. Capillary hypertension and abnormal pressure dynamics in patients with essential hypertension. *Clin Sci* 1990;79:5–8.

Wilson DM, Luetscher JA. Plasma prorenin activity and complications in children with insulin-dependent diabetes mellitus. *N Engl J Med* 1990;323:1101–1106.

Wisgerhof M, Brown RD. Increased adrenal sensitivity to angiotensin II in low-renin essential hypertension. *J Clin Invest* 1978;61:1456–1461.

Woo J, Cockram CS, Lau E, Chan A, Swaminathan R. Association between insulin and blood pressure in a community population with normal glucose tolerance. *J Hum Hypertens* 1992;6:343–347.

Woods KL, Walmsley D, Heagerty AM, Turner DL, Lian L-Y. ^{31}P nuclear magnetic resonance measurement of free erythrocyte magnesium concentration in man and its relation to blood pressure. *Clin Sci* 1988;74:513–517.

World Hypertension League. Alcohol and hypertension—implications for management. *J Hum Hypertens* 1991;5:227–232.

Wyss JM. The role of the sympathetic nervous system in hypertension. *Curr Opin Nephrol Hypertens* 1993;2:265–273.

Xie JX, Sasaki S, Joossens JV, Kesteloot H. The relationship between urinary cations obtained from the INTERSALT study and cerebrovascular mortality. *J Hum Hypertens* 1992;6:17–21.

Xie P, McDowell TS, Chapleau MW, Hajduczok G, Abboud FM. Rapid baroreceptor resetting in chronic hypertension. Implications for normalization of arterial pressure. *Hypertension* 1991;17:72–79.

Yanagisawa M, Kurihara H, Kimura S, et al. A novel potent vasoconstrictor peptide produced by vascular endothelial cells. *Nature* 1988;332:411–415.

Yang YJ, Hope ID, Ader M, Bergman RN. Insulin transport across capillaries is rate limiting for insulin action in dogs. *J Clin Invest* 1989;84:1620–1628.

Yarnell JWG, Baker IA, Sweetnam PM, et al. Fibrinogen, viscosity, and white blood cell count are major risk factors for ischemic heart disease. The Caerphilly and Speedwell Collaborative Heart Disease Studies. *Circulation* 1991;83:836–844.

Yin FCP, Ting C-T. Compliance changes in physiological and pathological states. *J Hypertens* 1992;10(Suppl 6):S31–S33.

Yokokawa K, Tahara H, Kohno M, et al. Hypertension associated with endothelin-secreting malignant hemangioendothelioma. *Ann Intern Med* 1991;114:213–215.

Zannad F, Stoltz J-F. Blood rheology in arterial hypertension. *J Hypertens* 1992;10(Suppl 5):S69–S78.

Zavaroni I, Mazza S, Dall'aglio E, Gasparini P, Passeri M, Reaven GM. Prevalence of hyperinsulinaemia in patients with high blood pressure. *J Intern Med* 1992;231:235–240.

Zimmermann S, Phillips RA, Dunaif A, et al. Polycystic ovary syndrome: lack of hypertension despite profound insulin resistance. *J Clin Endocrinol Metab* 1992;75:508–513.

4 Primary Hypertension: Natural History, Special Populations, and Evaluation

Now that the possible causes of primary hypertension have been considered, we turn to its clinical course and complications. We will first view the natural history of the disease if left untreated, examining the specific manner by which hypertension leads to premature cardiovascular damage and the ways such damage is clinically expressed. Additional coverage is provided for special populations—women, the elderly, diabetics, blacks and other ethnic groups—who may follow somewhat different courses. Based on this background, guidelines for the evaluation of the newly diagnosed hypertensive patient are possible.

OVERVIEW

A model of the natural history of hypertension is presented in Figure 4.1. The model indicates that some combination of hereditary and environmental factors sets into motion transient but repetitive perturbations of cardiovascular homeostasis (*prehypertension*), not enough to raise the pressure to levels defined as abnormal but enough to begin the cascade that, over many years, leads to pressures that usually are elevated (*early hypertension*). Some people, abetted by lifestyle changes, may abort the process and return to normotension. The majority, however, progress into *established hypertension*, which, as it persists, may induce a variety of complications identifiable as target organ damage and disease.

The higher the blood pressure (BP) and the longer it remains elevated, the greater the mor-

bidity and mortality. Though some patients with very high untreated BP never have trouble, we have no way to identify in advance those who will have an uncomplicated course, the few who will enter a rapidly accelerating phase (malignant hypertension), or the many who will more slowly, but progressively, develop cardiovascular complications.

The role of hypertension probably is underestimated from morbidity and mortality statistics, which largely are based on death certificates. When a patient dies from a stroke, a heart attack, or renal failure—all directly attributable to uncontrolled hypertension—the stroke, the heart attack, or the renal failure, but not the hypertension, often is listed on the death certificate.

PREHYPERTENSION

As those pathogenetic mechanisms discussed in Chapter 3 start the process that leads to hypertension, certain clues may predict that the patient is in the prehypertensive phase. These include:

—Low birth weight, particularly with large placental size (Law et al., 1993);
—Exaggerated rises of BP during stress (Light et al., 1992) or exercise (Molineux and Steptoe, 1988). Among a group of 341 people who had normal (less than 140/90 mm Hg) resting BP but a rise during a treadmill exercise test to above 225/90 mm Hg, the relative risk of developing a high resting BP over the next 32 months was 2.28 times higher than among those with a lesser rise during the exercise test (Wilson and Meyer, 1981);
—Pressures that are in the higher ranges of normal. As perhaps best seen in data from the Framingham

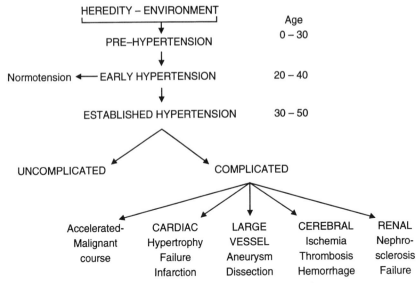

Figure 4.1. Representation of the natural history of untreated essential hypertension.

cohort (Kotchen et al, 1982), the BP tends to "track" over many years, remaining in the same relative position over time (Fig. 4.2). After an initial regression toward the mean between the first examination and the second, 2 years later, those in each segment of BP tend to remain in that segment, with a slow, gradual rise over the 14 years of follow-up.
—Presence of a number of causal or coincidental features. In the 30-year observation of the Framingham offspring, the major contributors to the incidence of hypertension beyond age were adiposity, heart rate, alcohol intake, hematocrit, blood sugar, serum protein, triglyceride, and phosphorus, the last having a negative correlation (Garrison et al., 1987). As described in Chapter 3, the distribution of body fat played a significant role, with a markedly higher incidence of hypertension among those with more upper body fat as determined by subscapular skinfold thickness. As in all other populations, the strongest predictor was the previous level of BP.

EARLY HYPERTENSION

Course of the BP

In most who become hypertensive, the hypertension persists, but in some, the BP returns to normal, presumably not to rise again. As emphasized in Chapter 2, hypertension should be confirmed by multiple readings before the diagnosis is made and therapy is begun. If the second set of readings is considerably lower and the patient is free of obvious vascular complications, the patient should be advised to adhere to a healthy lifestyle and to return every few months for repeat measurement or to self-monitor the BP at home. If the tendency toward a falling pressure

continues, the patient should be simply followed as (one would hope) he or she becomes and remains normotensive.

The wisdom of this course is shown by the Australian Therapeutic Trial (Management Committee, 1982): 12.8% of their patients whose diastolic BPs (DBPs) averaged above 95 on two sets of initial readings had a subsequent fall in DBP to below 95—a fall that persisted over the next year so that they could not be entered into the trial. An even larger portion (47.5%) of those who entered the trial with DBP above 95 and who received only placebo tablets for the next 3 years maintained their average DBP below 95 mm Hg. A significant portion remained below 90 while on placebo, including 11% of those whose initial DBP was as high as 105 to 109 mm Hg.

ESTABLISHED HYPERTENSION

As delineated in Chapter 1, the long-term effects of progressively higher levels of BP on the incidence of stroke and coronary heart disease are clear: In nine prospective observational studies involving 420,000 people with DBP from 70 to 110 mm Hg who were followed from 6 to 25 years, the associations were "positive, continuous and apparently independent" (MacMahon et al., 1990) (see Fig. 1.2).

Uncontrolled Long-Term Observations

In addition to these major studies, smaller groups of hypertensives were followed by single investigators before effective therapies became available (Ranges, 1949; Bechgaard, 1983). Perera (1955) followed 500 patients with casual DBP of 90 mm Hg or higher—150 from before onset and 350 from an uncomplicated phase—until their death. The incidence of complications is given in Table 4.1. The mean age of onset was 32, and the mean survival time was 20 years. Perera summarized his survey of the natural history of hypertension:

... as a chronic illness, more common in women, beginning as a rule in early adult life, related little if at all to pregnancy, and persisting for an average period of two decades before its secondary complicating pathologic features cause death at an average age fifteen to twenty years less than the normal life expectancy. Hypertensive vascular disease may progress at a highly variable rate, but on the whole the patient with this disorder spends most of his hypertensive life with insignificant symptoms and without complications.

Age of Onset

One additional point about Perera's data is worth emphasis: few of his patients experienced the onset of hypertension after age 45. A similar finding was observed in the Cooperative Study of Renovascular Hypertension, wherein the diagnosis of primary hypertension was made with even greater certainty on 1128 patients. Of these, the onset of an elevated BP was documented to be below age 20 in 12% and above age 50 in only 7% (Maxwell, 1975). Thus, hypertension appearing after age 50 should be suspected of being secondary.

On the other hand, in a more recent prospective study of a large, more representative population than the more severely hypertensive patients followed by Perera or seen in the Cooperative Study, 20% of people aged 40 to 69 who developed diastolic BP of 90 mm Hg or higher over

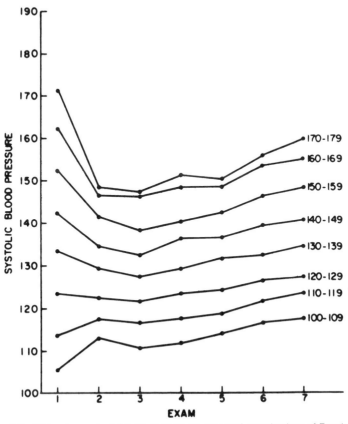

Figure 4.2. Mean systolic BP levels measured every 2 years on repeated examinations of Framingham Study men, aged 30 to 59 years, divided into groups by their initial levels of BP. Those taking antihypertensive drugs are excluded. (From Kotchen JM, McKean HE, Kotchen TA. BP trends with aging. *Hypertension* 1982;4(Suppl 3):128, and by permission of the American Heart Association.)

Table 4.1. Complications in 500 Untreated Hypertensives[a]

Complication	% Affected	Mean Survival after Onset (Years)
Cardiac		
Hypertrophy (seen by radiograph)	74	8
Hypertrophy (seen by ECG)	59	6
Congestive failure	50	4
Angina pectoris	16	5
Cerebral		
Encephalopathy	2	1
Stroke	12	4
Renal		
Proteinuria	42	5
Elevated blood urea nitrogen	18	1
Accelerated phase	7	1

[a]From Perera GA. Hypertensive vascular disease: description and natural history. *J Chron Dis* 1955;1:33–42.

Table 4.2. Five-Year Occurrence of Cardiovascular Events in Newly Diagnosed Hypertensive Subjects and Normotensive Subjects by Age at Baseline[a]

Age Group (Years)	Rate (per 100)		Odds Ratio
	New Hypertensive	Normotensive	
40–49	4.6 (239)	0.9 (4677)	5.2
50–59	5.6 (288)	3.2 (3655)	1.8
60–65	6.5 (153)	5.7 (1301)	1.2

[a]Number of subjects shown in parentheses.
From Buck C, Baker P, Bass M, Donner A. The prognosis of hypertension according to age at onset. *Hypertension* 1987;9:204–208, and by permission of the American Heart Association.

a 5-year period were 60 years of age or older (Buck et al., 1987). Moreover, the rate of developing a significant cardiovascular event among the newly discovered hypertensives was almost as high among those in their 40s as those aged 60 to 65 (Table 4.2). Note that the middle-aged hypertensives were much more likely to develop an event than normotensives of the same age but, as the authors state, "age overtakes hypertension as a cause of cardiovascular disease," so that among those aged 60 to 65, the rate was little different.

Prognosis in Women

In all of these series, women have shown a better prognosis: fewer women enter the accelerated-malignant phase or suffer from coronary artery disease. This lesser incidence of coronary heart disease (CHD) is almost certainly the main reason for the longer survival of women (Isles et al., 1992).

Untreated Patients in Clinical Trials

To those patients left untreated during the 1940s and 1950s when no effective therapy was

readily available, we can add those patients who served as the control populations in the trials of the therapy of hypertension performed in the 1960s, 1970s, and 1980s. Though these trials were not designed to observe the natural history of hypertension, their data can help to further define the course of untreated disease (Table 4.3). Those trials involving elderly patients will be considered separately, under "Hypertension in the Elderly."

The types of patients included in these trials and the manner in which they were followed differed considerably, so comparisons between them are largely inappropriate.

Veterans Administration Cooperative Study Group on Antihypertensive Agents

The publications on these data (Veterans Administration [VA] Cooperative Study Group on Antihypertensive Agents, 1967, 1970, and 1972) are landmarks in the field of clinical hypertension. The VA Study involved a selected population—male veterans who were reliable and cooperative—but the data probably are applicable to most moderately severe hypertensives.

DBP Between 115 and 129. The first VA study described the course of 70 men with initial DBP between 115 and 129 mm Hg who received only placebo. During their follow-up, which averaged 16 months and ranged up to 3 years, these complications were noted:

—6% (4 patients) died, 3 from ruptured aortic aneurysms;

—24% (17 patients) developed accelerated hypertension, cerebral hemorrhage, severe congestive heart failure, or azotemia;

—9% (6 patients) developed myocardial infarction, milder congestive failure, cerebral thrombosis, or transient ischemic attacks.

Thus, in less than 3 years, almost 40% of the patients with DBP between 115 and 129 mm Hg, *initially without severe target organ damage*, developed complications.

DBP Between 90 and 114. As surprising as the results described above were at the time, even more dramatic were the findings in the 194 patients with initial DBP of 90 to 114 mm Hg, a group considered to have mild to moderate hypertension (Veterans Administration Cooperative Study, 1970, 1972). Their initial BPs averaged 157/101, and just over half had some evidence of preexisting hypertensive complications. Maximal follow-up was 5.5 years and averaged 3.3 years. The overall risk to these

patients of developing a morbid event in a 5-year period was 55%.

All of the various complications except progression into accelerated hypertension occurred more frequently in the patients over age 60: 63% developed a serious complication during this short interval, compared to 15% of the patients under age 50. Another 14% of these younger patients had a significant rise in their DBP to above 124 mm Hg, so that without therapy they would be expected to develop complications quickly.

These results showed a more serious and rapidly progressive course of untreated mild to moderate essential hypertension than had been suggested by most previously reported studies. Even among those who had no preexisting target organ damage, 16% developed a complication in only 5 years.

United States Public Health Service Hospital Study

In this study (Smith, 1977), 389 patients with hypertension milder than that of the patients in the VA study were randomly divided into placebo and drug treatment groups and were followed for as long as 7 years. At the onset, none of the patients had evidence of target organ damage, and their mean BP was only 148/99. During the 7-year follow-up, the complications listed in Table 4.3 were noted among the placebo-treated

Table 4.3. Complications Among Control Groups in Trials of Antihypertensive Therapy

	Veterans Administration Cooperative		USPHS (Smith, 1977)	Australian (Management Committee, 1980)	Oslo (Helgeland, 1980)	Medical Research Council (1985)
	1967	1970				
Mean age	51	52	44	50	45	52
Range of diastolic blood pressure	115–129	90–114	90–115	95–109	90–110	95–109
No. on placebo	70	194	196	1617	379	8654
Average follow-up (years)	1.3	3.3	7	3	5.5	5.5
Rate/100 patients for entire trial						
Coronary disease						
Fatal	1	6	2	0.4	0.5	1.1
Nonfatal	3	1	26	4.9	2.9	1.6
Congestive heart failure	3	6	1	0.1	0.2	
Cerebrovascular disease	16	11	3	1.5	1.8	1.3
Renal insufficiency	4	2	1	0.1		
Progression of hypertension	4	10	12	12.2	17.2	11.7
Total mortality	6	10	2	1.2	2.4	2.9

group of truly mild hypertensives, confirming the conclusions of the VA study.

Australian Therapeutic Trial

Over 1600 adults with DBP of 95 to 109 mm Hg, initially free of known cardiovascular disease, were kept on placebo for an average of 3 years (Management Committee, 1980). Over this relatively short period, significantly increased morbidity and mortality occurred only in those whose DBP averaged 100 or higher during this interval.

When the course of the BP among these patients is examined, one sees something interesting. Figure 4.3, which I have constructed from the data in Table 10 of the 1980 *Lancet* paper, divides the patients given placebo into three groups by their DBP at entry (95 to 99, 100 to 104, and 105 to 109). The *horizontal bars* represent the percentage of each entry group whose average DBP during the 3 years of observation was below 90, 90 to 94, 95 to 99, and 100 or above, respectively. Note that even among those whose entry DBP was 105 to 109, 61% had a DBP under 100 while on placebo. For all three groups, 80% had average DBP below 100, and no excess morbidity or mortality occurred in that 80%. The average fall in BP over 3 years of placebo therapy was 14/11 mm Hg, and the DBP was below 95 in 47.5% of the patients at the end of the trial (Management Committee, 1982). Though the fall was greatest in those who lost weight, there was a significant decrease in the average BP even among those who gained weight while on placebo. Another 12.8% of the patients originally screened for this trial whose DBP had averaged above 95 on two occasions had a spontaneous fall in their BP to

below 95 during the year before the trial began. On the other hand, recall from Table 4.3 that 12.2% of these patients had a progressive rise in the DBP to above 110 mm Hg.

A number of implications can be drawn from these observations:

—Many patients not given antihypertensive drugs will have a significant fall in their BP, often to levels considered ''safe'' and not requiring therapy;
—Patients who are free of target organ damage and whose DBPs are below 100 and certainly below 95 can safely be left off active drug therapy for at least a few years;
—If not treated, patients should be kept under close observation.

These conclusions form part of the basis of the approach toward initial management of patients with relatively mild hypertension, which is presented in the next chapter.

Oslo Trial

This trial (Helgeland, 1980) was similar to the Australian trial in that it included only uncomplicated patients free of target organ damage with a DBP below 110 and randomly divided them into nontherapy and drug therapy groups. It differed in being smaller in size, involving only men below 50 years of age, and providing no placebo pills to the control group.

The results were quite similar to those of the Australian trial. About half of the nontreated group had a fall in DBP during the first 3 years. Few complications developed among those whose DBP was initially below 100 mm Hg, whereas 16.4% of those within initial DBP between 100 and 110 mm Hg had a cardiovascular complication.

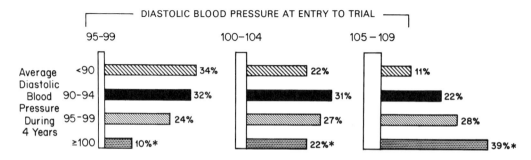

* Excess morbidity and mortality seen only among those with DBP ≥ 100 (22% of the total group), compared to drug treated patients

Figure 4.3. The average diastolic BP over 4 years in the 1617 hypertensive patients treated without drugs in the Australian Therapeutic Trial. Note that the majority of those with initial DBP from 95 all the way up to 109 ended with DBP below 100 and that excess complications were noted only in those whose end DBP was above 100. (Composed from data in Management Committee: *Lancet* 1980;1:1261.)

Medical Research Council Trial (1985)

Half of a much larger group of men and women, aged 35 to 64 years and whose DBP ranged from 90 to 109 mm Hg, were randomly assigned to placebo tablets for an average of 5.5 years. Their rates of subsequent events and progression to more severe hypertension were similar to those in the other trials of mild-to-moderate hypertension (Table 4.3).

From these multiple sources is derived the picture of the natural history of hypertension shown in Figure 4.1. We now will examine the various complications shown at the bottom of that figure.

COMPLICATIONS OF HYPERTENSION

The end of the natural history of untreated hypertension is an increased likelihood of premature disability or death from cardiovascular disease. Before considering the specific types of organ damage and the causes of death related to hypertension, the underlying basis for the arterial pathology caused by hypertension and the manner in which this pathology is expressed clinically will be examined.

As described in Chapter 3, the pathogenesis of hypertension involves structural changes in the resistance arterioles subsumed under the terms "remodeling" and "hypertrophy." These same changes almost certainly are also involved intimately in the development of the small vessel arteriosclerosis that is responsible for most of the target organ damage seen in long-standing hypertension. At the same time, the high pressure accelerates large vessel atherosclerosis (Fig. 4.4). Such arterial and arteriolar sclerosis may be considered the secondary consequence of typical combined systolic-diastolic hypertension, whereas it is the mechanism primarily responsible for the predominantly systolic hypertension so common among the elderly. Atherosclerotic plaques appear most commonly where the pressure is highest, such as in the abdominal aorta, rather than in the low-pressure pulmonary arteries.

Mechanisms of Arterial Damage

The translation of chronically elevated BP into vascular damage involves three interrelated mechanisms: pulsatile flow, endothelial cell changes, and the remodeling and growth of smooth muscle cells. It should be noted that the higher systolic blood pressures (SBPs) are likely more involved in these processes than are the lower diastolic levels, which accounts for the closer approximation of cardiovascular risk to SBP noted in Chapter 1.

Pulsatile Flow

O'Rourke (1992) has summarized the evidence concerning the importance of pulsatile phenomena:

Hypertension-related changes occur in large artery structure and function both in experimental animals and in man. Arteries are stiffer, as a consequence of higher pressure and accelerated age-related changes in the media. Pulse wave velocity in the arterial wall is faster, so that the impulse generated by ventricular ejection returns from the peripheral arteriolar terminations much earlier than in young normotensive subjects. This reflected wave can usually be discerned as a discrete event. Instead of returning during diastole, the wave returns during systole, and increases systolic pressure in the central aorta and left ventricle. Thus, in hypertension, left ventricular (LV) load is increased by three factors, an increase in peripheral resistance, a decrease in aortic distensibility and early wave reflection from the periphery of the body [Fig. 4.5]. . . . In hypertension, cardiac hypertrophy is attributable to a sustained increase in LV afterload. Longstanding hypertension and hypertrophy lead to age-related degenerative changes, caused by the effects of cyclic stress on the arterial walls. In hypertension, these stresses are increased and the degenerative changes progress more rapidly.

Endothelial Cell Changes

The increasing awareness of the probable multiple active roles of the endothelium in the pathogenesis of hypertension described in Chapter 3 has been accompanied by increasing evidence that hypertension, in turn, affects the endothelial cells and that these endothelial changes may be involved intimately in intimal thickening and atherosclerosis (Chobanian, 1990) (Fig. 4.6). In particular, the responses of vascular endothelium to fluid shear stresses that primarily are manifested near arterial branching obviously are involved in the focal occurrence of atherosclerosis in such regions of disturbed flow (De Paola et al., 1992).

In experimental animals, hypertension is associated with a decreased basal and stimulated release of endothelium-derived nitric oxide (Lüscher et al., 1992). In humans using high-resolution ultrasonography over superficial arteries, similar endothelial dysfunction is present even in children with risk factors for atherosclerosis before anatomic evidence of plaque formation can be found in the arteries studied (Celermajer et al., 1992).

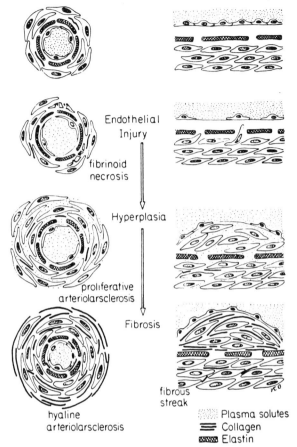

Endothelial
Injury

fibrinoid
necrosis

Hyperplasia

proliferative
arteriolarsclerosis

Fibrosis

fibrous
streak

hyaline
arteriolarsclerosis

▧ Plasma solutes
≡ Collagen
▨ Elastin

Figure 4.4. Small vessel arteriosclerosis, or arteriolosclerosis (*left*), has many features in common with large vessel atherosclerosis (*right*). This diagram outlines mechanisms whereby both lesions might originate from a common source (endothelial injury), which leads to entry of serum factors that stimulate replication of smooth muscle cells. In the large vessel, the result is accumulation of smooth muscle cells in the intima and formation of an atherosclerotic plaque. In small vessels, the result is hypertrophy, hyperplasia, and fibrosis of the vascular media. (From Schwartz SM, Ross R. Cellular proliferation in atherosclerosis and hypertension. *Prog Cardiovasc Dis* 1984;26:355.)

Smooth Muscle Cell Remodeling and Growth

The effects of hypertension on the growth of smooth muscle were shown indirectly by Bierman et al. (1981), who cultured arterial smooth muscle cells from tissue both proximal to and distal from aortic coarctations that had been resected from patients. Cells from the proximal area had a shorter in vitro life span (fewer replications) and a slower growth rate. These findings suggest that the accelerated rate of atherosclerosis typically found in the aorta proximal to the coarctation is secondary to an increased number of previous replications of smooth muscle cells in response to high arterial pressure. Such stimulation of arterial smooth muscle migration and proliferation by hypertension has been demonstrated (Chobanian, 1990). A number of stimuli

are likely involved in smooth muscle proliferation, some arising from platelets and other circulating cells, some arising from the endothelium, and some arising from the smooth muscle cells themselves (Bondjers et al., 1991).

Types of Arterial Lesions

Aggravation of atherosclerosis is only one of the pathologic consequences of hypertension. None is specific: Charcot-Bouchard cerebral aneurysms, which were believed to be relatively specific for hypertension, are found in normotensive older people. The more common vascular lesions found in hypertension are described below:

—Hyperplastic or proliferative arteriolosclerosis (Fig. 4.4), a proliferative reaction of the vessel wall to injury, seen most commonly with DBP levels above 120 mm Hg;

—Hyaline arteriolosclerosis (Fig. 4.4) with thickening and hyalinization of the intima and media that results in narrowing of the lumen;

—Miliary aneurysms in small cerebral penetration arterioles, usually at their first branching, representing poststenotic dilations beyond areas of intimal thickening. When they rupture, they cause the cerebral hemorrhages so typical of hypertension;

—Atherosclerosis or nodular arteriosclerosis that produces plaques where thrombi form that likely are responsible for the ischemia and infarction of heart, brain, kidney, and other organs that occur more frequently among hypertensives;

—Other defects in the media of arteries (such as those at the circle of Willis causing subarachnoid hemorrhages) may be accentuated by hypertension

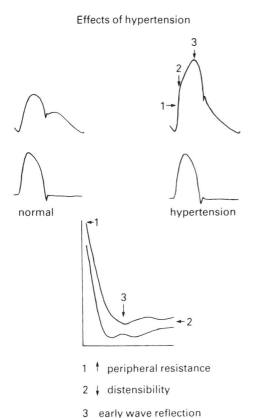

Effects of hypertension

normal   hypertension

1 ↑ peripheral resistance

2 ↓ distensibility

3 early wave reflection

Figure 4.5. Effect of hypertension on contour of the ascending aortic pressure wave (*top*) generated by the same ventricular ejection wave (*center*) and on the modulus of ascending aortic impedance (*bottom*). Aortic stiffening increases the pressure at peak systolic flow and increases characteristic impedance. Early wave reflection causes a late systolic pressure wave and shifts impedance curves to the right. The term "modulus" refers to a coefficient pertaining to a physical property; "impedance" is the ratio of the force on a system undergoing motion to the velocity of the particles in the system. (From O'Rourke M. Systolic blood pressure: arterial compliance and early wave reflection, and their modification by antihypertensive therapy. *J Hum Hypertens* 1989;3:47.)

but probably are congenital. Medial damage in the wall of the aorta may lead to the formation of large plaques with eventual aneurysmal dilation and rupture. The process of cystic medial necrosis that is responsible for some aortic dissections also occurs more frequently in hypertensives.

Causes of Death

Untreated Hypertension

Death may result when these arterial lesions either rupture or become occluded enough to cause ischemia or infarction of the tissues they supply. The overall increase in mortality associated with hypertension was examined in Chapter 1; Table 4.4 provides a more detailed look at the causes of death in hypertensives. The series in the table include different types of patients, so comparisons between them should be avoided. The following conclusions can be drawn from these data:

—As shown in the data from Smith et al. (1950), cardiovascular diseases are responsible for a higher proportion of deaths as the severity of the hypertension worsens;

—In general, patients with severe, resistant disease die of strokes; those presenting with advanced retinopathy and renal damage die of renal failure; the majority, with moderately high pressure, die of the complications of ischemic heart disease;

—Heart disease remains the leading cause of death.

Treated Hypertension

Considerable data show that since the advent of effective antihypertensive therapy, the nature of the heart disease has changed from congestive heart failure to coronary artery disease. As Doyle (1988) stated:

Data indicate that antihypertensive treatment has greatly reduced the incidence of complications of hypertension that are directly due to the raised BP, most notably congestive heart failure. By contrast, the percentage of deaths due to coronary events has risen since the introduction of antihypertensive drug treatment, leaving it as the major cause of death in treated hypertension. Presumably the removal of other causes of death, and the lengthened survival time in hypertensive patients, allows the development of coronary artery disease, which is apparently little affected if at all by control of BP.

Consider survival rather than mortality: Figure 4.7 shows the probability of surviving over an average 9.5-year interval for the persons aged 50 years and older selected as a representative sample of the adult United States population for the 1971 to 1975 National Health and Nutrition Examination Survey I (Cornoni-Huntley et al.,

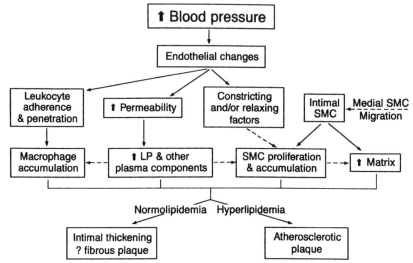

Figure 4.6. Diagram summarizing the effects of hypertension on the arterial intima. *SMC,* smooth muscle cell; *LP,* lipoprotein; ↑, increased. (From Chobanian AV. 1989 Corcoran Lecture: adaptive and maladaptive responses of the arterial wall to hypertension. *Hypertension* 1990;15:666.)

Table 4.4. Causes of Death in Primary Hypertension

			Percentage of Deaths			
	Year	No of Deaths	Heart Disease[a]	Stroke	Renal Failure	Nonvascular Causes
Untreated						
Janeway, 1913	1903–1912	212	33	14	23	30
Hodge and Smirk, 1967	1959–1964	173	48	22	10	20
Bechgaard, 1976	1932–1938	293	45	16	10	29
Smith et al., 1950	1924–1948	376				
Group 1[b]		100	28	9	3	60
Group 2		100	46	17	2	35
Group 3		76	52	18	16	14
Group 4		100	22	16	59	3
Bauer, 1976	1955–1974	144	41	34	15	10
Treated						
Breckenridge, 1970	1952–1959	87	18	28	44	10
Breckenridge et al., 1970	1960–1967	203	38	21	29	11
Strate et al., 1986	1970–1980	132	42	7	7	44
Bulpitt et al., 1986	1971–1981	410	51	18	3	28
Isles et al., 1986	1968–1983	750	52	23	?	25

[a]Includes ischemic heart disease and congestive failure.
[b]Grouping according to Keith-Wagener classification of hypertensive retinopathy.

1989). It is obvious that more hypertensive women but fewer blacks survive, further pointing out the need to consider the makeup of the population in examining the consequences of hypertension.

Specific Organ Involvement

Having tabulated the major causes of death resulting from the arterial pathology related to hypertension, let us examine in more detail the pathophysiology and consequences of these various complications. Thereafter, the clinical and laboratory manifestations of the target organ damage will be incorporated into guidelines for the evaluation of the hypertensive patient.

In general, the complications of hypertension can be considered either ''hypertensive'' or ''atherosclerotic'' (Table 4.5). Those listed as hypertensive are caused more directly by the increased level of the BP per se, whereas the atherosclerotic complications have multiple causes, hypertension playing a variable role (Birkenhägẹr and de Leeuw, 1992). However, the major contribution of hypertension to the atherosclerotic diseases is shown clearly by the epidemiologic data (Fig. 4.8).

Hypertensive Heart Disease

Hypertension both accelerates the development of coronary artery disease (CAD) and puts increased tension on the myocardium, causing it to hypertrophy. These conditions in turn may result in myocardial ischemia, and this ischemia coupled with LV hypertrophy (LVH) may lead to congestive heart failure (CHF), arrhythmias, and sudden death (Massie et al., 1989) (Fig. 4.9). Each of these conditions will now be covered in more detail.

Systolic and Diastolic Dysfunction. The earliest changes in the heart in the presence of hypertension are functional, either supernormal systolic function (de Simone et al., 1988) or,

more commonly, impaired diastolic function manifested by slow diastolic filling that reflects decreased diastolic relaxation (Rosenthal, 1992). An increase in late diastolic filling reflects an increased contribution by atrial contraction as a result of reduced atrial emptying during the early filling phase caused by the reduced LV compliance (Fagard, 1992). By itself, impaired diastolic function may interfere with maximal exercise capacity and, over time, is associated with heart failure and coronary disease (Brogan et al., 1992).

LV Hypertrophy. The most common effect of hypertension on the heart is hypertrophy of the left ventricle. Hypertrophy as a response to the increased afterload of elevated systemic vascular resistance can be viewed as compensatory or protective up to a certain point. Beyond that point, LVH is a powerful predictor of serious cardiovascular sequelae (Devereux et al., 1992).

Some increase in LV mass can be seen among children with pressures that are in the upper

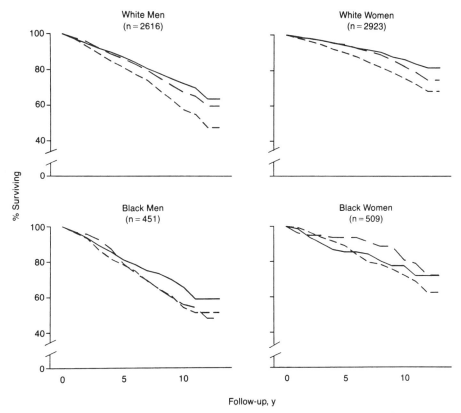

Figure 4.7. Probability of survival for up to 12 years according to BP category—normal (*solid line*), borderline hypertension (*long dashes*), and definite hypertension (*short dashes*)—among persons aged 50 years and over (National Health Epidemiologic Follow-up Study [NHEFS]). (From Cornoni-Huntley J, LaCroix AZ, Havlik RJ. Race and sex differentials in the impact of hypertension in the United States. The National Health and Nutrition Examination Survey I Epidemiology Follow-up Study. *Arch Intern Med* 1989;149:780.)

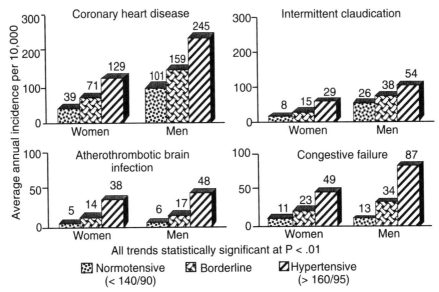

Figure 4.8. The age-adjusted risk of cardiovascular morbidity according to hypertensive status in the Framingham Heart Study. (From Kannel WB, Sorli P. Hypertension in Framingham. In: Paul O [ed]. *Epidemiology and Control of Hypertension.* New York: Stratton International Medical Books, 1975;553.)

Table 4.5. Complications of Hypertension

Hypertensive
  Accelerated-malignant hypertension (grades III and IV retinopathy)
  Encephalopathy
  Cerebral hemorrhage
  Left ventricular hypertrophy
  Congestive heart failure
  Renal insufficiency
  Aortic dissection

Atherosclerotic
  Cerebral thrombosis
  Myocardial infarction
  Coronary artery disease
  Claudication syndromes

From Smith WM. Treatment of mild hypertension: results of a ten-year intervention trial. *Circ Res* 1977;40(Suppl 1):98–105, and by permission of the American Heart Association.

20 percentiles, but not elevated (Hansen et al., 1992). In normotensive adults, LV mass is directly related to the risk for developing subsequent hypertension (de Simone et al., 1991b), suggesting that LVH may be involved in the genetic or other factors responsible for the pathogenesis of hypertension.

Prevalence. Whereas LVH is identified by electrocardiography in only 5 to 10% of hypertensives, LVH is found in about half of untreated hypertensives by echocardiography (Ganau et al., 1992). In Ganau et al.'s study of 165 patients, 13% had increased relative wall thickness with

normal ventricular mass (concentric remodeling), 27% had increased mass with normal relative wall thickness (eccentric hypertrophy) and only 8% had the typical hypertensive pattern of increased mass and relative wall thickness (concentric hypertrophy) (Fig. 4.10).

Pathogenesis. Independent of the BP, the hemodynamic volume load on the heart is an important determinant of LVH. Devereux et al. (1992) found a closer correlation between LV mass and LV stroke volume (0.60 vs. 0.40) than between LV stroke volume and SBP. This involvement of volume load likely explains the strong correlation between LVH and dietary sodium intake (Liebson et al., 1993). Other postulated stimuli for LVH include increased body size (both height and weight), increased whole blood viscosity, and increased sympathetic nervous and renin-angiotensin system activity (Devereux et al., 1992).

The basic signals that initiate and maintain myocardial hypertrophy likely include a number of growth factors whose effects may be transmitted via the α_1-adrenergic receptor to activate intracellular transducing proteins and ribonucleic acid (RNA) transcription factors (Frohlich et al., 1992). An important role of the renin-angiotensin system is suggested by the impressive effect of angiotensin-converting enzyme (ACE) inhibitors in causing regression of LVH and preventing remodeling after a myocardial infarction (MI) (Pfeffer et al., 1992), particularly since all components of the system are in cardiac tissue (Paul and Ganten, 1992). Elevated levels of aldosterone are associated with myocardial fibrosis (Weber and Brilla, 1991). A soluble factor identified from hypertrophic hearts, termed "myotrophin," induces early response genes and may be a biochemical link between hemodynamic stress and hypertrophy (Mukherjee et al., 1993).

Consequences. Hypertensives with LVH are more likely to experience cardiovascular morbidity and mortality than are those without LVH (Levy et al., 1990; Ghali et al., 1992). The pattern of LVH was found to significantly influence mortality over an average of 10.2 years in a group of 253 hypertensives without preexisting cardiac disease (Koren et al., 1991) (Fig. 4.11). These findings likely reflect the known associations of LVH with ventricular ectopy and sudden death (Schmieder and Messerli, 1992), as well

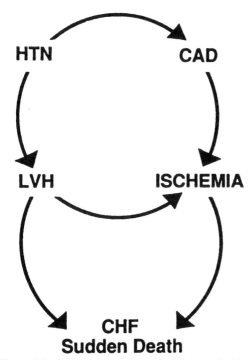

Figure 4.9. Schematic representation of the probable interrelationships between hypertension *(HTN)*, left ventricular hypertrophy *(LVH)*, and the various manifestations of hypertensive heart disease. The probable synergism between LVH and myocardial ischemia related to coronary artery disease *(CAD)* is emphasized and is likely to be responsible for many of the cases of congestive heart failure *(CHF)* and sudden death. (From Massie BM, Tubau JF, Szlachcic J, O'Kelly BF. Hypertensive heart disease: the critical role of left ventricular hypertrophy. *J Cardiovasc Pharmacol* 1989;13[suppl 1]:18.)

as with subendocardial ischemia because of the greater transmural resistance to microvascular perfusion (Fujii et al., 1992).

Patients with substantial concentric LVH may have high ejection fractions, reflecting small LV end-diastolic cavity dimensions. A group of such patients with "hypertensive hypertrophic cardiomyopathy," all elderly and mostly female and black, presented with dyspnea or chest pain suggesting heart failure (Topol et al., 1985; Karam et al., 1989). Their status was worsened by vasodilator medications that reduced afterload and caused hypotension by further increasing the already excessive LV emptying and reducing diastolic filling.

Regression. Since the presence of LVH may connote a number of deleterious effects of hypertension on cardiac function, a great deal of effort has been expended in showing that treatment of hypertension will cause LVH to regress. This will be explored further in Chapter 7, in which various agents are covered. With regression, LV function may or may not improve, but the long-term risk of cardiovascular events appears to be reduced (Kannel et al., 1988; Koren et al., 1991).

Congestive Heart Failure. The various alterations of systolic and diastolic function seen with LVH obviously could progress into LV pump failure or CHF. Hypertension is present in 75% of patients who develop CHF, tripling the risk of normotensives (Levy et al., 1993). Hypertension remains the major preventable factor in the disease that is involved in over 200,000 deaths and almost 2 million events each year in the United States, a number that will increase with the increasing number of elderly people (Schocken et al., 1992). Data suggest that antihypertensive treatment does not completely prevent CHF but postpones its development by several decades (Yusuf et al., 1989).

Most episodes of CHF in hypertensive patients are associated with dilated cardiomyopathy and a reduced ejection fraction. However, about 40% of episodes of CHF are associated with preserved LV systolic function but with diastolic dysfunction induced by LVH, fibrosis, and ischemia and increased afterload (Bonow and Udelson, 1992). Since all of these factors are common to hypertension, the common presence of hypertension in such patients is easy to understand.

Coronary Artery Disease. As described in Chapter 1, hypertension is quantitatively the largest risk factor for CAD. The development of myocardial ischemia reflects an imbalance

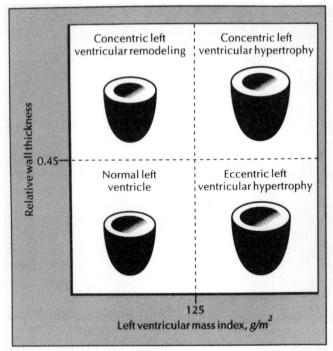

Figure 4.10. Identification of patterns of left ventricular geometry in hypertensive patients according to increases in left ventricular mass (*horizontal axis*) and relative wall thickness (*vertical axis*). Relative wall thickness is measured as posterior wall thickness times two divided by left ventricular internal dimension. *Dotted lines* denote cutpoints. (From Koren MJ, Devereux RB. Mechanism, effects, and reversal of left ventricular hypertrophy in hypertension. *Curr Opin Nephrol Hypertens* 1993;28:87.)

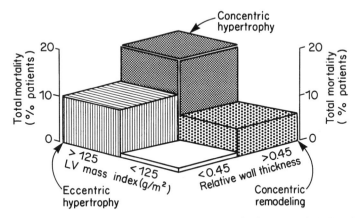

Figure 4.11. The relation of total mortality to patterns of left ventricular *(LV)* geometry in 253 patients with essential hypertension. Mortality rates were highest in patients with concentric hypertrophy, lowest in patients with normal ventricular geometry, and intermediate in patients with eccentric hypertrophy and concentric remodeling (P < .001 by analysis of variance). (Adapted from Koren MJ, Devereux RB, Casale PN, Savage DD, Laragh JH. Relation of left ventricular mass and geometry to morbidity and mortality in uncomplicated essential hypertension. *Ann Intern Med* 1991;114:345.)

between myocardial oxygen supply and demand. Hypertension, by reducing the supply and increasing the demand, can easily tip the balance. As noted in Chapter 1, mortality from CAD rises progressively with increasing BP and, as seen in Figure 4.8, the presence of hypertension markedly increases the incidence of MI.

Mechanisms. Hypertension is associated with multiple factors that accelerate CAD, including the following:

—Acceleration of atherosclerotic narrowing of larger coronary arteries (French et al., 1993);

—Abnormally high resistance of the coronary microvasculature, both in the absence of LVH (Brush et al., 1988) and (even more so) in the presence of LVH (Houghton et al., 1992);

—"Limited coronary reserve" (i.e., reduced capacity for the coronary bed to vasodilate), which reduces the expected increase in coronary blood flow in response to various stimuli (Polese et al., 1991). This impairment is ordinarily related to three conditions: (1) myocardial hypertrophy that outstrips the vascular bed; (2) thickened coronary arteries that are less able to dilate and; (3) the higher cavitary pressures within the left ventricle that impede blood flow through these vessels. As will be noted in Chapter 7, this limited reserve may be responsible for additional ischemia when perfusion pressure is lowered by antihypertensive therapy;

—Increased frequency of both symptomatic and asymptomatic myocardial ischemia, often accompanied by malignant ventricular arrhythmias (Zehender et al., 1992).

Clinical Manifestations. These multiple mechanisms render hypertensives more susceptible to silent ischemia (Hedblad and Janzon, 1992), unrecognized myocardial infarction, and sudden death (Kannel et al., 1985). Hypertension may play an even greater role in the pathogenesis of CAD than is commonly realized, since preexisting hypertension may go unrecognized in patients first seen after an MI. Although acute rises in BP may follow the onset of ischemic pain (McAlpine et al., 1988), the BP often falls immediately after the infarct and may never return to its prior high level. Of 58 hypertensives who had experienced an MI, 37 showed a transient normalization of their BP, although most redeveloped hypertension by 3 months (Astrup et al., 1978).

Once an MI occurs, the prognosis is affected by both the preexisting and the subsequent BP. The total mortality over the first year after an acute MI was 35% in those with preexisting hypertension, compared to 25% in those who were normotensive; furthermore, reinfarctions were twice as common in the first group (Herlitz et al., 1992). An increase in post-MI mortality has been noted among those whose BP fell significantly, presumably a reflection of poor pump function (Kannel et al., 1980). On the other hand, among these subjects, if the BP remained elevated, the prognosis was even worse, presumably representing a severe load on a damaged myocardium so that care must be taken with patients having either lower or higher BP after an infarction.

Large Vessel Disease

Hypertension is a risk factor for the development of peripheral vascular disease that usually is manifested as intermittent claudication (Fig. 4.8). Large vessel disease is accompanied by a high risk of death from cardiovascular causes (Criqui et al., 1992).

Abdominal Aortic Aneurysm. The incidence of abdominal aortic aneurysms is increasing, likely a consequence of the increasing number of elderly people (Grand Round, 1993). The majority of patients with aortic aneurysm are hypertensive (Reed et al., 1992). Among 201 hypertensive men over age 60, 9% were found to have an aortic aneurysm by ultrasonography, with the size varying from 3.6 to 5.9 cm (Lederle et al., 1988).

Aortic Dissection. As many as 80% of patients with aortic dissection have hypertension (Lindsay, 1992). The mechanism of dissection likely involves the combination of high pulsatile wave stress and accelerated atherosclerosis described under "Mechanisms of Arterial Damage," since the higher the pressure, the greater the likelihood of dissection.

Aortic dissection may occur either in the ascending aorta (proximal, or Type A) or in the descending aorta (distal, or Type B). Hypertension is more frequently a factor with distal dissections, whereas Marfan's syndrome and cystic medial necrosis are seen more frequently with the proximal lesion (Lindsay, 1992).

Takayasu's Disease. Hypertension is present in about half of patients with Takayasu's arteriopathy, a chronic inflammatory disease of large arteries reported most frequently in Japan and India (Ishikawa, 1988).

Cerebrovascular Disease

Each year over 400,000 people in the United States have a stroke, and about one-third of them die, making stroke the third most common cause of death after heart disease and cancer. In industrialized countries, strokes are responsible for 10% to 12% of all deaths (Bonita, 1992) with higher rates in places where coronary disease is less common, such as Japan (Reed, 1990). The stroke death rate is even higher, by about 50%, among United States blacks, a rate similar to that noted in numerous other groups with low per capita income (Modan and Wagener, 1992). Mortality rates from stroke have fallen markedly over the past 35 years in most industrialized countries, but the incidence has risen, likely because of the larger number of elderly people and the introduction of computed tomography, which increases the detection of smaller strokes. However, in the Framingham cohort, a higher incidence has been noted in subjects aged 55 to 64 in three successive decades beginning in 1953 (Wolf et al., 1992); thus, other factors likely are involved.

About 70% of strokes are ischemic, caused by either arterial thrombosis or embolism; 10% to 15% are caused by intraparenchymal hemorrhage; another 5% are caused by subarachnoid hemorrhage; and 5% to 15% are of unknown cause (Anderson et al., 1993). Transient ischemic attacks (TIAs)—acute episodes of focal loss of cerebral or visual function lasting less than 24 hours and attributed to inadequate blood supply—with symptoms of sudden onset that last for less than 24 hours may arise from emboli from atherosclerotic plaques and are closely associated with CAD (Scheinberg, 1991).

Role of Hypertension. Even more than with heart disease, hypertension is the major cause of stroke. As noted by Phillips and Whisnant (1992):

A wealth of epidemiological evidence indicates that hypertension is the most important modifiable risk factor for TIA, ischemic stroke, and focal intracerebral hemorrhage. Epidemiological observation and laboratory experimentation have shown that hypertension predisposes to stroke by (1) aggravating atherosclerosis in the aortic arch and cervicocerebral arteries; (2) causing arteriosclerosis and lipohyalinosis in the small-diameter penetrating cerebral end arteries; and (3) promoting heart disease that may be complicated by stroke.

The risk of stroke is even greater in hypertensives with other risk factors, including diabetes, smoking, prior cardiovascular disease, atrial fibrillation and LVH (Wolf et al., 1991), blood hyperviscosity (Coull et al., 1991), and a high hematocrit (Perry et al., 1992).

As noted in Chapter 1, isolated systolic hypertension in the elderly is associated with a 2 to 4 times greater incidence of strokes than seen in normotensive people of the same age. Elderly hypertensives more often have silent cerebrovascular disease (Hougaku et al., 1992), which eventually may lead to brain atrophy and vascular dementia (Salerno et al., 1992). Even in neurologically asymptomatic, middle-aged hypertensives, regional and global reductions in cerebral blood flow are found in one-third (Nobili et al., 1993).

Whether hypertensive or normotensive before their stroke, the majority of stroke patients at the time they are first seen will have a transient elevation of BP that spontaneously falls within a few days (Carlberg et al., 1993). Therefore, caution is advised in lowering the BP in the immediate poststroke period, as noted further in Chapter 7.

Extracranial Carotid Disease. Perhaps of greatest importance, because more can be done to prevent progression of the disease to stroke, is the recognition of extracranial carotid disease, which also is more common in hypertensives (Lusiani et al., 1990). Atherosclerotic disease in extracranial carotid arteries, often identified by bruits, is associated with a greater likelihood of TIAs and other cerebrovascular events. As identified by ultrasonography, both geometric and functional changes within the common carotid artery often are associated with LVH, both reflecting adaptations to hypertension and both associated with a higher risk of cardiovascular complications (Roman et al., 1992).

Renal Disease

Renal dysfunction, both structural and functional, is almost always demonstrable in hypertensive patients, even those with minimally elevated pressures. Pathologically, the main changes of milder degrees of hypertension are hyalinization and sclerosis of the walls of the afferent arterioles, referred to as "arteriolar nephrosclerosis." Renal involvement usually is asymptomatic and not demonstrable by usual clinical testing. Microalbuminuria, which reflects intraglomerular hypertension (Harvey et al., 1992), is the earliest manifestation. Any degree of proteinuria poses a risk of death (Damsgaard et al., 1990). The elevated serum uric acid level present in up to half of untreated hypertensives likely reflects nephrosclerosis (Messerli et al., 1980).

The loss of renal function grows progressively as the BP increases and the elevation continues (Perneger et al., 1993), but only a minority of hypertensives die as a result of renal failure (Table 4.4). Nonetheless, hypertension remains a leading risk for end-stage renal disease (ESRD), and is partly responsible for the much higher incidence of ESRD in blacks than in whites in the United States (Perneger and Whelton, 1993). Blacks suffer greater renal damage than whites with equal degrees of hypertension;

despite good control of their hypertension, their renal function may worsen (Walker et al., 1992).

Conclusion

In every patient, the damage from hypertension to the various target organs that have been described should be assessed in order to determine the need for therapy and to ensure that therapy primarily protects the most vulnerable parts of the cardiovascular system. Before turning to evaluation, however, I will describe groups of people whose hypertension, for various reasons, may have a different course than that seen in the predominately male, white, middle-aged populations observed in the clinical trials and long-term observational studies that have been reviewed.

SPECIAL POPULATIONS

Special populations include a major part of the hypertensive population: the elderly, women, diabetics, the obese, and blacks and other ethnic groups.

Hypertension in the Elderly

Two patterns of hypertension are seen in the elderly: combined systolic and diastolic, the carryover of primary (essential) hypertension common to middle age; and isolated systolic hypertension (ISH), the more frequent form in those over age 65. However, since the major consequences and, as is noted in Chapter 7, the therapy for both are quite similar, most of this discussion will not make a distinction between the two.

Prevalence

As noted in Chapter 1, whereas diastolic pressures tend to plateau before age 60 and drop thereafter, systolic pressures rise progressively (Fig. 1.4). Therefore, the incidence of ISH—defined as systolic $\geq$ 160, diastolic $\leq$ 90—progressively rises with age: In a recent meta-analysis of diverse, industrialized populations, the prevalence of ISH rose from 5% at age 60 to 12.6% at 70 and 23.6% at 80 (Staessen et al., 1990). The problem of "white coat" hypertension is just as common in the elderly so that out-of-the-office readings should be obtained if possible (Wittenberg et al., 1992).

Pseudohypertension. In addition to white coat hypertension, the elderly may have artifactually elevated pressures by usual indirect cuff measurements because of medial calcification of the large arteries, which precludes compression and collapse of the brachial artery. Therefore,

the manometer shows much higher pressures in the balloon than are present within the artery, giving rise to pseudohypertension (Oster and Materson, 1992).

Risks

At all ages, systolic pressures are better predictors of cardiovascular risk than are diastolic pressures. Those with ISH have more coronary disease and strokes, with an approximate 1% increase in the rate of mortality from all causes for each 1-mm rise in systolic pressure (Silagy and McNeil, 1992). Data from multiple populations are remarkably consistent: ISH is associated with increased mortality.

A possible exception to the progressive risks of every increment in systolic pressure has been claimed for the very old, people over age 85. In a 3-year follow-up of 724 noninstitutionalized 84- to 88-year-old people in Finland, the lowest mortality rates were noted in those with systolic pressure of 140 to 169 and diastolic pressure of 70 to 99 (Heikinheima et al., 1990). Table 4.6 summarizes data from six controlled trials of treatment of elderly hypertensives, showing the high rates of morbidity and mortality among the half left on placebo during the 2 to 5 years of follow-up. Total mortality, both from coronary disease and from stroke, is much higher in this group than in the middle-aged populations listed in Table 4.3.

Pathophysiology

The basic mechanism for the progressive rise in SBP with age is the loss of distensibility and elasticity in the large capacitance arteries, a process that was nicely demonstrated over 50 years ago (Hallock and Benson, 1937) (Fig. 4.12). Increasing volumes of saline were infused into the tied-off aortas taken from patients at death whose ages ranged from the 20s to the 70s. The pressure within the aortas from the elderly subjects rose much higher with very small increases in volume compared to younger subjects, reflecting the rigidity of the vessels.

Hemodynamically, ISH is characterized by a decreased compliance of the large arteries, high peripheral resistance, abnormal diastolic filling, well preserved to increased systolic function, and increased LV mass (Pearson et al., 1991). Cardiac output and blood volume may be diminished. The decreased volume, combined with the run-off from the smaller reservoir provided by the rigid large arteries, lowers diastolic pressure and further widens the pulse pressure.

Table 4.6 Complications Among Control Groups in Trials of Elderly Hypertensives

Complication	Australian (Management) 1981	EWPHE (Amery) 1985	Coope & Warrender 1986	SHEP 1991	STOP-HT (Dahlöf) 1991	MRC 1992
Mean age	64	72	69	72	76	70
Blood pressure at entry						
Systolic	<200	160–239	190–230	160–219	<180–230	160–209
Diastolic	95–109	90–119	105–120	<90	90–120	<115
Mean	165/101	182/101	197/100	170/77	195/102	185/91
No. on placebo	289	424	465	2371	815	2113
Average follow-up (years)	3	4.6	4.4	4.5	2.1	5.7
Rate/100 patients for entire trial:						
Coronary disease						
Fatal	1.3	11.8	6.0	3.4	2.5	5.2
Nonfatal	8.3	2.8	2.2	3.4	2.7	2.3
Congestive heart failure		5.4	7.7	4.5	4.8	
Cerebrovascular disease	4.2	13.7	9.4	6.8	6.6	6.4
Progression of hypertension		6.8		15.0	9.3	8.3
Total mortality	3.1	35.1	14.8	10.2	7.9	15.0

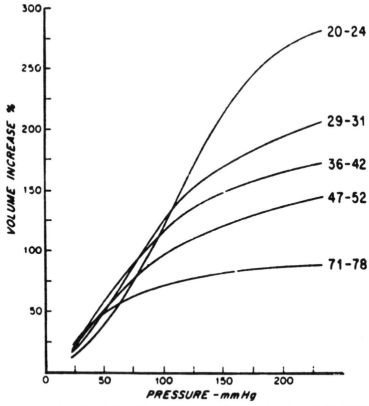

Figure 4.12. These curves show the relation of the percentage of increase in volume to the increase in pressure for five different age groups and were constructed from the mean values obtained from a number of aortas excised at autopsy. (From Hallock P, Benson IC. Studies of the elastic properties of human isolated aorta. *J Clin Invest* 1937;16:595.)

Elderly patients with combined systolic and diastolic hypertension (compared to younger hypertensives) have lower cardiac output, intravascular volume, renal blood flow, and plasma renin activity, and higher peripheral vascular resistance, LV wall thickness, and mass (Messerli et al., 1983).

If an abrupt rise in both systolic and diastolic pressure is noted in an elderly patient, atherosclerotic renovascular disease should be suspected. Less commonly, showers of cholesterol emboli into the kidneys from an aortic aneurysm (usually after arteriography) give rise to hypertension (Preston and Materson, 1992).

Postural Hypotension

Definition and Incidence. A fall in systolic pressure of 20 mm Hg after 1 minute of quiet standing usually is taken as an abnormal response indicative of postural hypotension. In the generally healthy population of elderly men and women enrolled in the Systolic Hypertension in the Elderly Program, postural hypotension was found in 10.4% at 1 minute after arising from a seated position and in 12.0% at 3 minutes, with 17.3% having hypotension at one or both intervals (Applegate et al., 1991). The prevalence would likely have been higher if the patients had been tested after rising from a supine position.

Mechanism. Normal aging is associated with various changes that may lead to postural hypotension. Cardiac output falls with age; in the elderly with hypertension, it is even lower. When elderly subjects are put under passive postural stress (60° upright tilt), their stroke volume and cardiac index fall further because of an inability to reduce end-systolic volume (Shannon et al., 1991). These ''normal'' changes obviously predispose the elderly to postural hypotension from any process that further reduces fluid volume or vascular integrity. Splanchnic pooling of blood after eating may lead to profound postprandial hypotension.

Moreover, as systolic pressure rises from atherosclerosis, baroreceptor sensitivity and vascular compliance are reduced further, increasing the likelihood of postural hypotension (Fig. 4.13). In addition, chronic hypertension shifts the threshold for cerebral autoregulation so that a small fall in systemic BP may precipitate a significant fall in cerebral blood flow.

Once postural hypotension is managed (see Chapter 7), the hypertension can then be treated. Evidence of the value of therapy of hypertension

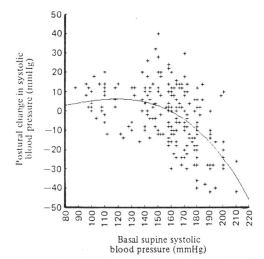

Figure 4.13. Relationship between basal supine systolic BP and postural change in systolic BP for aggregate data from old subjects. (From Lipsitz LA, Storch HA, Minaker KL, Rowe JW. Intra-individual variability in postural blood pressure in the elderly. *Clin Sci* 1985;69:337.)

in the elderly is provided in Chapter 5; details about therapy are given in Chapter 7.

Hypertension in Women

Women have about the same prevalence of hypertension as men (Fig. 1.4), and hypertension is an independent risk factor for stroke and coronary disease among them (Fiebach et al., 1989). Moreover, since there are more elderly women than elderly men, and since hypertension is both more common and deadly in the elderly, more women than men will eventually suffer a cardiovascular complication attributable to hypertension (Anastos et al., 1991). On the other hand, women are somehow protected against death from CHD when compared to men with comparable coronary risk profiles (Isles et al., 1992) (Fig. 4.14); this is likely the most important cause for the longer life span of women.

A number of possible explanations for this protection have been offered, including the following:

—A protective effect of estrogens, perhaps mediated through higher HDL-cholesterol levels;

—Reduction of blood viscosity and body iron stores by regular menses;

—Less insulin resistance and hyperinsulinemia because of less upper body fat (Wingard, 1990);

—A lower rate of cigarette smoking, an advantage that soon will be lost, as women have almost reached equality in this pernicious habit.

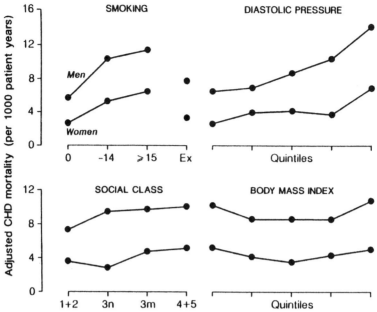

Figure 4.14. Adjusted CHD mortality in deaths per thousand patient years for both sexes by cigarette smoking, diastolic pressure, social class, and body mass index during a 15-year follow-up of over 7000 men and 8000 women in Scotland. (From Isles CG, Hole DJ, Hawthorne VM, Lever AF. Relation between coronary risk and coronary mortality in women of the Renfrew and Paisley survey: comparison with men. *Lancet* 1992;339:702.)

Hemodynamics

Hypertension in women is associated with higher resting heart rate and cardiac index and lower total peripheral resistance than in men with similar BP levels (Messerli et al., 1987). Older hypertensive women tend to have larger LV chambers and better LV function, higher levels of atrial natriuretic factor, and lower levels of plasma renin activity than men, all compatible with a greater degree of fluid volume expansion (de Simone et al., 1991a).

Hypertension in Blacks

In brief, blacks have more hypertension and suffer more from it, largely because of their lower socioeconomic status and resultant reduced access to needed health care. Their higher prevalence of hypertension likely reflects both genetic and environmental factors. If appropriate therapy is provided, most of their excessive morbidity and mortality related to hypertension can be relieved.

Prevalence

Adult blacks in the United States have higher BP levels, and therefore, more hypertension than do nonblacks (Figs. 1.4 and 1.8). These higher readings develop during childhood and adolescence and are established by early adulthood;

most of the higher readings in the young blacks are attributed to a larger body weight and size (Shear et al., 1987). In the baseline examination of a longitudinal study involving 5116 young black and white men and women aged 18 to 30, blacks had higher mean systolic and diastolic pressures than nonblacks did (Liu et al., 1989). As this population was followed for 5 years, the black-white differences increased, partly because of changes in lifestyle and body weight. Adjustments for age, education, body mass index, physical activity, and alcohol intake reduced the differences by 40% (Liu et al., 1992).

In addition to higher pressures as measured in the office, blacks in America (but not in Africa) usually have higher sleeping pressures as recorded by ambulatory monitoring (Fumo et al., 1992), suggesting that the American black-white difference is not racial but environmental.

Non-U.S. Blacks. Blacks from the West Indies working in Birmingham, England factories had pressures comparable to nonblacks, perhaps "due to the similarity in social class" (Cruickshank et al., 1985). As with other primitive populations, blacks in rural areas of Africa have lower pressures, which rise when they migrate to urban areas (Poulter et al., 1990).

Pathogenesis

Table 4.7 lists some of the numerous possible explanations for the higher prevalence of hypertension in U.S. blacks that have been proposed (Falkner, 1990). As in nonblacks, multiple factors are likely involved.

Genetics. Members of a single ethnic group would be expected to share more genes than would people of different origins. Data support genetic associations of hypertension among blacks (Savage et al., 1990), but they do not appear to differ quantitatively from those reported in nonblacks. This may reflect the genetic admixture that has occurred within black populations, which clearly differ within and between themselves.

Slavery Hypothesis. An interesting extension of the genetic role has been popularized by Wilson and Grim (1991). They first confirmed that the BP of blacks in the northern portion of the Western hemisphere was significantly higher than the pressure of blacks in sub-Sahara Africa, the area from which the former had come (Wilson et al., 1991).

These differences between U.S. and African blacks have generally been attributed to the psychosocial stresses of living as an oppressed minority in the United States with concomitant low socioeconomic status (James et al., 1992). However, U.S. blacks also display a tendency to retain sodium more avidly and thereby experience a greater rise in BP than do nonblacks when given salt loads (Luft et al., 1991). Helmer, the first to note lower plasma renin levels in U.S. blacks than in nonblacks, speculated that such

low renin levels could reflect a maladaptation of an enhanced ability of the kidney to conserve salt, an ability that was of great survival value to their African progenitors who lived in a hot environment and had little access to salt (Helmer, 1967). This presumably genetic trait, of value to African blacks, was of no value to U.S. blacks who lived in a cooler environment and who had more than ample access to salt. To the contrary, their more avid renal sodium retention could serve as the instigator of volume expansion and hypertension.

Blackburn and Prineas (1983) suggested that the transatlantic voyage involved in the slave trade that brought most blacks to the Western hemisphere could have introduced another genetic maladaptation. They conjectured that those African natives who could best conserve salt would be more likely to survive the exigencies of a long, hot journey beset with vomiting, diarrhea, and limited food and fluid intake. Since the survivors were better salt retainers, they would also develop more hypertension when salt was plentiful.

As attractive as the slavery hypothesis seems to be, it has been vigorously denied in all of its major parts by a Johns Hopkins historian (Curtin, 1992).

Sodium Sensitivity. Regardless of whether the slavery hypothesis is valid or not, a higher degree of responsiveness of the BP to abrupt (Luft et al., 1991) and chronic (Falkner and Kushner, 1990) manipulations of sodium intake has been noted in normotensive and hypertensive blacks compared to nonblacks. In those who had a pressor response to a sodium load, the renal excretion of the sodium was delayed and correlated with lower plasma renin levels.

The primary problem in sodium sensitivity generally is looked upon as retention of sodium because of abnormal renal hemodynamics (Campese et al., 1991), but an increased sensitivity to retained sodium also may be involved (Krishna et al., 1992).

Sodium Transport. As detailed in Chapter 3, abnormalities in sodium transport across vascular smooth muscle cells may be involved in the pathogenesis of most hypertension. Black normotensives and hypertensives have been found to have multiple differences from nonblacks in various cell transport measures, including the following:

—Higher intracellular sodium content (Cooper et al., 1990);

Table 4.7. Pathogenesis of Hypertension in Blacks

Genotype
 Candidate genes unique to blacks

Intermediate phenotype
 Sodium sensitivity
 Cation transport
 Renin-angiotensin-aldosterone
 Kallikrein-kinin, prostaglandin
 Adrenergic activity
 Insulin resistance

Phenotype
 Left ventricular hypertrophy
 Peripheral vascular resistance
 Nephrosclerosis

From Falkner B. Differences in blacks and whites with essential hypertension: biochemistry and endocrine. State of the art lecture. *Hypertension* 1990;15:681–686.

—Reduced RBC sodium-potassium cotransport (Canessa et al., 1990);

—Increased fibroblast sodium-hydrogen antiport activity (Hatori et al., 1990).

These and other differences may be either secondary to volume expansion arising from a defect in renal excretory capacity or primary cellular defects that induce peripheral vascular constriction (Aviv and Aladjem, 1990).

Stress. As described in Chapter 3, a large body of literature attests to an association between the stresses of low socioeconomic status and hypertension. As applied to U.S. blacks, the association likely explains a considerable portion of the increased prevalence of hypertension, but not all. A good example of the likely interaction between low socioeconomic status and a genetic trait is the finding that BP levels were significantly associated with darker skin color but only in those blacks in the lower levels of socioeconomic status (Klag et al., 1991).

Beyond low socioeconomic status, James and co-workers (1992) have long held to an influence of a coping strategy involving an active effort to manage the stressors of life by hard work and determination to succeed. They call this coping strategy ''John Henryism'' after a legendary uneducated black folk hero who defeated a mechanical steam drill in an epic battle but then dropped dead from complete exhaustion.

Sympathetic Nervous Activity. Despite the association of hypertension with the stress of low socioeconomic status, aborted educational achievement, and minority status in a prejudiced society, blacks do not display biochemical and hormonal evidences of heightened sympathetic nervous system activity (Pratt et al., 1992).

Increased Vascular Responsiveness. The apparent paradox of increased exposure to stress but unraised levels of sympathetic nervous activation may be explained by a greater degree of vascular responsiveness to pressor stimuli. Examples include higher peak BPs in black adolescents than in nonblack adolescents during treadmill exercise testing (Hohn et al., 1983), increased BP response to various active coping tests in blacks with borderline hypertension (Light et al., 1987), and increased pressor sensitivity to exogenous norepinephrine in blacks but not in nonblacks on a high sodium intake (Dimsdale et al., 1987).

Diet. Particularly among older black women, the higher prevalence of hypertension is correlated closely with obesity (Anderson et al., 1989). Although they have greater sensitivity to sodium, blacks do not appear to ingest more sodium than do nonblacks (Veterans Administration Cooperative, 1987). However, their intake of both potassium and calcium is lower (McCarron et al., 1982). One possible way that reduced calcium intake could raise BP is by a lower serum calcium level causing a secondary stimulation of parathyroid hormone (PTH) release, since higher PTH levels have been identified in black hypertensive patients (Brickman et al., 1993) and chronically elevated PTH levels raise the BP (Reichel et al., 1992). Moreover, if, as appears to be true, the hypertension of blacks is associated with volume expansion, a resultant increased excretion of calcium would further lower serum calcium levels and provoke increased PTH secretion.

Insulin Resistance. Insulin resistance, as noted in Chapter 3, may be important in the overall pathophysiology of hypertension. Few data are available on how insulin resistance relates to hypertension in blacks. Falkner et al. (1992) found that the increased resistance to exogenous insulin in hypertensive blacks was similar to that observed in nonblacks. This resultant hyperinsulinemia was closely correlated with their BP sensitivity to sodium.

Responsiveness to Growth Factors. Dustan (1992) attempted to explain the increased prevalence of severe hypertension in blacks by hypothesizing an increased responsiveness to vascular growth factors comparable to that noted in fibroblasts that form keloids. She relates such hypertrophy to the observation by Muirhead and Pitcock (1989) of a different histologic pattern in renal tissue from blacks with severe hypertension (myointimal hyperplasia) compared to the typical fibrinoid necrosis seen in nonblacks.

Complications

Hypertension not only is more common in blacks, it also is more severe, less well managed and, therefore, more deadly. As best as can be ascertained, blacks at any given level of BP do not suffer more vascular damage than nonblacks; rather, they display a shift to the right of the pressure distribution, yielding a higher overall prevalence and a higher proportion of severe disease (Cooper and Liao, 1992).

Much of the excess morbidity and mortality found in U.S. blacks compared to U.S. nonblacks is related to their lower socioeconomic status, but at every level of income, blacks have a higher mortality rate than whites (Sorlie et al., 1992). Despite the continued inequities, cardiovascular disease mortality rates have fallen dramatically for U.S. blacks, falls largely attributable to decreases in the prevalence of risk factors, including more control of hypertension (Folsom et al., 1987).

Cardiac Disease. Both by ECG (Taylor et al., 1983) and by echocardiography (Hammond et al., 1986), blacks have more LVH than nonblacks with equal levels of BP. Although the overall prevalence of CHD may be lower among U.S. blacks than among nonblacks, mortality rates from CHD are similar, likely reflecting more severe disease and less adequate health care (Curry, 1991).

Cerebrovascular Disease. Blacks have more strokes and die more frequently from them than do nonblacks. Age-specific stroke mortality rates among U.S. blacks were 3 to 4 times higher than for nonblacks in all age groups less than 65 years old (Caplan, 1991). All forms of cerebrovascular disease are more frequent in blacks, with even greater differences in those strokes that are more tightly connected with hypertension (i.e., subarachnoid and intracerebral hemorrhages) (Broderick et al., 1992).

Renal Disease. Although quantitatively only the third most common serious consequence of hypertension, progressive renal damage that results in ESRD is even more disproportionately represented among black hypertensives than are coronary or cerebrovascular diseases. ESRD associated with hypertension occurs as much as 17 times more often in U.S. blacks than among nonblacks (Shulman and Hall, 1991). When various known precursors are taken into account, including age, prevalence of hypertension, severity of hypertension, diabetes, and level of education, blacks still have a 4.5 times greater risk for ESRD than do nonblacks (Whittle et al., 1991). Moreover, even when they are treated as effectively, renal function in black hypertensives may continue to deteriorate, whereas it remains stable or improves in nonblacks (Walker et al., 1992).

Hypertension in Other Ethnic Groups

Blacks in the United States and other ethnic groups likely share both genetic and environmental exposures similarly. However, much less is known about the special characteristics of other ethnic groups, so only a few generalizations will be made about them.

Primitive Versus Acculturated

Groups of any race living a rural, more primitive lifestyle tend to ingest less sodium, remain less obese, and have less hypertension. When they migrate into urban areas and adapt more modern lifestyles, they ingest more sodium, gain weight, and develop more hypertension (Poulter et al., 1990). Rather dramatic changes in the prevalence of hypertension and the nature of cardiovascular complications have been seen when formerly isolated ethnic groups adopt modern lifestyles. Examples include the rises in pressure among Asians who move to the United States (Munger et al., 1991) and, more specifically, Japanese who move to Hawaii (Kagan et al., 1974).

Persistence of Ethnic Differences

Although environmental changes often alter BP and other cardiovascular traits, some ethnic groups preserve characteristics that presumably reflect stronger genetic influences. Examples include Bedouins in Israel (Paran et al., 1992) and Amerindians in the United States (Weiss et al., 1984). Amerindian descendants, such as Mexican-Americans in San Antonio, have a lesser prevalence of hypertension despite their high prevalence of obesity, diabetes, and insulin resistance (Haffner et al., 1990). Thus, ethnic origins may work both ways, to increase the propensity toward hypertension or to protect against the threat.

Hypertension with Diabetes

Prevalence

Diabetes mellitus and hypertension coexist more commonly than predicted by chance, perhaps 3 times more commonly. Of the 10% of diabetics with the insulin-dependent form (type I), hypertension is seen in most of the 40% who develop nephropathy, but is seen no more frequently in those who escape nephropathy than in the nondiabetic population (Nørgaard et al., 1990). In the 90% of diabetics with the insulin-independent form (type II), almost all of whom are obese, hypertension is more common than among obese people without diabetes (Hypertension in Diabetes Study Group, 1993). The connection between hypertension, diabetes, and obesity is even stronger in those whose obesity is predominantly in the upper body, comprising the major components of the insulin resistance syndrome described in Chapter 3.

Mechanisms

In both type I and type II diabetics, hyperinsulinemia is present; in type I because larger amounts of exogenous insulin are given than normal endogenous levels, in type II because of obesity-induced insulin resistance with resultant increased secretion of insulin in the eventually futile attempt to maintain euglycemia. Hyperinsulinemia may cause or at least aggravate hypertension in a number of ways (Epstein and Sowers, 1992) (Fig. 4.15).

The hypertension seen in type II diabetics is characterized by both volume expansion and increased vascular resistance, the latter related to the accelerated atherosclerosis that is common with longstanding hyperglycemia. Hyperglycemia per se inhibits endothelium-derived relaxation (Gupta et al., 1992) and stimulates transcription of the genes for growth factors acting on vascular smooth muscle cells (McClain et al., 1992).

Complications

Accelerated atherosclerosis gives rise to the cardiovascular complications that are so common in diabetics. Over 16 years, the diabetics in Framingham suffered almost twice as many strokes, 3 times more peripheral vascular disease and heart failure, and twice the number of coronary events than did nondiabetics (Kannel et al., 1990). All of these are increased further when hypertension accompanies diabetes.

The microvascular complications, retinopathy in particular, also are increased by hypertension (Cignarelli et al., 1992). The course and management of diabetic nephropathy, now second only to coronary disease as the cause of death in diabetic hypertensives, is covered in Chapter 9; details about the treatment of hypertension in diabetics is covered in Chapter 7.

Hypertension with Obesity

Even in the absence of type II diabetes, obesity is one of the major acquired factors responsible for hypertension, as described in Chapter 3, wherein the mechanisms and hemodynamic features of obesity-induced hypertension are covered.

Although some obese hypertensives have been found to have a more benign course than lean hypertensives (Barrett-Connor and Khaw, 1985), the majority of comparisons find little difference in the risk of major coronary disease events between lean and obese hypertensives (Phillips and Shaper, 1989). Two features must be considered in examining the risks of obesity-related hypertension: first, the distribution of the obesity, with a significantly greater cardiovascular risk among those whose obesity is predominately in the upper body (Folsom et al., 1993); second, factors that are responsible for leanness such as smoking and alcohol abuse which, independent of the hypertension, increase the risks of the lean (Stamler et al., 1991).

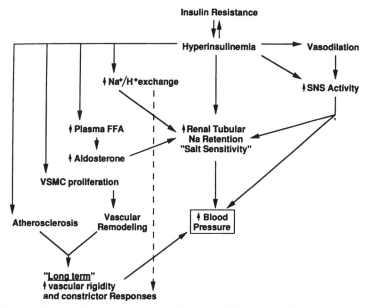

Figure 4.15. Schematic diagram of the proposed mechanisms by which hyperinsulinemia may contribute to hypertension. *SNS,* sympathetic nervous system; *FFA,* free fatty acids; *VSMC,* vascular smooth muscle cell. (From Epstein M, Sowers JR. Diabetes mellitus and hypertension. *Hypertension* 1992;19:403.)

Even after controlling for BP, obesity puts a load on the left ventricle, increasing LV mass (both wall thickness and internal dimension) (Lauer et al., 1991). The double burden of obesity and hypertension leads to a higher prevalence of CHF and CHD (Messerli, 1984).

ALTERING THE NATURAL HISTORY

Now that the possible mechanisms, natural history, major consequences, and special populations of untreated primary hypertension have been covered, an additional word about prevention is in order.

Most efforts to alter the natural history of hypertension involve therapy, both nondrug and drug. However, attempts to *prevent* hypertension must also be promoted more widely and followed. Without knowledge of the specific cause(s), no single preventive measure can be promoted with the assurance that it will work. However, to insist that specific causes be known before prevention is attempted is akin to saying that John Snow should not have closed the pump because he had no proof that *Vibrio cholera* organisms were the cause of death in those who drank the polluted water. The preventive measures likely to help—moderation in sodium, reduction of obesity, maintenance of physical conditioning, avoidance of stress, and greater attention to the other coexisting risk factors for premature cardiovascular disease—will do no harm and may do a great deal of good. These measures are covered in detail in Chapter 6.

EVALUATION OF THE HYPERTENSIVE PATIENT

Having examined the natural history of various hypertensive populations, we will now incorporate these findings into a game-plan for the evaluation of the individual hypertensive patient.

There are three main reasons to evaluate patients with hypertension: (1) to determine the type of hypertension, specifically looking for secondary causes; (2) to assess the impact of the hypertension on target organs; and (3) to estimate the patient's overall risk profile for the development of premature cardiovascular disease. Such evaluation can be accomplished with relative ease and should be part of the initial examination of every newly discovered hypertensive. The younger the patient and the higher the BP, the more aggressive the search for secondary causes should be. Among middle-aged and older persons, greater attention should be directed to the overall cardiovascular risk profile, since these populations are more susceptible to immediate catastrophes unless preventive measures are taken.

History

The history should focus on the duration of the BP and any prior treatment, the current use of various drugs that may cause it to rise, and symptoms of target organ dysfunction (Table 4.8). Though not usually considered part of the initial workup, attention should also be directed toward the patient's psychosocial status, looking for such information as the degree of knowledge about hypertension, the willingness to make necessary changes in lifestyle and to take medication, and the family and job situations. An area of great importance is sexual function, often neglected until it arises after antihypertensive therapy is given. Impotence, often attributed to antihypertensive drugs, may be present in as many as one-third of untreated hypertensive men and is most likely related to their underlying vascular disease (see Chapter 7).

Headaches and Hyperventilation

Most hypertension is asymptomatic even after it becomes persistent. This is in a way unfortunate: without symptoms, hypertension is often detected only after overt organ damage has occurred, years after the onset of the disease.

Of the symptoms that are reported, headache is the most common, but those who complain of headache are more likely to have their BP taken and hypertension discovered. Stewart (1953) found that only 17% of patients unaware of their hypertension complained of headache, but among patients with similar levels of BP who were aware of their diagnosis, 71% had headaches. This is in keeping with my belief that many of the symptoms described by hypertensives are secondary to anxiety over having ''the silent killer,'' as hypertension is frequently described, anxiety that is often expressed as recurrent acute hyperventilation episodes. Many of the symptoms described by hypertensives, such as band-like headaches, dizziness and light-headedness, fatigue, palpitations, and chest discomfort, reflect recurrent hyperventilation, a common problem among all patients (DeGuire et al., 1992), but likely even more common among hypertensives who are anxious over their diagnosis and its implications.

This belief that most symptoms, headache in particular, are related not to the level of BP but

Table 4.8. Important Aspects of the History

Duration of the hypertension
Last known normal blood pressure
Course of the blood pressure

Prior treatment of the hypertension
Drugs: types, doses, side effects

Intake of agents that may cause hypertension
Estrogens
Sympathomimetics
Adrenal steroids
Excessive sodium intake

Family history
Hypertension
Premature cardiovascular disease or death
Familial diseases: pheochromocytoma, renal disease, diabetes, gout

Symptoms of secondary causes
Muscle weakness
Spells of tachycardia, sweating, tremor
Thinning of the skin
Flank pain

Symptoms of target organ damage
Headaches
Transient weakness or blindness
Loss of visual acuity
Chest pain
Dyspnea
Claudication

Presence of other risk factors
Smoking
Diabetes
Dyslipidemia
Physical inactivity

Dietary history
Sodium
Alcohol
Saturated fats

Psychosocial factors
Family structure
Work status
Educational level

Sexual function

Features of sleep apnea
Early morning headaches
Daytime somnolence
Loud snoring
Erratic sleep

rather to anxiety over the diagnosis of hypertension is strengthened by the fact that the prevalence of headache among *newly diagnosed* hypertensives varies little in relation to the level of BP, with 15% to 20% having headaches whether their DBPs were as low as 95 mm Hg or as high as 125 mm Hg (Cooper et al., 1989). Moreover, neither headaches nor epistaxis, tinnitus, dizziness, or fainting were more common among *previously unrecognized* hypertensives than among those with normal BP (Weiss, 1972).

With very high BP, headaches do become more common. The headache is usually present upon awakening, is felt in the back of the head, may or may not be throbbing in character, and often lasts only a few hours even without analgesic therapy. It should also be noted that sleep apnea is common among even minimally obese hypertensives, as described in Chapter 15, so early morning headaches may reflect not hypertension but nocturnal hypoxia.

Physical Examination

The physical examination should include a careful search for damage to target organs and for features of various secondary causes (Table 4.9).

Fundoscopic

Only in the optic fundi can small blood vessels be seen with ease, but this requires dilation of the pupil, a procedure that should be more commonly practiced. With the short-acting mydriatic tropicamide 1%, excellent dilation can be achieved in almost 90% of patients within 15 minutes (Steinmann et al., 1987). Retinopathy is an independent indicator of mortality (Schouten et al., 1986) and should be determined in every hypertensive patient as part of the initial examination and yearly thereafter.

Keith, Wagener, and Barker (1939) classified the funduscopic changes. Two separate but

Table 4.9. Important Aspects of the Physical Examination

Accurate measurement of blood pressure

General appearance: distribution of body fat, skin lesions, muscle strength, alertness

Funduscopy

Neck: palpation and auscultation of carotids, thyroid

Heart: size, rhythm, sounds

Lungs: rhonchi, rales

Abdomen: renal masses, bruits over aorta or renal arteries, femoral pulses

Extremities: peripheral pulses, edema

Neurologic assessment

related vascular diseases are demonstrable: hypertensive neuroretinopathy (hemorrhages, exudates, and papilledema) and arteriosclerotic retinopathy (arteriolar narrowing, arteriovenous nicking, silver wiring) (Sapira, 1984). The original Keith-Wagener-Barker grouping mixed the two. The retinopathy of diabetes—punctate hemorrhages and hard exudates—is seen in twice as many hypertensive as nonhypertensive diabetics (Knowler et al., 1980). Spontaneous subconjunctional hemorrhages may be a sign of hypertension (Pitts et al., 1992).

Mild and Moderate Hypertension. When fundal photographs were carefully examined for increased light reflex, arteriolar narrowing, and arteriovenous crossing defects in 28 previously untreated hypertensive middle-aged men, the retinal vascular changes were significantly correlated with LVH by echocardiography, vascular resistance in the calf, and BP levels (Dahlöf et al., 1992). Similar findings have been described in most adolescents with hypertension (Daniels et al., 1991), but others have not been able to relate fundal changes to levels of BP or LVH detected by echocardiography (Dimmitt et al., 1989).

Severe Hypertension. The group III and IV changes—flame-shaped hemorrhages, soft exudates, and papilledema—are clearly indicative of very severe hypertension (Harnish and Pearce, 1973). The same initial vasoconstriction followed by ''breakthrough'' dilation shown to occur in the cerebral vessels has been held responsible for the retinal hemorrhages and exudates (Garner and Ashton, 1979).

Laboratory Findings

Routine

For most patients, a hematocrit, a urine analysis, an automated blood chemistry (glucose, creatinine, electrolytes), a lipid profile (total and high-density lipoprotein [HDL] cholesterol, triglycerides) and an ECG are all of the routine procedures needed. None of these usually yields abnormal results in the early, uncomplicated phases of essential hypertension.

Hypertriglyceridemia and, even more threatening, hypercholesterolemia are found twice more frequently in untreated hypertensives as in normotensives; the prevalence increases with the BP level (Fig. 4.16) (Bønaa and Thelle, 1991). The association may, in turn, reflect the quartet of upper body obesity, hyperlipidemia, glucose intolerance, and hypertension related to hyperinsulinemia (see Chapter 3).

Hyperuricemia is found in up to half of untreated hypertensives (Breckenridge, 1966) and reflects underlying nephrosclerosis (Messerli et al., 1980). Not only is gout more common in hypertensives (Roubenoff et al., 1991), but so are kidney stones, which likely are a consequence of increased urinary calcium excretion (Cappuccio et al., 1990). Incipient renal disease may be heralded by microalbuminuria.

Additional Testing for Target Organ Damage

Cardiac. Evidence of cardiac involvement includes the following:

—A forceful and sustained apical impulse with a fourth heart sound (Frohlich et al., 1992);
—Left atrial enlargement as detected by ECG or echocardiography (Miller et al., 1988);
—LV enlargement as detected by radiography;
—LVH as detected by ECG, which is much less sensitive and less specific than echocardiography, particularly in blacks (Lee et al., 1992). Nonetheless, ECG is useful in demonstrating rhythm and conduction disturbances, as well as ischemia (Prisant and Carr, 1993);
—LVH as detected by echocardiography;
—Changes in LV function, usually as measured by echocardiography. These include reductions in early diastolic filling related to decreased ventricular relaxation, higher systolic ejection phase indices, and subnormal functional response to exercise stress (Frohlich et al., 1992);
—Deficits in myocardial perfusion caused by hypertensive microvascular disease without obstructive epicardial coronary artery disease, which may give rise to positive exercise tests (Frohlich et al., 1992).

All hypertensives should have an ECG. Some believe that a limited echocardiograph (only two two-dimensional views and a brief M-mode scan) should be obtained, which costs less than half of the full procedure (Black et al., 1991). A limited echocardiograph will diagnose LVH and might provide a useful prognostic and therapeutic guide. However, most authorities recommend echocardiography only ''in selected cases'' (Joint National Committee, 1993).

Hypertensive patients have more CAD than nonhypertensives and may have symptoms of myocardial ischemia because of limited coronary reserve from ventricular hypertrophy and systolic wall stress (Strauer, 1992). The differential diagnosis between the two processes may require thallium-201 stress imaging (Prisant et al., 1992).

Cerebral. Although sensitive testing may show that neurobehavioral function is reduced (Blumenthal et al., 1993), it is not possible to

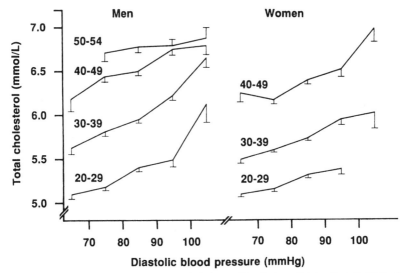

Figure 4.16. Plot of mean concentrations of serum total cholesterol levels (mmol/L) by diastolic BP in 8081 men 20 to 54 years old and in 7663 women 20 to 49 years old. T bars are SEM. (From Bønaa KH, Thelle DS. Association between blood pressure and serum lipids in a population. The Tromsø *Circulation* 1991;83:1305.)

relate cerebral dysfunction to the severity of the BP unless hypertension has become accelerated, with resultant encephalopathy. In the presence of symptoms of cerebral ischemia, particularly TIAs, the finding of a carotid bruit indicates the need for carotid ultrasonography in the hope of finding a correctable lesion. Hypertensives with subtle neuropsychological deficits have been found to have white matter lesions by brain magnetic resonance imaging (MRI) (Schmidt et al., 1991); also, vascular forms of dementia are seen more frequently in those with hypertension (Salerno et al., 1992).

Renal. The earliest symptom is nocturia, and the most commonly identifiable markers of renal involvement are hyperuricemia and microalbuminuria (Harvey et al., 1992)—which can, though rarely, progress to nephrotic-stage proteinuria (Narvarte et al., 1987). Later, serum creatinine begins to rise (Perneger et al., 1993), but the relationship between loss of renal function and rise of serum creatinine is asymptotic; thus, little absolute increase in serum creatinine will occur until more than 50% of renal function is lost (Perrone et al., 1992).

Vascular. Hypertension is a risk factor for aortic aneurysm; thus, abdominal palpation should be performed, particularly in thin, elderly hypertensives with evidence of vascular disease elsewhere (Lederle et al., 1988). Ultrasonography is needed for diagnostic certainty (Grand Round, 1993). Peripheral vessels should be pal-

pated for diminished pulse and auscultated for bruits.

Arterial Compliance. Far beyond these simple clinical examinations, increasing awareness of the importance of pulsatile phenomena in the pathogenesis of cardiovascular damage has led to attempts to measure arterial compliance, a quantitative measure of the distensibility of the arterial system, defined as the change in volume per unit change in pressure or the slope of the pressure-volume relationship (Safar et al., 1990; Simon and Levenson, 1991). With currently available noninvasive techniques, decreased compliance can be shown to be an early feature of hypertension that likely will prove useful in the future for assessment and prediction of cardiovascular complications (Gudbrandsson et al., 1992).

Search for Secondary Causes

The frequencies of various causes of secondary hypertension shown in Table 1.7 are likely much too high for the larger population with mild, asymptomatic hypertension. Nonetheless, even though only a few can be cured, every patient should receive a certain basic workup for these forms when feasible (Mueller and Laragh, 1991). This assumption is based on the following points: First, there is fulfillment in the search since, despite significant advances in drug therapy of hypertension, a lifetime of taking pills is an unattractive prospect; drugs cost money and

Table 4.10. Overall Guide to Workup for Secondary Causes of Hypertension

Diagnosis	Diagnostic Procedure	
	Initial	Additional
Chronic renal disease	Urinalysis, serum creatinine, renal sonography	Isotopic renogram, renal biopsy
Renovascular disease	Plasma renin before and 1 hour after captopril	Aortogram, isotopic renogram 1 hour after captopril
Coarctation	Blood pressure in legs	Aortogram
Primary aldosteronism	Plasma potassium, plasma renin and aldosterone (ratio)	Urinary potassium, plasma or urinary aldosterone after saline load; adrenal computed tomography (CT) and scintiscans
Cushing's syndrome	AM plasma cortisol after 1 mg dexamethasone at bedtime	Urinary cortisol after variable doses of dexamethasone; adrenal CT and scintiscans
Pheochromocytoma	Spot urine for metanephrine	Urinary catechols; plasma catechols, basal and after 0.3 mg clonidine; adrenal CT and scintiscans

produce side effects, and many patients will not keep taking them. Second, both physicians and patients are attracted to the drama of a cure. Certainly, the immediate correction of a renal arterial lesion is a more attractive prospect than a lifetime of taking pills. Third, the search for curable or secondary forms of hypertension may also involve uncovering information of value in establishing prognosis and the need for therapy. The minimal workup needed to rule out the secondary causes of hypertension also helps to determine the degree of target organ damage.

A great deal more concerning the workup of these various secondary diseases is included in their respective chapters. Table 4.10 is an overall guide to the work-up for secondary causes of hypertension. These diagnostic procedures are needed only if there is evidence from the history, physical examination, or initial urinalysis and blood chemistries that a secondary disease may be present, or if the patient is deemed at special risk because of features of "inappropriate hypertension" (Table 4.11). If so, the studies listed as "initial" will usually serve as adequate screening procedures. They are readily available to every practitioner. If they are abnormal, the "additional" procedures should be performed along with whatever other tests are needed to confirm the diagnosis.

Table 4.11. Features of "Inappropriate" Hypertension

Age of onset: before 20 or after 50

Level of blood pressure > 180/110 mm Hg

Organ damage
Funduscopy grade II or beyond
Serum creatinine > 1.5 mg/dl
Cardiomegaly or left ventricular hypertrophy as determined by electrocardiography

Presence of features indicative of secondary causes
Unprovoked hypokalemia
Abdominal bruit
Variable pressures with tachycardia, sweating, tremor
Family history of renal disease

Poor response to generally effective therapy

Need for Limitation

The application of decision analysis to clinical screening tests is a powerful tool in judging their value, a dimension rarely considered when the tests are ordered. This approach is based on Bayes' theorem (Blinowska et al., 1991; Coughlin et al., 1992). The concept not only involves the sensitivity and specificity of the test but also the prevalence of the disease to provide an answer as to the statistical likelihood that a positive or negative test result confirms or refutes the presence of the disease being screened. The main lesson is that with diseases with low prevalence rates, such as all secondary forms of hypertension, a positive screening test is neither proof nor even strong evidence for the existence of the disease.

When applied to the use of isotopic renography to screen for renovascular disease, the results are revealing (Table 4.12): Assuming a 2% prevalence of renovascular hypertension in the hypertensive population, a positive renogram has a predictive value of only 10.4%—that is, only 10.4% of hypertensives with a renogram suggestive of renovascular hypertension will have the disease. If the prevalence is 4%, as it might be in young hypertensives, a positive renogram has a 19.1% predictive value. If the prevalence is 10%, as it might be in a very selected population such as young women with an abdominal bruit, the predictive value rises to 38.6%. With any of these prevalence figures, a negative renogram is 98% to 99.6% predictive that renovascular hypertension is not present. A nomogram for Bayes' formula can be used to determine these predictive values if the sensitivity (i.e., false-negatives), specificity (i.e., false-positives), and prevalence of the disease are known (Møller-Petersen, 1985).

Plasma Renin Assays

For many years, John Laragh and coworkers have emphasized the value of ascertaining the plasma renin level coupled with the level of 24-hour urine sodium excretion, the renin-sodium profile. I, like most investigators, do not include this profile in the routine evaluation of all hypertensives, but use it only if other features of low-renin states (e.g., primary aldosteronism) or high-renin states (e.g., renovascular disease) are present. Nonetheless, a persuasive argument can

be made for the test as a useful tool for diagnosis, prognosis, and therapy. In the words of Mueller and Laragh (1991):

The test has its greatest strength for identifying sizable numbers of otherwise unrecognizable patients with very high or very low renin concentrations who might have curable disorders and who likely reflect different pathophysiologic vasoconstrictive mechanisms for which entirely different drug therapies are appropriate. However, the baseline renin test is also useful for assessing prognosis and the likelihood of a heart attack and it is valuable for deciding whether to use an anti-renin system drug (for medium and high renin concentrations) as opposed to natriuretic agents (low-renin patients) such as a diuretic or calcium antagonists as the primary step.

Ambulatory Monitoring and Echocardiography

Two more complicated and expensive procedures—ambulatory BP monitoring (ABPM) and echocardiography—likely will be performed more frequently as part of the workup of some hypertensives. Neither should be routine but, as noted in Chapter 2, ABPM performed under appropriate circumstances may provide very useful information not provided by any other technique and may save money by avoiding unnecessary therapy. As noted earlier in this chapter, echocardiography may also be more widely used, but a great deal more information about the meaning of its results is needed before it can be recommended as a routine procedure.

Assessment of Overall Cardiovascular Risk

Once the cause and consequences of the hypertension have been documented, it is necessary to assess the patient's overall cardiovascular risk status. The proper management of hypertension should involve attention to all of the risk factors that can be altered. Patients at high risk should be counseled and helped to reduce all of their risks. Since, for most patients, the BP is the easiest of the risks to control, this may be the first priority. As described more fully in the next chapter, the overall risk profile provides a more rational basis for determining the need for treatment and the goal of therapy than an arbitrary BP level. For now, the need for a complete assessment of cardiovascular risk—a simple and inexpensive undertaking—should be obvious in the proper management of all hypertensives. The ingredients for the most precise assessment, based upon the 26-year follow-up data from Framingham, are these: age, gender,

Table 4.12. Predictive Value of the Renogram for Renovascular Hypertension

Prevalence of Renovascular Hypertension	Predictive Value of Renogram	
	Positive Test	Negative Test
2%	0.104	0.996
4%	0.191	0.992
10%	0.386	0.980

Sensitivity = 0.85; specificity = 0.85.

SBP, serum total cholesterol and HDL cholesterol, cigarette smoking, glucose tolerance, fibrinogen levels, heart rate, body weight, and the presence of LVH as shown by ECG or echocardiography (Kannel, 1991). Using some of these measurements, it is possible to obtain a specific rate indicating the likelihood of a major cardiovascular event within the next 8 years (Anderson et al., 1991). Booklets for determining the risk of CHD and stroke are available from the American Heart Association. Figure

4.17 presents an example of the data for 50-year-old men. Notice that as each additional risk factor is added, the probability of a major cardiovascular catastrophe rises progressively for all three levels of SBP.

We will now turn from the mechanisms and natural history of hypertension to its management, next considering the rationale for its treatment, and thereafter the practical issues of non-drug and drug therapies.

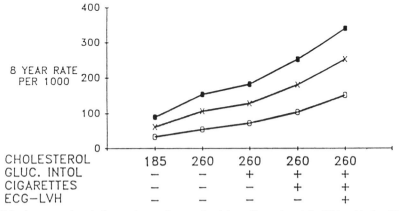

Figure 4.17. Risk of coronary heart disease by cardiovascular risk profile and systolic BP level in the 26-year follow-up of 50-year-old men in the Framingham Study. Systolic pressure (mm Hg): ■ 180, x 150, □ 105; *ECG-LVH,* left ventricular hypertrophy by electrocardiography. (From Kannel WB. The clinical heterogeneity of hypertension. *Am J Hypertens* 1991;4:283.)

References

Ammon S, Tubau JF, Szlachcic J, Tom J, Massie BM. Stress ^{201}Tl scintigraphy predicts cardiovascular morbidity in asymptomatic hypertensive men with multiple risk factors [Abstract]. *J Am Coll Cardiol* 1993;21:287A.

Anderson CS, Jamrozik KD, Burvill PW, Chakera TMH, Johnson GA, Stewart-Wynne EG. Determining the incidence of different subtypes of stroke: results from the Perth Community Stroke Study, 1989–1990. *Med J Aust* 1993;158:85–89.

Anderson KM, Wilson PWF, Odell PM, Kannel WB. An updated coronary risk profile. A statement for health professionals. *Circulation* 1991;83:356–362.

Anderson NB, Myers HF, Pickering T, Jackson JS. Hypertension in blacks: psychosocial and biological perspectives. *J Hypertens* 1989;7:161–172.

Applegate WB, Davis BR, Black RH, Smith WM, Miller ST, Burlando AJ. Prevalence of postural hypotension at baseline in the Systolic Hypertension in the Elderly Program (SHEP) Cohort. *J Am Geriatr Soc* 1991;39:1057–1065.

Astrup J, Bisgaard-Frantzen HO, Kvetny J. Masked hypertension in myocardial infarction. *Dan Med Bull* 1978; 25: 206–208.

Aviv A, Aladjem M. Essential hypertension in blacks: epidemiology, characteristics,

and possible roles of racial differences in sodium, potassium, and calcium regulation. *Cardiovasc Drug Ther* 1990;4: 335–342.

Barrett-Connor E, Khaw K-T. Is hypertension more benign when associated with obesity? *Circulation* 1985;72:53–60.

Bechgaard P. The natural history of arterial hypertension in the elderly. A fifty year follow-up study. *Acta Med Scand* 1983; (Suppl 676):9–14.

Bierman EL, Brewer C, Baum D. Hypertension decreases replication potential of arterial smooth muscle cells: aortic coarctation in humans as a model (41070). *Proc Soc Exper Biol Med* 1981;166:335–338.

Birkenhäger WH, de Leeuw PW. Determining hypertensive end-organ damage in trials: a review of current methodologies and techniques. *J Cardiovasc Pharmacol* 1992; 19(Suppl 5):43–50.

Black HR, Weltin G, Jaffe CC. The limited echocardiogram: a modification of standard echocardiography for use in the routine evaluation of patients with systemic hypertension. *Am J Cardiol* 1991;67: 1027–1030.

Blackburn H, Prineas R. Diet and hypertension: anthropology, epidemiology, and public health implications. *Prog Biochem Pharmacol* 1983;19:31–79.

Blinowska A, Chatellier G, Bernier J, Lavril M. Bayesian statistics as applied to hypertension diagnosis. *IEEE Trans Biochem Eng* 1991;38:699–706.

Blumenthal JA, Madden DJ, Pierce TW, Siegel WC, Appelbaum M. Hypertension affects neurobehavioral functioning. *Psychosomat Med* 1993;55:44–50.

Bønaa KH, Thelle DS. Association between BP and serum lipids in a population. The Tromsø Study. *Circulation* 1991;83: 1305–1314.

Bondjers G, Glukhova M, Hansson GK, Postnov YV, Reidy MA, Schwartz SM. Hypertension and atherosclerosis. Cause and effect, or two effects with one unknown cause? *Circulation* 1991;84(Suppl 6): 2–16.

Bonita R. Epidemiology of stroke. *Lancet* 1992;339:342–344.

Bonow RO, Udelson JE. LV diastolic dysfunction as a cause of congestive heart failure. Mechanisms and management. *Ann Intern Med* 1992;117:502–510.

Breckenridge A. Hypertension and hyperuricaemia. *Lancet* 1966;1:15–18.

Brickman AS, Nyby MD, Griffiths RF, von Hungen K, Tuck ML. Racial differences in platelet cytosolic calcium and calcitropic hormones in normotensive subjects. *Am J Hypertens* 1993;6:46–51.

Broderick JP, Brott T, Tomsick T, Huster G, Miller R. The risk of subarachnoid and intracerebral hemorrhages in blacks as compared with whites. *N Engl J Med* 1992;326:733–736.

Brogan WC III, Hillis LD, Flores ED, Lange RA. The natural history of isolated LV diastolic dysfunction. *Am J Med* 1992;92:627–630.

Brush JE Jr, Cannon RO III, Schenke WH, Bonow RO, Leon MB, Maron BJ, Epstein SE. Angina due to coronary microvascular disease in hypertensive patients without LV hypertrophy. *N Engl J Med* 1988; 319:1302–1307.

Buck C, Baker P, Bass M, Donner A. The prognosis of hypertension according to age at onset. *Hypertension* 1987;9:204–208.

Campese VM, Parise M, Karubian F, Bigazzi R. Abnormal renal hemodynamics in black salt-sensitive patients with hypertension. *Hypertension* 1991;18:805–812.

Canessa M, Laski C, Falkner B. Red blood cell Na$^+$ transport as a predictor of BP response to Na$^+$ load in young blacks and whites. *Hypertension* 1990;16:508–514.

Caplan LR. Strokes in African-Americans. *Circulation* 1991;83:1469–1471.

Cappuccio FP, Strazzullo P, Mancini M. Kidney stones and hypertension: population based study of an independent clinical association. *Br Med J* 1990;300: 1234–1236.

Carlberg B, Asplund K, Hägg E. The prognostic value of admission blood pressure in patients with acute stroke. *Stroke* 1993;24:1372–1375.

Celermajer DS, Sorensen KE, Gooch VM, Spiegelhalter DJ, Miller OI, Sullivan ID, Lloyd JK, Deanfield JE. Non-invasive detection of endothelial dysfunction in children and adults at risk of atherosclerosis. *Lancet* 1992;340:1111–1115.

Chobanian AV. 1989 Corcoran Lecture: adaptive and maladaptive responses of the arterial wall to hypertension. *Hypertension* 1990;15:666–674.

Cignarelli M, De Cicco ML, Damato A, Paternostro A, Pagliarini S, Santoro S, Cardia L, De Pergola G, Giorgino R. High systolic BP increases prevalence and severity of retinopathy in NIDDM patients. *Diabetes Care* 1992;15:1002–1008.

Cooper RS, Aina O, Chaco L, Shamsi N, Achilihu A, Islam N, Hsieh S-C, Feinberg H. Cell cations and BP in US whites, US blacks, and West African blacks. *J Hum Hypertens* 1990;4:477–484.

Cooper RS, Liao Y. Is hypertension among blacks more severe or simply more common [Abstract]? *Circulation* 1992;85:12.

Cooper WD, Glover DR, Hormbrey JM, Kimber GR. Headache and BP: evidence of a close relationship. *J Hum Hypertens* 1989;3:41–44.

Cornoni-Huntley J, LaCroix AZ, Havlik RJ. Race and sex differentials in the impact of hypertension in the United States. The National Health and Nutrition Examination Survey I Epidemiology Follow-up Study. *Arch Intern Med* 1989;149: 780–788.

Coughlin SS, Trock B, Criqui MH, Pickle LW, Browner D, Tefft MC. The logistic modeling of sensitivity, specificity, and predictive value of a diagnostic test. *J Clin Epidemiol* 1992;45:1–7.

Coull BM, Beamer N, de Garmo P, Sexton G, Nordt F, Knox R, Seaman VF. Chronic BP hyperviscosity in subjects with acute stroke, transient ischemic attack, and risk factors for stroke. *Stroke* 1991;22: 162–168.

Criqui MH, Langer RD, Fronek A, Feigelson HS, Klauber MR, McCann TJ, Browner D. Mortality over a period of 10 years in patients with peripheral arterial disease. *N Engl J Med* 1992;326:381–386.

Cruickshank JK, Jackson SHD, Beevers DG, Bannan LT, Beevers M, Stewart VL. Similarity of BP in blacks, whites and Asians in England: the Birmingham Factory Study. *J Hypertens* 1985;3:365–371.

Curry CL. Coronary artery disease in African-Americans. *Circulation* 1991;83: 1474–1475.

Curtin PD. The slavery hypothesis for hypertension among African Americans: the historical evidence. *Am J Public Health* 1992;82:1681–1686.

Dahlöf B, Stenkula S, Hansson L. Hypertensive retinal vascular changes: relationship to LV hypertrophy and arteriolar changes before and after treatment. *BP* 1992;1: 35–44.

Damsgaard EM, Froland A, Jorgensen OD, Mogensen CE. Microalbuminuria as predictor of increased mortality in elderly people. *Br Med J* 1990;300:297–300.

Daniels SR, Lipman MJ, Burke MJ, Loggie JMH. The prevalence of retinal vascular abnormalities in children and adolescents with essential hypertension. *Am J Ophthalmol* 1991;111:205–208.

de Simone G, Devereux RB, Roman MJ, Ganau A, Chien S, Alderman MH, Atlas S, Laragh JH. Gender differences in LV anatomy, blood viscosity and volume regulatory hormones in normal adults. *Am J Cardiol* 1991a;68:1704–1708.

de Simone G, Devereux RB, Roman MJ, Schlussel Y, Alderman MH, Laragh JH. Echocardiographic LV mass and electrolyte intake predict arterial hypertension. *Ann Intern Med* 1991b;114:202–209.

de Simone G, Di Lorenzo L, Costantino G, Moccia D, Buonissimo S, de Divitiis O. Supernormal contractility in primary hypertension without LV hypertrophy. *Hypertension* 1988;11:457–463.

DeGuire S, Gevirtz R, Kawahara Y, Maguire W. Hyperventilation syndrome and the assessment of treatment for functional cardiac symptoms. *Am J Cardiol* 1992; 70:673–677.

DePaola N, Gimbrone MA Jr, Davies PF, Dewey CF Jr. Vascular endothelium responds to fluid shear stress gradients. *Arteriosclerosis Thrombosis* 1992;12: 1254–1257.

Devereux RB. Echocardiographic insights into the pathophysiology and prognostic significance of hypertensive cardiac hypertrophy. *Am J Hypertens* 1989;2: 186S–195S.

Devereux RB, Koren MJ, de Simone G, Roman MJ, Laragh JH. LV mass as a measure of preclinical hypertensive disease. *Am J Hypertens* 1992;5:175S–181S.

Dimmitt SB, West JNW, Eames SM, Gibson JM, Gosling P, Littler WA. Usefulness of ophthalmoscopy in mild to moderate hypertension. *Lancet* 1989;1:1103–1106.

Dimsdale JE, Graham RM, Ziegler MG, Zusman RM, Berry CC. Age, race, diagnosis, and sodium effects on the pressor response to infused norepinephrine. *Hypertension* 1987;10:564–569.

Doyle AE. Does hypertension predispose to coronary disease? Conflicting epidemiological and experimental evidence. *Am J Hypertens* 1988;1:319–324.

Dustan HP. Growth factors and racial differences in severity of hypertension and renal diseases. *Lancet* 1992;339:1339–1340.

Epstein M, Sowers JR. Diabetes mellitus and hypertension. *Hypertension* 1992;19: 403–418.

Fagard R. Hypertensive heart disease: pathophysiology and clinical and prognostic consequences. *J Cardiovasc Pharmacol* 1992;19(Suppl 5):59–66.

Falkner B. Differences in blacks and whites with essential hypertension: biochemistry and endocrine. State of the art lecture. *Hypertension* 1990;15:681–686.

Falkner B, Hulman S, Kushner H. Hyperinsulinemia and BP sensitivity to sodium in young blacks. *J Am Soc Nephrol* 1992; 3:940–946.

Falkner B, Kushner H. Effect of chronic sodium loading on cardiovascular response in young blacks and whites. *Hypertension* 1990;15:36–43.

Fiebach NH, Hebert PR, Stampfer MJ, Colditz GA, Willett WC, Rosner B, Speizer FE, Hennekens CH. A prospective study of high BP and cardiovascular disease in women. *Am J Epidemiol* 1989; 130:646–654.

Folsom AR, Gomez-Marin O, Sprafka JM, Prineas RJ, Edlavitch SA, Gillum RF. Trends in cardiovascular risk factors in an urban black population, 1973–74 to 1985: the Minnesota Heart Survey. *Am Heart J* 1987;114:1199–1207.

Folsom AR, Kaye SA, Sellers TA, Hong C-P, Cerhan JR, Potter JD, Prineas RJ. Body fat distribution and 5-year risk of death in older women. *JAMA* 1993;269:483–487.

French JK, Elliott JM, Williams BF, Nixon DJ, Denton MA, White HD. Association of angiographically detected coronary artery disease with low levels of high-density lipoprotein cholesterol and systemic hypertension. *Am J Cardiol* 1993;71:505–510.

Frohlich ED, Apstein C, Chobanian AV, Devereux RB, Dustan HP, Dzau V, Fauad-Tarazi F, Horan MJ, Marcus M, Massie B, Pfeffer MA, Re RN, Roccella EJ, Savage D, Shub C. The heart in hypertension. *N Engl J Med* 1992;327:998–1008.

Fujii M, Nuno DW, Lamping KG, Dellsperger KC, Eastham CL, Harrison DG. Effect of hypertension and hypertrophy on coronary microvascular pressure. *Circ Res* 1992;71:120–126.

Fumo MT, Teeger S, Lang RM, Bednarz J, Sareli P, Murphy MB. Diurnal BP variation and cardiac mass in American blacks and whites and South African blacks. *Am J Hypertens* 1992;5:111–116.

Ganau A, Devereux RB, Roman MJ, de Simone G, Pickering TG, Saba PS, Vargiu

P, Simongini I, Laragh JH. Patterns of LV hypertrophy and geometric remodeling in essential hypertension. *J Am Coll Cardiol* 1992;19:1550–1558.

Garner A, Ashton N. Pathogenesis of hypertensive retinopathy: a review. *J R Soc Med* 1979;72:362–365.

Garrison RJ, Kannel WB, Stokes J III, Castelli WP. Incidence and precursors of hypertension in young adults: the Framingham Offspring Study. *Prev Med* 1987; 16:235–251.

Ghali JK, Liao Y, Simmons B, Castaner A, Cao G, Cooper RS. The prognostic role of LV hypertrophy in patients with or without coronary artery disease. *Ann Intern Med* 1992;117:831–836.

Grand Round. Abdominal aortic aneurysm. *Lancet* 1993;341:215–220.

Gudbrandsson T, Julius S, Krause L, Jamerson K, Randall OS, Schork N, Weder A. Correlates of the estimated arterial compliance in the population of Tecumseh, Michigan. *BP* 1992;1:27–34.

Gupta S, Sussman I, McArthur CS, Tornheim K, Cohen RA, Ruderman NB. Endothelium-dependent inhibition of Na⁺-K⁺ ATPase activity in rabbit aorta by hyperglycemia. Possible role of endothelium-derived nitric oxide. *J Clin Invest* 1992; 90:727–732.

Haffner SM, Mitchell BD, Stern MP, Hazuda HP, Patterson JK. Decreased prevalence of hypertension in Mexican-Americans. *Hypertension* 1990;16:225–232.

Hallock P, Benson IC. Studies of the elastic properties of human isolated aorta. *J Clin Invest* 1937;16:595–602.

Hammond IW, Devereux RB, Alderman MH, Lutas EM, Spitzer MC, Crowley JS, Laragh JH. The prevalence and correlates of echocardiographic LV hypertrophy among employed patients with uncomplicated hypertension. *J Am Coll Cardiol* 1986;7:639–650.

Hansen HS, Nielsen JR, Froberg K, Hyldebrandt N. LV hypertrophy in children from the upper five percent of the BP distribution—the Odense school child study. *J Hum Hypertens* 1992;6:41–45.

Harnish A, Pearce ML. Evolution of hypertensive retinal vascular disease: correlation between clinical and postmortem observations. *Medicine* 1973;52:483–533.

Harvey JM, Howie AJ, Lee SJ, Newbold KM, Adu D, Michael J, Beevers DG. Renal biopsy findings in hypertensive patients with proteinuria. *Lancet* 1992; 340:1435–1436.

Hatori N, Gardner JP, Tomonari H, Fine BP, Aviv A. Na⁺-H⁺ antiport activity in skin fibroblasts from blacks and whites. *Hypertension* 1990;15:140–145.

Hedblad B, Janzon L. Hypertension and ST segment depression during ambulatory. Electrocardiographic recording. Results from the prospective population study ''men born in 1914'' from Malm , Sweden. *Hypertension* 1992;20:32–37.

Heikinheima RJ, Haavisto MV, Kaarela RH, Kanto AJ, Koivunen MJ, Rajala SA. BP in the very old. *J Hypertens* 1990;8:361–367.

Helgeland A. Treatment of mild hypertension: a five year controlled drug trial. The Oslo Study. *Am J Med* 1980;69:725–732.

Helmer OM. Hormonal and biochemical factors controlling BP. In: *Les Concepts de Claude Bernard sur le Milieu Interieur.* Paris: Masson & Cie 1967:115–128.

Herlitz J, Karlson BW, Richter A, Wiklund O, Jablonskiene D, Hjalmarson Å. Prognosis in hypertensives with acute myocardial infarction. *J Hypertens* 1992; 10:1265–1271.

Hohn AR, Riopel DA, Keil JE, Loadholt B, Margolius HS, Halushka PV, Privitera PJ, Webb JG, Medley ES, Schuman SH, Rubin MI, Pantell RH, Braunstein ML. Childhood familial and racial differences in physiologic and biochemical factors related to hypertension. *Hypertension* 1983;5:56–70.

Hougaku H, Matsumoto M, Kitagawa K, Harada K, Oku N, Itoh T, Maeda H, Handa N, Kamada T. Silent cerebral infarction as a form of hypertensive target organ damage in the brain. *Hypertension* 1992; 20:816–820.

Houghton JL, Carr AA, Prisant LM, Rogers WB, von Dohlen TW, Flowers NC, Frank MJ. Morphologic, hemodynamic and coronary perfusion characteristics in severe LV hypertrophy secondary to systemic hypertension and evidence for nonatherosclerotic myocardial ischemia. *Am J Cardiol* 1992;69:219–224.

Hypertension in Diabetes Study Group. Hypertension in diabetes study (HDS): I. prevalence of hypertension in newly presenting type 2 diabetic patients and the association with risk factors for cardiovascular and diabetic complications. *J Hypertens* 1993;11:309–317.

Ishikawa K. Diagnostic approach and proposed criteria for the clinical diagnosis of Takayasu's arteriopathy. *J Am Coll Cardiol* 1988;12:964–972.

Isles CG, Hole DJ, Hawthorne VM, Lever AF. Relation between coronary risk and coronary mortality in women of the Renfrew and Paisley survey: comparison with men. *Lancet* 1992;339:702–706.

James SA, Keenan NL, Strogatz DS, Browning SR, Garrett JM. Socioeconomic status, John Henryism, and BP in black adults. *Am J Epidemiol* 1992;135:59–67.

Kagan A, Harris BR, Winkelstein W, et al. Epidemiologic studies of coronary heart disease and stroke in Japanese men living in Japan, Hawaii, and California: demographic, physical, dietary, and biochemical characteristics. *J Chron Dis* 1974; 27:345–364.

Kannel WB. The clinical heterogeneity of hypertension. *Am J Hypertens* 1991; 4:283–287.

Kannel WB, D'Agostino RB, Levy D, Belanger AJ. Prognostic significance of regression of LV hypertrophy [Abstract]. *Circulation* 1988;78(Suppl 2):89.

Kannel WB, D'Agostino RB, Wilson PWF, Belanger AJ. Diabetes, fibrinogen, and risk of cardiovascular disease: the Framingham experience. *Am Heart J* 1990; 120:672–676.

Kannel WB, Dannenberg AL, Abbott RD. Unrecognized myocardial infarction and hypertension: the Framingham Study. *Am Heart J* 1985;109:581–585.

Kannel WB, Sorli P, Castelli WP, McGee D. BP and survival after myocardial infarction: the Framingham Study. *Am J Cardiol* 1980;45:326–330.

Karam R, Lever HM, Healy BP. Hypertensive hypertrophic cardiomyopathy or hypertrophic cardiomyopathy with hypertension? A study of 78 patients. *J Am Coll Cardiol* 1989;13:580–584.

Keith NM, Wagener HP, Barker NW. Some different types of essential hypertension: their course and prognosis. *Am J Med Sci* 1939;197:332–343.

Knowler WC, Bennett PH, Ballintine EJ. Increased incidence of retinopathy in diabetics with elevated BP. *N Engl J Med* 1980;302:645–650.

Koren MJ, Devereux RB. Mechanism, effects, and reversal of LV hypertrophy in hypertension. *Curr Opin Nephrol Hypertens* 1993;28:87–95.

Koren MJ, Devereux RB, Casale PN, Savage DD, Laragh JH. Relation of LV mass and geometry to morbidity and mortality in uncomplicated essential hypertension. *Ann Intern Med* 1991;114:345–352.

Kotchen JM, McKean HE, Kotchen TA. BP trends with aging. *Hypertension* 1982; 4(suppl 3)128–134.

Koren MJ, Ulin RJ, Laragh JH, Devereux RB. Reduction in LV mass during treatment of essential hypertension is associated with improved prognosis [Abstract]. *Am J Hypertens* 1991;4:1A.

Krishna GG, Anand S, Kapoor SC. Augmented hypertensive response to mineralocorticoids (MC) in blacks [Abstract]. J Am Soc Nephrol 1992;3:532.

Lauer MS, Anderson KM, Kannel WB, Levy D. The impact of obesity on LV mass and geometry. *JAMA* 1991;266:231–236.

Law CM, de Swiet M, Osmond C, Fayers PM, Barker DJP, Cruddas AM. Initiation of hypertension in utero and its amplification throughout life. *Br Med J* 1993; 306:24–27.

Lederle FA, Walker JM, Reinke DB. Selective screening for abdominal aortic aneurysms with physical examination and ultrasound. *Arch Intern Med* 1988;148: 1753–1756.

Lee DK, Marantz PR, Devereux RB, Kligfield P, Alderman MH. LV hypertrophy in black and white hypertensives. Standard electrocardiographic criteria overestimate racial differences in prevalence. *JAMA* 1992;267:3294–3299.

Levy D, Garrison RJ, Savage DD, Kannel WB, Castelli WP. Prognostic implications of echocardiographically determined LV mass in the Framingham Heart Study. *N Engl J Med* 1990;322:1561–1566.

Levy D, Ho KKL, Larson MG, Kannel WB. The progression from hypertension to overt heart failure [Abstract]. *J Am Coll Cardiol* 1993;21:101A.

Liebson PR, Grandits G, Prineas R, Dianzumba S, Flack JM, Cutler JA, Grimm R, Stamler J. Echocardiographic correlates of LV structure among 844 mildly hypertensive men and women in the Treatment of Mild Hypertension Study (TOMHS). *Circulation* 1993;87:476–486.

Light KC, Dolan CA, Davis MR, Sherwood A. Cardiovascular responses to an active coping challenge as predictors of BP patterns 10 to 15 years later. *Psychosom Med* 1992;54:217–230.

Light KC, Obrist PA, Sherwood A, James SA, Strogatz DS. Effects of race and marginally elevated BP on responses to stress. *Hypertension* 1987;10:555–563.

Lindsay J Jr. Aortic dissection. *Heart Disease and Stroke* 1992;March/April:69–76.

Lipsitz LA, Storch HA, Minaker KL, Rowe JW. Intra-individual variability in postural BP in the elderly. *Clin Sci* 1985; 69:337–341.

Liu K, Ballew C, Jacobs DR Jr, Sidney S, Savage PJ, Dyer A, Hughes G, Blanton MM. Ethnic differences in BP, pulse rate, and related characteristics in young adults. The CARDIA Study. *Hypertension* 1989;14:218–226.

Liu K, Ruth K, Flack J, Burke G, Savage P, Liang K-Y, Hardin M, Hulley S. Ethnic differences in 5-year BP change in young adults. The CARDIA Study [Abstract]. *Circulation* 1992;85:6.

Luft FC, Miller JZ, Grim CE, Fineberg NS, Christian JC, Daugherty SA, Weinberger MH. Salt sensitivity and resistance of BP. *Hypertension* 1991;17(Suppl 1):102–108.

Lüscher TF, Tanner FC, Dohi Y. Age, hypertension and hypercholesterolaemia alter endothelium-dependent vascular regulation. *Pharmacol Toxicol* 1992;70(Suppl 2):32–39.

Lusiani L, Visoñ A, Pagnan A. Noninvasive study of arterial hypertension and carotid atherosclerosis. *Stroke* 1990;21:410–414.

MacMahon S, Peto R, Cutler J, Collins R, Sorlie P, Neaton J, Abbott R, Godwin J, Dyer A, Stamler J. BP, stroke, and coronary heart disease. Part 1, prolonged differences in BP: prospective observational studies corrected for the regression dilution bias. *Lancet* 1990;335:765–774.

Management Committee. The Australian therapeutic trial in mild hypertension. *Lancet* 1980;1:1261–1267.

Management Committee. Untreated mild hypertension. *Lancet* 1982;1:185–191.

Massie BM, Tubau JF, Szlachcic J, O'Kelly BF. Hypertensive heart disease: the critical role of LV hypertrophy. *J Cardiovasc Pharmacol* 1989;13(Suppl 1):18–24.

Maxwell MH. Cooperative study of renovascular hypertension: current status. *Kidney Int Suppl* 1975;8:153–160.

McAlpine HM, Morton JJ, Leckie B, Rumley A, Gillen G, Dargie HJ. Neuroendocrine activation after acute myocardial infarction. *Br Heart J* 1988;60:117–124.

McCarron DA, Morris CD, Cole C. Dietary calcium in human hypertension. *Science* 1982;217:267–269.

McClain DA, Paterson AJ, Roos MD, Wei X, Kudlow JE. Glucose and glucosamine regulate growth factor gene expression in vascular smooth muscle cells. *Proc Natl Acad Sci U S A* 1992;89:8150–8154.

Medical Research Council. MRC trial of treatment of mild hypertension: principal results. *Br Med J* 1985;291:97–104.

Mengden T, Binswanger B, Weisser B, Vetter W. An evaluation of self-measured BP in a study with a calcium-channel antagonist versus a β-blocker. *Am J Hypertens* 1992;5:154–160.

Messerli FH, Ventura HO, Glade LB, Sundgaard-Riise K, Dunn FG, Frohlich ED. Essential hypertension in the elderly: haemodynamics, intravascular volume, plasma renin activity, and circulating catecholamine levels. *Lancet* 1983;2:983–985.

Messerli FH. Obesity in hypertension: how innocent a bystander? *Am J Med* 1984;77:1077–1082.

Messerli FH, Garavaglia GE, Schmieder RE, Sundgaard-Riise K, Nunez BD, Amodeo C. Disparate cardiovascular findings in men and women with essential hypertension. *Ann Intern Med* 1987;107:158–161.

Miller JT, O'Rourke RA, Crawford MH. Left atrial enlargement: an early sign of hypertensive heart disease. *Am Heart J* 1988;116:1048–1051.

Modan B, Wagener DK. Some epidemiological aspects of stroke: mortality/morbidity trends, age, sex, race, socioeconomic status. *Stroke* 1992;23:1230–1236.

Molineux D, Steptoe A. Exaggerated BP responses to submaximal exercise in normotensive adolescents with a family history of hypertension. *J Hypertens* 1988; 6:361–365.

Møller-Petersen J. Nomogram for predictive values and efficiencies of tests. *Lancet* 1985;1:348.

Mueller FB, Laragh JH. Clinical evaluation and differential diagnosis of the individual hypertensive patient. *Clin Chem* 1991; 37:1868–1879.

Muirhead EE, Pitcock JA. Histopathology of severe renal vascular damage in blacks. *Clin Cardiol* 1989;12(Suppl 4):58–65.

Mukherjee DP, McTiernan CF, Sen S. Myotrophin induces early response genes and enhances cardiac gene expression. *Hypertension* 1993;21:142–148.

Mulvany MJ. A reduced elastic modulus of vascular wall components in hypertension? *Hypertension* 1992;20:7–9.

Munger RG, Gomez-Marin O, Prineas RJ, Sinaiko AR. Elevated BP among Southeast Asian refugee children in Minnesota. *Am J Epidemiol* 1991;133:1257–1265.

Narvarte J, Priv· M, Saba SR, Ramirez G. Proteinuria in hypertension. *Am J Kidney Dis* 1987;10:408–416.

Nobili F, Rodriguez G, Marenco S, De Carli F, Gambaro M, Castello C, Pontremoli R, Rosadini G. Regional cerebral blood flow in chronic hypertension: a correlative study. *Stroke* 1993;24:1148–1153.

Nørgaard K, Feldt-Rasmussen B, Borch-Johnsen K, S lan H, Deckert T. Prevalence of hypertension in type 1 (insulin-dependent) diabetes mellitus. *Diabetologia* 1990; 33:407–410.

O'Rourke MF. Arterial mechanics and wave reflection with antihypertensive therapy. *J Hypertens* 1992;10(Suppl 5):43–49.

Oster JR, Materson BJ. Renal and electrolyte complications of congestive heart failure and effects of therapy with angiotensin2D-converting enzyme inhibitors. *Arch Intern Med* 1992;152:704 710.

Paran E, Galily Y, Abu-Rabia Y, Neuman L, Keynan A. Environmental and genetic factors of hypertension in a biracial Beduin population. *J Hum Hypertens* 1992; 6:107–112.

Paul M, Ganten D. The molecular basis of cardiovascular hypertrophy: the role of the renin-angiotensin system. *J Cardiovasc Pharmacol* 1992;19(Suppl 5):51–58.

Pearson AC, Gudipati C, Nagelhout D, Sear J, Cohen JD, Labovitz AJ, Mrosek D, St Vrain J. Echocardiographic evaluation of cardiac structure and function in elderly subjects with isolated systolic hypertension. *J Am Coll Cardiol* 1991;17:422–430.

Perera GA: Hypertensive vascular disease: description and natural history. *J Chron Dis* 1955;1:33–42.

Perneger TV, Nieto J, Whelton PK, Klag MJ, Comstock GW, Szklo M. A prospective study of BP and serum creatinine. *JAMA* 1993;269:488–493.

Perneger TV, Whelton PK. The epidemiology of hypertension-related renal disease. *Curr Opin Nephrol Hypertens* 1993;2:395–403.

Perrone RD, Madias NE, Levey AS. Serum creatinine as an index of renal function: new insights into old concepts. *Clin Chem* 1992;38:1933–1953.

Perry IJ, Wannamethee G, Shaper AG. Haematocrit, BP and stroke in middle-aged men [Abstract]. *J Hypertens* 1992; 10:1430.

Pfeffer MA, Braunwald E, Moyé LA, Basta L, Brown EJ Jr, Cuddy TE, Davis BR, Geltman EM, Goldman S, Flaker GC, Klein M, Lamas GA, Packer M, Rouleau J, Rouleau JL, Rutherford J, Wertheimer JH, Hawkins CM. Effect of captopril on mortality and morbidity in patients with LV dysfunction after myocardial infarction. Results of the Survival and Ventricular Enlargement Trial. *N Engl J Med* 1992;327:669–677.

Phillips A, Shaper AG. Relative weight and major ischaemic heart disease events in hypertensive men. *Lancet* 1989; 1:1005–1008.

Phillips SJ, Whisnant JP. Hypertension and the brain. The National High BP Education Program. *Arch Intern Med* 1992; 152:938–945.

Pitts JF, Jardine AG, Murray SB, Barker NH. Spontaneous subconjunctival haemorrhage—a sign of hypertension? *Br J Ophthalmol* 1992;76:297–299.

Polese A, De Cesare N, Montorsi P, Fabbiocchi F, Guazzi M, Loaldi A, Guazzi MD. Upward shift of the lower range of coronary flow autoregulation in hypertensive patients with hypertrophy of the left ventricle. *Circulation* 1991;83:845–853.

Poulter NR, Khaw KT, Hopwood BEC, Mugambi M, Peart WS, Rose G, Sever PS. The Kenyan Luo migration study: observations on the initiation of a rise in BP. *Br Med J* 1990;300:967–972.

Pratt JH, Manatunga AK, Bowsher RR, Henry DP. The interaction of norepinephrine excretion with BP and race in children. *J Hypertens* 1992;10:93–96.

Preston RA, Materson BJ. Renal cholesterol emboli: a cause of hypertension in the elderly. *Cardiovasc Risk Factors* 1992, 2:101–104.

Prisant LM, Carr AA. Beyond diagnosis of LV hypertrophy in patients with essential hypertension. *Am J Hypertens* 1993; 6:174–176.

Prisant LM, von Dohlen TW, Houghton JL, Carr AA, Frank MJ. A negative thallium (+ dipyridamole) stress test excludes significant obstructive epicardial coronary artery disease in hypertensive patients. *Am J Hypertens* 1992;5:71–75.

Ranges HA. Benign aspects of hypertensive disease. *Med Clin North Am* 1949; May:611–617.

Reed DM. The paradox or high risk of stroke in populations with low risk of coronary heart disease. *Am J Epidemiol* 1990; 131:579.

Reichel H, Liebethal R, Hense H–W, Schmidt-Gayk H, Ritz E. Disturbed calcium metabolism in subjects with elevated diastolic BP. *Clin Invest* 1992; 70:748–751.

Reichek N. Patterns of LV response in essential hypertension. *J Am Coll Cardiol* 1992;19:1559–1560.

Roman MJ, Saba PS, Pini R, Spitzer M, Pickering TG, Rosen S, Alderman MH, Devereux RB. Parallel cardiac and vascular adaptation in hypertension. *Circulation* 1992;86:1909–1918.

Rosenthal J. Systolic and diastolic cardiac function in hypertension. *J Cardiovasc Pharmacol* 1992;19(Suppl 5):112–115.

Roubenoff R, Klag MJ, Mead LA, Liang K-Y, Seidler AJ, Hochberg MC. Incidence and risk factors for gout in white men. *JAMA* 1991;266:3004–3007.

Safar ME, Levy BI, Laurent S, London GM. Hypertension and the arterial system: clinical and therapeutic aspects. *J Hypertens* 1990;8(Suppl 7):113–119.

Salerno JA, Murphy DGM, Horwitz B, DeCarli C, Murphy JV, Rapoport SI, Schapiro MB. Brain atrophy in hypertension. A volumetric magnetic resonance imaging study. *Hypertension* 1992;20:340–348.

Sapira JD. An internist looks at the fundus oculi. *Dis Mon* 1984;30:1–64.

Savage DD, Levy D, Dannenberg AL, Garrison RJ, Castelli WP. Association of echocardiographic LV mass with body size, BP and physical activity (the Framingham Study). *Am J Cardiol* 1990;65:371–376.

Savage DD, Watkins LO, Grim CE, Kumanyika SK. Hypertension in black populations. In: Laragh JH, Brenner BM, eds. *Hypertension: Pathophysiology, Diagnosis, and Management.* New York: Raven Press, 1990:1837–1852.

Scheinberg P. Transient ischemic attacks: an update. *J Neurol Sci* 1991;101:133–140.

Schmidt R, Fazekas F, Offenbacher H, Lytwyn H, Blematl B, Niederkorn K, Horner S, Payer F, Freidl W. Magnetic resonance imaging of white matter lesions and cognitive impairment in hypertensive individuals. *Arch Neurol* 1991;48:417–420.

Schmieder RE, Messerli FH. Determinants of ventricular ectopy in hypertensive cardiac hypertrophy. *Am Heart J* 1992;123:89–94.

Schmieder RE, Messerli FH, Garavaglia G, Nunez B. Glomerular hyperfiltration indicates early target organ damage in essential hypertension. *JAMA* 1990; 264:2775–2780.

Schocken DD, Arrieta MI, Leaverton PE, Ross EA. Prevalence and mortality rate

of congestive heart failure in the United States. *J Am Coll Cardiol* 1992; 20: 301–306.

Schouten EG, Vandenbroucke JP, van der Heide-Wessel C, van der Heide RM. Retinopathy as an independent indicator of all-causes mortality. *Int J Epidemiol* 1986;15:234–236.

Schwartz SM, Ross R. Cellular proliferation in atherosclerosis and hypertension. *Prog Cardiovasc Dis* 1984;26:355–372.

Shannon RP, Maher KA, Santinga JT, Royal HD, Wei JY. Comparison of differences in the hemodynamic response to passive postural stress in healthy subjects > 70 years and < 30 years of age. *Am J Cardiol* 1991;67:1110–1116.

Shear CL, Freeman DS, Burke GL, Harsha DW, Berenson GS. Body fat patterning and BP in children and young adults. The Bogalusa Heart study. *Hypertension* 1987;9:236–244.

SHEP Cooperative Research Group. Prevention of stroke by antihypertensive drug treatment in older persons with isolated systolic hypertension. Final results of the Systolic Hypertension in the Elderly Program (SHEP). *JAMA* 1991;265: 3255–3264.

Shulman NB, Hall WD. Renal vascular disease in African-Americans and other racial minorities. *Circulation* 1991;83: 1477–1479.

Silagy CA, McNeil JJ. Epidemiologic aspects of isolated systolic hypertension and implications for future research. *Am J Cardiol* 1992;69:213–218.

Simon A, Levenson J. Use of arterial compliance for evaluation of hypertension. *Am J Hypertens* 1991;4:97–105.

Smith DE, Odel HM, Kernohan JW. Causes of death in hypertension. *Am J Med* 1950;9:516–527.

Smith WM. Treatment of mild hypertension: results of a ten-year intervention trial. *Circ Res* 1977;40(Suppl 1):98–105.

Sorlie P, Rogot E, Anderson R, Johnson NJ, Backlund E. Black-white mortality differences by family income. *Lancet* 1992;340:346–350.

Staessen J, Amery A, Fagard R. Isolated systolic hypertension in the elderly. *J Hypertens* 1990;8:393–405.

Steinmann WC, Millstein ME, Sinclair SH. Pupillary dilation with tropicamide 1% for funduscopic screening. *Ann Intern Med* 1987;107:181–184.

Stewart IMcDG. Headache and hypertension. *Lancet* 1953;1:1261–1266.

Strauer BE. The concept of coronary flow reserve. *J Cardiovasc Pharmacol* 1992; 19(Suppl 5):67–80.

Taylor JO, Borhani NO, Entwisle G, Farber M, Hawkins CM (Hypertension Detection and Follow-up Program). Summary of the baseline characteristics of the hypertensive participants. *Hypertension* 1983;5(Suppl 4):44–50.

Topol EJ, Traill TA, Fortuin NJ. Hypertensive hypertrophic cardiomyopathy of the elderly. *N Engl J Med* 1985;312:277–283.

Veterans Administration Cooperative Study Group on Antihypertensive Agents. Effects of treatment on morbidity in hypertension. Results in patients with diastolic

BPs averaging 115 through 129 mm Hg. *JAMA* 1967;202:116–122.

Veterans Administration Cooperative Study Group on Antihypertensive Agents. Effects of treatment on morbidity in hypertension. Results in patients with diastolic BPs averaging 90 through 114 mm Hg. *JAMA* 1970;213:1143–1152.

Veterans Administration Cooperative Study Group on Antihypertensive Agents. Urinary and serum electrolytes in untreated black and white hypertensives. *J Chron Dis* 1987;9:839–847.

Walker WG, Neaton JD, Cutler JA, Neuwirth R, Cohen JD. Renal function change in hypertensive members of the Multiple Risk Factor Intervention Trial. Racial and treatment effects. *JAMA* 1992;268:3085–3091.

Weber KT, Brilla CG. Pathological hypertrophy and cardia interstitium. *Circulation* 1991;83:1849–1865.

Weiss KM, Ferrell RE, Hanis CL. A new world syndrome of metabolic diseases with a genetic and evolutionary basis. *Yearbook Phys Anthropol* 1984;27:153–178.

Weiss NS. Relation of high BP to headache, epistaxis, and selected other symptoms. The United States Health Survey of Adults. *N Engl J Med* 1972;287:631–633.

Whittle JC, Whelton PK, Seidler AJ, Klag MJ. Does racial variation in risk factors explain black-white differences in the incidence of hypertensive end-stage renal disease? *Arch Intern Med* 1991; 151:1359–1364.

Wilson NV, Meyer BM. Early prediction of hypertension using exercise BP. *Prev Med* 1981;10:62–68.

Wilson TW, Grim CE. Biohistory of slavery and BP differences in blacks today. *Hypertension* 1991;17(Suppl 1):122–128.

Wilson TW, Hollifield LR, Grim CE. Systolic BP levels in black populations in sub-Sahara Africa, the West Indies, and the United States: a meta-analysis. *Hypertension* 1991;18(Suppl 1):87–91.

Wingard DL. Sex differences and coronary heart disease. A case of comparing apples to pears? *Circulation* 1990;81:1710–1712.

Wittenberg C, Zabludowski JR, Rosenfeld JB. Overdiagnosis of hypertension in the elderly. *J Hum Hypertens* 1992; 6: 349–351.

Wolf PA, D'Agostino RB, Belanger AJ, Kannel WB. Probability of stroke: a risk profile from the Framingham Study. *Stroke* 1991;22:312–318.

Wolf PA, D'Agostino RB, O'Neal A, Sytkowski P, Kase CS, Belanger AJ, Kannel WB. Secular trends in stroke incidence and mortality. The Framingham Study. *Stroke* 1992;23:1551–1555.

Yusuf S, Thom T, Abbott RD. Changes in hypertension treatment and in congestive heart failure mortality in the United States. *Hypertension* 1989;13(Suppl 1):74–79.

Zehender M, Meinertz T, Hohnloser S, Geibel A, Gerisch U, Olschewski M, Just H. Prevalence of circadian variations and spontaneous variability of cardiac disorders and ECG changes suggestive of myocardial ischemia in systemic arterial hypertension. *Circulation* 1992;85:1808–1815.

5 Treatment of Hypertension: Rationale and Goals

In the preceding four chapters, the epidemiology, natural history, and pathophysiology of primary (essential) hypertension were reviewed. We will now turn to its treatment, examining the benefits and costs of therapy in this chapter and the use of nondrug and drug treatment in the two chapters that follow.

This chapter addresses a question that many have simply answered "on faith"—Is the treatment of hypertension beneficial? The answer is clearly "yes" for those people with more severe degrees of hypertension, severity defined by the level of blood pressure (BP), the extent of target organ damage, and the presence of other cardiovascular risk factors. The answer, I believe, is much less certain for those with milder degrees of hypertension, and for some, the answer is clearly "no." As we shall see, most experts and practitioners in the United States have been more willing to pursue therapy of mild hypertension aggressively, whereas those elsewhere tend to be more cautious.

ATTITUDES ABOUT THERAPY OF HYPERTENSION

Evolution of the Current U.S. Practice

We have witnessed a major therapeutic revolution, matched in this century only by the advent of antibiotics. Spurred by the recognition of the major role played by uncontrolled hypertension in accelerating premature cardiovascular disease, and encouraged by the success in treating the more severe forms of the disease, physicians have begun drug therapy for millions of patients with milder degrees of hypertension.

A mounting, almost unbridled enthusiasm for "early and aggressive" drug therapy of mild hypertension began in the late 1970s, so that in the United States the treatment of hypertension is now the major reason for office visits to physicians and for the use of prescription drugs (Schappert, 1993). As a result of this unbridled enthusiasm, antihypertensive medication was being taken by over 30% of all Americans aged 55 to 64 and by over 40% of those aged 65 to 74 in 1982 to 1984 (Havlik et al., 1989). Since then, the proportion of those being treated likely has risen further (Joint National Committee, 1993).

The label "therapeutic activist" applies more to physicians in the United States than to physicians elsewhere. In an incisive essay, Guttmacher and associates (1981) provide two major reasons for the widespread acceptance of active drug therapy for mild hypertension, even in advance of evidence of its benefits. The first is that it is *preventive*, again based on the demonstrated evidence for the benefit of therapy for more severe hypertension. The second is *sociologic*, related to two widely held attitudes: (*a*) "technological optimism—the disposition to employ technologies in the belief that the benefits that flow from them will outweigh whatever unforeseen and undesirable effects that might ensue, and that these effects will themselves be manageable by existing or potential technological means," and (*b*) "therapeutic activism—physicians prefer to take the risk of treating when intervention may not be called for to the potential error of not treating when treatment is needed" (Guttmacher et al., 1981).

Differences Between the United States and Elsewhere

There are major differences in the opinions of experts and the practices of physicians in the United States versus most of the rest of the world. These differences can be seen in two major reports written by experts in the United States and England. The U.S. Joint National Committee report (1993) states:

If BP remains at or above 140/90 mm Hg during a 3–6 month period despite vigorous encouragement of lifestyle modifications, antihypertensive medications should be started, especially in individuals with target organ damage (TOD) and/or other known risk factors for cardiovascular disease. In the absence of TOD and other major risk factors, some physicians may elect to withhold antihypertensive drug therapy from patients with DBP [diastolic BP] in the 90–94 mm Hg range and SBP [systolic BP] in the 140–149 mm Hg range. In these patients, careful follow-up is indicated at 3–6 month intervals because BP may rise to higher levels, and cardiac and vascular changes may occur. Clinical trial data strongly suggest that antihypertensive drug therapy should be initiated before the development of TOD.

Contrast that statement with that of the second working party of the British Hypertension Society (Sever et al., 1993):

The management of patients whose DBPs remain between 90 and 99 mm Hg on repeated measurements over three to six months is controversial. Although the risk of heart attack and stroke is increased in this BP range, the risks and hence potential benefit of drug treatment to individual patients may be relatively small. The evidence of benefit from therapeutic intervention in all classes of patients is not universally accepted.

In view of the distribution of BPs in the population as noted in Chapter 1, the application of the U.S. recommendations would translate into many more patients with hypertension being put on drug treatment in the United States than would be treated in England. In fact, surveys of physicians' practices in the two countries document such differences: the majority of U.S. practitioners do treat patients with DBPs well below 100 mm Hg (Bostick et al., 1991); the majority of English practitioners do not (Waller et al., 1990).

Advocates of More Limited Therapy

Outside the United States

The more conservative attitude outside the United States reflects, in part, ethical concerns about the use of drug intervention among large numbers of asymptomatic people with mild hypertension in an attempt to reduce the risk for a small portion of the entire group. These concerns were delineated by Geoffrey Rose (1981), who wrote:

In reality the care of the symptomless hypertensive person is preventive medicine, not therapeutics. . . . If a preventive measure exposes many people to a small risk, then the harm it does may readily . . . outweigh the benefits, since these are received by relatively few. . . . We may thus be unable to identify that small level of harm to individuals from long-term intervention that would be sufficient to make that line of prevention unprofitable or even harmful. Consequently we cannot accept long-term mass preventive medication.

Within the United States

Despite the general enthusiasm of U.S. physicians to treat early and for low levels of hypertension, voices of caution have been heard here. Among the most eloquent is Edward Freis (1990) who, as principal investigator of the original Veterans Administration (VA) Cooperative Trials, has been given a large share of the credit for documenting the value of therapy. Another advocate of caution in the United States is Dr. Allan Brett (1984), who wrote:

In medical practice, the duty to inflict no harm (nonmaleficence) continuously competes with the duty to benefit the patient (beneficence). It follows that equivocal data on interventional efficacy may be sufficient to justify a recommendation to change some habits, since the risk of doing harm is small. Conversely, reasonably certain data is necessary to justify pharmacologic interventions, since the risk of doing harm is relatively greater. This argument assumes importance for a medicalized society in which unbridled enthusiasm to medicate often precedes reasonable proof of efficacy.

Despite these different attitudes and practices, I believe there is enough middle ground to develop a consensus on indications for drug therapy. Before attempting to "synthesize" such a consensus, I will review the rationale behind the universal acceptance of the need for antihypertensive therapy for many (if not all) hypertensives.

RATIONALE FOR DRUG THERAPY

The acceptance of the need to reduce the BP with antihypertensive agents comes in part from epidemiologic and experimental evidence, but mainly from the results of large-scale therapeutic trials.

Epidemiologic Evidence: Relation of Disease and Death to Blood Pressure Levels

This evidence, covered in Chapter 1, provides a clear conclusion: the risks of cardiovascular morbidity and mortality rise progressively with increasing BP levels (MacMahon et al., 1990).

Interrupting the Progress of Hypertension

The 15- to 17-year longitudinal study of Welshmen by Miall and Chinn (1973) and the 24-year follow-up of American aviators by Oberman et al. (1967) showed that hypertension begets further hypertension. In both studies, the higher the pressure, the greater was the rate of change of pressure, pointing to an obvious conclusion: progressive rises in pressure can be prevented by keeping the pressure down. This conclusion is further supported by the results of the major placebo-controlled trials of the therapy of hypertension: whereas 10% to 17% of those on placebo progressed beyond the respective threshold levels of diastolic pressure above 110 mm Hg, only a small handful of those on drug treatment did so (see Chapter 4).

Evidence from Natural Experiments in Humans

Vascular damage and the level of BP can be closely correlated in three situations: unilateral renal vascular disease, coarctation, and pulmonary hypertension. These three experiments of nature provide evidence that what is important is the level of the pressure flowing through a vascular bed and not some other deleterious effect associated with systemic hypertension. Tissues with lower pressure are protected; those with higher pressure are damaged.

Unilateral Renal Vascular Disease

The kidney with renal artery stenosis is exposed to a lower pressure than the contralateral kidney without stenosis. Arteriolar nephrosclerosis develops in the high-pressure nonstenotic kidney, occasionally to such a degree that hypertension can be relieved only by removal of the nonstenotic kidney, along with repair of the stenosis (Thal et al., 1963).

Coarctation of the Aorta

The vessels exposed to the high pressure above the coarctation develop atherosclerosis to a much greater degree than do the vessels below the coarctation, where the pressure is low (Hollander et al., 1976).

Pulmonary Hypertension

The low pressure within the pulmonary artery ordinarily protects these vessels from damage. When patients develop pulmonary hypertension secondary to mitral stenosis or certain types of congenital heart disease, both arteriosclerosis and arteriolar necrosis often develop within the pulmonary vessels (Heath and Edwards, 1958).

Evidence from Animal Experiments

Just as hypertension accelerates and worsens atherosclerosis in humans, animals made hypertensive develop more atherosclerosis than normotensive animals fed the same high-cholesterol diet (Chobanian, 1990). In animals, the lesions caused by hypertension, including accelerated atherosclerosis, can be prevented by lowering the pressure with antihypertensive agents (Masson et al., 1958; Chobanian et al., 1992).

Evidence from Clinical Trials of Antihypertensive Therapy

The last piece of evidence—that there is benefit from lowering an elevated BP—is the most important. Over the past four decades—since oral antihypertensive therapy has become available—protection with antihypertensive therapy has been demonstrated at progressively lower levels of pressure, originally for patients with DBPs above 140 mm Hg, more recently down to levels of 95 mm Hg.

Trials in Malignant Hypertension

The benefits of drug therapy in malignant hypertension were easy to demonstrate in view of its predictable, relatively brief, and almost uniformly fatal course in untreated patients. Starting in 1958, a number of studies appeared showing a significant effect of medical therapy in reducing mortality in malignant hypertension (see Chapter 8).

Trials in Moderate and Severe Hypertension

Demonstrating that therapy made a difference in nonmalignant, essential hypertension took a great deal longer. However, during the late 1950s and early 1960s, reports began to appear that suggested that therapy of nonmalignant hypertension was helpful (Leishman, 1961; Hodge et al., 1961; Hood et al., 1963). The first controlled, albeit small, study by Hamilton et al. (1964) showed a marked decrease in complications over a 2- to 6-year interval for 26 effectively treated patients as compared to 31 untreated patients.

VA Cooperative Study. The first definitive proof of the protection provided by antihypertensive therapy in nonmalignant hypertension came from the VA Cooperative Study, begun in 1963. The value of therapy in the 73 men with DBPs of 115 to 129 mm Hg given hydrochlorothiazide, reserpine, and hydralazine became obvious after less than 1 1/2 years (Veterans Administration Cooperative Study Group, 1967) (Table 5.1).

Along with these men with DBPs of 115 to 129, another 380 with DBPs between 90 and 114 also were assigned randomly to either placebo or active therapy. It took a longer time—up to 5.5 years, with an average of 3.3 years—to demonstrate a statistically clear advantage of therapy in this group (Veterans Administration Cooperative Study Group, 1970). A total of 19 of the placebo group but only 8 of the treated group died of hypertensive complications, and serious morbidity occurred more often among the placebo group. Overall, major complications occurred in 29% of the placebo group and 12% of the treated group.

Further analysis showed that the difference in morbidity was highly significant for those 210 men with DBPs between 105 and 114 mm Hg, but only suggestively so for those 170 with DBPs between 90 and 104 (Veterans Administration Cooperative Study, 1972).

Trials in Mild Hypertension With Nontreated Controls

The promising results of the VA study prompted the initiation of a number of additional

Table 5.1. VA Cooperative Study: Mortality and Morbidity in Patients with Diastolic Blood Pressure Between 115 and 129 mm Hg

	Placebo	Anti-hypertensive Drug
No. in study	70	73
Deaths	4	0
Complications	23	2
Accelerated hypertension	12	0
Cerebrovascular accident	4	1
Coronary artery disease	2	0
Congestive heart failure	2	0
Renal damage	2	0
Treatment failure	1	1

From Veterans Administration Cooperative Study Group on Antihypertensive Agents: *JAMA* 1967;202:116.

controlled trials of therapy of hypertension. A meta-analysis was performed on the data published by early 1990 from all 14 randomized trials of therapy of patients with any degree of hypertension that were not confounded by additional interventions for other risk factors (Collins et al., 1990) (Table 5.2), such as the Multiple Risk Factor Intervention Trial. The combined results of these 14 trials of all degrees of hypertension show clear evidence of protection against strokes and vascular death (Fig. 5.1). The reduction in all coronary heart disease (CHD) events was less (14%) but still statistically significant. However, the reduction in CHD mortality was only 11%, which was statistically insignificant.

In addition to these 14 trials, the results of three trials of treatment of elderly hypertensives have been published. They will be described separately, as will four trials that have compared two forms of therapy—diuretics and beta blockers.

The 14 unconfounded randomized trials included a total of 36,908 patients, 30,000 with DBPs below 110 mm Hg, another 3000 with DBPs below 115, and the remainder with DBPs up to 130 mm Hg. A diuretic was the initial drug given to those who were treated in all trials but two: a beta blocker was given to half of the treated patients in the Medical Research Council (MRC) trial (1985) and to all of the treated patients in the Coope and Warrender trial (1986). In 9 of the 14 trials, a placebo was given to half of the patients, whereas less intensive (usual care) treatment was provided both the control groups in the three Hypertension Detection and Follow-Up Program Cooperative Group (1979) strata, and the stroke survivors in the Carter (1970) and Hypertension-Stroke Cooperative (1974) studies.

Over the mean 5-year follow-up of all 14 trials, the average difference in DBP between the treated and control groups was 5 to 6 mm Hg. This degree of BP reduction was predicted to provide a 35% to 40% decrease in strokes and a 20% to 25% decrease in CHD. As seen in Figure 5.1 (for all studies) and in Figure 5.2 (for the individual studies), the full amount of protection against strokes was seen, but only about half of the expected protection against CHD was noted. Total and vascular mortality were significantly reduced, mainly because of the decrease in strokes.

Before attempting to understand why full protection was seen against strokes but not against

Table 5.2. Population Trial Design in Unconfounded Randomized Trials of at Least 1 Year of Antihypertensive Drug Treatment

Trial of Stratum (Reference, Years)	No. of Patients	Entry DBP (mm Hg)	Mean Age (Years)	Male (%)	Mean Follow-Up (Years)	Main Drugs	Mean DBP Differences (mm Hg) in Attenders[a]
Trials in which all patients had entry DBP <110 mm Hg							
VA-NHLBI (1978)	1,012	85–105	38	81	1.5	CD	7
HDFP stratum I (1979)	7,825	90–104	51[b]	55[b]	5.0	CD	5
Oslo (Helgeland, 1980)	785	90–109[c]	45	100	5.5	HZ	10
ANBPS (Management Committee, 1980)	3,427	95–109	50	63	4.0	CZ	6
MRC (1985)	17,354	90–109	52	52	5.0	BF or PR	6
Trials in which all patients had entry DBP ≤115 mm Hg							
VA (1970)	380	90–114	51	100	3.3	HZ + RE + HD	19
USPHS (1977)	389	90–114	44	80	7.0	CZ + RU	10
HDFP stratum II (1979)	2,052	105–114	51[b]	55[b]	5.0	CD	7
HSCSG (1974)	452	90–115	59	41	2.3	MC + DS	12
Trials in which some or all patients had entry DBP >115 mm Hg							
VA (1967)	143	115–129	51	100	1.5	HZ + RE + HD	27
Wolff (1966)	87	100–130	49	32	1.4	RE	20
Barraclough (1973)	116	100–120	56	43	2.0	BF or MD	13
Carter (1970)	99	≥110	NR	57	4.0	TH	NR
HDFP stratum III (1979)	1,063	≥115	51[b]	55[b]	5.0	CD	6
EWPHE (Amery, 1985)	840	90–119	72	30	4.7	HZ + TT	10
Coope and Warrender (1986)	884	105–120	69	31	4.4	AT	11
Mean or total	39,908	99	52	53	5.0	—	6[a]

[a]The difference in mean DBP per person-year of follow-up, based on data from those who attended follow-up for blood pressure measurement, was 6.4 mm Hg. The difference between all those allocated treatment (irrespective of compliance) and all those allocated control is likely to have been somewhat smaller (e.g., 5–6 mm Hg).
[b]Mean for entire HDFP study (all strata).
[c]No lower limit of DBP if systolic BP ≥150 mm Hg.
AT = atenolol, BF = bendrofluazide, CD = chlorthalidone, CD = chlorothiazide, DS = deserpidine, HZ = hydrochlorothiazide, MC = methyclothiazide, MD = methyldopa, PR = propranolol, RE = reserpine, RU = rauwolfia, TH = thiazide, TT = triamterene, NR = not recorded. VA-NHLBI = Veterans, 1978; HDFP = Hypertension Detection and Follow-up Program; MRC = Medical Research Council, 1985; VA = Veterans, 1970; VA = Veterans, 1967; Wolff = Wolff and Linderman, 1966; EWPHE = Amery et al., 1985.
From Collins R, et al. Blood pressure, stroke, and coronary heart disease. Part 2: Short-term reductions in blood pressure: overview of randomised drug trials in their epidemiological context. *Lancet* 1990;335:827–838.

CHD, one should look more closely at the larger trials.

Australian Trial in Mild Hypertension. The 3427 men and women included in this trial had DBPs between 95 and 109 mm Hg on the second set of BP readings and were free of clinical evidence of cardiovascular disease (Management Committee of the Australian National Blood Pressure Study, 1980) (Table 5.2). One-half were given placebo; it took 3 years to show a significant 30% difference in trial end-points.

Medical Research Council Trial. In many ways similar in design to the Australian and Oslo trials, the MRC trial was much larger and utilized two types of drug therapy for the half assigned to active treatment, either a diuretic or a beta blocker (Medical Research Council Working Party, 1985, 1988). The results are sim-

ilar to those observed in the other placebo-controlled trials: strokes were decreased, but coronary disease and total mortality were not significantly reduced by therapy (Fig. 5.2).

The conclusions of the MRC investigators (1985) were as follows:

The trial has shown that if 850 mildly hypertensive patients are given active antihypertensive drugs for one year about one stroke will be prevented. This is an important but an infrequent benefit. Its achievement subjected a substantial percentage of the patients to chronic side effects, mostly but not all minor. Treatment did not appear to save lives or substantially alter the overall risk of coronary heart disease. More than 95% of the control patients remained free of any cardiovascular event during the trial.

Neither of the two drug regimens had any clear overall advantage over the other. The diuretic was perhaps

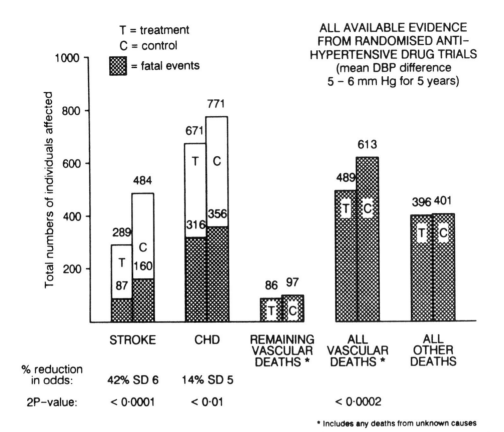

Figure 5.1. Combined results of the 14 unconfounded randomized trials of antihypertensive drug therapy in patients with all degrees of hypertension (total subjects = 37,000, mean DBP at entry = 99 mm Hg, mean DBP difference during follow-up = 6 mm Hg, mean time from entry to vascular event = 3 years). (From Collins R, Peto R, MacMahon S, et al. Blood pressure, stroke, and coronary heart disease. Part 2: Short-term reductions in blood pressure: overview of randomised drug trials in their epidemiological context. *Lancet* 1990;335:827).

better than the beta blocker in preventing stroke, but the beta blocker may have prevented coronary events in non-smokers.

European Working Party on High Blood Pressure in the Elderly (EWPHE) Trial.

This is the only major trial with untreated controls to show a statistically significant decrease in deaths from CHD (Amery et al., 1985). However, nonfatal myocardial infarctions (MIs) were more frequent in the treated group, and the overall effect on strokes was not significant.

Two features differentiate this study from the remainder: first, it involved only hypertensives over age 60; second, therapy included a potassium-sparing agent, triamterene, so that diuretic-induced hypokalemia (and hypercholesterolemia) were avoided. The protection against the biochemical alterations of the usually higher doses of naked diuretic used in the other trials (Table 5.2) could explain why CHD deaths were reduced in the EWPHE but not in the other trials.

Elderly Patients in Primary Care. This was the second published study on treatment of an elderly population (Coope and Warrender, 1986), but the patients in this study had more severe hypertension—DBPs between 105 and 120—than did those covered in the EWPHE trial. Treatment, largely with bendrofluazide and atenolol, was provided to half of the 884 patients aged 60 to 79 years at entry. Over a mean follow-up of 4.4 years, the treated group had an average fall of 18/11 mm Hg in pressure, a 30% reduction in fatal strokes, and a 58% decrease in all strokes, but no decrease in the incidence of MI or total mortality compared with the nontreated group.

Trials With Treated Controls

Although the data are more difficult to interpret as being purely related to either an overall difference in pressure or a specific difference of one mode of therapy versus another, we will now consider the large studies involving different forms and degrees of therapy in mild hypertension (Table 5.3).

Hypertension Detection and Follow-Up Program (HDFP).

The HDFP was designed to test the value of antihypertensive therapy for all degrees of hypertension among a representative sample of the American population aged 30 to 69 (Hypertension Detection and Follow-Up Program Cooperative Group, 1979). Of the 10,940 patients, over 7800 had DBPs between 90 and 104. Because patients with more severe hypertension also were included, it was considered inappropriate to leave any on placebo, so all patients were offered therapy. Half were referred to usual sources of medical care (i.e., Referred Care, or RC); the other half were given more intensive therapy using the stepped care (SC) drug regimen. Even though it was not placebo-controlled, this study was not confounded by other maneuvers beyond antihypertensive therapy, so it is included in the meta-analysis by Collins et al. (Table 5.2).

Over the 5 years of the study, more of the SC group received medication and reached the goal of therapy. Overall, 5-year mortality was reduced by 17% in the SC group (6.4 versus 7.7 per 100). Even more impressively, the SC half of the 7800 with "mild" hypertension (DBP 90 to 104) showed a 20% reduction in mortality. This was presumably a reflection of the higher proportion of the SC group who received medication and achieved the goal of therapy—a DBP below 90 or a reduction of the initial DBP of 10 mm Hg. The SC patients ended the trial with an average DBP some 5 mm Hg lower than that of the RC group—83 compared with 88 mm Hg. Equally impressive, the degree of protection was even greater among those with mildest hypertension: among the 5300 with DBPs between 90 and 104 who were not taking antihypertensive drugs and were free of end-organ damage on entry, the 5-year mortality rate was reduced 28.6% for the SC group (Hypertension Detection and Follow-up Cooperative Group, 1982a). When this population was subdivided further, the greatest degree of protection was found in those with entry DBPs of 90 to 94.

Questions about the HDFP Data. The 20% reduction in overall mortality among the mild hypertensives (5.9 versus 7.4 per 100) is highly significant statistically and has been accepted as

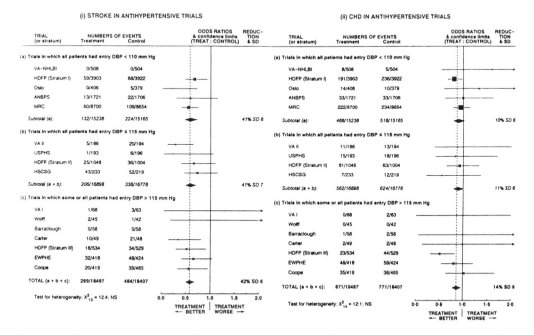

Figure 5.2. Effects on *(i)* stroke and *(ii)* coronary heart disease *(CHD)* in the unconfounded randomized trials of antihypertensive drug treatment. *Solid squares* represent the odds ratio (treatment:control) in each trial; the sizes of the squares are proportional to the amount of "information" contributed by that study. 99% confidence intervals (for individual trials) are denoted by *lines* and 95% confidence intervals (for overview of trials) by *diamonds*. (From Collins R, Peto R, MacMahon S, et al. Blood pressure, stroke, and coronary heart disease. Part 2: Short-term reductions in blood pressure: overview of randomised drug trials in their epidemiological context. *Lancet* 1990;335:827–838).

Table 5.3. Treatment Trials in Less Severe Hypertension With Treated Controls: Design and Blood Pressure Results

	Study and Year Reported			
	HDFP, 1979	MRFIT, 1982	IPPPSH, 1985	HAPPHY (Wilhelmsen, 1987)
Population				
Age (years)	30–69	35–57	40–64	40–64
% Male	54	100	50	100
% Black	45	7	—	—
Entry DBP (mm Hg)	I 90–104	≤115	100–125	100–130
	II 105–114 III ≥115	Hypertensives: 90–114 or on drug at entry		
End-organ damage	Included	Excluded	Excluded	Excluded
Total sample size ½ in each group	10,940	12,866 Hypertensives: 8012	6357	6569
Follow-up (years)	5	6–8	3–5	3.7 (mean)
Controls	Referred care	Usual Care	Placebo + nonβ-blocker drugs	Diuretic + nonβ-blocker drugs
Drugs (mg/dl)				
I	CTLD (25–100)	CTLD (25–100) or HCTZ (25–100)	OXPR (≥160)	Atenolol (100) or Metoprolol (200)
II	RES (0.1–0.25) or AMD (500–2000)	RES (0.1–0.25) or AMD (500–2000) or PROP (80–480)	AMIL, SPIR, TMTR, AMD, CLON, RES, GUAN, RESC, HDRZ, PRAZ, NFDP	Hydralazine (75–150)
III	HDRZ (30–200)	HDRZ (30–200)		SPIR (750–100)
DBP (mm Hg)				
Baseline	101	96	108	107
Change, study treated	– 17	– 14	– 19	– 19
Change, study control	– 12	– 10	– 18	– 18
Net change	– 5	– 4	– 1	– 1

CTLD, chlorthalidone; HCTZ, hydrochlorothiazide; OXPR, oxprenolol; RES, reserpine; AMD, alpha methyldopa; PROP, propranolol; AMIL, amiloride; SPIR, spironolactone; TMTR, triamterene; CLON, clonidine; GUAN, guanethidine; RESC, rescinnamide; HDRZ, hydralazine; PRAZ, prazosin; NFDP, nifedipine.
From MacMahon SW, Cutler JA, Furberg CD, Payne GH. The effects of drug treatment for hypertension on morbidity and mortality from cardiovascular disease: a review of randomized controlled trials. *Prog Cardiovasc Dis* 1986;29(Suppl 1):99–118.

strong evidence for the benefit of treating mild hypertension to achieve a DBP below the 90 mm Hg level.

However, the meaning of the HDFP results is not entirely clear, and doubts have been expressed as to whether the trial conclusively proved the benefit of active drug therapy for mild hypertension, particularly since the reduction in overall mortality included both a 20% decrease in cardiovascular deaths and a 13% decrease in noncardiovascular deaths. The former is likely attributable to the lowering of the pressure, but the 13% decrease in noncardiovascular deaths

likely reflects the more intensive overall medical care provided to the SC group. Thus, the reduced mortality has been attributed to the strong support system given the SC patients (Aagaard, 1981). However, the SC group had a lower incidence of strokes (Hypertension Detection and Follow-up Cooperative Group, 1982b), as well as a greater degree of both prevention and reversal of left ventricular hypertrophy (LVH) (Hypertension Detection and Follow-up Cooperative Group, 1985), both of which seem likely related to more effective antihypertensive therapy and not to overall medical care.

Multiple Risk Factor Intervention Trial (MRFIT). Unlike the other trials, MRFIT was designed to test the value of reductions of all three major risk factors for coronary disease— cigarette smoking, hypercholesterolemia, and hypertension in special intervention (SI) clinics (Multiple Risk Factor Intervention Trial, 1982). As with HDFP, the inclusion of patients with DBPs up to 114 led the investigators to offer therapy to the other half through usual sources of care in the community (Usual Care, or UC). Of the total of 12,866 enrollees, 8012 were hypertensive. Those given SI care ended with a fall in pressure at the end of the 6 years of 7/4 mm Hg more than did those given UC care.

The difference in coronary mortality, 7.1% lower in the SI group than in the UC group, was not statistically significant, most likely because the UC patients received so much care that they had a much lower mortality rate than expected. When the effects of the three SI programs were examined separately, the treatment of hypertension was the one that failed to result in any improvement and, in fact, was of apparent harm to some of the 62% of the total group who had hypertension. Those with initial DBPs of 90 to 94 who were treated more intensively with drugs (the SI group) had higher coronary and total mortality rates than did those less intensively treated (the UC group). No difference was observed in those with DBPs of 95 to 99 mm Hg, and protection was demonstrated by more intensive therapy in those with DBPs above 99.

Of additional concern was the higher coronary death rate in the more intensively treated SI hypertensives who had an abnormal baseline resting electrocardiogram (ECG). Subsequent analysis of these data showed an association between ECG abnormalities at entry and diuretic therapy: the relative risk of CHD mortality for those prescribed diuretics compared with those not prescribed diuretics was estimated as 3.34 among those with baseline ECG abnormalities at rest and as 0.95 among those without such abnormalities (Multiple Risk Factor Intervention Trial, 1985). This surprising finding prompted the Oslo and HDFP investigators to look at their participants in the same manner. Both found similar results: coronary morbidity in the Oslo trial (Holme et al., 1984) and coronary mortality in the HDFP trial (Hypertension Detection and Follow-up Cooperative Group, 1984) were higher in those who entered with an abnormal ECG and who received therapy (in the Oslo

trial) or more therapy (in the HDFP) (Table 5.4). Though these results did not reach statistical significance in either trial, the uniformity of the data strongly suggest that therapy *as it was given in these trials* could increase the likelihood of coronary events in patients with mild hypertension.

Trials Comparing Therapy With or Without a Beta Blocker

The remaining controlled studies in Table 5.3 differ from the others listed in Table 5.2 in that their purpose was not to determine the benefit of a reduction in BP but rather to compare the benefits of two forms of therapy. The first, the IPPPSH trial (International Prospective Primary Presentation Study in Hypertension, 1985), compared therapy with or without a specific beta blocker; the second, the HAPPHY (Heart Attack Primary Prevention in Hypertension) trial (Wilhelmsen et al., 1987), compared therapy with one of two beta blockers versus therapy with a diuretic. Together with the MRC trial (Medical Research Council Working Party, 1985), wherein the half of the patients given therapy were equally divided between a diuretic and a beta blocker, these trials can be used to examine the benefits of therapy with a beta blocker against therapy without a beta blocker.

The minimal difference (1 mm Hg in DBP) obtained in the IPPPSH trial resulted in no differences between the half given a beta blocker plus other drugs and the half given other drugs but no beta blocker.

HAPPHY and MAPHY. In the HAPPHY trial, 6569 men aged 40 to 64 were divided into two groups, half receiving a beta blocker, either metoprolol or atenolol, the other half receiving a diuretic, either bendrofluazide or hydrochlorothiazide. When the multicenter study was begun in March 1976, only metoprolol was used; in the third year of the trial, atenolol was added; eventually, an equal number of patients took either beta blocker. The HAPPHY trial was discontinued at the end of 1985, but the half of the patients who were in the metoprolol versus diuretic limb were followed for another 14 months. The slightly prolonged metoprolol limb was then analyzed separately and published as the Metoprolol Atherosclerosis Prevention in Hypertensives (MAPHY) Study (Wikstrand et al., 1988).

The overall HAPPHY data show no difference in the incidence of CHD or mortality between the diuretic and the beta blocker (metoprolol

Table 5.4. Coronary Event Rates per 1000 Person-Years With or Without ECG Abnormalities at Entry

Trial	No. of Subjects	Coronary Heart Disease Rate per 1000 Person-Years				End-Point
		Less Therapy	More Therapy	Difference (%)		
MRFIT, 1982						
Normal ECG	5593	3.4	2.6	−24		Death
Abnormal ECG	2418	2.9	4.9	+70		
HDFP, 1984b						
Normal ECG	3210	3.1	2.0	−35		Death
Abnormal ECG	1963	3.5	4.3	+23		
		No Therapy	Therapy	Difference (%)		
Oslo (Holme et al., 1984)						
Normal ECG	498	7.2	8.8	+22		Event
Abnormal ECG	287	6.4	12.0	+88		

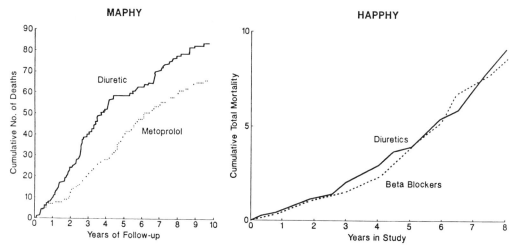

Figure 5.3. *Left,* Total cumulative mortality in the two groups in the MAPHY trial. *Solid line* indicates diuretic therapy (n = 1625); *broken line,* metoprolol (n = 1609) (P = .028). (From Wikstrand J, Warnold I, Olsson G, et al. Primary prevention with metoprolol in patients with hypertension. *JAMA* 1988;259:1976, copyright 1988, American Medical Association). *Right,* Cumulative total mortality in the two groups in the HAPPHY trial. (From Wilhelmsen L, Berglund G, Elmfeldt D, et al. Beta blockers versus diuretics in hypertensive men: main results from the HAPPHY Trial. *J Hypertens* 1987;5:561).

or atenolol) treatment groups (Fig. 5.3, *right*). However, the metoprolol half of the MAPHY group had significantly lower total mortality than did those on diuretics, with fewer deaths from both CHD and stroke (Fig. 5.3, *left*). The authors chose the median follow-up time of 4.2 years to demonstrate the greatest difference between the two groups because there was some admixture of the two forms of therapy toward the end of the 11 years of the study. The difference in total mortality was 48% at 4.2 years, but by the end of the study, the difference had shrunken to a statistically insignificant 22%.

Beyond the questionable use of the median time rather than the end of the study, as is the usual practice, numerous questions have been raised about the disparate data from the HAPPHY and MAPHY trials. Regardless, the MAPHY data have been defended as the first documentation of primary protection against coronary disease by one type of drug (metoprolol) compared with another (thiazide diuretic) (Wikstrand et al., 1988). Since there was no placebo group, the data cannot be used as evidence that metoprolol lowered the incidence of CHD below that of an untreated population, but only that it was superior to a diuretic. Moreover, the difference mainly reflects a *higher* coronary mortality rate in the diuretic-treated half of the MAPHY patients compared to that seen in the other trials.

Overall Impact of Beta Blocker Therapy. The data from the three trials that only compared beta blocker therapy with non–β–blocker therapy can be combined with that from the MRC trial, wherein the half of the subjects who received drug therapy were randomly allocated to either a diuretic (bendrofluazide) or a beta blocker (propranolol). A meta-analysis of these four sets of data, computing the differences between the therapies based on beta blockers and those not based on beta blockers for each trial and for the two sexes separately, shows that therapy with a beta blocker tended to decrease mortality in men but tended to increase mortality in women (Staessen et al., 1988) (Fig. 5.4). In two of the three trials, the beta blocker was more cardioprotective in those who did not smoke, whereas in the MAPHY trial, the beta blocker was more protective in those who did smoke.

Trials in the Elderly

In view of the rapidly increasing numbers of elderly people and their high prevalence of hypertension (see Chapter 1), it is noteworthy that three major clinical trials on the treatment of hypertension in the elderly have been completed and yet another is in progress as of this writing (Amery et al., 1991). These three trials markedly expand the data previously available (Table 5.5), which include a small trial from Japan (Kuramoto et al., 1981), two medium-sized trials in Europe (Amery et al., 1985) and England (Coope and Warrender, 1986), and the considerable numbers of people over age 60 who enrolled in the Australian (Management Committee, 1981) and HDFP trials.

A meta-analysis of the results of seven of these eight trials has been performed, excluding the Systolic Hypertension in the Elderly (SHEP) trial "because isolated systolic hypertension constitutes a separate pathophysiological entity" (Thijs et al., 1992). Although all-cause mortality was reduced only by 9% overall, cardiovascular mortality was significantly reduced

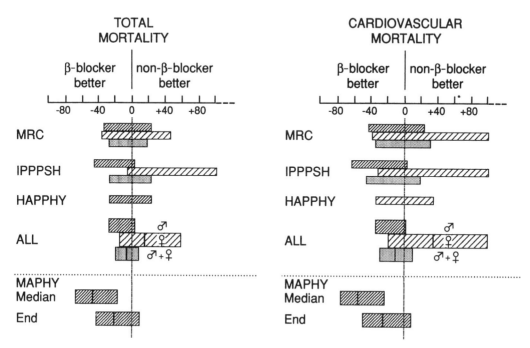

Figure 5.4. Percentage of differences (means and 95% confidence intervals) in total (*left*) and cardiovascular (*right*) mortality between antihypertensive treatment based on beta blockers and not based on beta blockers in various trials and two sexes. For the Metoprolol Atherosclerosis Prevention in Hypertensives (MAPHY) Study, statistics refer to median and total (end of study) follow-up. In meta-analysis *(ALL)*, results of three trials were combined (MRC, International Prospective Primary Prevention Study in Hypertension [IPPPSH], and Heart Attack Primary Prevention in Hypertensives [HAPPHY]) (From Staessen J, Fagard R, Amery A. Primary prevention with metoprolol in patients with hypertension [Letter]. *JAMA* 1988;260:1713, copyright 1988, American Medical Association).

Table 5.5. Population and Design of Randomized Placebo-Controlled Trials in the Elderly

Trials (References)	No. of Patients	Mean Entry BP (mm Hg)	Age Range (Years)	Male (%)	Mean Follow-Up (Years)	Main Drugs	Mean Difference in BP Reduction (mm Hg)
HDFP (1979)	2374	170/101	60–69	55	5	Chlorthalidone	?/5
Kuramoto (1981)	91	168/86	60–90+	55	4	Trichlomethiazide	5/2
Australian (Management, 1981)	582	165/101	60–69	55	4	Chlorothiazide	11/7
EWPHE (Amery, 1985)	840	182/101	60–96	30	4.6	Hydrochlorothiazide + trimterene	21/7
Coope and Warrender (1986)	884	197/100	60–79	30	4.4	Atenolol Bendrofluazide	16/10
SHEP (1991)	4736	170/77	60–80+	43	4.5	Chlorthalidone Atenolol	11/3
STOP-HT (Dahlöf, 1991)	1627	195/102	70–84	37	2	Hydrochlorothiazide + amiloride or 1 of 3 β-blockers	22/9
MRC (1992)	4396	185/91	65–74	42	5.8	Hydrochlorothiazide + amiloride or atenolol	16/7

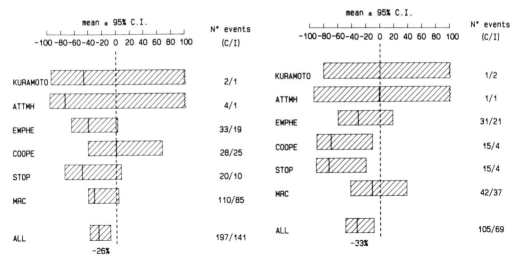

Figure 5.5. A meta-analysis of six trials of treatment of hypertension in the elderly, showing for each study the percentage of difference in coronary mortality (*left*) and stroke mortality (*right*) between the treated and control groups, together with the 95% confidence interval (*C.I.*) of this difference. A *negative sign* indicates a decrease in mortality in the treated group. The summary of all the data, calculated by the Mantel-Haenszel procedure, is at the bottom (*ALL*). For each study, the number of events in the control and intervention groups *(C/I)* is given on the right side of each set of bar graphs. The studies are denoted as follows: *Kuramoto,* Kuramoto et al., 1981; *ATTMH,* Australian Therapeutic Trial (Management Committee, 1981); *EWPHE,* European Working Party (Amery et al., 1985); *Coope,* Coope and Warrender, 1986; *STOP,* Swedish Trial in Old Patients (Dahlöf et al., 1991); *MRC,* Medical Research Council Working Party, 1992. (From Thijs L, Fagard R, Lijnen P, et al. A meta-analysis of outcome trials in elderly hypertensives. *J Hypertens* 1992;10:1103–1109).

by 22%, and both coronary and stroke mortality were significantly reduced (Fig. 5.5). In the SHEP trial (SHEP Cooperative Research Group, 1991), mortality was not significantly reduced, but the numbers of nonfatal myocardial infarction, stroke, and congestive heart failure (CHF) events were significantly lowered (Table 5.6).

The numbers of stroke, coronary, CHF, and all cardiovascular events, including all morbidity and mortality, were impressively reduced in nearly all of these trials. The impact of therapy on CHF was particularly striking in both the Swedish Trial in Old Patients with Hypertension (STOP-Hypertension) and the SHEP trial.

In view of the importance of these data, I now will take a closer look at the results of the three larger trials—SHEP, STOP-Hypertension, and MRC.

Systolic Hypertension in the Elderly Program (SHEP). This is the only trial that exclusively enrolled patients with isolated systolic hypertension (ISH), the most common form of hypertension in the elderly (see Chapter 4). Over 450,000 people were screened to enroll the 4736 patients with SBPs over 160 and DBPs under 90 and no limitations of daily activities or conditions that threatened their near-term survival (SHEP Cooperative Research Group, 1991).

The half who were started on drug therapy received a low dose (12.5 mg) of the diuretic chlorthalidone. If the pressure did not respond, the dose was increased to 25 mg, and then up to 50 mg of atenolol could be added. Thereby, BP fell slowly and gently, and was generally well tolerated. At the end of the 5 years, almost half of the drug-treated patients were receiving only a diuretic in order to reach the goal of either an SBP below 160 or, if the initial SBP was 160 to 179, a reduction of at least 20 mm Hg. The mean fall in BP was 27/9 mm Hg.

A large percentage of the half initially assigned to placebo had a rise in pressure above the pre-set limits and therefore were switched to active drug therapy—44% by the end of 5 years. This large conversion of placebo patients to active treatment means that the results—as impressive as they are—are diluted, since more morbidity would almost certainly have occurred in the placebo group if all had remained off active therapy. The mean fall in BP of the placebo group was 16/6 mm Hg, yielding only a difference of 11/3 mm Hg between the two groups. That difference was sufficient to provide

a significant difference in trial outcome measures.

Swedish Trial in Old Patients with Hypertension (STOP-Hypertension). This trial enrolled elderly patients with combined systolic and diastolic hypertension (Dahlöf et al., 1991). Unlike the multiple steps of therapy in the SHEP, these patients received either hydrochlorothiazide, 25 mg, plus amiloride, 2.5 mg, or a small dose of one of three beta blockers (atenolol, metoprolol, or pindolol) as a first step and a combination of the diuretic and one of the beta blockers as the second step. At the end of the trial, 77% of the placebo group and 84% of the active group were taking their originally assigned medication. Two-thirds of the active group were taking combined therapy to achieve the goal of a BP under 160/95.

MRC Trial in the Elderly. The last of the major trials in the elderly to be reported is also the weakest, likely because it was conducted by a network of 226 general practices throughout the United Kingdom (Medical Research Council Working Party, 1992). Of the 4396 subjects entered, 25% were lost to follow-up. Of those assigned to a specific therapy—either a diuretic or a beta blocker in the active half or a placebo in the other half—more than half were not taking their assigned therapy by the end of the study.

Despite these methodologic problems, there were significant reductions in strokes and all cardiovascular events, although mortality rates differed little between the treated and placebo groups. Perhaps of greatest interest were the differences in protection against stroke and coronary disease provided by the two drugs: whereas the beta blocker was only slightly less effective than the diuretic against stroke, it was totally ineffective against coronary disease. The better

Table 5.6. Effects of Therapy in Elderly Hypertensive Patients

	Australian Management (1981)	EWPHE Amery (1985)	Coope & Warrender (1986)	SHEP (1991)	STOP-HT (Dahlöf, 1991)	MRC (1992)
Mean BP at entry	165/101	182/101	197/100	170/77 (100% ISH)	195/102	185/91 (43% ISH)
Relative risk of events per 1000 patient years (treated versus placebo)						
Stroke	0.67	0.64*	0.58*	0.67*	0.53*	0.75*
Coronary disease	0.82	0.80	1.03	0.73*	0.87[b]	0.81
Congestive failure		0.78	0.68	0.45*	0.49*	
All cardiovascular	0.69	0.71*	0.76*	0.68*	0.60*	0.83*

[a]Statistically significant.
[b]MI only: sudden deaths decreased from 13 to 14.

effects noted in the diuretic-treated patients were not attributable to the somewhat greater and more rapid control of BP compared to the beta blocker group, leading the investigators to "raise the possibility that the diuretic confers benefit through another mechanism beside blood pressure lowering" (Medical Research Council Working Party, 1992).

Overview of the Trials in the Elderly. Beard et al. (1992) reviewed the six major trials shown in Table 5.5 and concluded that "There is convincing evidence that efforts should be made to reduce both systolic and diastolic pressures to below 160/90 mm Hg in patients up to the age of 80 years," since "there is now indisputable evidence that the active treatment of hypertension in the elderly is associated with significant improvements in cardiovascular morbidity and mortality." These authors point out that the benefits provided to the elderly in these six trials, as seen in Table 5.6 and Figure 5.5, are considerably greater than those provided to younger patients in the 12 trials described in Table 5.2 and Figure 5.2.

As impressive as these data are, caution has been advised about extrapolating them to the general population of often less healthy elderly people (Staessen et al., 1991) and to the population over 80 years old, in whom survival may be better at higher pressures, particularly since so few patients over 80 were included in the trials (Bulpitt and Fletcher, 1992).

Overview of All Trials

Both in the 12 trials involving middle-aged patients and to a lesser degree in the 6 involving the elderly, one fact is obvious: protection against stroke has been more impressive than protection against coronary disease. The difference observed in the trials in the elderly is about what the prospective epidemiologic evidence shown in Chapter 1, Figure 1.2 (MacMahon et al., 1990) would predict, but a shortfall remains in the middle-aged population (Figures 5.1 and 5.2). It should be noted that Figures 5.1 and 5.2 include the results of two trials in the elderly: the EWPHE trial, which showed some of the more positive effects on coronary disease, and the Coope and Warrender trial, which showed no protection.

The lesser degree of protection from coronary disease, the major cause of cardiovascular morbidity and mortality, than was expected from antihypertensive therapy has been observed not only in the controlled trials but also in clinical practice. One of the clearest demonstrations of the failure of therapy to reduce the risk of cardiovascular disease to that seen in untreated persons with similar levels of pressure is the experience of the Glasgow Blood Pressure Clinic, where 3783 patients were treated between 1968 and 1983, for an average of 6.5 years. The mortality rates for those patients, whose DBPs were reduced to less than 90 mm Hg, were compared with the rates for age- and sex-matched populations in two nearby communities, Renfrew and Paisley (Isles et al., 1986) (Fig. 5.6). It is obvious that mortality rates were higher in the treated groups than in those without hypertension whose DBPs were at the same level.

Why are the excess risks associated with elevated BP not removed by prolonged reduction of the pressure to the levels seen in untreated people? A number of possibilities exist.

Unresolved Risks of Treated Hypertension

Multifactorial Origin of Coronary Heart Disease

CHD, much more than stroke, is related causally to multiple factors including cholesterol, smoking, and diabetes. As shown in the Gothenberg trial (Samuelsson et al., 1987), which is described below under "Hazards of Therapy," it may not be possible to reduce CHD risk significantly by attacking only one risk factor. Most trials have done just that. Moreover, the extent of silent but significant coronary artery disease may have been more advanced among many participants in the therapeutic trials than generally was recognized (O'Kelly et al., 1989).

Short Duration of Intervention

Even when multiple risks are attacked, as in the MRFIT trial, the intervention may not have been begun early enough or continued long enough to have a meaningful impact on the atherosclerotic process.

Despite the added statistical power provided by combining multiple studies in a meta-analysis, the relatively short time of follow-up provides relatively few events. As Collins et al. (1990) note: "If chronic processes are involved so that the eventual effects of a 5–6 mm Hg difference in DBP are not fully seen during just the few years of treatment duration for those dying in the trials, then the power of even an overview of all trials might be inadequate to detect benefit."

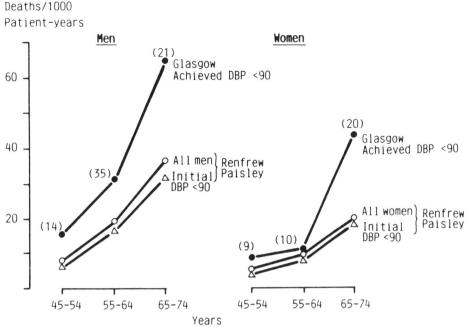

Figure 5.6. Age- and sex-specific mortality rates (deaths/1000 patient-years) in Glasgow Clinic patients whose diastolic blood pressures *(DBP)* were reduced to less than 90 mm Hg by treatment at their last clinic visit, compared with subjects in the Renfrew/Paisley control population. Deaths in the Glasgow Clinic are given in parentheses. (From Isles CG, Walker LM, Beevers GD, et al. Mortality in patients of the Glasgow Blood Pressure Clinic. *J Hypertens* 1986;4:141).

Methodologic Problems

Other problems with the analyses performed on the data in the clinical trials have been noted, in particular the use of the "intention-to-treat" method, wherein patients assigned initially to one group are kept in that group regardless of their subsequent experience (Maxwell, 1987). In addition, most patients were entered into studies too quickly, before their pressures had fallen to their true level. For these and other reasons (Simpson, 1990), data from large-scale trials may minimize the benefits conferred by therapy.

Hazards of Therapy

As will be delineated in Chapter 7, every anti-hypertensive drug can induce adverse effects. The two drugs almost exclusively used in the majority of patients in most of the trials—diuretics and beta blockers—are particularly prone to induce various metabolic changes that may adversely affect coronary risk. The high doses of diuretics used in most trials are particularly suspect since they may raise total and low-density lipoprotein (LDL) cholesterol, worsen glucose tolerance, lower serum potassium and, at the same time, fail to reduce the burden of LVH.

The potential impact of one of the adverse effects of diuretic and beta blocker therapy, the rise in serum cholesterol, is suggested by data from a 12-year study of 686 men in Gothenberg, Sweden, who were treated for up to 12 years with one or both antihypertensive agents without concomitant attempts to alter their lipid status. The CHD morbidity that developed during the 4th to 12th years of therapy was predicated closely on the combined changes in BP and serum cholesterol level (Samuelsson et al., 1987) (Fig. 5.7). Even with the maximal degree of BP reduction (20%), little impact on CHD morbidity was noted among those whose cholesterol levels rose by an average of 7%. Those whose cholesterol levels fell by an average of 11% achieved the maximal degree of protection.

The better coronary protection seen in the last three major trials in the elderly could reflect the avoidance of problems from the high doses of diuretics and beta blockers used in the previous trials. Rather than the equivalent of 50 to 100 mg of hydrochlorothiazide used previously, 12.5 to 25 mg were the starting doses in the SHEP, STOP-Hypertension, and MRC trials in the elderly. Also, in all three, care was taken to avoid hypokalemia through the use of potassium supplements in the SHEP and by potassium-sparers in the other two trials.

Lack of Adequate Control

In many trials, a significant portion (from 20% to almost 50%) of the study population was not treated successfully to the usual goal of a DBP below 90 mm Hg (Hansson and Dahlöf, 1990). As is well documented in the patients treated in the Glasgow Clinic, the mortality rates of treated patients are determined not by their initial BP but by the level of pressure achieved during therapy (Isles et al., 1986) (Fig. 5.8). Thus, inadequate or poorly sustained reductions in pressure may have been responsible for the persistence of higher risk during therapy.

Overtreatment of Susceptible Patients

Conversely, overtreatment also may have contributed, at least among the sizeable portion of the hypertensive population susceptible to myocardial ischemic injury by a reduction in coronary perfusion pressure. An association between reduction of BP and ischemic injury was first suggested by Stewart (1979), who reported a fivefold increase in MI among patients whose DBP was reduced to below 90 mm Hg. Stewart's report was largely neglected, but when Cruickshank et al. (1987) reported the same phenomenon, interest immediately focused on the problem and has intensified progressively.

The data from 13 studies that were available in mid-1990 were analyzed by Farnett et al. (1991). The summary curve model that best fits the data from the seven of these studies that evaluated cardiac events by levels of treated DBP clearly indicates a J or U curve (Fig. 5.9). Since that review, additional reports of a J curve have appeared (Cohen et al., 1991; McCloskey et al., 1992; Hypertension Follow-up Group, 1992).

Increased cardiovascular mortality also has been reported among nontreated persons whose natural DBP is below 90 mm Hg. This was reported in an analysis of the original Framingham data by Anderson (1978) and among elderly hypertensives who served as controls in the trials of Coope and Warrender (1986) and EWPHE (Staessen et al., 1989). Such increased mortality could reflect the presence of severe cardiac dysfunction unrelated to antihypertensive therapy. Thus, in the Framingham cohort, higher mortality rates at low DBPs were seen in survivors of myocardial infarction but not in low-risk subjects (D'Agostino et al., 1991).

Cruickshank (1988) postulates that the probable mechanism for the increase in coronary ischemia with treatment-induced falls in systemic pressure is an inability to maintain coronary blood flow as perfusion pressure falls because

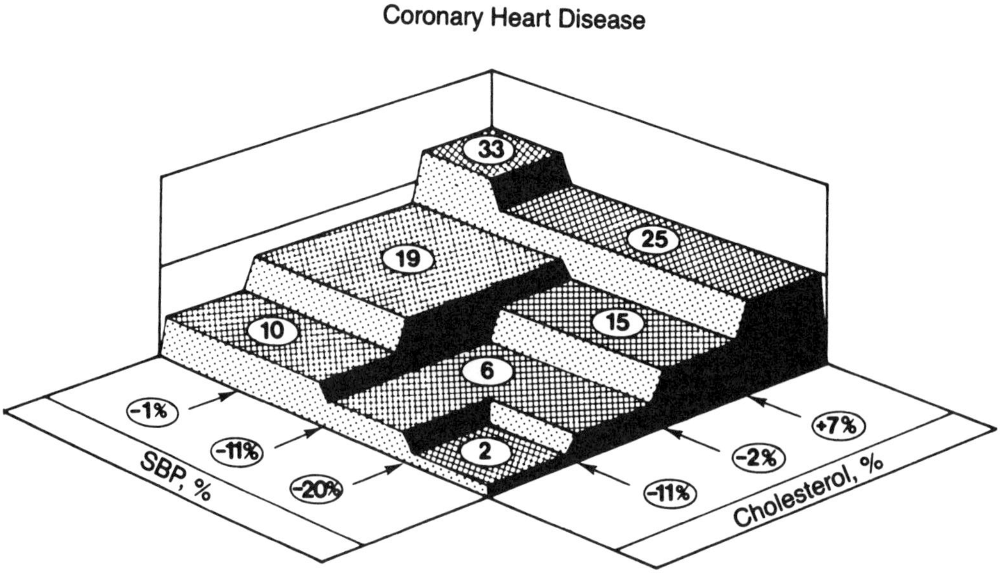

Coronary Heart Disease

Figure 5.7. Coronary heart disease morbidity during the 4th to 12th years of antihypertensive treatment in relationship to relative change (during initial 4 years of follow-up) of both systolic blood pressure (*SBP*) and serum cholesterol levels (*Cholesterol*) divided into quartiles. Rates are adjusted for risk at entry. (From Samuelsson O, Wilhelmsen L, Andersson OK, et al. Cardiovascular morbidity in relation to change in blood pressure and serum cholesterol levels in treated hypertension. Results from the Primary Prevention Trial in Göteborg, Sweden. *JAMA* 1987;258:1768, copyright 1989, American Medical Association).

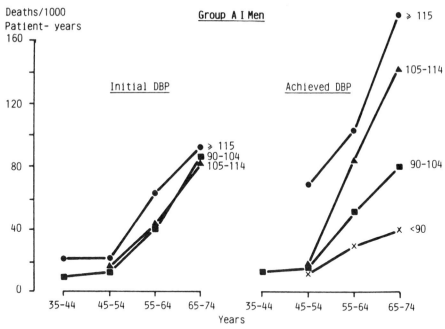

Figure 5.8. Age-specific mortality rates (death/1000 patient-years) for a subset of 1162 men not initially on therapy whose blood pressures were measured both at entry to the clinic and thereafter during treatment. At all ages, the influence of achieved blood pressure on mortality was greater than that of initial blood pressure. *DBP*, diastolic blood pressure. (From Isles CG, Walker LM, Beevers GD, et al. Mortality in patients of the Glasgow Blood Pressure Clinic. *J Hypertens* 1986;4:141).

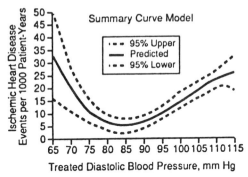

Figure 5.9. Relation between morbidity and mortality from coronary disease and the level of treated diastolic blood pressure in seven studies of hypertensive patients treated for over 1 year, mostly with diuretics and beta blockers. (From Farnett L, Mulrow CD, Linn WD, Lucey CR, Tuley MR. The J-curve phenomenon and the treatment of hypertension. *JAMA* 1991;265:489–495).

presence of myocardial hypertrophy (Polese et al., 1991).

As noted in Chapter 2, falls in pressure during sleep may be profound and further accentuated by inadvertent overtreatment. Mansour et al. (1993) have shown that hypertensives with LVH experience nocturnal ischemia in association with treatment-induced falls in diastolic pressure.

Cruickshank's presentation and concept have not gone unchallenged. In particular, questions have been raised as to the exactness of the critical level where the break in the curve appears and the relatively few events that make up the curves (Hansson, 1990). Moreover, a decrease in coronary events has been seen in patients with left ventricular dysfunction whose initially low pressures were reduced even further by angiotensin-converting enzyme (ACE) inhibitor therapy, well below the break of 85 to 90 mm Hg in the J curve (Yusuf et al., 1992). For these reasons, Fletcher and Bulpitt (1992), in their review of the available evidence, conclude that "the J-curve is probably a consequence, not a cause of coronary heart disease." The issue, one hopes, will be settled by a prospective large-scale study wherein patients will have their DBPs reduced

of impairment of autoregulation within atherosclerotic vessels (i.e., a fall in coronary flow reserve). As Strandgaard and Haunsø (1987) have demonstrated, the coronary circulation has poor autoregulatory reserve; since oxygen extraction is nearly maximal at rest, lowering of perfusion pressure can lead to myocardial ischemia. The problem is compounded in the to different levels below 90 (HOT Study Group, 1993).

Until those data are available, I remain persuaded by Cruickshank's arguments (1992). Simply stated, inadvertent overtreatment, particularly but not exclusively among patients with preexisting coronary disease, likely contributes to the failure to demonstrate a reduction in heart attacks in patients treated for hypertension.

There are, then, multiple reasons why antihypertensive therapy, as previously and currently provided, has not fulfilled the promise of protection against coronary disease.

Other Data on the Benefits of Antihypertensive Therapy

In addition to the multiple controlled trials that have looked primarily at the effects of therapy on CHD and stroke, many smaller studies have examined the influence of antihypertensive therapy on other end-points. These end-points include total mortality and the distribution of specific causes of death, as well as both morbidity and mortality from the damage induced by hypertension on the major end-organs as described in Chapter 4 (the heart, brain, kidneys, and large arteries).

Overall Mortality and Specific Causes of Death

Total mortality rates have fallen over the past 20 years, both for hypertensive and normotensive people in the United States and in most industrialized societies (see Chapter 1). Most of this fall is attributable to a decrease in deaths caused by cardiovascular diseases (stroke more than coronary disease).

However, the contribution made by antihypertensive therapy per se is uncertain. In the controlled trials, it seems likely that treatment is the major, if not exclusive, mechanism of reduction in death rates, with its predominant effect on stroke mortality. In the larger population, the control of hypertension is given much less credit by some analysts for the fall in stroke and in overall and coronary mortality; instead, an equal or larger role is attributed to decreases in cholesterol and smoking (Tsevat et al., 1991). Nonetheless, as shown in an analysis of the Framingham cohort, improvements in the control of hypertension have contributed to the decline in mortality from cardiovascular disease over the past 30 years (Sytkowski et al., 1990).

Coronary Heart Disease

The treatment of hypertension may be at least partly responsible for the major shift in the causes of death among hypertensive patients over the past 30 years (see Chapter 4). Whereas CHF was responsible for over half of the deaths in hypertensive patients before 1950, its role has diminished dramatically (Doyle, 1988). At the same time, deaths attributed to CHD have risen from less than 15% to over 40% of the total. This increased proportion of deaths from CHD likely reflects, in part, the lesser impact of antihypertensive therapy to reduce CHD mortality while it has reduced mortality from other cardiovascular causes (e.g., CHF and stroke).

Left Ventricular Hypertrophy and Function

LVH is a major marker for mortality, and hypertension clearly is a major mechanism for LVH (see Chapter 4). Reduction of pressure can cause regression of LVH, as demonstrated as long ago as 1945 following sympathectomy (White et al., 1945) and amply documented since then with various antihypertensive agents (Dahlöf et al., 1992b; Cruickshank et al., 1992).

Although the abrupt lowering of pressure may induce repolarization abnormalities (Pepi et al., 1988), growing evidence documents improvements in myocardial function and structure (Weber et al., 1992; Messerli et al., 1993) and in coronary vasodilator reserve (Motz et al., 1992) by antihypertensive therapy. Whether these changes in LVH will translate into reduced coronary morbidity and mortality remains to be documented, although two abstracts have claimed to show such reductions in concert with regression of LVH after prolonged antihypertensive therapy (Kannel et al., 1988; Koren et al., 1991).

The potential for even better cardioprotection than expected by reduction of preload and afterload with any type of antihypertensive therapy has been shown by studies that show how ACE inhibitors reduce the progression of left ventricular dysfunction and MI quite distinctly from their antihypertensive effects (SOLVD Investigators, 1992; Pfeffer et al., 1992).

Renal Function

Although proteinuria can be reduced by any drug that lowers BP (Erley et al., 1992), it has been difficult to demonstrate a long-term protective effect of antihypertensive therapy on renal function save in patients with diabetic nephropathy, wherein ACE inhibitors may provide benefits that extend beyond the reduction in BP (Kasiske et al., 1993). Since progressive glomerulosclerosis is the likely consequence of the direct transmission of high systemic pressures, the lowering of systemic pressure ought to slow the progression of hypertensive renal damage. This has been seen in nonblack patients but not in blacks, despite equal control of BP in both groups (Walker et al., 1992). At least in blacks, and perhaps in all hypertensives, greater reductions in systemic pressure than currently are considered adequate or the use of specifically renoprotective agents may be needed to preserve renal function.

Resistance Vessels

Following prolonged periods of antihypertensive therapy, remodeling of the hypertrophic changes within resistance vessels has been measured both directly (Heagerty et al., 1988) and indirectly (Hartford et al., 1988). This improvement does not restore all of the abnormal structural or functional responses seen within these vessels (Aalkjaer et al., 1989) but likely is responsible for the significant decrease in total peripheral resistance that accompanies successful reduction in BP (Agabiti-Rosei et al., 1989). Here again, the greatest benefit may follow the use of drugs that suppress the renin-aldosterone system, which may be a culprit beyond its influence on the pressure itself (Dahlöf et al., 1992a).

Overall Impact of Antihypertensive Therapy

As a last point, it should be noted that the analyses of the effect of antihypertensive therapy on the overall rates of cardiovascular disease in the population have shown that more extensive treatment and control of hypertension have had only a modest impact. Only 8% to 12% of the fall in coronary and stroke mortality over the past 15 years can be attributed to improved control of hypertension (see Chapter 1). Part of this arises from the fact that much of the population-wide risk for stroke and coronary disease is with people whose BPs are not ''hypertensive'' and therefore not currently considered in need of active (i.e., drug) therapy. According to data from the Australian population, more than a third of strokes and almost half of heart attacks occur in people with DBPs below 90 mm Hg (Hobbs et al., 1992).

Even if therapy could completely remove all of the risks associated with definite hypertension, cardiovascular diseases would remain rampant in our high-risk population of smoking, sedentary, dyslipidemic, obese people. Only by reducing all of these risks could meaningful pro-

longation of life expectancy be achieved (Tsevat et al., 1991) (Table 5.7).

Despite this rather pessimistic view, the treatment of hypertension is among the most cost-effective measures now available for prolonging quality of life (Maynard, 1992) (Table 5.8). The figures are for England in mid-1990 and may differ in exact amounts from those in the United States, but the relative positions should be comparable.

Having reviewed all of the evidence favoring the treatment of hypertension, we are left with the question: What level of BP should be treated, and what is the goal of therapy?

WHAT LEVEL OF BLOOD PRESSURE SHOULD BE TREATED?

Despite persistent differences, both in theory and in practice, on the level of BP that indicates the need for anithypertensive therapy (Swales, 1993), a consensus position can be stated: Most patients with BPs persistently above 150/95 should be treated; those with persistent pressures between 140/90 and 150/95 (who account for about 40% of the total) should be treated if they have other major risk factors for premature cardiovascular disease or significant target organ damage.

This is the position taken by an expert committee of the World Health Organization (WHO) and International Society of Hypertension (ISH) (Guidelines Subcommittee, 1993) (Fig. 5.10), as well as by the 1993 Joint National Committee, which recommends that ''physicians may elect to withhold antihypertensive drug therapy from patients with BP in the 140–149/90–94 range in the absence of target organ damage and other major risk factors.''

Problems with Using Blood Pressure Alone

The major problem with past clinical practice has been the use of the BP level alone in making the decision for institution of therapy (Alderman, 1993). Thus, in examples cited in a report from New Zealand (Consensus Development Conference, 1992; Jackson et al., 1993), ''this has led to the situation in which a 60 year old woman with a DBP of 100 mm Hg but no other risk factors (her absolute risk of cardiovascular disease is about 10% in 10 years) may meet the criteria for treatment, whereas a 70 year old man with multiple risk factors but a DBP of 95 mm Hg (his absolute risk is about 50% in 10 years) may not.''

Table 5.7. Gains in Life Expectancy in Years for 35-Year-Old Individuals

	Gain in Life Expectancy	
Intervention	Male	Female
Reduce cholesterol level:		
To 200 mg/dl if 200–239 mg/dl	0.5	0.4
To 200 mg/dl if 240–299 mg/dl	1.7	1.5
To 200 mg/dl if ≥300 mg/dl	4.2	6.3
Reduce number of cigarettes smoked:		
By 50%	1.2	1.5
Eliminate smoking	2.3	2.8
Reduce diastolic blood pressure:		
To 88 mm Hg if 90–94 mm Hg	1.1	0.9
To 88 mm Hg if 95–104 mm Hg	2.3	1.7
To 88 mm Hg if ≥105 mm Hg	5.3	5.7
Reduce weight:		
To ideal if <30% over ideal	0.7	0.5
To ideal if ≥30% over ideal	1.7	1.1

From Tsevet J. et al. Expected gains in life expectancy from various coronary heart disease risk factor modifications. *Circulation* 1991;83:1194–1201.

Table 5.8. Estimates of the Costs of Adding 1 Quality-Adjusted Life Year

Maneuver	Cost ($, 1990)
Cholesterol testing and diet therapy (all aged 40–69)	409
Advice to stop smoking	502
Antihypertensive therapy to prevent stroke (age 45–65)	1748
Pacemaker implantation for heart block	2046
Cholesterol testing and drug treatment	2753
Coronary bypass surgery, severe LMVD with angina	3887
Kidney transplant	8761
Coronary bypass surgery, one vessel disease, moderate angina	35024
Hospital hemodialysis	40864

Modified from Maynard A. The economics of hypertension control: some basic issues. *J Hum Hypertens* 1992;6:417–420.

On the basis of the results of the multiple clinical trials wherein reductions of BP by about 10/5 mm Hg resulted in reductions of overall cardiovascular risk by about one-third, the treatment of these two patients would be expected to reduce the absolute risk in the 60-year-old woman by about 3% in 10 years (30% of 10%) but in the 70-year-old man by about 17% (30% of 50%). As the report states: "In other words, if 100 women aged 60 with DBP of 100 mm Hg and no other risk factors were treated for 10 years, about 3 events would be prevented, whereas if 100 men aged 70 with a DBP of 95 mm Hg and multiple other risk factors were treated, about 17 events would be prevented."

Application of Overall Risk

The New Zealand panel proceeds to provide a management strategy that accomplishes what Alderman (1993) and others believe is essential. Although some may find this strategy a bit too conservative, withholding drug therapy from some who would benefit from it, I believe it deserves careful consideration as a sensible and practical overall approach to answer the critical question, which is not, "What level of blood pressure should be treated?" but rather, "Which patient should be treated?"

The panel's recommendations start with the objectives of reducing the absolute risk of premature death and disease by "treatment to lower blood pressure when the benefits are considered to outweigh the adverse effects of treatment and when the cost-effectiveness of treatment is considered acceptable" (Jackson et al., 1993). To determine the patient's approximate risk status before making the decision to treat, one must take into account age, gender, and the presence of other major risk factors and symptomatic cardiovascular disease (Table 5.9).

The report proceeds with the following recommendation:

... Individuals with an estimated absolute risk of cardiovascular disease of approximately 20% or more in 10 years [based on age, gender and the features listed in Table 5.9], plus a sustained systolic BP greater than 150 mm Hg or diastolic BP greater than 90 mm Hg, should be considered for individualized treatment to lower blood pressure [see Figure 5.11 to estimate risk]. It is estimated that, for these patients, lowering BP by 5 mm Hg diastolic or 10 mm Hg systolic would reduce the risk of cardiovascular disease by about one-third. In those with an absolute risk of 20% in 10 years, the risk would be reduced to about 13% in 10 years; this would mean that one event would be prevented for every 150 patients treated per year. Any adverse effects of treatment are unlikely to outweigh the benefits of treatment at this level of risk and treatment is likely to be relatively cost-effective.

The report proceeds to indicate that therapy should always be considered for those people aged 40 to 60 years with sustained BP above 170 mm Hg systolic or 100 mm Hg diastolic, regardless of their level of absolute risk. Referral for additional investigation is recommended for all people below age 40 with BP above 150/90.

According to Figure 5.11, treatment is advised for those patients with either high enough levels

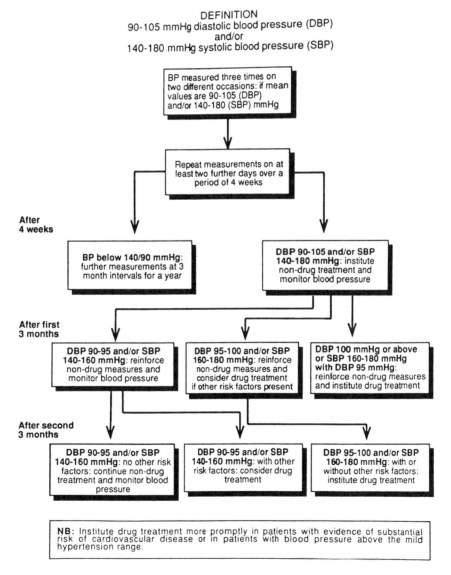

Figure 5.10. Recommendations for the definition and management of mild hypertension by the Guidelines Subcommittee of the World Health Organization and the International Society of Hypertension. *BP*, blood pressure. (From the Guidelines Subcommittee of the WHO/ISH Mild Hypertension Liaison Committee. 1993 guidelines for the management of mild hypertension. *Hypertension* 1993; 22:392–403.)

Table 5.9. Features Considered in the Decision to Treat

Other risk factors
Cigarette smoking
Total cholesterol/HDL cholesterol ratio > 6
Diabetes
Obesity (body mass index > 30)
Family history of premature cardiovascular
   disease (in parent or sibling before age 55)

Symptomatic cardiovascular disease
Angina or silent ischemia
Myocardial infarction
Coronary angioplasty or bypass surgery
Heart failure
Left ventricular hypertrophy demonstrated
   by ECG or echocardiography
Transient ischemic attacks
Stroke
Peripheral vascular disease
Familial hyperlipidemia
Other target organ damage such as renal
   disease

Adapted from Consensus Development Conference Report. A Consensus Development Conference Report to the National Advisory Committee on Core Health and Disability Support Services. In: *The Management of Raised Blood Pressure in New Zealand.* Wellington, New Zealand: National Advisory Committee on Core Health and Disability Support Services, 1992; and from Jackson R, et al. *Br Med J* 1993;397:107–110.

of pressure, or additional risk factors, or symptomatic cardiovascular disease that put them at a 20% or higher 10-year risk for cardiovascular disease with both age and gender taken into account. These recommendations could be considered too conservative since greater reductions in BP should result in greater reductions in absolute risk. Recall, however, that the average reduction of BP below that obtained in the placebo-treated patients in the various clinical trials was in the 10/5 mm Hg range. Clearly, greater reductions would be expected in those with higher degrees of hypertension, and the report recommends therapy for all with BP above 170/100.

Additional Considerations

Beyond the specifics in the New Zealand panel's report, additional considerations should be kept in mind:

—All patients should be kept under surveillance. In all of the trials for mild hypertension, a certain percentage of patients, varying from 10% to 17%, have experienced a progression of their BP to levels of imminent risk (see Chapter 4);

—Those at relatively low risk likely will not suffer from deferral of active drug therapy. Recall the experience of the placebo-treated half of the patients in the Australian Trial (Management Committee, 1980): over 4 years, the average DBP fell below 95 in 47.5% of patients whose baseline DBP was 95 to 109, and excess mortality and morbidity were seen only in those whose average DBP remained above 100;

—More detailed and accurate ways to ascertain individual patient's absolute risk are available, including computer programs based on the Framingham data as provided in the American Heart Association's Coronary Risk Handbook;

—When the decision to use drug therapy is rationally based on a balance between risk and benefit, more aggressive use of drugs may be indicated in some patients. This includes hypertensive diabetics with evidence of early renal damage, who are known to have a poor prognosis if left untreated and to benefit from reduction of their hypertension (Kasiske et al., 1993);

—All patients, regardless of risk status, should be offered and strongly encouraged to follow those lifestyle modifications that are likely to help, as described in Chapter 6.

The bottom line comes down to this: The majority of hypertensives have fairly mild, asymptomatic hypertension, and the benefits of treatment—measured as the reduction in complications—progressively fall the milder the degree of hypertension. Many patients receive relatively little benefit, yet are exposed both to adverse side effects and to the fairly large financial costs of therapy. Therefore, for maximal patient benefit, a management strategy based on overall risk is rational and appropriate.

Now that the rationale for the institution of therapy has been described, let us turn to the issue of how far to lower the pressure.

GOAL OF THERAPY

Until recently, the goal of therapy was simply to first reduce the DBP to lower than 90 mm Hg and then to a level below 85 mm Hg. This was based on the results of the HDFP, wherein fewer complications were seen in the SI group whose average DBP was 83 mm Hg, compared with the UC group, who averaged 88 mm Hg (HDFP, 1979). This approach is based on the premise that the lower the achieved pressure, the greater the protection from cardiovascular

| Blood pressure | SBP (mmHg) | 150 | 160 | 170* | | 150 | 160 | 170* |
| | DBP (mmHg) | 90 | 95 | 100* | | 90 | 95 | 100* |

Men / Women

Risk factor profile

Age 40 years

no risk factors			
1 risk factor			
2 risk factors			
3 risk factors			
Symptomatic CVD			

Age 50 years

no risk factors			
1 risk factor			
2 risk factors			
3 risk factors			
Symptomatic CVD			

Age 60 years

no risk factors			
1 risk factor			
2 risk factors			
3 risk factors			
Symptomatic CVD			

Age 70 years

no risk factors			
1 risk factor			
2 risk factors			
3 risk factors			
Symptomatic CVD			

KEY (10 year risk for CVD) <10% ▨▨▨ 10-20% ☐ 20-40% ■ >40% ▥▥▥

* treatment is advised in individuals with sustained average blood pressure above these levels, despite low absolute risk (see text).

Figure 5.11. Approximate 10-year risk of a cardiovascular disease event per 100 patients, by risk factor status. *CVD*, cardiovascular disease; *DBP*, diastolic blood pressure; *SBP*, systolic blood pressure. (From Consensus Development Conference Report. A Consensus Development Conference Report to the National Advisory Committee on Core Health and Disability Support Services. In: *The Management of Raised Blood Pressure in New Zealand*. Wellington, New Zealand: National Advisory Committee on Core Health and Disability Support Services, 1992.)

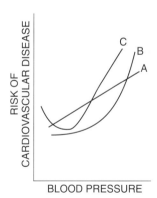

Figure 5.12. Three models of hypothetical relationships between levels of blood pressure and risk of cardiovascular disease. See text for detailed explanation of curves. (From Epstein FH. Primary prevention of coronary heart disease. Proceedings of the XVth International Congress of Therapeutics, Brussels, September 5–9, 1979, *Excerpta Medica*, 1980).

complications. This is described as line *A* in Figure 5.12 (Epstein, 1980).

However, the results of the multiple clinical trials, as described in the preceding pages, have suggested that the consequences of therapy are better portrayed as either line *B*, wherein little if any additional benefit is derived from increasingly greater reduction in pressure, or line *C*, wherein additional risks arise as the pressure is reduced further (i.e., line *C* is a J curve).

The situation remains uncertain. Some do not believe it is desirable to alter the goal of reducing DBP below 85 mm Hg (Hansson, 1990); others believe the wiser course is to bring the DBP only down to 90, particularly in those with known CHD, and then perhaps to 85 but no lower (Cruickshank, 1992). Concern also has been raised about the potential for inadvertent overtreatment during the hours of sleep, when pressures tend to fall even more.

Uncertainty also remains about the appropriate goal of therapy for the systolic level, particularly in the elderly with predominantly systolic hypertension. Since the mean systolic levels were brought down to around 145 mm Hg in the trials in the elderly, that seems to be a reasonable goal. To aim for much lower readings might expose the elderly to considerable postural hypotension and other manifestations of tissue hypoperfusion.

Despite these concerns, we should not lose sight of the fact that the reason for the lesser protection found among treated hypertensives could reflect not overtreatment, but undertreatment (Hansson, 1990). Clearly, it is essential that all patients have their DBP brought down to the 85 to 90 range in order to provide the demonstrated benefits of therapy. For some, such as diabetics with nephropathy, considerably lower levels may be needed. To ensure the adequacy of therapy, patients should monitor their own pressure out of the office (see Chapter 2).

Until a proper prospective study is done, we will remain uncertain as to how low the pressure should be reduced for maximal protection of most patients. At this time, knowing how common underlying coronary disease is in hypertensive patients, a goal of 140/85 seems appropriate. At the same time, we must not lose sight of the need, often greater than that of lowering the BP, of reducing other known cardiovascular risk factors. To neglect these by focusing only on the BP is to lose sight of the only reason for all of our efforts: the protection of the patient from premature cardiovascular disability and death while preserving the best possible quality of life.

Importance of Population Strategies

Most of our current efforts are directed at the individual patient with existing hypertension. Clearly, we also need to advise the larger population to do those things that may protect against the development of hypertension—an approach directed toward ''sick populations'' rather than only ''sick individuals'' (Rose, 1992). Such population strategies cannot include medications but rather utilize totally safe and easily applied lifestyle modifications. The next chapter describes these modifications.

References

Aagaard G. Hypertension Detection and Followup Program: an alternative interpretation. *Am Heart J* 1981;102:300–302.

Aalkjær, Eiskjær H, Mulvany MJ, Jespersen B, Kjær T, Sörenen SS, Pedersen EB. Abnormal structure and function of isolated subcutaneous resistance vessels in essential hypertensive patients despite antihypertensive treatment. *J Hypertens* 1989;7:305–310.

Agabiti-Rosei E, Muiesan ML, Muiesan G. Regression of structural alterations in hypertension. *Am J Hypertens* 1989; 2:70S–76S.

Alderman MH. Blood pressure management: indivudualized treatment based on absolute risk and the potential for benefit. *Ann Intern Med* 1993;119:329–335.

Amery A, Birkenhäger W, Brixko P, Bulpitt C, Clement D, Deruyttere M, De Schaepdryver A, Dollery C, Fagard R, Forette F, Forte J, Hamdy R, Henry JF, Joossens JV, Leonetti G, Lund-Johansen P, O'Malley K, Petrie J, Strasser T, Tuomilehto J. Mortality and morbidity results from the European Working Party on High Blood Pressure in the Elderly Trial. *Lancet* 1985; 1:1349–1354.

Amery A, Birkenhäger W, Bulpitt CJ, Clément D, De Leeuw P, Dollery CT, Fagard R, Fletcher A, Forette F, Leonetti G, O'Brien ET, O'Malley K, Rodicio JL, Rosenfeld J, Staessen J, Strasser T, Terzoli L, Thijs L, Tuomilehto J, Webster J. Syst-Eur. A multicentre trial on the treatment of isolated systolic hypertension in the elderly: objectives, protocol, and organization. *Aging* 1991;3:287–302.

Anderson TW. Re-examination of some of the Framingham blood-pressure data. *Lancet* 1978;2:1139–41.

Barraclough M, Joy MD, MacGregor GA, Foley TH, Lee MR, Rosendorff C, Holland WW, Cranston WI, Rea JN, Bainton D, Cochrane AL, Greene J, Kilpatrick GS, Weddell JM. Control of moderately raised blood pressure. Report of a co-operative randomized controlled trial. *Br Med J* 1973;3:434–436.

Beard K, Bulpitt C, Mascie-Taylor H, O'Malley K, Sever P, Webb S. Management of elderly patients with sustained hypertension. *Br Med J* 1992;304:412–416.

Bostick RM, Luepker RV, Kofron PM, Pirie PL. Changes in physician practice for the prevention of cardiovascular disease. *Arch Intern Med* 1991;151:478–484.

Brett AS. Ethical issues of risk factor intervention. *Am J Med* 1984;76:557–561.

British Hypertension Society. Treating mild hypertension. Agreement from the large trials. *Br Med J* 1989;298:694–698.

Bulpitt CJ, Fletcher AE. Aging, blood pressure and mortality. *J Hypertens* 1992; 10(Suppl 7):45–49.

Carter AB. Hypotensive therapy in stroke survivors. *Lancet* 1970;1:485–489.

Chobanian AV. 1988 Corcoran Lecture: adaptive and maladaptive responses of the arterial wall to hypertension. *Hypertension* 1990;15:666–674.

Chobanian AV, Haudenschild CC, Nickerson C, Hope S. Trandolapril inhibits atherosclerosis in the Watanabe heritable hyperlipidemic rabbit. *Hypertension* 1992; 20:473–477.

Cohen JD, Butler SM, Cutler JA, Neaton JD. Relationship between blood pressure change and mortality among MRFIT hypertensives [Abstract]. *Circulation* 1991;84(Suppl 2):37.

Collins R, Peto R, MacMahon S, Hebert P, Fiebach NH, Eberlein KA, Godwin J, Qizilbash N, Taylor JO, Hennekens CH. Blood pressure, stroke, and coronary heart disease. Part 2: Short-term reductions in blood pressure: overview of randomised drug trials in their epidemiological context. *Lancet* 1990;335:827–838.

Consensus Development Conference Report. A Consensus Development Conference Report to the National Advisory Committee on Core Health and Disability Support Services. In: *The Management of Raised Blood Pressure in New Zealand*. Wellington, New Zealand: National Advisory Committee on Core Health and Disability Support Services, 1992.

Coope J, Warrender TS. Randomised trial of treatment of hypertension in elderly patients in primary care. *Br Med J* 1986; 293:1145–1151.

Cruickshank JM. Coronary flow reserve and the J curve relation between diastolic blood pressure and myocardial infarction. *Br Med J* 1988;297:1227–1230.

Cruickshank JM. Letter to the editor. *N Engl J Med* 1992;327:55.

Cruickshank JM, Lewis J, Moore V, Dodd C. Reversibility of left ventricular hypertrophy by differing types of antihypertensive therapy. *J Hum Hypertens* 1992; 6:85–90.

Cruickshank JM, Thorp JM, Zacharias FJ. Benefits and potential harm of lowering high blood pressure. *Lancet* 1987; 1:581–584.

D'Agostino RB, Belanger AJ, Kannel WB, Cruickshank JM. Relation of low diastolic blood pressure to coronary heart disease death in presence of myocardial infarction: the Framingham study. *Br Med J* 1991; 303:385–389.

Dahlöf B, Herlitz H, Aurell M, Hansson L. Reversal of cardiovascular structural changes when treating essential hypertension. The importance of the renin-angiotensin-aldosterone system. *Am J Hypertens* 1992a;5:900–911.

Dahlöf B, Lindholm LH, Hansson L, Scherstén B, Ekbom T, Wester P-O. Morbidity and mortality in the Swedish Trial in Old Patients with Hypertension (STOP-Hypertension). *Lancet* 1991;338:1281–1285.

Dahlöf B, Pennert K, Hansson L. Reversal of left ventricular hypertrophy in hypertensive patients. A metaanalysis of 109 treatment studies. *Am J Hypertens* 1992b; 5:95–110.

Doyle AE. Does hypertension predispose to coronary disease? Conflicting epidemiological and experimental evidence. *Am J Hypertens* 1988;1:319–324.

Epstein FH. Primary prevention of coronary heart disease. Proceedings of the XVth International Congress of Therapeutics, September 5–9, 1979. Brussels: *Excerpta Medica*, 1980:1–11.

Erley CM, Haefele U, Heyne N, Braun N, Risler T. Reduction of microalbuminuria in essential hypertension by different antihypertensive drugs regardless of changes in renal hemodynamics [Abstract]. *J Am Soc Nephrol* 1992;3:531.

Farnett L, Mulrow CD, Linn WD, Lucey CR, Tuley MR. The J-curve phenomenon and the treatment of hypertension. Is there a point beyond which pressure reduction is dangerous? *JAMA* 1991;265:489–495.

Fletcher AE, Bulpitt CJ. How far should blood pressure be lowered? *N Engl J Med* 1992;326:251–254.

Freis ED. Rationale against the drug treatment of marginal diastolic systemic hypertension. *Am J Cardiol* 1990;66:368–371.

Guidelines Subcommittee of the WHO/ISH Mild Hypertension Liaison Committee. 1993 guidelines for the management of mild hypertension. *Hypertension* 1993; 22:392–403.

Guttmacher S, Teitelman M, Chapin G, Garbowski G, Schnall P. Ethics and preventive medicine. The case of borderline hypertension. *Hastings Center Report* 1981; 11:12–20.

Hamilton M, Thompson EN, Wisniewski TKM. The Role of blood-pressure control in preventing complications of hypertension. *Lancet* 1964;1:235–238.

Hansson L. How far should blood pressure be lowered? What is the role of the J-curve? *Am J Hypertens* 1990;3:726–729.

Hansson L, Dahlöf B. What are we really achieving with long-term antihypertensive drug therapy? In: Laragh JH, Brenner BM, eds. *Hypertension: Pathophysiology, Diagnosis, and Management.* New York: Raven Press, 1990:2131–2141.

Hartford M, Wendelhag I, Berglund G, Wallentin I, Ljungman S, Wikstrand J. Cardiovascular and renal effects of long-term antihypertensive treatment. *JAMA* 1988;259:2553–2557.

Havlik RJ, LaCroix AZ, Kleinman JC, Ingram DD, Harris T, Cornoni-Huntley J. Antihypertensive drug therapy and survival by treatment status in a national survey. *Hypertension* 1989;13(Suppl 1): 28–32.

Heagerty AM, Bund SJ, Aalkjaer C. Effects of drug treatment on human resistance arteriole morphology in essential hypertension: direct evidence for structural remodelling or resistance vessels. *Lancet* 1988;2:1209–1212.

Heath D, Edwards JE. The pathology of hypertensive pulmonary vascular disease. A description of six grades of structural changes in the pulmonary arteries with special reference to congenital cardiac septal defects. *Circulation* 1958;18:533–547.

Helgeland A. Treatment of mild hypertension: a five year controlled drug trial. *Am J Med* 1980;69:725–732.

Hobbs M, Hockey R, Jamrozik K. Review of the benefits of treating hypertension. *J Hum Hypertens* 1992;6:427–435.

Hodge JV, McQueen EG, Smirk H. Results of hypotensive therapy in arterial hypertension: based on experience with 497 patient treated and 156 controls, observed for periods of one to eight years. *Br Med J* 1961;1:1–7.

Hollander W, Madoff I, Paddock J, Kirkpatrick B. Aggravation of atherosclerosis by hypertension in a subhuman primate model with coarctation of the aorta. *Circ Res* 1976;38(Suppl 2):631–672.

Holme I, Helgeland A, Hjermann I, Leren P, Lund-Larsen PG. Treatment of mild hypertension with diuretics. The importance of ECG abnormalities in the Oslo Study and in MRFIT. *JAMA* 1984;251:1298–1299.

Hood D, Bjork S, Sannerstedt R, Angervall G. Analysis of mortality and survival in actively treated hypertensive disease. *Acta Med Scand* 1963;174:393–402.

HOT Study Group. The hypertension optimal treatment study (the HOT Study). *Blood Pressure* 1993;2:62–68.

Hypertension Detection and Follow-Up Program Cooperative Group. Five-year findings of the Hypertension Detection and Follow-Up Program. I. Reduction in mortality of persons with high blood pressure, including mild hypertension. *JAMA* 1979;242:2562–2571.

Hypertension Detection and Follow-Up Program Cooperative Group. Five-year findings of the Hypertension Detection and Follow-Up Program. III. Reduction in stroke incidence among persons with high blood pressure. *JAMA* 1982a; 247:633–638.

Hypertension Detection and Follow-Up Program Cooperative Group. The effect of treatment on mortality in "mild" hypertension. *N Engl J Med* 1982b; 307:976–980.

Hypertension Detection and Follow-Up Program Cooperative Group. The effect of antihypertensive drug treatment on mortality in the presence of resting electrocardiographic abnormalities at baseline: the HDFP experience. *Circulation* 1984; 70:996–1003.

Hypertension Detection and Follow-Up Program Cooperative Group. Five-year findings of the Hypertension Detection and Follow-Up Program. Prevention and reversal of left ventricular hypertrophy with antihypertensive therapy. *Hypertension* 1985;7:105–112.

Hypertension Follow-Up Group of the Japan Federation of Democratic Medical Institutions. Effect of cigarette smoking on the J-shaped relationship between treated blood pressure and cardiovascular disease. *J Hum Hypertens* 1992;6:359–365.

Hypertension-Stroke Cooperative Study Group. Effect of antihypertensive treatment on stroke recurrence. *JAMA* 1974; 229:409–418.

IPPPSH Collaborative Group. Cardiovascular risk and risk factors in a randomized trial of treatment based on the beta-blocker oxprenolol: the International Prospective Primary Prevention Study in Hypertension (IPPPSH). *J Hypertens* 1985;3:379–392.

Isles CG, Walker LM, Beevers GD, Brown I, Cameron HL, Clarke J, Hawthorne V, Hole D, Lever AF, Robertson JWK, Wapshaw JA. Mortality in patients of the Glasgow Blood Pressure Clinic. *J Hypertens* 1986;4:141–156.

Joint National Committee. The fifth report of the Joint National Committee on Detection, Evaluation, and Treatment of High Blood Pressure (JNC V). *Arch Intern Med* 1993;153:154–183.

Kannel WB, D'Agostino RB, Levy D, Belanger AJ. Prognostic significance of regression of left ventricular hypertrophy [Abstract]. *Circulation* 1988;78(Suppl 2):89.

Kasiske BL, Kalil RSN, Ma JZ, Liao M, Keane WF. Effect of antihypertensive therapy on the kidney in patients with diabetes: a meta-regression analysis. *Ann Intern Med* 1993;118:129–138.

Koren MJ, Ulin RJ, Laragh JH, Devereux RB. Reduction in left ventricular mass during treatment of essential hypertension is associated with improved prognosis [Abstract]. *Am J Hypertens* 1991;4:1A–2A.

Kuramoto K, Matsushita S, Kuwajima I, Murakami M. Prospective study on the treatment of mild hypertension in the aged. *Jpn Heart J* 1981;22:75–85.

Leishman AWD: Hypertension—treated and untreated—a study of 400 cases. *Br Med J* 1961;1:1–5.

MacMahon S, Peto R, Cutler J, Collins R, Sorlie P, Neaton J, Abbott R, Godwin J, Dyer A, Stamler J. Blood pressure, stroke, and coronary heart disease. Part 1: Prolonged differences in blood pressure: prospective observational studies corrected for the regression dilution bias. *Lancet* 1990;335:765–774.

MacMahon SW, Cutler JA, Furberg CD, Payne GH. The effects of drug treatment for hypertension on morbidity and mortality from cardiovascular disease: a review of randomized controlled trials. *Prog Cardiovasc Dis* 1986;29(Suppl 1):99–118.

Management Committee. The Australian therapeutic trial in mild hypertension. *Lancet* 1980;1:1261–1267.

Management Committee. Treatment of mild hypertension in the elderly. A study initiated and administered by the National Heart Foundation of Australia. *Med J Aust* 1981;2:398–402.

Mansour P, Boström P-Å, Mattiasson I, Lilja B, Berglund G. Low blood pressure levels and signs of myocardial ischaemia: importance of left ventricular hypertrophy. *J Hum Hypertens* 1993;7:13–18.

Masson GMC, McCormack LJ, Dustan HP, Corcoran AC. Hypertensive vascular disease as a consequence of increased arterial pressure. Quantitative study in rats with hydralazine-treated renal hypertension. *Am J Pathol* 1958;34:817–832.

Maxwell C. Clinical trials in hypertension: some general thoughts and some particular controversies. *Nephron* 1987;47(Suppl 1):1–4.

Maynard A. The economics of hypertension control: some basic issues. *J Hum Hypertens* 1992;6:417–420.

McCloskey LW, Psaty BM, Koepsell TD, Aagaard GN. Level of blood pressure and risk of myocardial infarction among treated hypertensive patients. *Arch Intern Med* 1992;152:513–520.

Medical Research Council Working Party. Medical Research Council trial of treatment of hypertension in older adults: principal results. *Br Med J* 1992;304:405–412.

Medical Research Council Working Party. MRC trial of treatment of mild hypertension: principal results. *Br Med J* 1985;291:97–104.

Medical Research Council Working Party. Stroke and coronary heart disease in mild hypertension: risk factors and the value of treatment. *Br Med J* 1988;296:1565–1570.

Messerli FH, Aristizabal D, Soria F. Reduction of left ventricular hypertrophy—how beneficial? *Am Heart J* 1993;125(Part 2):1520–1524.

Miall WE, Chinn S. Blood pressure and ageing; results of a 15–17 year follow-up study in South Wales. *Clin Sci Mol Med* 1973;45(Suppl):23–33.

Motz WH, Scheler S, Strauer BE. Medical repair of hypertensive left ventricular remodeling. *J Cardiovasc Pharmacol* 1992;20(Suppl 1):32–36.

Multiple Risk Factor Intervention Trial Research Group. Baseline rest electrocardiographic abnormalities, antihypertensive treatment, and mortality in the Multiple Risk Factor Intervention Trial. *Am J Cardiol* 1985;55:1–15.

Multiple Risk Factor Intervention Trial Research Group. Multiple risk factor intervention trial. Risk factor changes and mortality results. *JAMA* 1982;248:1465–1477.

O'Kelly BF, Massie BM, Tubau JF, Szlachcic J. Coronary morbidity and mortality, preexisting silent coronary artery disease, and mild hypertension. *Ann Intern Med* 1989;110:1017–1026.

Oberman A, Lane NE, Harlan WR, Graybiel A, Mitchell RE. Trends in systolic blood pressure in the thousand aviator cohort over a twenty-four-year period. *Circulation* 1967;36:812–822.

Pepi M, Alimento M, Maltagliati A, Guazzi MD. Cardiac hypertrophy in hypertension. Repolarization abnormalities elicited by rapid lowering of pressure. *Hypertension* 1988;11:84–91.

Pfeffer MA, Braunwald E, Moye LA, et al. Effect of captopril on mortality and morbidity in patients with left ventricular dysfunction after myocardial infarction: results of the Survival and Ventricular Enlargement Trial. *N Engl J Med* 1992; 327:669–677.

Polese A, De Cesare N, Montorsi P, Fabbiocchi F, Guazzi M, Loaldi A, Guazzi MD. Upward shift of the lower range of coronary flow autoregulation in hypertensive patients with hypertrophy of the left ventricle. *Circulation* 1991;83:845–853.

Rose G. Strategy of prevention: lessons from cardiovascular disease. *Br Med J* 1981; 282:1847–1851.

Rose G. *The Strategy of Preventive Medicine.* Oxford: Oxford University Press, 1992.

Samuelsson O, Wilhelmsen L, Andersson OK, Pennert K, Berglund G. Cardiovascular morbidity in relation to change in blood pressure and serum cholesterol levels in treated hypertension. Results from the Primary Prevention Trial in Göteborg, Sweden. *JAMA* 1987;258:1768–1776.

Schappert SM. National ambulatory medical care survey: 1991 summary. Hyattsville, Maryland: National Center for Health Statistics. *Advanced Data* 1993;230:1–20.

Sever P, Beevers G, Bulpitt C, Lever A, Ramsay L, Reid J, Swales J. Management guidelines in essential hypertension: report of the second working party of the British Hypertension Society. *Br Med J* 1993;306:983–987.

SHEP Cooperative Research Group. Prevention of stroke by antihypertensive drug treatment in older persons with isolated systolic hypertension. Final results of the Systolic Hypertension in the Elderly Program (SHEP). *JAMA* 1991;266: 3255–3264.

Simpson FO. Fallacies in the interpretation of the large-scale trials of treatment of mild to moderate hypertension. *J Cardiovasc Pharmacol* 1990;16(Suppl 7):92–95.

SOLVD Investigators. Effect of enalapril on mortality and the development of heart failure in asymptomatic patients with reduced left ventricular ejection fractions. *N Engl J Med* 1992;327:685–691.

Staessen J, Bulpitt C, Clement D, De Leeuw P, Fagard R, Fletcher A, Forette F, Leonetti G, Nissinen A, O'Malley K, Tuomilehto J, Webster J, Williams BO. Relation between mortality and treated blood pressure in elderly patients with hypertension: report of the European Working Party on High Blood Pressure in the elderly. *Br Med J* 1989;298:1552–1556.

Staessen J, Fagard R, Amery A. Isolated systolic hypertension in the elderly: implications of SHEP for clinical practice and for the ongoing trials. *J Hum Hypertens* 1991;5:469–474.

Staessen J, Fagard R, Amery A. Primary prevention with metoprolol in patients with hypertension [Letter]. *JAMA* 1988;260: 1713–1714.

Stewart IMG. Relation of reduction in pressure to first myocardial infarction in patients receiving treatment for severe hypertension. *Lancet* 1979;1:861–865.

Strandgaard S, Haunsø S. Why does antihypertensive treatment prevent stroke but not myocardial infarction? *Lancet* 1987;2: 658–661.

Swales JD. Guidelines on guidelines. *J Hypertens* 1993;11:899–903.

Sytkowski PA, Kannel WB, D'Agostino RB. Changes in risk factors and the decline in mortality from cardiovascular disease. The Framingham Heart Study. *N Engl J Med* 1990;322:1635–1641.

Thal AP, Grage TB, Vernier RL. Function of the contralateral kidney in renal hypertension due to renal artery stenosis. *Circulation* 1963:27:36–43.

Thijs L, Fagard R, Lijnen P, Staessen J, Van Hoof R, Amery A. A meta-analysis of outcome trials in elderly hypertensives. *J Hypertens* 1992;10:1103–1109.

Tsevat J, Weinstein MC, Williams LW, Tosteson ANA, Goldman L. Expected gains in life expectancy from various coronary heart disease risk factor modifications. *Circulation* 1991;83:1194–1201.

US Public Health Service Hospitals Cooperative Study Group (Smith WM). Treatment of mild hypertension: results of a ten-year intervention trial. *Circ Res* 1977; 40(Suppl 1):98–105.

Veterans Administration Cooperative Study Group on Antihypertensive Agents. Effects of treatment on morbidity in hypertension. Result in patients with diastolic blood pressures averaging 115 through 129 mm Hg. *JAMA* 1967;202:1028–1034.

Veterans Administration Cooperative Study Group on Antihypertensive Agents. Effects of treatment on morbidity in hypertension. Result in patients with diastolic blood pressures averaging 90 through 114 mm Hg. *JAMA* 1970;213:1143–1152.

Veterans Administration Cooperative Study Group on Antihypertensive Agents. Effects of treatment on morbidity in hypertension. III. Influence of age, diastolic pressure, and prior cardiovascular disease; further analysis of side effects. *Circulation* 1972;45:991–1004.

Veterans Administration/National Heart, Lung, and Blood Institute Study Group for Evaluating Treatment in Mild Hypertension. Evaluation of drug treatment in mild hypertension: VA-NHLBI feasibility trial. *Ann N Y Acad Sci* 1978;304:267–288.

Waller PC, McInnes GT, Reid JL. Policies for managing hypertensive patients: a survey of the opinions of British specialists. *J Hum Hypertens* 1990;4:509–515.

Walker WG, Neaton JD, Cutler JA, Neuwirth R, Cohen JD. Renal function change in hypertensive members of the Multiple Risk Factor Intervention Trial. *JAMA* 1992;268:3085–3091.

Weber KT, Anversa P, Armstrong PW, Brilla CG, Burnett JC Jr, Cruickshank JM, Devereux RB, Giles TD, Korsgaard N, Leier CV, Mendelsohn FAO, Motz WH, Mulvany MJ, Strauer BE. Remodeling and reparation of the cardiovascular system. *J Am Coll Cardiol* 1992;20:3–16.

Weinberger MH. Do no harm. Antihypertensive therapy and the "J" curve [Editorial]. *Arch Intern Med* 1992;152:473–476.

White PD, Smithwick RH, Mathews MW, Evans E. The electrocardiogram in hypertension. II. The effect of radical lumbodorsal sympathectomy. *Am Heart J* 1945;30:165–188.

Wikstrand J, Warnold I, Olsson G, Tuomilehto J, Elmfeldt D, Berglund G. Primary prevention with metoprolol in patients with hypertension. Mortality results from the MAPHY study. *JAMA* 1988;259: 1976–1982.

Wilhelmsen L, Berglund G, Elmfeldt D, Fitzsimons T, Holzgreve H, Hosie J, Hörnkvist P-E, Pennert K, Tuomilehto J, Wede H. Beta-blockers versus diuretics in hypertensive men: main results from the HAPPHY Trial. *J Hypertens* 1987;5:561–572.

Wolff FW, Lindeman RD. Effects of treatment in hypertension. Results of a controlled study. *J Chron Dis* 1966;19: 227–240.

Yusuf S, Pepine CJ, Garces C, Pouleur H, Salem D, Kostis J, Benedit C, Rousseau M, Bourassa M, Pitt B. Effect of enalapril on myocardial infarction and unstable angina in patients with low ejection fractions. *Lancet* 1992;340:1173–1178.

6 Treatment of Hypertension: Nondrug Therapy

With an appreciation of the benefits and costs of antihypertensive therapy, we now will consider the practical aspects of accomplishing a reduction in blood pressure (BP). In this chapter, the use of nondrugs to treat hypertension will be examined, followed by evidence that hypertension might be prevented by four lifestyle interventions. The next chapter covers the use of drugs.

The use of nondrug therapies, preferably referred to as *lifestyle modifications*, as initial therapy for most patients—at least for the first 3 to 6 months after recognition of their hypertension—is advocated by experts in the United States (Joint National Committee, 1993), in Britain (Sever et al., 1993) and worldwide (World Hypertension League, 1993). Such therapy may lower pressure to a level considered safe, particularly among the large number of patients with minimally elevated pressures. For the remainder, nondrug therapy may not be enough, but it can aid in reducing the pressure without risk, so that less drug therapy will be needed.

The following nondrug ''prescription'' should be practical for most hypertensives:

—Stop smoking;
—If body weight is excessive, reduce weight;
—Restrict dietary sodium intake to 100 mmol/day (2.3 g of sodium or 6 g of sodium chloride), with caution not to reduce the intake of calcium-rich foods (i.e., low-fat milk and cheese products);
—Increase dietary potassium intake by replacing processed foods with natural foods;
—Supplement with calcium and magnesium only if deficient;
—Increase fiber and restrict saturated fat;
—No limits on caffeine-containing beverages;
—Limit alcohol to 1 ounce per day, as contained in two usual portions of wine, beer, or spirits;
—Increase physical activity;
—Use relaxation therapy if indicated.

ISSUE OF EFFICACY

Many practitioners, though they recognize the potential benefits of these lifestyle modifications, do not advise their patients to use them (Silagy et al., 1992). There are two main reasons: first, it is too much trouble; second, many patients do not respond. More time and effort undoubtably are needed to instruct and motivate patients than to write out a prescription. However, various nonphysician practitioners—nurses, dieticians, psychologists—are available in most places to help in the effort. Although it is true that many patients do not adhere to these nondrug therapies, poor compliance is a major problem with drug treatment as well. The same techniques to improve patient adherence to drug therapy that are described in the next chapter should help with both.

Nonspecific Effects

An antihypertensive effect has been claimed for virtually everything that has been tried, including some therapies that almost certainly are ineffective, such as dilute hydrochloric acid

(Ayman, 1930) and cholecystectomy (Volini and Flaxman, 1939). As is obvious from the repeated observation that BPs tend to fall spontaneously for the first 6 to 12 weeks of observation, as noted in Chapter 2, studies must be properly designed with adequate run-in periods or parallel observations of groups either randomly allocated to nondrug therapy or left untreated.

Protection Against Cardiovascular Disease

The larger issue of whether these nondrug therapies will, in fact, reduce morbidity and mortality in hypertensive patients may never be settled. The difficulty of demonstrating such protection in the various therapeutic trials using antihypertensive drugs was described in Chapter 5. There is likely no way to document the efficacy of nondrug therapies, which are less potent and more difficult to monitor than drug treatment. Nondrug therapies must be accepted on the evidence they will lower the BP without risk, and with a reasonable chance of adherence by most patients.

COMBINED THERAPIES

A number of studies of mild hypertension have shown that combinations of nondrug therapies will lower BP while they reduce the amount of antihypertensive drugs needed to control the hypertension (Dodson et al., 1985; Aberg and Tibblin, 1989; Jula et al., 1990; Little et al., 1991). Others have compared single or multiple lifestyle modifications with antihypertensive drugs (Wassertheil-Smoller et al., 1992; Kostis et al., 1992; Fagerberg et al., 1992; Nilsson et al., 1992; Neaton et al., 1993).

The overall message of these studies is clear: With nondrug therapies over 6 months to 5 years of follow-up, most hypertensives achieve a significant fall in BP and are able to further reduce their overall cardiovascular risk status, mainly by improvements in lipid status. However, the degree of BP reduction with nondrug therapies was less than that achieved with drugs in these studies. This observation is tempered by the relatively modest degree of weight loss or sodium restriction achieved in most trials despite assiduous attempts to motivate patients to alter diets and activity (Elmer et al., 1991). On the other hand, impressive reductions in hyperinsulinemia, a likely major cardiovascular risk factor and promoter of hypertension, have been observed with lifestyle changes (Nilsson et al., 1992; Fagerberg et al., 1992).

A relatively large and long trial, The Treatment of Mild Hypertension Study (TOMHS), documented a significant antihypertensive effect (average -8.6/-8.6 mm Hg) from multiple nondrug therapies along with a placebo pill (average weight loss of 6.6 lbs, sodium reduction of 10%, increased exercise and moderation of alcohol) (Neaton et al., 1993). Those subjects who took an antihypertensive drug while following the nutritional-exercise regimen had a further fall in BP of -4.8/-2.5 mm Hg.

Despite these impressive effects, we are left with no definitive evidence of the overall effects of lifestyle modifications on morbidity or mortality, the type of information that is clearly needed to prove their value. Moreover, the economic costs of nutritional-exercise regimens often are greater than those of drug therapy (Johannesson and Fagerberg, 1992). Nonetheless, these modalities seem to improve both blood pressure and cardiovascular risk status enough to support their use as the initial approach to the management of virtually all hypertensives.

The effects of individual lifestyle modifications on hypertension now will be examined, to be followed by consideration of their potential for prevention of the disease. Although the initial results of the Trials of Hypertension Prevention (TOHP-I) (1992) will be covered in the last part of this chapter, since this study was designed as a preventive trial in subjects who have only high-normal blood pressure, they deserve mention here since the TOHP-I is the largest and best-controlled study comparing the effects of most of the individual nondrug maneuvers on blood pressure. Altogether, 2182 men and women, aged 30 to 54, with diastolic blood pressure from 80 to 89 mm Hg, were randomly assigned to one of three lifestyle changes (weight reduction, sodium restriction, or stress management) for 18 months or to one of four nutritional supplements (calcium, magnesium, potassium, or fish oil) for 6 months, with placebo controls for both groups. The results document a significant effect of weight loss (average of 3.9 kg) and sodium restriction (average of 44 mmol/day) but no effect of the other modalities (Fig. 6.1).

TOBACCO

The previous five editions of this book stated that smoking did not affect blood pressure significantly since tolerance to the acute pressor effect of nicotine quickly develops and because the chronic smoker may have a lower BP, since

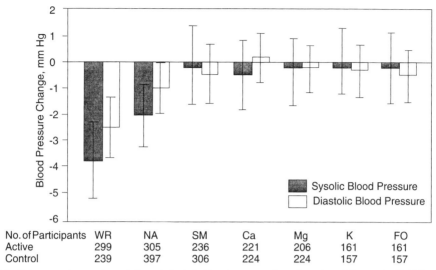

Figure 6.1. Net mean changes in systolic and diastolic blood pressure (baseline minus follow-up), with 95% confidence intervals. WR, weight reduction; Na, sodium reduction; SM, stress management; Ca, calcium supplementation; Mg, magnesium supplementation; K, potassium supplementation; FO, fish oil supplementation. (From Trials of Hypertension Prevention Collaborative Research Group. The effects of nonpharmacologic interventions on blood pressure of persons with high normal levels. Results of the Trials of Hypertension Prevention, Phase I. JAMA 1992;267:1213–1220.)

smokers weigh less than nonsmokers. That statement is incorrect. The error arose because of the almost universal practice of having smokers abstain from smoking for some time before their blood pressures are measured, usually because medical facilities always are "smoke-free." Thus, the significant and immediate and repetitive pressor effect of smoking has been missed because it only lasts for 15 to 30 minutes after each cigarette has been smoked. Only recently have studies using ambulatory blood pressure monitoring recognized the major pressor effect of smoking (Mann et al., 1991; De Cesaris et al., 1991; Groppelli et al., 1992) (Fig. 6.2). Smokeless tobacco (Bolinder et al., 1992) and cigars, if their smoke is inhaled (Kaufman et al., 1987), also may raise blood pressure.

This pressor effect must be at least partly responsible for the major increase in strokes (Shinton and Beevers, 1989) and coronary disease (Rosengren et al., 1992) among smokers as well as for their apparent resistance to antihypertensive therapy (Materson et al., 1988). The noxious cardiovascular effects of smoking also involve a worsening of lipid status (Craig et al., 1989); an increase in central obesity (Daniel et al., 1992), which in turn may be involved in a worsening of insulin resistance (Facchini et al., 1992); and an attenuation of endothelium-dependent arteriolar dilatation (Rubinstein et al., 1991).

Thus, hypertensives who use tobacco must be repeatedly and unambiguously told to quit and given assistance in doing so (Lee and D'Alonzo, 1993). Nicotine patches may be effective and usually do not raise the blood pressure (Fiore et al., 1992). If the patient cannot quit smoking, $alpha_1$-receptor blocking drugs, but not beta-blockers, may attenuate the smoking-induced rise in blood pressure (Groppelli et al., 1990).

WEIGHT REDUCTION

As noted in Chapter 3, obesity, in particular that located in the upper body, commonly is associated with hypertension, and the combination may in turn be related to hyperinsulinemia secondary to insulin resistance (Kaplan, 1989). Despite claims of fewer complications in the obese (Carman et al., 1992), obese persons have at least as much coronary and cerebrovascular disease as do lean hypertensives (Phillips and Shaper, 1989; Kannel et al., 1990); the excess mortality in lean hypertensives is due to their excessive smoking and alcohol intake (Stamler et al., 1991).

Clinical Experience

Staessen et al. (1989) plotted the effect of varying degrees of weight loss on the systolic and diastolic blood pressures of almost 650 patients in 11 studies published from 1954 to 1985 (Fig. 6.3). When only the adequately con-

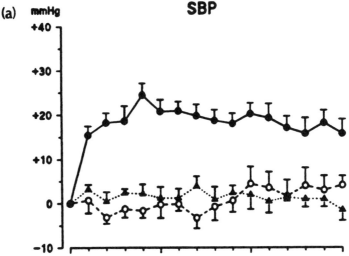

Figure 6.2. Changes in systolic blood pressure *(SBP)* over 15 minutes after smoking the first cigarette of the day within the first 5 minutes *(solid circles),* during no activity *(open circles),* and during sham-smoking *(triangles)* in 10 normotensive smokers. (From Groppelli A, Giorgi DMA, Omboni S, Parati G, Mancia G. Blood pressure and heart rate response to repeated smoking before and after beta blockade and selective α_1 inhibition. *J Hypertens* 1992;10:495–499.)

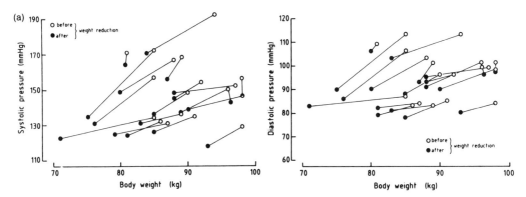

Figure 6.3. Systolic and diastolic blood pressure before and after body weight reduction. (From Staessen J, Fagard R, Lijnen P, Amery A. Body weight, sodium intake and blood pressure. *J Hypertens* 1989;7(Suppl 1):19–23.)

trolled studies were considered, the mean effect of a 1-kg fall in body weight was a fall in systolic and diastolic pressures of 1.6/1.3 mm Hg. More recent studies have further documented the efficacy of weight reduction in lowering blood pressure, as recorded by readings taken throughout the day and night by ambulatory monitors (Das-Gupta et al., 1991).

A significant fall in blood pressure has been noted with only modest weight reduction (Schotte and Stunkard, 1990). With more weight loss, as achieved by 400- to 600-calorie formula diets, even greater falls in blood pressure are seen (Wadden et al., 1992).

After a review of the pertinent data, Prineas (1991) concluded that the effect of weight reduc-

tion is independent of sodium restriction. In clinical practice, it is likely that the two measures will work together to achieve a greater fall in blood pressure than either could achieve alone (Gillum et al., 1983). Caution is needed in the use of sympathomimetic agents to reduce the appetite since they may raise the blood pressure (Silverstone, 1992), but either serotonin blockers (e.g., fluoxetine)(Gray et al., 1992) or serotoninergic compounds (e.g., dexfenfluramine) (Kolanowski et al., 1992) may be safe and helpful in further lowering the blood pressure while increasing weight loss.

Mechanisms

With very low calorie intake, a massive natriuresis initially causes significant weight loss and a fall in blood pressure (Krieger and Landsberg, 1989). Thereafter, two factors appear to be responsible for the continued fall in blood pressure: a fall in sympathetic nervous activity (Andersson et al., 1991) and a fall in plasma insulin (Franssila-Kallunki et al., 1992) that is associated with a reduction in sodium sensitivity (Rocchini et al., 1989). Weight loss also has been shown to reduce free cytosolic calcium in platelets, which could cause a fall in blood pressure if the same reduction occurs in vascular smooth muscle (Scherrer et al., 1991).

SODIUM RESTRICTION

Although dietary sodium restriction had been shown to lower blood pressure by Ambard in 1906 and Allen in 1920, it was Kempner (1948) who popularized rigid sodium restriction at a time when little else was available for therapy of hypertension. Kempner's rice diet was shown to be effective because it was so low in sodium (Watkin et al., 1950).

After thiazides were introduced during the late 1950s and their mode of action was shown to involve a mild state of sodium depletion, both physicians and patients eagerly adopted this form of therapy in place of dietary sodium restriction. In discarding rigid salt restriction, physicians disregarded the benefits of modest restriction both for its inherent antihypertensive effect and for its potential of reducing diuretic-induced hypokalemia. Moreover, the amount of salt ingested by some patients—15 to 20 g per day—may completely overcome the antihypertensive effectiveness of diuretics (Winer, 1961).

Clinical Experience

Antihypertensive Effect

Modest restriction of dietary sodium intake, by about one-third of the usual intake down to a level of around 100 mmol/day, has been shown in an analysis of all 20 well-controlled studies published through early 1990 to lower the blood pressure an average of 4.9 ± 1.3 mm Hg systolic and 2.6 ± 0.08 mm Hg diastolic (Cutler et al., 1991). Even greater average effects of moderate sodium restriction were noted by Law et al. (1991) in their analysis of 68 crossover trials and 10 randomized controlled trials of sodium restriction. Although their analysis has been criticized for its inclusion of poorly controlled data (Swales, 1991), Law et al. (1991) documented that the effectiveness of sodium restriction increases with increasing initial BP levels and increasing age; they also documented the need

for patients to remain on the restricted diet for at least 5 weeks to observe the full effect. Elderly hypertensive subjects respond particularly well (Weinberger and Fineberg, 1991) (Fig. 6.4), perhaps because their hypertension is more volume dependent in keeping with their lower plasma renin levels (Niarchos et al., 1984). Although the maneuver used by Weinberger and Fineberg to assess sodium sensitivity involved a 1-day rigid restriction of sodium plus a diuretic, their results likely reflect the more chronic response to modest sodium restriction.

Dose Response. The analyses by Cutler et al. (1991) and Law et al. (1991) supported a dose-response relation. MacGregor et al. (1989) gave three levels of sodium—50, 100, or 200 mmol/day each for 4 weeks—to 20 mild hypertensives in a double-blind, randomized, crossover study. Compared with the level on 200 mmol/day, the average supine BP fell 8/5 mm Hg on the 100-mmol/day intake and 16/9 mm Hg on the 50-mmol/day intake. The authors concluded:

> The study showed an apparently linear dose response to sodium restriction in this group of patients. This graded response suggests that at least over the range of sodium intakes studied, there is no threshold value below which sodium intake needs to be reduced. Therefore, to obtain the maximum effect, sodium intake should be reduced as far as is practicable.

These same investigators reported an additive effect of moderate sodium restriction in patients on an angiotensin-converting enzyme (ACE) inhibitor and a diuretic, suggesting that sodium restriction is valuable even when antihypertensive drugs are needed (Singer et al., 1991).

Protection from Diuretic-Induced Potassium Loss

Unlimited access to dietary sodium and the daily intake of a diuretic make every patient vulnerable to the major side effect of diuretic therapy—hypokalemia. The diuretic inhibits sodium reabsorption at the cortical diluting segment of the nephron, proximal to that part of the distal convoluted tubule wherein exchange of potassium ion (K^+) for sodium (Na^+) occurs. When a diuretic is given daily while the patient ingests large amounts of sodium, the initial diuretic-induced sodium depletion shrinks plasma volume, activating renin release and secondarily increasing aldosterone secretion. As the diuretic continues to inhibit sodium reabsorption proximal to the K^+-Na^+ exchange site, more Na^+ is delivered to this distal site. The increased

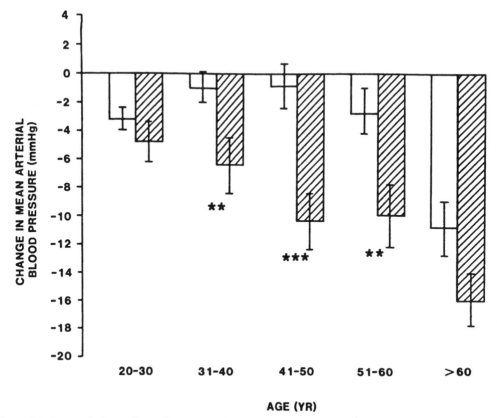

Figure 6.4. Bar graph shows change in mean arterial pressure used to define salt responsivity as a function of age in normotensive *(open bars)* and hypertensive *(hatched bars)* subjects. *Brackets* represent standard deviation of the mean. Significance values between hypertensive and normal subjects are indicated by ** (p < 0.01) and *** (p < 0.001). Sodium sensitivity is greater in hypertensives and increases progressively with age. (From Weinberger MH, Fineberg NS. Sodium and volume sensitivity of blood pressure. Age and pressure change over time. *Hypertension* 1991;18:67–71.)

amounts of aldosterone act to increase sodium reabsorption at the distal exchange site, thereby increasing potassium secretion, and the potassium is swept into the urine.

With modest sodium restriction (70 to 100 mmol/day), less sodium would be delivered to the distal exchange site, and therefore less potassium would be swept into the urine. This modest restriction should not further activate the renin-angiotensin-aldosterone mechanism to cause more distal tubular sodium-for-potassium exchange since that usually occurs only with more rigid sodium restriction. This postulate was confirmed in a test of 12 hypertensive patients (Ram et al., 1981). The patients were given one of three diuretics for 4-week intervals while ingesting a diet with either 72 or 195 mmol per day of sodium. While on the modestly restricted diet, total body potassium levels fell only half as much.

Additional Benefits

Beyond the documented effects on BP and diuretic-induced potassium waste, moderate sodium restriction has been shown to reduce left ventricular hypertrophy (Jula et al., 1992a), correct a defect in beta-adrenergic responsiveness in older people (Feldman, 1992), and prevent renal glomerular damage in experimental animals (Benstein et al., 1990).

Mechanisms

Most of the detailed studies on the responses to sodium restriction have used much more rigid deprivation (usually 10 mmol/day) over short intervals. Though such studies simply may amplify what happens with more modest sodium restriction, caution is advised in interpolating the data from rigid to modest sodium restriction, as noted in relation to potassium waste.

With that caveat in mind, the effects of sodium restriction have been shown to include (*a*) a fall in cardiac output (Omvik and Lund-Johansen, 1986) and perhaps a fall in peripheral resistance (Benetos et al., 1992), (*b*) a reduction in left ventricular wall thickness (Jula et al., 1992a; Liebson et al., 1992), (*c*) a rise in plasma norepinephrine that involves an increase in renal norepinephrine release (Friberg et al., 1990), (*d*) a decrease in atrial natriuretic peptide secretion (Jula et al., 1992b), and (5) activation of the renin-aldosterone mechanism (Egan et al., 1991). Neither the sympathetic nervous system nor the renin-aldosterone mechanism should be markedly stimulated by the moderate degree of sodium restriction advocated for the treatment of hypertension.

The fall in BP tends to be greater in those with low plasma renin levels that rise little during sodium restriction (Sullivan, 1991). Such patients may be the ''nonmodulators'' described by Williams and Hollenberg (1991) (see Chapter 3). Beyond the influence of the renin-aldosterone mechanism, sodium sensitivity may also be related to a variety of influences including the presence of hypertension, obesity, black race, and older age (Rocchini et al., 1989; Weinberger and Fineberg, 1991).

Problems in Practice

In various trials, the majority of patients have restricted dietary sodium intake by an average of about 30% (Elmer et al., 1991). Less success has been reported in less well controlled studies of dietary counseling (Alli et al., 1992) or in community-wide mass media campaigns (Staessen et al., 1988). On the other hand, Forte et al. (1989) have described a successful community intervention trial among people in rural Portugal who were previously on a very high salt intake. Ellison et al. (1989) have shown that a 15% to 20% reduction in sodium intake can easily be achieved by changes in food purchasing and preparation, with a resultant significant fall in overall BP levels.

Processed and Fast Foods. As we increasingly use processed and fast foods instead of home-prepared fresh foods, the major impediment to sodium restriction has become the high sodium content in processed foods, to which salt is added as a taste enhancer, tenderizer, color preserver, or leavener. More than 75% of average sodium consumption comes from processed foods and is, in that sense, nondiscretionary (Mattes and Donnelly, 1991). One hopes that as

mandatory labeling requirements are implemented after 1993 in the United States, consumers will become more aware of the literal mines of salt that are hidden in many processed foods, and that food processors will continue to reduce the amounts of sodium they add.

Additional problems may make even modest sodium restriction difficult to achieve:

—One out of five Americans eats at a fast-food restaurant every day, where most choices contain large amounts of sodium (Massachusetts Medical Society, 1989);
—Sodium is present in large amounts in many antacids (Drake and Hollander, 1981): Alka-Seltzer, Bromo Seltzer, and Biosodol have 500 to 1540 mg per tablet. Lower-sodium preparations are available: Tums, Titralac, and Maalox Plus have only 1 to 2 mg per tablet;
—The high sodium content of some injectable antibiotics may add as much as 140 mmol/day (Baron et al., 1984);
—Some beverages (e.g., Vichy water, tomato juice, V8 vegetable juice) are high in sodium content;
—The elderly may lose some of their perception of the saltiness of food and therefore add even more to satisfy their taste (Schiffman, 1983).

Putative Dangers

Despite the concerns raised (Muntzel and Drüeke, 1992), there is virtually no danger with moderate sodium restriction. Rigid sodium restriction, down to levels of 10 to 20 mmol/day, may cause a variety of problems, although these have been seen mostly in vulnerable experimental animals and hardly ever in humans. These problems include a lesser ability to respond to volume losses from heat exposure and other major environmental stresses (Ely et al., 1990), a decrease in the intake of other needed nutrients (Engstrom and Tobelmann, 1983), rises in serum lipids and insulin (Ruppert et al., 1991), and decreased renal perfusion (Warren and O'Connor, 1981). A few hypertensives with renal disease, particularly those with analgesic nephropathy, waste considerable amounts of sodium. In such patients, overly rigid sodium restriction may worsen renal function and, by activating renin release, aggravate hypertension.

None of these problems has been documented with the moderate degree of sodium restriction that is advocated and—more to the point—that is attainable by free-living people. Specifically, moderate sodium restriction does not impair the ability to exercise vigorously in hot environments (Hargreaves et al., 1989), does not reduce the intake of other nutrients (Nowson and Morgan, 1988), does not affect blood lipids (Grimm et al., 1992), and does not cause hypoperfusion of any vital organ.

Conclusions

For the overwhelming majority of hypertensives, moderate sodium restriction is worthwhile and feasible. The reduction of BP possible with a universal reduction in sodium intake of 50 mmol/day has been estimated to translate into a 22% reduction of the incidence of stroke and a 16% reduction in the incidence of coronary disease (Law et al., 1991). Such estimates may be valid: repeated surveys from 1966 to 1986 in Belgium show a progressive decrease in average sodium intake from 203 mmol/day to 144 mmol/day; these falls correlate closely with lesser rises in BP with increasing age and decreased stroke mortality in the population (Joosens and Kesteloot, 1991). The real potential for benefit, with the very remote possibility of harm, makes moderate sodium restriction a desirable goal both for the individual hypertensive patient and for the population at large.

POTASSIUM SUPPLEMENTS

Many of the benefits of reduced sodium intake could reflect an increased potassium intake. To achieve even a modest reduction in sodium intake, high-sodium/low-potassium processed foods usually are replaced with low-sodium/high-potassium natural foods. Epidemiologic evidence supports an inverse relationship between potassium intake and BP (Linas, 1991) particularly among blacks (Veterans Administration, 1987), and short-term potassium depletion exacerbates hypertension (Krishna and Kapoor, 1991).

Clinical Experience

In a meta-analysis of 19 clinical trials involving 412 hypertensive and 174 normotensive subjects published between 1980 and 1989, oral potassium supplements were shown to significantly lower both systolic and diastolic BP, by an average of -8.2/-4.5 mm Hg among the hypertensives (Cappuccio and MacGregor, 1991) (Fig. 6.5). Studies published since that analysis further document an antihypertensive effect of increased dietary potassium intake (Siani et al., 1991) or potassium supplements (Patki et al., 1990; Fotherby and Potter, 1992).

Mechanisms

Supplemental potassium may not lower the BP of patients already on a sodium-restricted diet (Smith et al., 1985; Grimm et al., 1990). This likely reflects the major mechanism by which potassium appears to lower BP, a natriuresis (Linas, 1991). Numerous other mechanisms have been supported, including decreases in renin-angiotensin and norepinephrine and an increase in vasodilatory prostaglandins (Barden et al., 1991).

Protection Against Strokes

Increased potassium intake may protect against strokes. This was suggested by Acheson and Williams (1983) and supported by the finding that an increase in potassium intake of 10 mmol/day was associated with a 40% reduction in stroke mortality among 859 older people (Khaw and Barrett-Conner, 1987). These findings are supported by studies that demonstrate protection against vascular damage in the brain and kidneys of susceptible rats by high-potassium diets (Volpe et al., 1990; Tobian et al., 1992). This vascular protection may involve an inhibition of various processes involved in atherosclerosis, including free radical formation, platelet aggregation, and smooth muscle proliferation (Young and McCabe, 1992).

Practical Aspects

Even though potassium supplements may lower the BP, they are too costly and potentially hazardous for routine use in the treatment of hypertension in normokalemic patients. They are indicated for diuretic-induced hypokalemia, and the use of potassium-containing salt substitutes (e.g., Co-Salt) will add little expense. For the larger population, a reduction of high-sodium/low-potassium processed foods with an increase of low-sodium/high-potassium natural foods is all that is likely needed to achieve the potential benefits. Fruits and beans provide the largest quantity of potassium per serving.

CALCIUM SUPPLEMENTS

Calcium intake may be lower among hypertensive patients than among normotensive people (McCarron, 1982; Witteman et al., 1989; Ascherio et al., 1992), increased calcium intake may reduce the incidence of hypertension (Dwyer et al., 1992), and calcium supplements may lower the BP of some hypertensive patients (McCarron and Morris, 1985) and prevent pre-eclampsia (Belizan et al., 1991) (see Chapter 11).

Clinical Experience

The report by McCarron and Morris (1985) that calcium supplements may lower the BP of

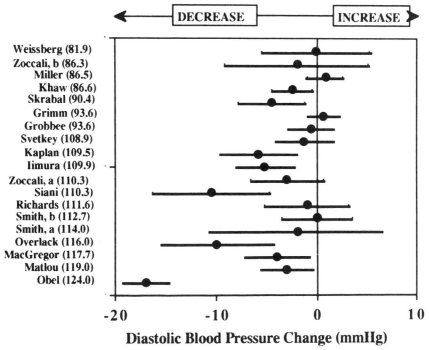

Figure 6.5. Mean and 95% confidence intervals of the differences in supine diastolic blood pressure after oral potassium supplementation in published series, identified by the first author. Values in parentheses represent the average mean blood pressure during control or placebo period. (From Cappuccio FP, MacGregor GA. Does potassium supplementation lower blood pressure? A meta-analysis of published trials. *J Hypertens* 1991;9:465–473.)

some hypertensive patients provoked a steady stream of studies on the antihypertensive efficacy of calcium supplements. Three meta-analyses of 15 to 19 randomized controlled trials through 1990 came to the same conclusion: daily calcium supplements of 1 to 2 g for weeks to years have a small and inconsistent effect on BP (Cappuccio et al., 1989; Grobbee and Waal-Manning, 1990; Cutler and Brittain, 1990). Data from 10 trials involving hypertensive patients demonstrate the lack of significant effects (Fig. 6.6). A similar lack of efficacy has been noted in elderly (Morris and McCarron, 1992) and previously untreated (Galle et al., 1993) hypertensives. In most studies, some hypertensives do respond, although their response may reflect the expected scatter of change with any maneuver.

Mechanisms

If some patients do respond, they likely are those who have a mild degree of secondary hyperparathyroidism that arises to compensate for increased urinary calcium excretion that, in turn, reduces plasma ionized calcium levels. The entire sequence may very well begin with high sodium intake, which causes volume expansion in sodium-sensitive, low-renin patients and leads

to increased urinary calcium excretion (Kaplan, 1988) (Fig. 6.7). Support for this concept comes from the finding that those who respond to supplemental calcium tend to be those with low serum calcium and high parathyroid (PTH) levels (Lyle et al., 1988; Resnick, 1989).

Beyond what is shown in Figure 6.7, there is no logical explanation for a hypotensive effect of additional calcium intake, since a rise in extracellular calcium should, if anything, tend to raise intracellular calcium levels and raise the BP further.

Practical Aspects

As shown in Figure 6.6, calcium supplements may raise the BP in some patients and lower the pressure in others. Moreover, as shown in Figure 6.7, calcium supplements may increase further the hypercalcuria responsible for the development of "calcium sensitivity" and thereby lead to kidney stones and urinary tract infection (Peleg et al., 1992). Until there is a simple way to determine calcium sensitivity, the best course seems to be to ensure a reasonable dietary calcium intake but not to give calcium supplements to either prevent or treat hypertension.

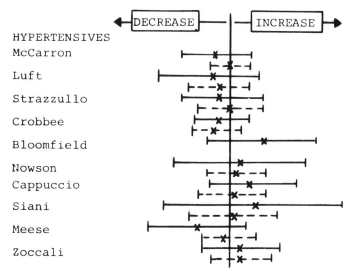

Figure 6.6. Mean *(X)* and 95% confidence intervals of the differences in supine systolic (⎯⎯⎯) and diastolic (- - -) blood pressure after oral calcium supplementation in 10 randomized controlled studies of hypertensive subjects. Studies are identified by the first author. (From Cappuccio FP, Siani A, Strazzullo P. Oral calcium supplementation and blood pressure: an overview of randomized controlled trials. *J Hypertens* 1989;7:941–946.)

Sodium-sensitive, Low-renin Hypertension

Volume
expansion ---> ↑U$_{Ca}$ ---> ↓plasma $_{Ca}$ ---> ↑PTH ---> ↑BP

↑Ca
intake ---> [further ↑U$_{Ca}$] ---> ↑plasma $_{Ca}$ ---> ↓PTH ---> ↓BP

Figure 6.7. A potential explanation for a hypotensive action of increased dietary calcium intake. (From Kaplan NM. Calcium and potassium in the treatment of essential hypertension. *Semin Nephrol* 1988;8:176–184.)

MAGNESIUM SUPPLEMENTS

The same advice seems to be appropriate in regard to magnesium. The theoretical connection between magnesium deficiency and hypertension is more direct and logical than that of calcium and hypertension (Gilbert D'Angelo et al., 1992), but serum and intracellular magnesium levels are normal in most untreated hypertensives. However, low muscle magnesium concentration has been found in half of patients on chronic diuretic therapy (Drup et al., 1993), and magnesium deficiency usually is responsible when hypokalemia is not corrected by potassium repletion (Whang et al., 1992). Moreover, intravenous magnesium has been said to reduce arrhythmias and mortality in acute myocardial infarction (Horner, 1992).

The antihypertensive effect of supplemental magnesium has been less well studied than the antihypertensive effects of potassium or calcium. Although some studies report that magnesium has an antihypertensive effect (Motoyama et al., 1989; Witteman et al., 1992; Widman et al., 1993), most do not (Whelton and Klag, 1989; Patki et al., 1990), except in hypomagnesemic patients (Lind et al., 1991). Therefore, magnesium supplements should only be given to patients found to be magnesium deficient. For those patients, 15 mmol/day of magnesium may lower BP, enable potassium to be repleted, and improve glucose metabolism (Paolisso et al., 1992).

MACRONUTRIENTS

The BP may fall in response to the type of macronutrients in the diet. Vegetarians tend to have low BP, which may be attributable to a lower glycemic index of their diet (Sciarrone et al., 1993). When hypertensives consumed a vegetarian diet under controlled conditions for 6 weeks, an average fall in systolic BP of 5 mm Hg was observed (Margetts et al., 1988).

Fiber

One feature of a vegetarian diet is the increased amount of fiber. Studies in which plant fiber has been given, either alone (Eliasson et al., 1992) or with a low-fat, low-sodium diet (Dodson et al., 1989), have shown that it lowers the BP by about 5 mm Hg in hypertensive patients but not in normotensives (Swain et al., 1990). Moreover, fiber intake of less than 12 g/day was associated with a 1.57 increased relative risk for developing hypertension over a 4-year follow-up compared to the risk associated with an intake of more than 24 g/day (Ascherio et al., 1992).

Dietary Fat

Little if any effect on BP has been noted in multiple controlled trials of varying the amount of total dietary fat or of the ratio of polyunsaturated, monounsaturated, and saturated fatty acids (Sacks, 1989; Shinton et al., 1989; Singer et al., 1990).

Fish Oil

On the other hand, increasingly strong evidence supports a modest antihypertensive effect of relatively large amounts of the omega-3 polyunsaturated fatty acids found in highest concentrations in cold water fish, confirming the benficial effect of a diet of mackerel and herring reported by Singer et al. (1983). For example, Knapp and FitzGerald (1989) examined the effects of small (3 g) and large (15 g) amounts of n-3 fatty acids from fish oil versus such amounts of n-6 fatty acids from safflower oil and a mixture of oils that approximated the fats present in the American diet; each of these regimens was administered to eight men with mild hypertension. They noted a fall of BP of 6.5/4.4 mm Hg in those given the high dose of fish oil but not in the other groups.

A meta-analysis of 31 placebo-controlled trials involving 1356 subjects found a dose-response effect of fish oil on BP of -0.66/-0.35 mm Hg per gram of omega-3 fatty acids (Morris et al., 1993). The mechanism by which fish oils lower BP may involve an increase in vasodilatory prostaglandins (Chin et al., 1992), attenuation of vascular responsiveness to angiotensin and norepinephrine (Chin et al., 1993), modula-

tion of L-type calcium channels (Hallaq et al., 1992), or activation of cell membrane sodium pumps (Miyajima et al., 1993).

Protein

Little is known about the effects of protein on the BP of people other than a lack of difference between meat and nonmeat protein (Prescott et al., 1988). Protein intake was inversely related to BP levels among 8000 Japanese men in Hawaii (Reed et al., 1985) and in over 2000 people from 12 countries in the Intersalt study (Dyer et al., 1992).

Carbohydrate

In rats, high-sucrose diets raise BP (Preuss et al., 1992). In man, high carbohydrate intake for brief periods causes sodium retention but no increase in BP (Affarah et al., 1986). However, plasma insulin levels, already high in hypertensives, are driven even higher by such diets and may interfere with the antihypertensive effect of weight reduction if such reduction involves the use of high-carbohydrate/low-fat diets (Parillo et al., 1988).

Other Dietary Changes

Claims of a BP lowering effect have been made for crude onion extract (Louria et al., 1985) and for garlic powder (Auer et al., 1990). Vitamin C (Hemilä, 1991) and other antioxidants (Ceriello et al., 1991; Sunman et al., 1993) may have a hypotensive effect but have not been adequately tested.

CAFFEINE

The amount of caffeine contained in 2 cups of coffee will raise the BP about 5 mm Hg in infrequent users of caffeine but not in habitual users, indicating tolerance (Sharp and Benowitz, 1990). Ambulatory recordings confirm this pressor effect (Myers and Reeves, 1991), which may accentuate the hemodynamic responses to stress, either mental (van Dusseldorp et al., 1992) or physical (Pincomb et al., 1991). On the other hand, little if any effect has been seen when hypertensives abstain from coffee (MacDonald et al., 1991).

ALCOHOL

As detailed in Chapter 3, the consumption of more than 1 to 2 ounces of ethanol per day is associated with a higher prevalence of hypertension and has been shown to produce an acute pressor action in controlled studies (World

Hypertension League, 1991). On the other hand, most large-scale surveys find no higher BPs among those who consume less than three drinks per day (MacMahon, 1987; Shaper et al., 1988). Since consumption of that amount clearly has been associated with a lower mortality and morbidity rate from coronary disease than seen with either abstinence or higher amounts (Marmot and Brunner, 1991; Klatsky, 1992), the following guidelines seem appropriate:

—Carefully assess alcohol intake;
—If intake is more than two drinks per day, equivalent to about 1 ounce of ethanol, advise a reduction to that level;
—If a significant pressor effect seems likely from even that amount, advise abstinence;
—For most persons who consume no more than two drinks per day, no change seems necessary. Since women may be more sensitive to the pressor and other deleterious effects of alcohol (Gapstur et al., 1992), their intake may need to be limited to only one drink per day.

In a controlled study, a reduction in weekly alcohol intake from 440 ml to 66 ml was associated with a 4.8/3.3 mm Hg fall in pressure; if an average weight loss of 7.5 kg also was accomplished by caloric restriction, the fall in pressure averaged 10.2/7.5 mm Hg (Puddey et al., 1992). In a subsequent study, concomitant vigorous exercise did not add to the antihypertensive effect of alcohol restriction (Cox et al., 1993). Physicians should always advise persons who drink too much to reduce consumption since a significant number will follow that advice (Maheswaran et al., 1992) and achieve a fall in BP (Ueshima et al., 1993).

PHYSICAL ACTIVITY

Clinical Experience

After regularly repeated aerobic (isotonic) exercise, the resting BP usually is lowered. Although most of the 22 studies on exercise and BP published from 1980 to 1990 have major design faults, they almost uniformly show a reduction of 5 to 7 mm Hg for both systolic and diastolic pressures, independent of weight loss (Arroll and Beaglehole, 1992). The validity of the overwhelmingly positive findings is supported by the significant association between the degree of fall in systolic pressure and the change in exercise capacity noted in 29 studies of both normotensive and hypertensive subjects (Fagard et al., 1990) (Fig. 6.8). Elderly hypertensives also obtain an antihypertensive effect from physical activity (Reaven et al., 1991). Moreover,

the degree of rise in BP during exercise is blunted after regular physical training (World Hypertension League, 1991b).

Mechanisms

Immediately after strenuous dynamic exercise, vasodilation persists (Cléroux et al., 1992), and the systolic BP remains well below the pre-exercise level for a period that may be as long as 13 hours (Pescatello et al., 1991). After enough repetitive exercise to reach the "conditioned" state, resting and ambulatory BP and heart rate usually are lower (Somers et al., 1991). These lasting effects reflect a number of changes (Arakawa, 1993): an increase in arterial compliance (Cameron et al., 1992), a decrease in sympathetic activity coupled with favorable changes in the baroreflex (Kingwell et al., 1992), decreased activity in the endogenous Na^+-K^+ pump inhibitor (Koga et al., 1992), and improved glucose/insulin relationships. These last changes in glucose/insulin relationships include increased glucose transporter levels in muscle (Houmard et al., 1991), increased glucose utilization independent of insulin action (Wasserman et al., 1991), increased insulin sensitivity, and reduced insulin secretion (De Fronzo et al., 1987). In view of the likely prohypertensive effects of hyperinsulinemia, these changes may be the most important benefits of exercise (Després et al., 1991).

Isometric Exercise

Despite the reflex-mediated vasoconstriction during isometric or static exercise (Perez-Gonzalez, 1981), a fall in resting BP has been observed after repetitive isometric contractions equal to 30% of maximal capacity (Wiley et al., 1992). Better effects follow circuit weight training involving aerobic effects by a continuing series of repetitive moderate weight lifts (Stewart, 1992).

Another activity that involves isometric activity is sexual intercourse, which is accompanied by significant rises in pulse and BP (Nemec et al., 1976) (Table 6.1). The responses in 10 normal young men (Table 6.1) were essentially the same whether the man was on the top or on the bottom, despite the presumably greater isometric activity with man-on-the-top position.

Effects of Antihypertensive Therapy

Hypertensive patients have, on average, a decreased exercise capacity compared to normotensives (Missault et al., 1992). When hypertensives exercise, they may experience problems

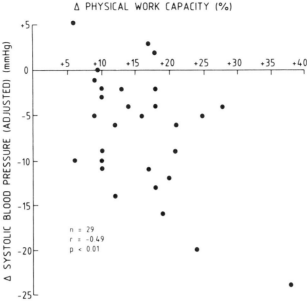

Figure 6.8. Change in systolic blood pressure with training, adjusted for control data, versus change in physical work capacity. Each point represents the average for one group of subjects. (From Fagard R, Bielen E, Hespel P, Lijnen P, Staessen J, Vanhees L, Van Hoof R, Amery A. Physical exercise in hypertension. In: Brenner B, Laragh J, eds. *Hypertension: Pathophysiology, Diagnosis and Management.* New York: Raven Press 1990:1985–1998.)

Table 6.1. Blood Pressure and Pulse Responses During Sexual Intercourse in 10 Normal Men

	Rest	Intromission	Orgasm	2 Minutes Later
Blood pressure				
Man on top	112/66	148/79	163/81	118/69
Man on bottom	113/70	143/74	161/77	121/71
Heart rate				
Man on top	67	136	189	82
Man on bottom	65	125	183	77

From Nemec ED, Mansfield L, Kennedy JW. Heart rate and blood pressure responses during sexual activity in normal males. *Am Heart J* 1976;92:274–277.

with various antihypertensive drugs: diuretics may limit the plasma volume expansion that is needed for aerobic training (Nadel, 1985); beta-blockers blunt exercise-mediated increases in heart rate and cardiac output and may reduce performance (Vanhees et al., 1991). Nonetheless, the hemodynamic responses to both static and dynamic exercise can break through beta-blockade, and a training effect can be achieved (Radaelli et al., 1992). Neither ACE inhibitors nor calcium entry blockers reduce exercise capacity (Vanhees et al., 1991). The rise in BP during isometric exercise may be blunted better by an alpha-blocker (Hamada et al., 1987) and during isotonic exercise by a beta- or an alpha-blocker (Klaus, 1989).

Potential for Prevention

Among a large group of Harvard alumni, Paffenbarger et al. (1983) found that those who did not engage in vigorous physical activity were at 35% greater risk of developing hypertension, whether they had high BPs while at Harvard, a family history of hypertension, or obesity, all of which increased further the risk of hypertension. Similarly, in a 1- to 12-year follow-up of 6039 men and women, those who had low levels of physical fitness at the initial examination had a 1.52 greater relative risk for the development of hypertension than did those with higher levels of physical fitness after appropriate adjustment for age, sex, baseline BP, and body mass index (Blair et al., 1984). Even among schoolchildren, lower levels of BP are found in those who maintain high levels of leisure time physical activity (Hansen et al., 1991).

These studies, as hopeful as they are, obviously do not prove that regular performance of physical activity or the attainment of high levels of physical fitness will prevent the development of hypertension in view of the possible influence of multiple confounding factors. Regardless, among multiple populations, higher levels of physical activity and physical fitness have been associated with a lower rate of cardiovascular disease and mortality (Paffenbarger et al., 1993).

RELAXATION

Relaxation of skeletal muscles has been known for a long time to lower the BP (Jacobson, 1939). More recently, a variety of relaxation therapies—including transcendental meditation (TM), yoga, biofeedback, and psychotherapy—have been shown to reduce the BP of hypertensive patients at least transiently (Patel and Marmot, 1988; McGrady and Higgins, 1989). Though each therapy has its advocates, none has been shown conclusively to be either practical for the majority of hypertensives or effective in maintaining a significant long-term effect (Eisenberg et al., 1993). In two of the few controlled long-term trials, hypertensives who practiced muscle relaxation had BPs that were no lower than those of control groups (van Montfrans et al., 1990; Johnston et al., 1993).

If it is available and acceptable to the patient, one or another form of relaxation therapy may be tried, since such techniques may provide additional benefits in reducing coronary risk beyond any effect on BP (Johnston, 1991). Patients should be forewarned that short-term effects may not be maintained, so continued surveillance is needed.

MISCELLANEOUS

Chinese herbal combinations may work (Wong et al., 1991), and acupuncture has its advocates (Tam and Yiu, 1975), but no controlled studies have been done. Pet owners have demonstrated significantly lower systolic pressures and blood lipid levels than nonowners, effects not attributable to differences in obvious confounding factors (Anderson et al., 1992).

Bed Rest and Sedatives

When patients, even those as difficult to control as outpatients, are hospitalized, their BP almost always comes down, mainly because the sympathetic nervous system becomes less active (Hossmann et al., 1981).

The BP usually falls considerably during sleep. However, there is no evidence that sedatives or tranquilizers lower BP (US Public Health, 1965). Monoamine oxidase (MAO) inhibitors will lower the BP, but their use is limited by the potential for bad pressor reactions with tyramine-containing foods.

Surgical Procedures

From about 1935 through the 1950s, surgical sympathectomy, along with a rigid low-salt diet, was about all that was available for treating hypertension. Sympathectomy was shown to be beneficial for those with severe disease (Thorpe et al., 1950). With current medical therapy, there seems to be no place for sympathectomy. Similarly, implantation of an electric stimulator on the carotid sinus nerve has been shown to lower the BP (Brest et al., 1972), but modern medical therapy has made the procedure unnecessary.

A totally uncontrolled study has reported remarkable success by decompression of one or another intracranial artery, supposedly compressing the left lateral medulla oblongata (Jannetta et al., 1985). Compression of the area is demonstrable at autopsy in patients with primary hypertension, but neither gross nor microscopic damage is seen (Naraghi et al., 1992).

CONCLUSIONS: THE POTENTIAL FOR PREVENTION

These various lifestyle modifications will reduce the BP of most hypertensives, in some to a level that is safe enough to obviate drug therapy. As discussed earlier, one or more of these nondrug therapies should be tried in all patients. Those with mild hypertension may thereby be able to stay off drugs; those with more severe hypertension may need less medication.

Caution is obviously needed in accepting the short- and long-term efficacy of the various nondrug therapies. Part of their antihypertensive effect may be attributable to the "natural" fall in BP seen when repeated readings are taken. Such falls may reflect a statistical regression toward the mean, a placebo effect, or a relief of anxiety and stress with time. The same phenomenon likely is responsible for much of the initial response to drug therapy as well, so both drugs and nondrugs may be given credit deserved by neither.

An even greater possible value for nondrug therapies is their potential for lowering the BP even a small amount in the broader community, delaying if not preventing the development of hypertension and thereby having a much greater impact than the "high-risk" approach of treating only those with established disease (Stamler et al., 1993).

In three well controlled preventive trials involving subjects with "high-normal" BP (Stamler et al., 1989; Hypertension Prevention Trial, 1990; Trials of Hypertension Prevention, 1992) individual and combined lifestyle modifications lowered the BP and reduced the incidence of overt hypertension.

When the development of hypertension over a 4-year follow-up was related to baseline intake of various foods and drink and initial body weight in over 30,000 males in the United States, the following potential reductions in the inci-

dence of hypertension were calculated: 46.7% by weight reduction to a Quetelet index of less than 23; 3.8% by reduction of alcohol to less than two drinks per day; 11.1% by increase of dietary fiber to 24 g/day (Ascherio et al., 1992).

On the basis of these considerations, a group of U.S. experts has called for the widespread application of a multifaceted approach to prevent hypertension through weight loss, reduced sodium intake and alcohol consumption, and increased physical activity (National High Blood Pressure Education Program Working Group, 1993). Lifestyle modifications should be enthusiastically promoted for everyone. However, they will not be enough for most persons with significant hypertension, who will likely need one or more of the drugs described in the next chapter.

References

Aberg H, Tibblin G. Addition of non-pharmacological methods of treatment in patients on antihypertensive drugs: results of previous medication, laboratory tests and life quality. *J Intern Med* 1989;226:39–46.

Acheson RM, Williams DRR. Does consumption of fruit and vegetables protect against stroke? *Lancet* 1983;1:1191–1193.

Affarah HB, Hall WD, Heymsfield SB, Kutner M, Wells JO, Tuttle EP Jr. High-carbohydrate diet: antinatriuretic and blood pressure response in normal men. *Am J Clin Nutr* 1986;44:341–348.

Alli C, Avanzini F, Bettelli G, Bonati M, Colombo F, Corso R, Di Tullio M, Gentile MG, Sangalli L, Taioli E, Tognoni G. Feasibility of a long-term low-sodium diet in mild hypertension. *J Hum Hypertens* 1992;6:281–286.

Anderson WP, Reid CM, Jennings GL. Pet ownership and risk factors for cardiovascular disease. *Med J Aust* 1992;157:298–301.

Andersson B, Elam M, Wallin BG, Björntorp P, Andersson OK. Effect of energy-restricted diet on sympathetic muscle nerve activity in obese women. *Hypertension* 1991;18:783–789.

Arakawa K. Antihypertensive mechanism of exercise. *J Hypertens* 1993;11:223–229.

Arroll B, Beaglehole R. Does physical activity lower blood pressure? A critical review of the clinical trials. *J Clin Epidemiol* 1992;45:439–447.

Ascherio A, Rimm EB, Giovannucci EL, Colditz GA, Rosner B, Willett WC, Sacks F, Stampfer MJ. A prospective study of nutritional factors and hypertension among US men. *Circulation* 1992;86:1475–1484.

Auer W, Eiber A, Hertkorn E, Hoehfeld E, Koehrle U, Lorenz A, Mader F, Merx W, Otto G, Schmidt-Otto B, Taubenheim H. Hypertension and hyperlipidaemia: garlic helps in mild cases. *Br J Clin Pract* 1990;69(Suppl):3–6.

Ayman D. An evaluation of therapeutic results in essential hypertension. I. The interpretation of symptomatic relief. *JAMA* 1930;95:246–249.

Barden A, Beilin LJ, Vandongen R, Puddey IB. A double-blind placebo-controlled trial of the effects of short-term potassium supplementation on blood pressure and atrial natriuretic peptide in normotensive women. *Am J Hypertens* 1991;4:206–213.

Baron DN, Hamilton-Miller JMT, Brumfitt W. Sodium content of injectable β-lactam antibiotics. *Lancet* 1984;1:1113–1114.

Belizan JM, Villar J, Gonzalez L, Campodonico L, Bergel E. Calcium supplementation to prevent hypertensive disorders of pregnancy. *N Engl J Med* 1991; 325:1399–1405.

Benetos A, Yang-Yan X, Cuche J-L, Hannaert P, Safar M. Arterial effects of salt restriction in hypertensive patients. A 9-week, randomized, double-blind, crossover study. *J Hypertens* 1992;10:355–360.

Benstein JA, Feiner HD, Parker M, Dworkin LD. Superiority of salt restriction over diuretics in reducing renal hypertrophy and injury in uninephrectomized SHR. *Am J Physiol* 1990;258:F1675–F1681.

Blair SN, Goodyear NN, Gibbons LW, Cooper KH. Physical fitness and incidence of hypertension in healthy normotensive men and women. *JAMA* 1984;252:487–490.

Blaufox MD, Lee HB, David B, Oberman A, Wassertheil-Smoller S, Langford H. Renin predicts diastolic blood pressure response to nonpharmacologic and pharmacologic therapy. *JAMA* 1992;267:1221–1225.

Bolinder GM, Ahlborg BO, Lindell JH. Use of smokeless tobacco: Blood pressure elevation and other health hazards found in a large-scale population survey. *J Intern Med* 1992;232:327–334.

Brest AN, Wiener L, Bachrach B. Bilateral carotid sinus nerve stimulation in the treatment of hypertension. *Am J Cardiol* 1972;29:821–826.

Cameron JD, Dart AM, Topham S. Effects of 4 weeks exercise training on arterial compliance in man [Abstract]. *Circulation* 1992;86(Suppl 1):276.

Cappuccio FP, MacGregor GA. Does potassium supplementation lower blood pres-

sure? A meta-analysis of published trials. *J Hypertens* 1991;9:465–473.

Cappuccio FP, Siani A, Strazzullo P. Oral calcium supplementation and blood pressure: an overview of randomized controlled trials. *J Hypertens* 1989;7:941–946.

Carman WJ, Barrett-Connor E, Sowers M, Khaw K-T. Are lean hypertensives at greater risk of cardiovascular mortality than obese hypertensives? [Abstract]. *Circulation* 1992;85:5.

Ceriello A, Giugliano D, Quatraro A, Lefebvre PJ. Anti-oxidants show an anti-hypertensive effect in diabetic and hypertensive subjects. *Clin Sci* 1991;81:739–742.

Chin J, Gust A, Kaye D, Angus J, Dart A, Jennings G. Effects of N-3 fatty acids on vascular reactivity in vivo and in vitro in man [Abstract]. *J Hypertens* 1992; 10(Suppl 4):16.

Chin JPF, Gust AP, Nestel PJ, Dart AM. Marine oils dose-dependently inhibit vasoconstriction of forearm resistance vessels in humans. *Hypertension* 1993;21:22–28.

Cléroux J, Kouamé N, Nadeau A, Coulombe D, Lacourcière Y. Aftereffects of exercise on regional and systemic hemodynamics in hypertension. *Hypertension* 1992; 19:183–191.

Craig WY, Palomaki GE, Haddow JE. Cigarette smoking and serum lipid and lipoprotein concentrations: an analysis of published data. *Br Med J* 1989;298:784–788.

Cox KL, Puddey IB, Morton AR, Beilin LJ, Vandongen R, Masarei JRL. The combined effects of aerobic exercise and alcohol restriction on blood pressure and serum lipids: a two-way factorial study in sedentary men. *J Hypertens* 1993;11:191–201.

Cutler JA, Brittain E. Calcium and blood pressure. An epidemiologic perspective. *Am J Hypertens* 1990;3:137–146.

Cutler JA, Follmann D, Elliott P, Suh IL. An overview of randomized trials of sodium reduction and blood pressure. *Hypertension* 1991;17(Suppl 1):27–33.

Daniel M, Martin AD, Faiman C. Sex hormones and adipose tissue distribution in premenopausal cigarette smokers. *Int J Obesity* 1992;16:245–254.

DasGupta P, Brigden G, Ramhamdany E, Lahiri A, Baird IM, Raftery EB. Circadian variation and blood pressure: response to rapid weight loss by hypocaloric hyponatraemic diet in obesity. *J Hypertens* 1991;9:441–447.

De Cesaris R, Ranieri G, Andriani A, Filitti V, Bonfantino MV. Effects of cigarette-smoking on blood pressure and heart rate. *J Hypertens* 1991;9(Suppl 6):122–123.

DeFronzo RA, Sherwin RS, Kraemer N. Effect of physical training on insulin action in obesity. *Diabetes* 1987;36:1379–1385.

Després J-P, Pouliot M-C, Moorjani S, Nadeau A, Tremblay A, Lupien PJ, Thériault G, Bouchard C. Loss of abdominal fat and metabolic response to exercise training in obese women. *Am J Physiol* 1991;261:E159–E167.

Dodson PM, Pacy PJ, Cox EV. Long-term follow-up of the treatment of essential hypertensin with a high-fibre, low-fat and low-sodium dietary regimen. *Hum Nutr Clin Nutr* 1985:39C:213–220.

Dodson PM, Stephenson J, Dodson LJ, Kurnik D, Kritzinger EE, Taylor KG, Fletcher RF. Randomised blind controlled trial of a high fibre, low fat and low sodium dietary regimen in mild essential hypertension. *J Hum Hypertens* 1989;3:197–202.

Drup I, Skajaa K, Thybo NK. Oral magnesium supplementation restores the concentrations of magnesium, potassium and sodium-potassium pumps in skeletal muscle of patients receiving diuretic treatment. *J Int Med* 1993;233:117–123.

Drake D, Hollander D. Neutralizing capacity and cost effectiveness of antacids. *Ann Intern Med* 1981;94:215–217.

Dwyer JH, Curtin LR, Davis IJ, Dwyer KM, Feinleib M. Dietary calcium and 10 year incidence of treated hypertension in the NHANES I epidemiologic follow-up [Abstract]. *Circulation* 1992;86(Suppl 1):678.

Dyer A, Elliott P, Kesteloot H, Stamler J, Stamler R, Freeman J, Shipley M, Marmot M, Rose G. Urinary nitrogen excretion and blood pressure in INTERSALT [Abstract]. *J Hypertens* 1992;10(Suppl 4):122.

Egan BM, Weder AB, Petrin J, Hoffman RG. Neurohumoral and metabolic effects of short-term dietary NaCl restriction in men. Relationship to salt-sensitivity status. *Am J Hypertens* 1991;4:416–421.

Eisenberg DM, Delbanco TL, Berkey CS, Kaptchuk TJ, Kupelnick B, Kuhl J, Chalmers TC. Cognitive behavioral techniques for hypertension: are they effective? *Ann Intern Med* 1993;118:964–972.

Eliasson K, Ryttig KR, Hylander B, Rössner S. A dietary fibre supplement in the treatment of mild hypertension. A randomized, double-blind, placebo-controlled trial. *J Hypertens* 1992;10:195–199.

Ellison RC, Capper AL, Stephenson WP, Goldberg RJ, Hosmer DW Jr, Humphrey KF, Ockene JK, Gamble WJ, Witsch JC, Stare FJ. Effects on blood pressure of a decrease in sodium use in institutional food preparation: the Exeter-Andover Project. *J Clin Epidemiol* 1989;42:201–208.

Elmer PJ, Grimm RH Jr, Flack J, Laing B. Dietary sodium reduction for hypertension prevention and treatment. *Hypertension* 1991;17(Suppl 1):182–189.

Ely DL, Folkow B, Paradise NF. Risks associated with dietary sodium reduction in the spontaneous hypertensive rat model of hypertension. *Am J Hypertens* 1990;3:650–660.

Engstrom AM, Tobelmann RC. Nutritional consequences of reducing sodium intake. *Ann Intern Med* 1983;98(Part 2):870–872.

Facchini FS, Hollenbeck CB, Jeppesen J, Chen YDI, Reaven GM. Insulin resistance and cigarette smoking. *Lancet* 1992;339:1128–1130.

Fagard R, Bielen E, Hespel P, Lijnen P, Staessen J, Vanhees L, Van Hoof R, Amery A. Physical exercise in hypertension. In: Brenner B, Laragh J, eds. *Hypertension: Pathophysiology, Diagnosis and Management.* New York: Raven Press 1990: 1985–1998.

Fagerberg B, Berglund A, Andersson OK, Berglund G. Weight reduction versus anti-hypertensive drug therapy in obese men with high blood pressure: Effects upon plasma insulin levels and association with changes in blood pressure and serum lipids. *J Hypertens* 1992;10:1053–1061.

Feldman RD. A low-sodium diet corrects the defect in β-adrenergic response in older subjects. *Circulation* 1992;85:612–618.

Fiore MC, Jorenby DE, Baker TB, Kenford SL. Tobacco dependence and the nicotine patch. Clinical guidelines for effective use. *JAMA* 1992;268:2687–2694.

Forte JG, Pereira Miguel JM, Pereira Miguel MJ, de Padua F, Rose G. Salt and blood pressure: a community trial. *J Hum Hypertens* 1989;3:178–184.

Fotherby MD, Potter JF. Potassium supplementation reduces clinic and ambulatory blood pressure in elderly hypertensive patients. *J Hypertens* 1992;10:1403–1408.

Franssila-Kallunki A, Rissanen A, Ekstrand A, Ollus A, Groop L. Effects of weight loss on substrate oxidation, energy expenditure, and insulin sensitivity in obese individuals. *Am J Clin Nutr* 1992;55:356–361.

Friberg P, Meredith I, Jennings G, Lambert G, Fazio V, Esler M. Evidence for increased renal norepinephrine overflow during sodium restriction in humans. *Hypertension* 1990:16:121–130.

Galløe AM, Graudal N, Møller J, Bro H, Jørgensen M, Christensen HR. Effect of oral calcium supplementation on blood pressure in patients with previously untreated hypertension: a randomized, double-blind, placebo-controlled, crossover study. *J Hum Hypertens* 1993;7:43–45.

Gapstur SM, Potter JD, Sellers TA, Folsom AR. Increased risk of breast cancer with alcohol consumption in postmenopausal women. *Am J Epidemiol* 1992;136:1221–1231.

Gilbert D'Angelo EK, Singer HA, Rembold CM. Magnesium relaxes arterial smooth muscle by decreasing intracellular Ca^{2+} without changing intracellular Mg^{2+}. *J Clin Invest* 1992;89:1988–1994.

Gillum RF, Prineas RJ, Jeffery RW, Jacobs DR, Elmer PJ, Gomez O, Blackburn H.

Nonpharmacologic therapy of hypertension: the independent effects of weight reduction and sodium restriction in overweight borderline hypertensive patients. *Am Heart J* 1983;105:128–133.

Gray DS, Fujioka K, Devine W, Bray GA. Fluoxetine treatment of the obese diabetic. *Int J Obesity* 1992;16:193–198.

Grimm RH, Elmer P, Svendsen K, Launer C, Van Hell N, Neaton J. A low sodium diet does not affect blood lipids/lipoproteins in men with mild hypertension (HT): analysis of the Minneapolis Mount Sinai Hypertension Trial (MSHT) [Abstract]. *Am J Hypertens* 1992;5:21a–22a.

Grimm RH Jr, Neaton JD, Elmer PJ, Svendsen KH, Levin J, Segal M, Holland L, Witte LJ, Clearman DR, Kofron P, LaBounty RK, Crow R, Prineas RJ. The influence of oral potassium chloride on blood pressure in hypertensive men on a low-sodium diet. *N Engl J Med* 1990;322:569–574.

Grobbee DE, Waal-Manning HJ. The role of calcium supplementation in the treatment of hypertension. *Drugs* 1990;39:7–18.

Groppelli A, Giorgi DMA, Omboni S, Parati G, Mancia G. Persistent blood pressure increase induced by heavy smoking. *J Hypertens* 1992;10:495–499.

Groppelli A, Omboni S, Parati G, Mancia G. Blood pressure and heart rate response to repeated smoking before and after β-blockade and selective $α_1$ inhibition. *J Hypertens* 1990;8(Suppl 5):35–40.

Hallaq H, Smith TW, Leaf A. Modulation of dihydropyridine-sensitive calcium channels in heart cells by fish oil fatty acids. *Proc Natl Acad Sci* 1992;89:1760–1764.

Hamada M, Kazatani Y, Shigematsu Y, Ito T, Kokubu T, Ishise S. Enhanced blood pressure response to isometric handgrip exercise in patients with essential hypertension: effects of propranolol and prazosin. *J Hypertens* 1987;5:305–309.

Hansen HS, Froberg K, Hyldebrandt N, Nielsen JR. A controlled study of eight months of physical training and reduction of blood pressure in children: the Odense schoolchild study. *Br Med J* 1991;303:682–685.

Hargreaves M, Morgan TO, Snow R, Guerin M. Exercise tolerance in the heat on low and normal salt intakes. *Clin Sci* 1989;76:553–557.

Hemilä H. Vitamin C and lowering of blood pressure: Need for intervention trials? *J Hypertens* 1991;9:1076–1077.

Horner SM. Efficacy of intravenous magnesium in acute myocardial infarction in reducing arrhythmias and mortality. Meta-analysis of magnesium in acute myocardial infarction. *Circulation* 1992;86:774–779.

Hossmann V, FitzGerald GA, Dollery CT. Influence of hospitalization and placebo therapy on blood pressure and sympathetic function in essential hypertension. *Hypertension* 1981;3:113–118.

Houmard JA, Egan PC, Neufer PD, Friedman JE, Wheeler WS, Israel RG, Dohm GL. Elevated skeletal muscle glucose transporter levels in exercise-trained middle-aged men. *Am J Physiol* 1991;261:E437–E443.

Hypertension Prevention Trial Research Group. The Hypertension Prevention Trial:

three-year effects of dietary changes on blood pressure. *Arch Intern Med* 1990; 150:153–162.

Jacobson E. Variation of blood pressure with skeletal muscle tension and relaxation. *Ann Intern Med* 1939;12:1194–1212.

Jannetta PJ, Segal R, Wolfson SK Jr. Neurogenic hypertension: Etiology and surgical treatment. I. Observations in 53 patients. *Ann Surg* 1985;201:391–398.

Johannesson M, Fagerberg B. A health-economic comparison of diet and drug treatment in obese men with mild hypertension. *J Hypertens* 1992;10:1063–1070.

Johnston DW. Stress management in the treatment of mild primary hypertension. *Hypertension* 1991;17(Suppl 3):63–68.

Johnston DW, Gold A, Kentish J, Smith D, Vallance P, Shah D, Leach G, Robinson B. Effect of stress management on blood pressure in mild primary hypertension. *Br Med J* 1993;306:963–966.

Joint National Committee on Detection, Evaluation, and Treatment of High Blood Pressure (JNC V). The Fifth Report of the Joint National Committee on Detection, Evaluation, and Treatment of High Blood Pressure (JNC V). *Arch Intern Med* 1993; 153:154–183.

Joossens JV, Kesteloot H. Trends in systolic blood pressure, 24-hour sodium excretion, and stroke mortality in the elderly in Belgium. *Am J Med* 1991;90(Suppl 3A):5.

Jula A, Karanko H, Rönnemaa T. Effects of long-term sodium restriction on left ventricular hypertrophy in mild to moderate essential hypertension. [Abstract]. *J Hypertens* 1992a;10(Suppl 4):104.

Jula R, Rönnemaa T, Rastas M, Karvetti R-L, Mäki J. Long-term nopharmacological treatment for mild to moderate hypertension. *J Intern Med* 1990;227:413–421.

Jula A, Rönnemaa T, Tikkanen I, Karanko H. Responses of atrial natriuretic factor to long-term sodium restriction in mild to moderate hypertension. *J Intern Med* 1992b;231:521–529.

Kannel WB, Zhang T, Garrison RJ. Is obesity-related hypertension less of a cardiovascular risk? The Framingham study. *Am Heart J* 1990;120:1195–1201.

Kaplan NM. Calcium and potassium in the treatment of essential hypertension. *Semin Nephrol* 1988;8:176–184.

Kaplan NM. The deadly quartet. Upper-body obesity, glucose intolerance, hypertriglyceridemia, and hypertension. *Arch Intern Med* 1989;149:1514–1520.

Kaufman DW, Palmer JR, Rosenberg L, Shapiro S. Cigar and pipe smoking and myocardial infarction in young men. *Br Med J* 1987;294:1315–1316.

Kempner W. Treatment of hypertensive vascular disease with rice diet. *Am J Med* 1948;4:545–577.

Khaw K-T, Barrett-Connor E. Dietary potassium and stroke-associated mortality. A 12-year prospective population study. *N Engl J Med* 1987;316:235–240.

Kingwell BA, Dart AM, Jennings GL, Korner PI. Exercise training reduces the sympathetic component of the blood pressure-heart rate baroreflex in man. *Clin Sci* 1992;82:357–362.

Klatsky AL, Armstrong MA, Friedman GD. Alcohol and mortality. *Ann Intern Med* 1992;117:646–654.

Klaus D. Management of hypertension in actively exercising patients. Implications for drug selection. *Drugs* 1989;37: 212–218.

Knapp HR, FitzGerald GA. The antihypertensive effects of fish oil. A controlled study of polyunsaturated fatty acid supplements in essential hypertension. *N Engl J Med* 1989;320:1037–1043.

Koga M, Ideishi M, Matsusaki M, Tashiro E, Kinoshita A, Ikeda M, Tanaka H, Shindo M, Arakawa K. Mild exercise decreases plasma endogenous digitalis-like substance in hypertensive individuals. *Hypertension* 1992;19(Suppl 2):231–236.

Kolanowski J, Younis LT, Vanbutsele R, Detry J-M. Effect of dexfenfluramine treatment on body weight, blood pressure and noradrenergic activity in obese hypertensive patients. *Eur J Clin Pharmacol* 1992;42:599–606.

Kostis JB, Rosen RC, Brondolo E, Taska L, Smith DE, Wilson AC. Superiority of nonpharmacologic therapy compared to propranolol and placebo in men with mild hypertension: a randomized, prospective trial. *Am Heart J* 1992;123:466–474.

Krieger DR, Landsberg L. Neuroendocrine mechanisms in obesity-related hypertension. In: Laragh JH, Brenner BM, Kaplan NM, eds. *Perspectives in Hypertension, vol 2: Endocrine Mechanisms in Hypertension*. New York: Raven Press, 1989: 105–128.

Krishna GG, Kapoor SC. Potassium depletion exacerbates essential hypertension. *Ann Intern Med* 1991;115:77–83.

Law MR, Frost CD, Wald NJ. III—Analysis of data from trials of salt reduction. *Br Med J* 1991;302:819–824.

Lee EW, D'Alonzo GE. Cigarette smoking, nicotine addiction, and its pharmacologic treatment. *Arch Intern Med* 1993; 153:34–48.

Liebson P, Prineas R, Grandits G, Dianzumba S, Grimm R. Variables associated with regression of left-ventricular mass in the treatment of mild hypertension study (TOMHS) [Abstract]. *Circulation* 1992;86:499.

Linas SL. The role of potassium in the pathogenesis and treatment of hypertension. *Kidney Int* 1991;39:771–786.

Lind L, Lithell H, Pollare T, Ljunghall S. Blood pressure response during long-term treatment with magnesium is dependent on magnesium status. A double-blind, placebo-controlled study in essential hypertension and in subjects with high-normal blood pressure. *Am J Hypertens* 1991; 4:674–679.

Little P, Girling G, Hasler A, Trafford SA. A controlled trial of a low sodium, low fat, high fibre diet in treated hypertensive patients: Effect on antihypertensive drug requirement in clinical practice. *J Human Hypertens* 1991;5:175–181.

Louria DB, McAnally JF, Lasser N, Lavenhar M, Perri NA, Noto G. Onion extract in treatment of hypertension and hyperlipidemia: a preliminary communication. *Curr Ther Res* 1985;37:127–131.

Lyle RM, Melby CL, Hyner CG. Metabolic differences between subjects whose blood pressure did or did not respond to oral calcium supplementation. *Am J Clin Nutr* 1988;47:1030–1035.

MacDonald TM, Sharpe K, Fowler G, Lyons D, Freestone S, Lovell HG, Webster J, Petrie JC. Caffeine restriction: effect on mild hypertension. *Br Med J* 1991; 303:1235–1238.

MacGregor GA, Markandu ND, Sagnella GA, Singer DRJ, Cappuccio FP. Double-blind study of three sodium intakes and long-term effects of sodium restriction in essential hypertension. *Lancet* 1989; 2:1244–1247.

MacMahon S. Alcohol consumption and hypertension. *Hypertension* 1987; 9:111–121.

Maheswaran R, Beevers M, Beevers DG. Effectiveness of advice to reduce alcohol consumption in hypertensive patients. *Hypertension* 1992;19:79–84.

Mann SJ, James GD, Wang RS, Pickering TG. Elevation of ambulatory systolic blood pressure in hypertensive smokers. A case-control study. *JAMA* 1991;265: 2226–2228.

Margetts BM, Beilin LJ, Armstrong BK, Vandongen R. Vegetarian diet in mild hypertension: effects of fat and fiber. *Am J Clin Nutr* 1988;48:801–805.

Marmot M, Brunner E. Alcohol and cardiovascular disease: the status of the U shaped curve. *Br Med J* 1991;303:565–568.

Massachusetts Medical Society Committee on Nutrition. Sounding board. Fast-food fare—Consumer guidelines. *N Engl J Med* 1989;321:752–756.

Materson BJ, Reda D, Freis ED, Henderson WG. Cigarette smoking interferes with treatment of hypertension. *Arch Intern Med* 1988;148:2116–2119.

Mattes RD, Donnelly D. Relative contributions of dietary sodium sources. *J Am Coll Nutr* 1991;10:383–393.

McCarron DA. Calcium, magnesium, and phosphorus balance in human and experimental hypertension. *Hypertension* 1982;4(Suppl 3):27–33.

McCarron DA, Morris CD. Blood pressure response to oral calcium in persons with mild to moderate hypertension. *Ann Intern Med* 1985;103:825–831.

McGrady A, Higgins JT Jr. Prediction of response to biofeedback-assisted relaxation in hypertensives: development of a hypertensive predictor profile (HYPP). *Psychosomatic Med* 1989;51:277–284.

Miyajima T, Saito K, Lin C, Hsieh S, Kawahara J, Sano H, Yokoyama M. Effects of eicosapentaenoic acid (epa) on cell membrane lipids, sodium transport and blood pressure in essential hypertension [Abstract]. *Am J Hypertens* 1993;6(Part 2):120A.

Missault L, Duprez D, de Buyzere M, de Backer G, Clement D. Decreased exercise capacity in mild essential hypertension: non-invasive indicators of limiting factors. *J Hum Hypertens* 1992;6:151–155.

Morris CD, McCarron DA. Effect of calcium supplementation in an older population with mildly increased blood pressure. *Am J Hypertens* 1992;5:230–237.

Morris MC, Sacks F, Rosner B. Does fish oil lower blood pressure? A meta-analysis of controlled trials. *Circulation* 1993; 88:523–533.

Motoyama T, Sano H, Fukuzaki H. Oral magnesium supplementation in patients with essential hypertension. *Hypertension* 1989;13:227–232.

Muntzel M, Drüeke T. A comprehensive review of the salt and blood pressure relationship. *Am J Hypertens* 1992;5:1S–42S.

Myers MG, Reeves RA. The effect of caffeine on daytime ambulatory blood pressure. *Am J Hypertens* 1991;4:427–431.

Nadel ER. Physiological adaptations to aerobic training. *American Scientist* 1985; 73:334–343.

Naraghi R, Gaab MR, Walter GF, Kleineberg B. Arterial hypertension and neurovascular compression at the ventrolateral medulla. *J Neurosurg* 1992;77:103–112.

National High Blood Pressure Education Program Working Group. National high blood pressure education program working group report on primary prevention of hypertension. *Arch Intern Med* 1993;153:186–208.

Neaton JD, Grimm RH Jr, Prineas RJ, Stamler J, Grandits GA, Elmer PJ, Cutler JA, Flack JM, Schoenberger JA, McDonald R, Lewis CE, Liebson PR. Treatment of mild hypertension study (TOMHS): final results. *JAMA* 1993;270:713–724.

Nemec ED, Mansfield L, Kennedy JW. Heart rate and blood pressure responses during sexual activity in normal males. *Am Heart J* 1976;92:274–277.

Niarchos AP, Weinstein DL, Laragh JH. Comparison of the effects of diuretic therapy and low sodium intake in isolated systolic hypertension. *Am J Med* 1984; 77:1061–1068.

Nilsson PM, Lindholm LH, Scherstén BF. Life style changes improve insulin resistance in hyperinsulinaemic subjects: a one-year intervention study of hypertensives and normotensives in Dalby. *J Hypertens* 1992;10:1071–1078.

Nowson CA, Morgan TO. Change in blood pressure in relation to change in nutrients effected by manipulation of dietary sodium and potassium. *Clin Exp Pharmacol Physiol* 1988;15:225–242.

Omvik P, Lund-Johansen P. Is sodium restriction effective treatment of borderline and mild essential hypertension? A long-term haemodynamic study at rest and during exercise. *J Hypertens* 1986;4:535–541.

Paffenbarger RS Jr, Hyde RT, Wing AL, Lee I-M, Jung DL, Kampert JB. The association of changes in physical-activity level and other lifestyle characteristics with mortality among men. *N Engl J Med* 1993; 328:538–545.

Paffenbarger RS Jr, Wing AL, Hyde RT, Jung DL. Physical activity and incidence of hypertension in college alumni. *Am J Epidemiol* 1983;117:245–257.

Paolisso G, Di Maro G, Cozzolino D, Salvatore T, D'Amore A, Lama D, Varricchio M, D'Onofrio F. Chronic magnesium administration enhances oxidative glucose metabolism in thiazide treated hypertensive patients. *Am J Hypertens* 1992; 5:681–686.

Parillo M, Coulston A, Hollenbeck C, Reaven G. Effect of a low fat diet on carbohydrate metabolism in patients with hypertension. *Hypertension* 1988;11:244–248.

Patel C, Marmot M. Can general practitioners use training in relaxation and management of stress to reduce mild hypertension? *Br Med J* 1988;296:21–24.

Patki PS, Singh J, Gokhale SV, Bulakh PM, Shrotri DS, Patwardhan B. Efficacy of potassium and magnesium in essential hypertension: a double blind, placebo controlled, crossover study. *Br Med J* 1990;301: 521–523.

Peleg I, McGowan JE, McNagny SE. Dietary calcium supplementation increases the risk of urinary tract infection [Abstract]. *Clin Res* 1992;40:562A.

Perez-Gonzalez JF. Factors determining the blood pressure responses to isometric exercise. *Circ Res* 1981;48(Suppl 1):76–86.

Pescatello LS, Fargo AE, Leach CN Jr, Scherzer HH. Short-term effect of dynamic exercise on arterial blood pressure. *Circulation* 1991;83:1557–1561.

Phillips A, Shaper AG. Relative weight and major ischaemic heart disease events in hypertensive men. *Lancet* 1989;1: 1005–1008.

Pincomb GA, Wilson MF, Sung BH, Passey RB, Lovallo WR. Effects of caffeine on pressor regulation during rest and exercise in men at risk for hypertension. *Am Heart J* 1991;122:1107–1115.

Prescott SL, Jenner DA, Beilin LJ, Margetts BM, Vandongen R. A randomized controlled trial of the effect on blood pressure of dietary non-meat protein versus meat protein in normotensive omnivores. *Clin Sci* 1988;74:665–672.

Preuss HG, Knapka JJ, MacArthy P, Yousufi AK, Sabnis SG, Antonovych TT. High sucrose diets increase blood pressure of both salt-sensitive and salt-resistant rats. *Am J Hypertens* 1992;5:585–591.

Prineas RJ. Clinical interaction of salt and weight change on blood pressure level. *Hypertension* 1991;17(Suppl 1):143–149.

Puddey IB, Parker M, Beilin LJ, Vandongen R, Masarei JRL. Effects of alcohol and caloric restrictions on blood pressure and serum lipids in overweight men. *Hypertension* 1992;20:533–541.

Radaelli A, Piepoli M, Adamopoulos S, Pipilis A, Clark SJ, Casadei B, Meyer TE, Coats AJS. Effects of mild physical activity, atenolol and the combination on ambulatory blood pressure in hypertensive subjects. *J Hypertens* 1992;10:1279–1282.

Ram CVS, Garrett BN, Kaplan NM. Moderate sodium restriction and various diuretics in the treatment of hypertension. Effects of potassium wastage and blood pressure control. *Arch Intern Med* 1981;141: 1015–1019.

Reaven PD, Barrett-Connor E, Edelstein S. Relation between leisure-time physical activity and blood pressure in older women. *Circulation* 1991;83:559–565.

Reed D, McGee D, Yano K, Hankin J. Diet, blood pressure, and multicollinearity. *Hypertension* 1985;7:405–410.

Resnick LM. Calcium metabolism in the pathophysiology and treatment of clinical hypertension. *Am J Hypertens* 1989;2: 179s–185s.

Rocchini AP, Key J, Bondie D, Chico R, Moorehead C, Katch V, Martin M. The effect of weight loss on the sensitivity of blood pressure to sodium in obese adolescents. *N Engl J Med* 1989;321:580–585.

Rosengren A, Wilhelmsen L, Wedel H. Coronary heart disease, cancer and mortality in male middle-aged light smokers. *J Intern Med* 1992;231:357–362.

Rubinstein I, Yong T, Rennard SI, Mayhan WG. Cigarette smoke extract attenuates endothelium-dependent arteriolar dilation in vivo. *Am J Physiol* 1991;261: H1913–H1918.

Ruppert M, Diehl J, Kolloch R, Overlack A, Kraft K, Göbel B, Hittel N, Stumpe KO. Short-term dietary sodium restriction increases serum lipids and insulin in salt-sensitive and salt-resistant normotensive adults. *Klin Wochenschr* 1991;69(Suppl 25):51–57.

Sacks FM. Dietary fats and blood pressure: a critical review of the evidence. *Nutr Rev* 1989;47:291–300.

Scherrer U, Nussberger J, Torriani S, Waeber B, Darioli R, Hofstetter J-R, Brunner HR. Effect of weight reduction in moderately overweight patients on recorded ambulatory blood pressure and free cytosolic platelet calcium. *Circulation* 1991; 83:552–558.

Schiffman SS. Taste and smell in disease. *N Engl J Med* 1983;308:1337–1342.

Schotte DE, Stunkard AJ. The effects of weight reduction on blood pressure in 301 obese patients. *Arch Intern Med* 1990; 150:1701–1704.

Sciarrone SEG, Strahan MT, Beilin LJ, Burke V, Rogers P, Rouse IR. Ambulatory blood pressure and heart rate responses to vegetarian meals. *J Hypertens* 1993; 11:277–285.

Sever P, Beevers G, Bulpitt C, Lever A, Ramsay L, Reid J, Swales J. Management guidelines in essential hypertension: report of the second working party of the British hypertension society. *Br Med J* 1993; 306:983–987.

Shaper AG, Wannamethee G, Whincup P. Alcohol and blood pressure in middle-aged British men. *J Hum Hypertens* 1988; 2:71–78.

Sharp DS, Benowitz NL. Pharmacoepidemiology of the effect of caffeine on blood pressure. *Clin Pharmacol Ther* 1990; 47:57–60.

Shinton R, Beevers G. Meta-analysis of relation between cigarette smoking and stroke. *Br Med J* 1989;298:789–794.

Shinton RA, Dodson PM, Beevers DG. Hypertension and dietary fat. *J Hum Hypertens* 1989;3:73–78.

Siani A, Strazzullo P, Giacco A, Pacioni D, Celentano E, Mancini M. Increasing the dietary potassium intake reduces the need for antihypertensive medication. *Ann Intern Med* 1991;115:753–759.

Silagy C, Muir J, Coulter A, Thorogood M, Yudkin P, Roe L. Lifestyle advice in general practice: rates recalled by patients. *Br Med J* 1992;305:871–874.

Silverstone T. Appetite suppressants. *Drugs* 1992;43:820–836.

Singer P, Jaeger W, Berger I, Barleben H, Wirth M, Richter-Heinrich E, Voigt S, Gödicke W. Effects of dietary oleic, linoleic and -linolenic acids on blood pressure, serum lipids, lipoproteins and the formation of eicosanoid precursors in patients with mild essential hypertension. *J Hum Hypertens* 1990;4:227–233.

Singer P, Jaeger W, Wirth M, Voigt S, Naumann E, Zimontkowski S, Hajdu I, Goedicke W. Lipid and blood pressure-lowering effect of mackerel diet in man. *Atherosclerosis* 1983;49:99–108.

Singer DRJ, Markandu ND, Sugden AL, Miller MA, MacGregor GA. Sodium restriction in hypertensive patients treated with a converting enzyme inhibitor and a thiazide. *Hypertension* 1991;17:798–803.

Smith SJ, Markandu ND, Sagnella GA, MacGregor GA. Moderate potassium chloride supplementation in essential hypertension: is it additive to moderate sodium restriction? *Br Med J* 1985;290:110–113.

Somers VK, Conway J, Johnston J, Sleight P. Effects of endurance training on baroreflex sensitivity and blood pressure in borderline hypertension. *Lancet* 1991;337: 1363–1368.

Staessen J, Bulpitt CJ, Fagard R, Joossens JV, Lijnen P, Amery A. Salt intake and blood pressure in the general population: A controlled intervention trial in two towns. *J Hypertens* 1988;6:965–973.

Staessen J, Fagard R, Lijnen P, Amery A. Body weight, sodium intake and blood pressure. *J Hypertens* 1989;7(Suppl 1):19–23.

Stamler J, Stamler R, Neaton JD. Blood pressure, systolic and diastolic, and cardiovascular risks. U.S. population data. *Arch Intern Med* 1993;153:598–615.

Stamler R. Implications of the INTERSALT study. *Hypertension* 1991;17(Suppl 1): 16–20.

Stamler R, Ford CE, Stamler J. Why do lean hypertensives have higher mortality rates than other hypertensives? Findings of the Hypertension Detection and Follow-Up Program. *Hypertension* 1991;17:553–564.

Stamler R, Stamler J, Gosch FC, Civinelli J, Fishman J, McKeever P, McDonald A, Dyer AR. Primary prevention of hypertension by nutritional-hygienic means. Final report of a randomized, controlled trial. *JAMA* 1989;262:1801–1807.

Stewart KJ. Weight training in coronary artery disease and hypertension. *Prog Cardiovasc Dis* 1992;35:159–168.

Sullivan JM. Salt sensitivity. Definition, conception, methodology, and long-term issues. *Hypertension* 1991;17(Suppl 1):61–68.

Sunman W, Hughes AD, Sever PS. Free-radical scavengers, thiol-containing reagents and endothelium-dependent relaxation in isolated rat and human resistance arteries. *Clin Sci* 1993;84:287–295.

Swain JF, Rouse IL, Curley CB, Sacks FM. Comparison of the effects of oat bran and low-fiber wheat on serum lipoprotein levels and blood pressure. *N Engl J Med* 1990;322:147–152.

Swales JD. Dietary salt and blood pressure: the role of meta-analyses. *J Hypertens* 1991;9(Suppl 6):42–46.

Sullivan JM. Salt sensitivity. Definition, conception, methodology, and long-term issues. *Hypertension* 1991;17(Suppl 1): 61–68.

Tam K-Ch, Yiu H-H. The effect of acupuncture on essential hypertension. *Am J Chinese Med* 1975;3:369–375.

Thorpe JJ, Welch WJ, Poindexter CA. Bilateral thoracolumbar sympathectomy for hypertension. *Am J Med* 1950;9:500–515.

Tobian L, Sugimoto T, Everson T. High K diets protect arteries, possibly by lowering renal papillary Na and thereby increasing interstitial cell secretion [Abstract]. *Hypertension* 1992;20:403.

Trials of Hypertension Prevention Collaborative Research Group. The effects of nonpharmacologic interventions on blood pressure of persons with high normal levels. Results of the Trials of Hypertension Prevention, Phase I. *JAMA* 1992; 267:1213–1220.

Ueshima H, Mikawa K, Baba S, Sasaki S, Ozawa H, Tsushima M, Kawaguchi A, Omae T, Katayama Y, Kayamori Y, Ito K. Effect of reduced alcohol consumption on blood pressure in untreated hypertensive men. *Hypertension* 1993;21:248–252.

US Public Health Service Cooperative Study. Evaluation of antihypertensive therapy. II. Double-blind controlled evaluation of mebutamate. *JAMA* 1965;193:103–105.

van Dusseldorp M, Smits P, Lenders JWM, Temme L, Thien T, Katan MB. Effects of coffee on cardiovascular responses to stress: a 14-week controlled trial. *Psychosom Med* 1992;54:344–353.

Vanhees L, Fagard R, Lijnen P, Amery A. Effect of antihypertensive medication on endurance exercise capacity in hypertensive sportsmen. *J Hypertens* 1991; 9:1063–1068.

van Montfrans GA, Karemaker JM, Wieling W, Dunning AJ. Relaxation therapy and continuous ambulatory blood pressure in mild hypertension: a controlled study. *Br Med J* 1990;300:1368–1372.

Veterans Administration Cooperative Study Group on Antihypertensive Agents. Urinary and serum electrolytes in untreated black and white hypertensives. *J Chron Dis* 1987;40:839–847.

Volini IF, Flaxman N. the effect of nonspecific operations on essential hypertension. *JAMA* 1939;112:2126–2128.

Volpe M, Camargo MJF, Mueller FB, Campbell WG Jr, Sealey JE, Pecker MS, Sosa RE, Laragh JH. Relation of plasma renin to end organ damage and to protection of K+ feeding in stroke-prone hypertensive rats. *Hypertension* 1990;15:318–326.

Wadden TA, Foster GD, Letizia KA, Stunkard AJ. A multicenter evaluation of a proprietary weight reduction program for the treatment of marked obesity. *Arch Intern Med* 1992;152:961–966.

Warren SE, O'Connor DT. The antihypertensive mechanism of sodium restriction. *J Cardiovasc Pharmacol* 1981;3:781–790.

Wasserman DH, Geer RJ, Rice DE, Bracy D, Flakoll PJ, Brown LL, Hill JO, Abumrad NN. Interaction of exercise and insulin action in humans. *Am J Physiol* 1991; 260:E37–E45.

Wassertheil-Smoller S, Oberman A, Blaufox MD, Davis B, Langford H. The Trial of Antihypertensive Interventions and Management (TAIM) Study. Final results with regard to blood pressure, cardiovascular risk, and quality of life. *Am J Hypertens* 1992;5:37–44.

Watkin DM, Froeb HF, Hatch FT, Gutman AB. Effects of diet in essential hypertension. II. Results with unmodified Kempner rice diet in fifty hospitalized patients. *Am J Med* 1950;9:441–491.

Weinberger MH, Fineberg NS. Sodium and volume sensitivity of blood pressure. Age and pressure change over time. *Hypertension* 1991;18:67–71.

Whang R, Whang DD, Ryan MP. Refractory potassium repletion. A consequence of magnesium deficiency. *Arch Intern Med* 1992;152:40–45.

Whelton PK, Klag MJ. Magnesium and blood pressure: review of the epidemiologic and clinical trial experience. *Am J Cardiol* 1989;63:26G–30G.

Widman L, Wester PO, Stegmayr BK, Wirell M. The dose-dependent reduction in blood pressure through administration of magnesium. *Am J Hypertens* 1993;6:41–45.

Wiley RL, Dunn CL, Cox RH, Hueppchen NA, Scott MS. Isometric exercise training lowers resting blood pressure. *Med Sci Sports Exerc* 1992;24:749–754

Williams GH, Hollenberg NK. Non-modulating hypertension. A subset of sodium-sensitive hypertension. *Hypertension* 1991;17(Suppl 1):81–85.

Winer BM. The antihypertensive mechanism of salt depletion induced by hydrochlorothiazide. *Circulation* 1961;24:788–796.

Witteman JCM, Grobbee DE, Derkx FHM, Bouillon R, de Bruijn AM, Hofman A. Reduction of blood pressure with oral magnesium supplementation in women with mild to moderate hypertension [Abstract]. *Circulation* 1992;86(Suppl 1):672.

Witteman JCM, Willett WC, Stampfer MJ, Colditz GA, Sacks FM, Speizer FE, Rosner B, Hennekens CH. A prospective study of nutritional factors and hypertension among US women. *Circulation* 1989; 80:1320–1327.

Wong ND, Ming S, Hong-Yan Z, Black HR. A comparison of Chinese traditional and Western medical approaches for the treatment of mild hypertension. *Yale J Biol Med* 1991;64:79–87.

World Hypertension League. Alcohol and hypertension—Implications for management. *J Hum Hypertens* 1991a;5:227–232.

World Hypertension League. Nonpharmacological interventions as an adjunct to the pharmacological treatment of hypertension: a statement by WHL. *J Hum Hypertens* 1993;7:159–164.

World Hypertension League. Physical exercise in the management of hypertension. *J Hypertens* 1991b;9:283–287.

Young DB, McCabe RD. Potassium's vascular protective mechanisms: inhibition of free radical formation, platlet aggregation and smooth muscle proliferation [Abstract]. *Hypertension* 1992;20:429.

7 Treatment of Hypertension: Drug Therapy

In the previous two chapters, I reviewed the evidence for the need for blood pressure (BP) reduction and the use of lifestyle modifications to lower the pressure. This chapter first provides general guidelines for the drug treatment of hypertension with emphasis on achieving adherence to therapy. Then each drug currently available is described. An analysis of initial drug choice and of the subsequent order of additional therapy follows, along with considerations of the management of special populations and of hypertensives with various other conditions.

GENERAL GUIDELINES

Since the treatment of hypertension is now the leading indication for the use of drugs in the United States (Schappert, 1993), new agents constantly are being introduced and heavily promoted. Although the results of major clinical trials do influence medical practice (Lamas et al., 1992), therapeutic choices often are based on promotional activities that are biased (Kessler, 1991). In this chapter, I constantly attempt to maintain an objective view, both about the use of drugs overall and about the relative value of individual agents. Although specific choices are favored often, the coverage in this chapter is based on scientifically valid data to allow individual clinicians the opportunity to develop their own approach.

Comparisons Between Drugs: Efficacy

Group Trials

The individual practitioner's choice of drug is often based on perceived differences in efficacy and the likelihood of side effects. In fact, efficacy varies little between the various available drugs; in order to gain Food and Drug Administration (FDA) approval for marketing in the United States, the drug must have been shown to be effective in reducing the BP in a large portion of the 1500 or more patients given the drug during its clinical investigation. Moreover, the dose and formulation of drug are chosen so as not to lower the pressure too much or too fast to avoid hypotensive side effects. Virtually all oral drugs are designed to do the same thing: lower the pressure at least 10% in the majority of patients with mild to moderate hypertension (Herxheimer, 1991).

Not only must each new drug be shown to be effective in large numbers of hypertensive patients, but also the drug must have been tested against currently available agents to show at least equal efficacy. When comparisons between various drugs are made, they almost always come out very close to one another. The best such comparison was performed in the Treatment of Mild Hypertension Study (TOMHS), designed as a pilot for a much larger and longer trial comparing the effects of a representative of all five major classes of drugs on morbidity and mortality (Treatment of Mild Hypertension Research Group, 1991; Neaton et al., 1993). The study involved random allocation of five drugs (chlorthalidone, acebutolol, doxazosin, amlodipine, enalapril), each given to almost 200 mild hypertensives, while another group took a placebo and all patients remained on a nutritional-hygienic program. The overall antihypertensive efficacy of the five drugs over 5 years was virtually equal (Neaton et al., 1993).

Despite the fairly equal overall efficacy of various antihypertensive drugs, individual patients may vary considerably in their response to different drugs. Some of this variability can be accounted for by patient characteristics, including age and race. This was seen in a Veterans Administration (VA) cooperative 1-year trial in which 1292 men were randomly given one of six drugs from each major class: overall and in the black patients, the calcium blocker was most effective, but the angiotensin-converting enzyme (ACE) inhibitor was best in younger whites, and the beta blocker was best in older whites (Materson et al., 1993).

Individual Patient Trials

Since individual patients do vary in their response, individual patient randomized clinical trials, referred to as "n of 1" (Guyatt et al., 1990), have been proposed to ascertain the best drug for each patient. The idea is simple: the patient undergoes successive treatment periods, each providing an active drug and a matched placebo assigned at random with both the patient and the physician blinded to the choice, which is made by the pharmacist. The process can go on as long as needed until an effective and well-tolerated agent is found for each individual patient.

Although the concept is simple, I doubt whether many practitioners (or their patients) will go to that much trouble. Fortunately, the physician can make a fairly exact ascertainment, if not of the "best" drug, certainly of an effective and well-tolerated one. This simply requires an open mind, a willingness to try one drug after another (each chosen from the major classes of available antihypertensive agents with careful monitoring of the patient, preferably by using home BP readings), and a thorough ascertainment of side effects (Brunner et al., 1990). This approach—the individualized choice of therapy with substitution for drugs found to be ineffec-

tual or bothersome—is preferable to the rigid "diuretic-first step-care" approach widely practiced in the past. More about this will follow the description of the various choices now available.

Prediction of Response

In the future, it may be possible to determine a patient's response to long-term therapy by short-term concentration-effect analysis measuring the falls in BP after the first dose, corrected for previously determined placebo effects, in relation to repetitive measurements of plasma drug concentration (Donnelley et al., 1992). The analysis, although not practical now for routine use, "has potential application in clinical practice as a means of quickly identifying poor or non-responders and for determining individual dose requirements for optimum long-term BP control" (Donnelley et al., 1992).

Dose-Response Relationships

Avoiding Overdosing

Beyond the individual variabilities in response to drugs, there is a more generalized problem with the use of antihypertensive agents: they often are prescribed in doses that are too high (Kaplan, 1992). The problem of overdosing has been obvious with virtually every new drug introduced, wherein the initial recommended doses have been gradually reduced because, after widespread clinical experience, they proved to be too high. Whereas 100 to 200 mg of hydrochlorothiazide were initially used, 12.5 mg is now recognized as enough for many patients. The initial recommended daily dose of captopril was up to 600 mg; now 50 to 100 mg is usually prescribed.

The problem arises in the preapproval testing of new drugs, as described by Andrew Herxheimer (1991):

For a new drug to penetrate the market quickly, it should be rapidly effective in a high proportion of patients and simple to use. To achieve this, the dosage of the first prescription is therefore commonly set at about the ED_{90} level—i.e., the dose which the early clinical (phase II) studies have shown to be effective in 90% of the target population, provided that the unwanted effects at this dose are considered acceptable. In 25% of patients a smaller, perhaps much smaller, dose (the ED_{25}) will be effective. The patients in this quartile are the most sensitive to the drug and are liable to receive far more than they need if they are given the ED_{90}. They are also likely to be more sensitive to the dose-related side-effects of the drug.

The problem is visualized in Figure 7.1, which shows the idealized dose-response curve (John-

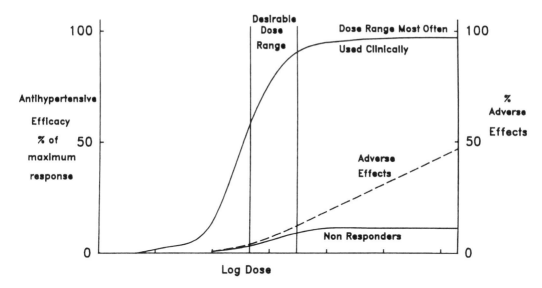

Figure 7.1. A stylized diagram of the relationship between the efficacy, adverse effects, and dose of an antihypertensive agent plotted on a logarithmic scale. (From Johnston GD. Dose-response relationships with antihypertensive drugs. *Pharmacol Ther* 1992;55:53–93.)

ston, 1992). Most doses used clinically are near or beyond the desirable dose range. Therefore, patients who are more responsive will receive excessive doses and thereby will be exposed to more adverse effects.

One solution to this problem is the marketing of tablets that contain less than the usual maximal effective dose. Practitioners must be willing to start patients with doses that will not be fully effective and to gradually titrate the dose to the desired response. As Herxheimer (1991) notes, ''The disadvantage from the marketing standpoint is that for the majority of patients the dose must be titrated. That is time-consuming for doctors and patients and more difficult to explain to them. A drug requiring dose titration cannot be presented as the quick fix, the instant good news that marketing departments love.''

The Need to Lower the Pressure Gradually

The ''quick fix'' is inappropriate for most patients. The fall in pressure should be relatively small and gradual to allow for maintenance of blood flow to vital organs in keeping with what is known about the autoregulation of cerebral and coronary blood flow (Strandgaard and Haunso, 1987) (Fig. 7.2). Normally, cerebral blood flow (CBF) remains relatively constant at about 50 ml/minute/100 g of brain (Strandgaard and Paulson, 1989). When the systemic BP falls, the vessels dilate; when the pressure rises, the vessels constrict. The limits of cerebral autoreg-

ulation in normal people are between mean arterial pressures of about 60 and 120 mm Hg (e.g., 80/50 to 160/100).

In hypertensives without neurologic deficits, the CBF is not different from that found in normotensives. This constancy of the CBF reflects a shift in the range of autoregulation to the right to a range of mean pressure from about 100 to 180 mm Hg (e.g., 130/85 to 240/150) (Fig. 7.2). This shift maintains a normal CBF despite the higher pressure but makes the hypertensive vulnerable to cerebral ischemia when the pressure falls to a level that is well tolerated by normotensives.

Note that the lower limit of autoregulation capable of preserving CBF in hypertensive patients is at a mean BP around 110 mm Hg. Thus, acutely lowering the pressure from 160/ 100 (mean = 127) to 140/85 (mean = 102) may induce cerebral hypoperfusion, although hypotension in the usual sense has not been induced. This likely explains why many patients experience manifestations of cerebral hypoperfusion (weakness, easy fatigability, and postural dizziness) at the start of antihypertensive therapy, even though BP levels do not seem inordinately low.

Fortunately, with effective control of the BP by medication, the curve drifts back toward normal, explaining the eventual ability of hypertensive patients to tolerate falls in pressure to levels that initially produced symptoms of cerebral

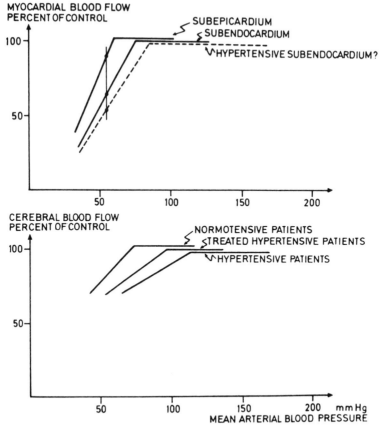

Figure 7.2. Autoregulation of myocardial (*above*) and cerebral (*below*) blood flow. Mean myocardial blood flow autoregulation curves are shown for subepicardium and corresponding subendocardial layers of the left ventricle in canine hearts. The autoregulatory curve of subendocardial blood flow in hypertensive hearts is suggested. During low arterial pressure (*vertical line*), when autoregulation is exhausted in both myocardial layers, subendocardial blood flow is lower than in the more superficial layers of the left ventricle. Mean cerebral blood flow autoregulation curves from normotensive, severely hypertensive, and effectively treated hypertensive patients are shown. (From Strandgaard S, Haunsø S. Why does antihypertensive treatment prevent stroke but not myocardial infarction? *Lancet* 1987;2:658–661.)

ischemia. Not all patients show a readaptation toward normal; presumably their structural changes are not reversible. Thus, older patients with more cerebral atherosclerosis may remain susceptible to cerebral ischemia when their BP is lowered even gently (Jansen et al., 1986).

The coronary circulation, particularly in those with extensive atherosclerosis, may also autoregulate very poorly, and patients with preexisting coronary artery disease may be particularly prone to subendocardial ischemia as their BP is lowered (Strandgaard and Haunsø, 1987; Cruickshank, 1988). Since the hypertrophied myocardium often found in chronic hypertensives can extract little additional oxygen beyond what is removed under normal conditions, the vulnerability of patients to myocardial ischemia when their BP is lowered below the critical level

needed to maintain adequate perfusion is easily understood (Polese et al., 1991) (see Chapter 5).

The Need for 24-Hour Coverage

As noted in Chapter 2, self-recorded measurements (Ménard et al., 1988) and ambulatory automatic BP monitoring (White, 1989) are being increasingly used to ensure the 24-hour duration of action of antihypertensive agents. This is particularly critical with the increasing use of once-a-day medications that often do not provide 24-hour efficacy (Neutel et al., 1990; Donnelley et al., 1992). Thereby, the patient is exposed to the full impact of the early morning abrupt rise in pressure that is almost certainly involved in the increased incidence of various cardiovascular events immediately after arising.

Although ambulatory monitoring is not available for most patients, self-recorded measurements with inexpensive semiautomatic devices should be possible for most, thereby assuring the adequacy of control throughout the waking hours—particularly the early morning hours. Caution is advised against having patients take their medication late in the evening or before retiring, since virtually every formulation has its maximal effect within 3 to 4 hours and, as noted in Chapter 2, BP usually falls considerably for the first 5 to 6 hours of sleep. Hypotension and tissue ischemia could thereby be induced (Mancia, 1993). In the future, formulations may become available that release the medication only after a 4- to 6-hour interval, so bed-time dosing would be appropriate. For now, if patients awake because of nocturia, some 2 or 3 hours before rising for the day, they can be instructed to take their medication at that time.

Comparisons Between Drugs: Side Effects

As to the issue of differences in side effects between different agents, two points are obvious: first, no drug that causes dangerous side effects beyond a rare idiosyncratic reaction when given in usual doses will remain on the market even if it slips by the approval process, as witnessed by the uricosuric diuretic ticrynafen; second, drugs that cause frequent bothersome though not dangerous side effects, such as guanethidine, will likely no longer be used now that so many other choices are available.

The various antihypertensive agents vary significantly, both in the frequency of side effects and, to an even greater degree, in their nature. The only currently available comparisons of a representative drug from all major classes given as monotherapy to sizeable numbers of patients are the Treatment of Mild Hypertension Study (Neaton et al., 1993) and the VA Cooperative Study (Materson et al., 1993). Side effects differed between the drugs, but no one drug was markedly more or less acceptable than the others.

Over the past 20 years, a number of studies have examined the side effects of antihypertensive agents on the quality of life (QOL) (Guyatt et al., 1993). Only nine of those published through 1991 met the criteria of comparing active treatment to baseline measures with the patients as their own control in blinded, randomized trials, but these involved 1620 patients in 27 groups using 14 drugs from 6 of the 7 major classes (Beto and Bansal, 1992). Beto and Bansal's meta-analysis assessed the effects of drugs

on five specific QOL measures: sexual function, sleep, psychomotor abilities, mood, and general well-being. The overall effect size, computed for each study by dividing the mean change between baseline and treatment by the average of the standard deviations, was found in all nine studies to be significantly positive for all measures except sexual function (Fig. 7.3) and differed little between the six types of drugs.

These results confirm the general impression: although 10% to 20% of patients will experience bothersome side effects from virtually any and every antihypertensive drug, the overall impact of therapies upon QOL over 2 to 6 months of observation is positive (Croog et al., 1990; Fletcher et al., 1992). However, different drugs do have different profiles of side effects, and only by such thorough and carefully constructed questionnaires can subtle differences be detected, particularly those involving mood and psychologic functioning (Dimsdale, 1992). For instance, equipotent doses of two ACE inhibitors induced different effects on QOL: captopril, positive; enalapril, negative (Testa et al., 1993).

The Problem of Noncompliance

Interference with the QOL by therapy surely is one factor responsible for the fact that fewer than half of hypertensives put on treatment have their pressure well controlled (Joint National Committee, 1993). Multiple other factors are also involved (Table 7.1).

Patient and Disease Characteristics

Hypertensives have special problems related to the nature of their disease. Many are largely unaware of the definition, possible causes, sequelae, and therapeutic needs of hypertension. Being asymptomatic, patients have little motivation to seek or follow treatment. Many are found to have high BP at the age (late 30s and early 40s) when the threat of a loss of vigor and vitality is insidiously beginning, and the recognition of hypertension often provokes a strong denial reaction (McClellan et al., 1988). Moreover, the diagnosis carries considerable economic and social threats—loss of job, insurance, and sexual potency—that may further inhibit people from accepting the diagnosis and dealing with the problem.

Treatment Characteristics

The therapy of hypertension has all the wrong characteristics for compliance, and these are often compounded by clinical practices such as

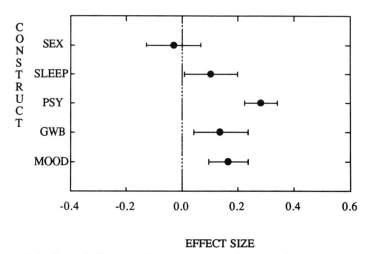

EFFECT SIZE

Figure 7.3. Meta-analysis of overall effects of antihypertensive drug therapy on five measures (constructs) of quality of life, showing generally positive effects. *Sex*, sexual function; *Psy*, psychomotor; *GWB*, general well-being. (From Beto JA, Bansal VK. Quality of life in treatment of hypertension. A metaanalysis of clinical trials. *Am J Hypertens* 1992;5:125–133.)

Table 7.1. Factors That Reduce Compliance to Therapy

Patient and disease characteristics
Asymptomatic
Chronic condition
Condition suppressed, not cured
No immediate consequences of stopping
 therapy
Social isolation
Disrupted home situation
Psychiatric illness

Treatment characteristics
Long duration of therapy
Complicated regimens
Expensive medications
Side effects of medications
Multiple behavioral modifications
Lack of specific appointment times
Long waiting time in office

the use of multiple daily doses of medications (Eisen et al., 1990). Side effects discourage compliance, and side effects are common. As with impotence in the use of diuretics, the symptoms that follow institution of drug therapy may not be expected from the known pharmacologic effects of the drug. As noted earlier, subtle effects on mood and psychologic functioning may develop (Dimsdale, 1992), which can only be identified by careful assessments.

Assessment of Compliance

Unfortunately, most physicians, though confident that they can predict the compliance of their patients with therapy, make predictions no more accurate than can be obtained by the toss of a coin (Stephenson et al., 1993). Although there are multiple ways to assess patients' compliance, none has been found to be particularly accurate (Pullar, 1991). More sophisticated techniques, such as electronic medication monitors (Rudd et al., 1992), are being developed but are not currently feasible in clinical practice.

Ways to Improve Compliance

Haynes (1983) summarized the situation by saying that "the two outstanding features of most successful compliance interventions [are] the level of supervision of, or attention paid to, the patient and the extent to which compliance is reinforced, rewarded or encouraged." Guidelines to improve patient compliance are given in Table 7.2. A few of these deserve more emphasis.

Educate and Maintain Contact with the Patient. Information about medications, when written in simple language and attractively presented, is useful (Baker et al., 1991). Broken appointments to clinics have been reduced by mail, telephone, and physician reminders (Macharia et al., 1992).

Keep Care Inexpensive and Simple. The minimum effective doses should be prescribed, generic brands should be used (Neal, 1989), and larger doses of tablets should be broken in half with readily available pill cutters. Fortunately, more and more once-a-day formulations are available so that fewer tablets are needed.

The use of less expensive medications is being emphasized in an attempt to reduce the costs of health care and to ensure that the indigent are not denied needed medications whenever there is no safety net in place to assure care for the poor. Although the indigent can often be provided medications through pharmaceutical company programs (Dustan et al., 1992), the cost of therapy remains a barrier to the management of hypertension (Shulman et al., 1991). On the other hand, simplistic comparisons of costs based purely on the costs per tablet (Hebert et al., 1993) are misleading. For example, a generic thiazide diuretic that costs 5 cents a tablet ends up costing, on average, 30 cents a day; the additional 25 cents arises from the need (in one-third of diuretic-treated patients) for supplemental potassium, which costs 75 cents a day. The need for additional laboratory testing to recognize hypokalemia, hypercholesterolemia, and similar conditions largely removes any real savings between a diuretic and many other agents (Hilleman et al., 1993).

SPECIFICS ABOUT ANTIHYPERTENSIVE DRUGS

The modern era of antihypertensive therapy began only a little over 40 years ago with the pioneering work of Ed Freis in the United States (Freis, 1990b) and Sir Horace Smirk in New Zealand (Doyle, 1991). The remainder of this chapter will examine the large panoply of drugs that have been developed since then. Some that are used extensively elsewhere but that are not now available in the United States will also be covered, along with newer agents that are on the horizon. Drugs that have outlived their usefulness will be disregarded.

We will consider the drugs in the order shown in Table 7.3. It is of interest to notice the changes in their relative frequency of use in the United States from 1986 through 1992 (Fig. 7.4). Diuretics remain the most popular, but their use is falling; beta-blockers were the second most popular, but their use, too, is diminishing, whereas the newer classes—ACE inhibitors and calcium entry blockers—are rising rapidly. The

---

Table 7.2. General Guidelines to Improve Patient Adherence to Antihypertensive Therapy

- Be aware of the problem and be alert to signs of patient nonadherence.
- Establish the goal of therapy: to reduce blood pressure to near normotensive levels with minimal or no side effects.
- Educate the patient about the disease and its treatment.
    - Involve the patient in decision making.
    - Encourage family support.
- Maintain contact with the patient.
    - Encourage visits and calls to allied health personnel.
    - Allow the pharmacist to monitor therapy.
    - Give feedback to the patient via home BP readings.
    - Make contact with patients who do not return.
- Keep care inexpensive and simple.
    - Do the least work-up needed to rule out secondary causes.
    - Obtain follow-up laboratory data only yearly unless indicated more often.
    - Use home blood pressure readings.
    - Use nondrug, no-cost therapies.
    - Use the fewest daily doses of drugs needed.
    - Use generic drugs and break larger doses of tablets in half.
    - If appropriate, use combination tablets.
    - Tailor medication to daily routines.
- Prescribe according to pharmacologic principles.
    - Add one drug at a time.
    - Start with small doses, aiming for 5- to 10-mm Hg reductions at each step.
    - Have medication taken immediately upon awakening in the morning or after 4 A.M. if patient awakens to void.
    - Prevent volume overload with adequate diuretic and sodium restriction.
- Be willing to stop unsuccessful therapy and try a different approach.
- Anticipate side effects.
- Adjust therapy to ameliorate side effects that do not spontaneously disappear.
- Continue to add effective and tolerated drugs, stepwise, in sufficient doses to achieve the goal of therapy.

Table 7.3. Antihypertensive Drugs Available in the United States

Diuretics		Adrenergic Inhibitors		Vasodilators	
Thiazides	**Peripheral**	**Beta receptor**	**Direct**	**ACE inhibitors**	
Chlorthalidone	**inhibitors**	**blockers**	Hydralazine	Benazepril	
Indapamide	Guanadrel	Acebutolol	Minoxidil	Captopril	
Metolazone	Guanethidine	Atenolol		Enalapril	
Thiazides	Reserpine	Betaxolol	**Calcium blockers**	Fosinopril	
		Bisoprolol	Amlodipine	Lisinopril	
Loop diuretics	**Central alpha₂**	Carteolol	Diltiazem	Quinapril	
Bumetanide	**agonists**	Metoprolol	Felodipine	Ramipril	
Furosemide	Clonidine	Nadolol	Isradipine		
Torsemide	Guanabenz	Penbutolol	Nicardipine		
	Guanfacine	Pindolol	Nifedipine		
Potassium	Methyldopa	Propranolol	Verapamil		
sparers		Timolol			
Amiloride	**Alpha₁ receptor**				
Spironolactone	**blockers**	**Combined**			
Triamterene	Doxazosin	**alpha and**			
	Prazosin	**beta blocker**			
	Terazosin	Labetalol			

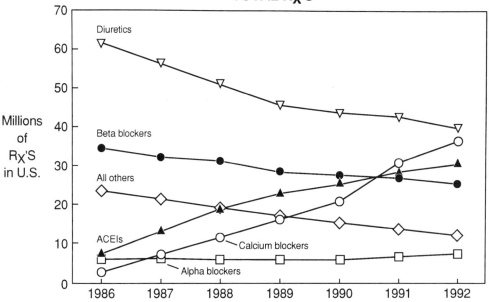

Figure 7.4. Numbers of prescriptions written for antihypertensive drugs in millions in the United States from 1986 to 1992 (National Prescription Audit. Ambler, Pennsylvania: IMS, 1993.)

reasons for these changes should become obvious in the remainder of this chapter.

After a description of some of the basic pharmacology and clinical usefulness of each agent, we will consider the choice of first and second drugs, the selection of specific drugs for various types of hypertensive patients, the use of combinations, and conditions wherein special care is advised in the choice of drugs. The use of drugs in various secondary forms of hypertension (e.g., ACE inhibitors in renovascular hypertension and spironolactone in primary aldosteronism) is considered in the respective chapters on these secondary states.

DIURETICS

Diuretics are still the drugs most frequently prescribed to treat hypertension, but their use has been decreasing over the past 5 years (Fig. 7.4). This trend may be reversed because of the recognition that, despite a variety of biochemical side effects, they and beta-blockers are the only classes of drugs that have been tested and shown to reduce overall cardiovascular morbidity and mortality (Joint National Committee, 1993).

As noted earlier, in a world increasingly concerned about the costs of health care, diuretics may also be advocated because, purely on the basis of cost per tablet, they are cheaper (Hebert et al., 1993). That simplistic view, though misleading (Hilleman et al., 1993), greatly attracts health care managers.

Classification

Diuretics differ in structure and major site of action within the nephron (Fig. 7.5). These differences determine their relative efficacy, as expressed in the maximal percentage of filtered sodium chloride excreted (Rose, 1991). Agents acting in the proximal tubule (Site I) are seldom used to treat hypertension. Treatment is usually initiated with a thiazide-type diuretic (acting at Site III). Chlorthalidone and indapamide are structurally different, though still related to the thiazides, and will be covered with them. If renal function is severely impaired (i.e., serum creatinine above 2.5 mg/dl), a loop diuretic (acting at Site II) or metolazone is needed. A potassium-sparing agent (acting at Site IV) may be given with the diuretic to reduce the likelihood of hypokalemia. By themselves, potassium-sparing agents are relatively weak antihypertensives.

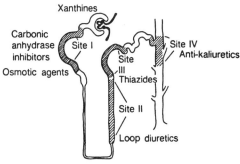

Figure 7.5. Diagrammatic representation of the nephron showing the four main tubular sites where diuretics interfere with sodium reabsorption. The main action of xanthines on the kidney is on vascular perfusion of the glomerulus, though some effect on sodium reabsorption at site I also is likely. (From Lant A. Diuretic drugs. Progress in clinical pharmacology. *Drugs* 1986;31[Suppl 4]:40–55.)

The specific agents now available in the United States are listed in Table 7.4. New diuretic agents such as mefruside and xipamide are being investigated, including at least one that does not increase urinary potassium loss (Kau et al., 1992).

Thiazide Diuretics

Mode of Action

The thiazide diuretics act by inhibiting sodium and chloride cotransport across the luminal membrane of the early segment of the distal convoluted tubule, where 5% to 8% of filtered sodium is normally reabsorbed (Rose, 1991) (Site III, Fig. 7.5). Plasma and extracellular fluid volume are thereby shrunken, and cardiac output falls (Wilson and Freis, 1959). Humoral and intrarenal counter-regulatory mechanisms rapidly reestablish the steady state so that sodium intake and excretion are balanced within 3 to 9 days in the presence of a decreased body fluid volume (Rose, 1991). With chronic use, plasma volume returns partially toward normal, but at the same time, peripheral resistance decreases (Conway and Lauwers, 1960) (Fig. 7.6).

Determinants of Response

A number of interrelated hemodynamic changes may influence the degree of BP reduction with continued diuretic therapy. Those who respond less well, with a fall in mean BP of less than 10%, were found to have a greater degree of plasma volume depletion and greater stimulation of renin and aldosterone, contributing to a persistently high peripheral resistance (van Brummelen et al., 1980). In those whose BP responds better, the renin levels may rise equally, but the responders may have a lesser response of aldosterone secretion to the same degree of renin-angiotensin stimulation (Weber et al., 1977). Blockage of the reactive rise in renin-angiotensin-aldosterone by addition of an ACE inhibitor will potentiate the antihypertensive action even though there is little additional fluid volume loss (van Schaik et al., 1987).

In addition, diuretics cause a modest rise in plasma norepinephrine levels (Lake et al., 1979). On the other hand, the fall in resistance could be secondary to activation of vasodepressor mechanisms: both plasma prostacyclin levels (Wilson, 1986) and urine kallikrein activity (O'Connor et al., 1981) are raised in those whose BP responds to diuretics. Moreover, inhibitors of prostaglandin synthesis will blunt the effect of most diuretics (Ellison, 1991).

Table 7.4. Diuretics and Potassium-Sparing Agents

	Daily Dosage (mg)	Duration of Action (hr)
Thiazides		
Bendroflumethiazide (Naturetin)	2.5–5.0	More than 18
Benzthiazide (Exna)	12.5–50	12–18
Chlorothiazide (Diuril)	125–500	6–12
Cyclothiazide (Anhydron)	0.5–2	18–24
Hydrochlorothiazide (Esidrix, HydroDIURIL, Oretic)	12.5–50	12–18
Hydroflumethiazide (Saluron, Diucardin)	12.5–50	18–24
Methyclothiazide (Enduron, Aquatensen)	2.5–5.0	More than 24
Polythiazide (Renese)	1–4	24–48
Trichlormethiazide (Metahydrin, Naqua)	1–4	24
Related sulfonamide compounds		
Chlorthalidone (Hygroton, Thalitone)	12.5–50	24–72
Indapamide (Lozol)	1.25–2.5	24
Metolazone (Zaroxolyn, Mykrox)	0.5–10	24
Quinethazone (Hydromox)	25–100	18–24
Loop diuretics		
Bumetanide (Bumex)	0.5–5	4–6
Ethacrynic acid (Edecrin)	25–100	12
Furosemide (Lasix)	20–480	4–6
Potassium-sparing agents		
Amiloride (Midamor)	5–10	24
Spironolactone (Aldactone)	25–100	8–12
Triamterene (Dyrenium)	50–150	12

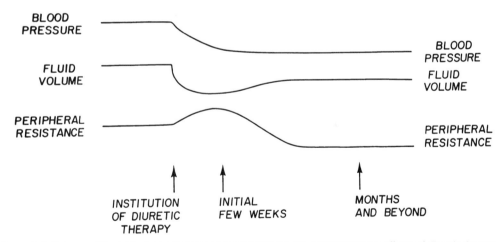

Figure 7.6. Scheme of the hemodynamic changes responsible for the antihypertensive effects of diuretic therapy.

Thiazide Congeners

Indapamide. Indapamide (Lozol) is also a chlorobenzene sulfonamide that differs in having a methylindoline moiety, which may provide additional antihypertensive actions beyond its diuretic effect by decreasing vascular reactivity and resistance (Campbell and Brackman, 1990). It is as effective in reducing the BP as are thia-zides and maintains a 24-hour effect (Ocon and Mora, 1990).

Unlike thiazides, the majority of studies show that it does not adversely alter blood lipids (Aubert et al., 1990). Moreover, it has antioxidant properties that have been shown to increase prostacyclin generation in vitro (Uehara et al., 1990) and inhibit the peroxidation of low-density lipoprotein (LDL) (Breugnot et al., 1992), effects that could translate into better cardiovascular protection than seen with other diuretics.

Metolazone. This long-acting and more potent quinazoline thiazide derivative maintains its effect in the presence of renal insufficiency (Paton and Kane, 1977). Small doses, 0.5 to 1.0 mg/day, of a new formulation (Mykrox) (Miller et al., 1988) may be equal to ordinary long-acting thiazide diuretics; the agent is particularly useful in patients with azotemia and resistant hypertension.

Efficacy

When used alone, thiazide diuretics provide efficacy similar to that of other classes of drugs (Neaton et al., 1993). Blacks and the elderly respond better to diuretics than do nonblacks and younger patients (Materson et al., 1993).

Diuretics potentiate the effect of all other antihypertensive agents including calcium entry blockers (Burris et al., 1990). This potentiation depends on the contraction of fluid volume by the diuretic (Finnerty et al., 1970) and the prevention of fluid accumulation that frequently follows the use of other antihypertensive drugs. Because of the altered pressure-natriuresis curve of essential hypertension (described in Chapter 3), whenever the BP is lowered, fluid retention is expected (Fig. 7.7). The need for a diuretic may be lessened with ACE inhibitors, which inhibit the renin-aldosterone mechanism, and calcium entry blockers, which have some intrinsic natriuretic activity.

Duration of Action

The times listed in Table 7.4 under "Duration of Action" relate to the diuretic effect. There are few data to document whether the antihypertensive effect lasts beyond the diuretic effect. In one study, 25 mg of hydrochlorothiazide (HCTZ) plus the potassium-sparer amiloride taken daily at 7:00 a.m. lowered ambulatory BP only a few millimeters for the next 10 hours and none at all for the remainder of the 24 hours (Otterstad et al., 1992). On the other hand, 25- and 50-mg doses of HCTZ once daily persistently reduced BP during the next 14 hours as measured by ambulatory monitoring and after 24 hours as measured in the office (Lacourciere and Provencher, 1989).

Dosage

Monotherapy. The recommended daily dose of thiazide diuretics has been progressively falling from as high as 200 mg of HCTZ or equivalent doses of other thiazides in the early 1960s (Cranston et al., 1963) to as little as 6.25 to 12.5 mg today.

In hypertensives with good renal function, most of the antihypertensive effect will be obtained from such small doses, with less hypokalemia and other side effects (Carlsen et al., 1990; Johnston et al., 1991). Carlsen et al. (1990) used bendrofluazide, which is somewhat longer acting than HCTZ and approximately 10 times more potent, milligram for milligram. The 1.25-mg dose (equivalent to 12.5 mg of HCTZ) provided an antihypertensive effect equal to that of

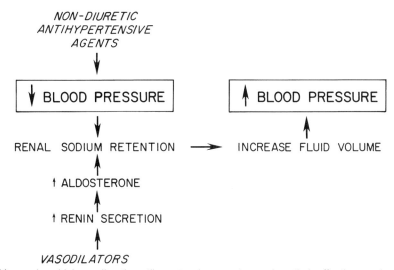

Figure 7.7. Manner by which nondiuretic antihypertensive agents may lose their effectiveness by reactive renal sodium retention.

the full 10-mg dose (equivalent to 100 mg of HCTZ). Johnston et al. (1991) found that 125 μg of cyclopenthiazide (equivalent to 10 mg of HCTZ) provided equally significant reductions in BP compared to 500 μg after 1 year. Less fall of serum potassium and no increases of serum urate or cholesterol were seen with the lower doses in both studies.

In the massive Systolic Hypertension in the Elderly Program (SHEP Cooperative Research Group, 1991), 12.5 mg of chlorthalidone was the starting dose and was adequate to bring the systolic pressures down to the goal in almost half of the subjects. Larger doses may provide some additional antihypertensive effect, but the degree is limited (i.e., the dose-response curve with thiazides is fairly flat). In the Medical Research Council (MRC) trials (Medical Research Council Working Party, 1987), 5.0 mg of bendrofluazide or 25 mg of HCTZ provided equal antihypertensive efficacy as did twice-larger doses. With chlorthalidone, 15 mg provided almost the same effect as 25 mg (Vardan et al., 1987).

Even though the average patient will have a good response to such small doses, some patients will require more, even up to 200 mg of HCTZ a day (Freis et al., 1988). In another study, 12.5 mg of HCTZ did not lower BP over a 4-week interval, but 25 mg did thereafter (Borghi et al., 1992). However, as shown by Carlsen et al. (1990), the full antihypertensive effect of low doses of diuretic may not become apparent in 4 weeks, so patience is advised when low doses are prescribed.

Combination Therapy

Even more convincing data confirm a significant effect from small doses, even below 12.5 mg/day of HCTZ, when diuretics are added to a variety of other drugs to enhance their antihypertensive efficacy (DeQuattro and Weir, 1993). MacGregor et al. (1983) and Dahlöf et al. (1988) reported that 12.5 mg of HCTZ provided an additional effect equivalent to 25 or 50 mg/day when added to 400 mg of acebutolol or 20 mg of enalapril, respectively. Andrén et al. (1983) found equivalent additive effects of 6.25, 12.5, and 25 mg of HCTZ added to 10 or 40 mg/day of enalapril. Again, not all agree: Magee and Freis (1986) found no effect of 12.5 mg of HCTZ added to 80 mg of the beta blocker nadolol; however, 25 mg did provide additional lowering of systolic pressure.

Conclusion. The overall evidence indicates that most hypertensives will respond over time to very small doses of thiazide diuretic (i.e., 12.5 to 25 mg of HCTZ), and that the relatively little additional effect that will be achieved by raising the daily dose beyond 50 mg/day comes at a high price in terms of side effects. Persons who are taking larger doses may be able to reduce the dose with no loss of antihypertensive efficacy but with improvement in biochemical abnormalities (Weisser and Ripka, 1992).

Resistant Patients

Resistance to the natriuretic and antihypertensive action of diuretics may occur for numerous reasons (Ellison, 1991):

—Excessive dietary sodium intake may overwhelm the diuretic's ability to maintain a shrunken fluid volume (Winer, 1961);
—For those with renal impairment (i.e., serum creatinine above 2.5 mg/dl or creatinine clearance below 30 ml/minute), thiazides likely will not work. Since these drugs must get into the renal tubules to work and since endogenous organic acids that build up in renal insufficiency compete with diuretics for transport into the proximal tubule, the renal response progressively falls with increasing renal damage (Brater, 1988) (see Chapter 9);
—Food affects the absorption and bioavailability of different diuretics to variable degrees (Neuvonen and Kivisto, 1989), so the drugs should be taken in a uniform pattern as to the time of day and food ingestion;
—Nonsteroidal anti-inflammatory drugs (NSAIDs) will blunt the effect of most diuretics (Pope et al., 1993), partly by their prevention of diuretic-induced changes in renal hemodynamics through their inhibition of prostaglandin synthesis (Ellison, 1991).

Relation to Renin Levels

As noted previously, the degree of BP response to diuretics is predicated on their capacity to activate the counter-regulatory defenses to a lower BP and a shrunken fluid volume—in particular, a reactive rise in renin levels. Those who start with low, suppressed plasma renin activity (PRA) levels and who are capable of mounting only a weak rise in these levels after diuretics are begun have been shown to be more "diuretic responsive" (Niarchos et al., 1984). As logical as this finding seems to be, some researchers find no relation between response to either HCTZ (Wyndham et al., 1987) or chlorthalidone (Salvetti et al., 1987) to either pretreatment PRA levels or their rise after therapy.

Side Effects (Fig. 7.8)

The likely pathogenesis for most of the more common complications related to diuretic use arise from the intrinsic activity of the drugs, and most are therefore related to the dose and duration of diuretic use. Logically, side effects occur with about the same frequency and severity with equipotent doses of all diuretics, and their occurrence will diminish with lower doses. In general, the longer the diuretic action, the more the various complications: more hypokalemia occurs when two doses of 50 mg of hydrochlorothiazide are given 12 hours apart than when a single does of 100 mg is given once a day (McInnes et al., 1982); hypokalemia was 3 times more common with the longer-acting chlorthalidone than with HCTZ in the Multiple Risk Factor Intervention Trial (MRFIT) (Grimm et al., 1985).

Hypokalemia. Urinary potassium wasting occurs with diuretics because they increase delivery of sodium and water to the distal nephron where high levels of aldosterone (stimulated by increased angiotensin II) increase potassium secretion (Nader et al., 1988).

Magnitude. In a review of published series, the fall in serum potassium with diuretic therapy of hypertension was found to average 0.67 mmol/L (Morgan and Davidson, 1980). The plasma contains less than 1% of total body potassium (TBK), most of the remainder being within cells. The majority of isotopic measurements of TBK in hypertensive patients receiving diuretics find only about a 200- to 300-mmol decrease, somewhat less than 10% of body stores, though almost all show a more significant fall in plasma K^+ (Nader et al., 1988).

Potassium loss may be partially compensated in time: both the degree of hypokalemia and the fall in TBK (Leemhuis et al., 1976) are lessened after a few months despite continued therapy. This may reflect a decrease in the secretion of potassium after the higher initial fluid flow rate down the nephron has caused more potassium to be swept into the urine (Wright, 1987), as well as a depression of distal nephron K^+ excretion and of aldosterone secretion by the lower serum K^+ levels.

Incidence. In various series, the percentage of diuretic-treated patients who develop hypokalemia varies from zero to as many as 40%, reflecting various factors that influence potassium wastage. More will be wasted the higher the dose of diuretic and the longer duration of

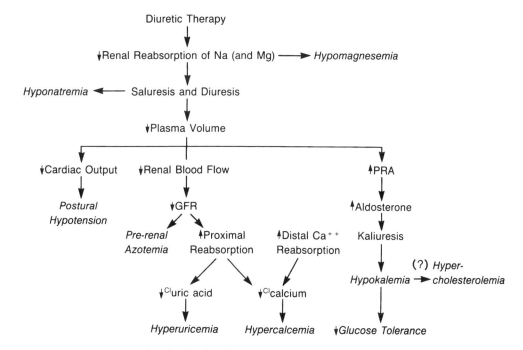

Figure 7.8. Mechanisms by which chronic diuretic therapy may lead to various complications. The mechanism for hypercholesterolemia remains in question, although it is shown as arising via hypokalemia. *GFR,* glomerular filtration rate.

its action, and the greater the intake of sodium (Ram et al., 1981). The elderly are more susceptible because of their lower total body potassium (Flynn et al., 1989).

Consequences. With relatively mild hypokalemia, muscle weakness, polyuria, and a propensity toward arrhythmias may appear. Patients on digitalis may develop toxicity (Packer, 1990), perhaps because both digitalis and hypokalemia inhibit the Na^+,K^+–ATPase pump, whose activity is essential to normal intracellular electrolyte balance and membrane potential (Nørgaard and Kjeldsen, 1991). Most of the overt hazards of diuretic-induced hypokalemia have been seen only with fairly marked K^+ depletion (Knochel, 1984).

Ventricular Arrhythmias and Stress. A controversy has arisen about whether diuretic-induced hypokalemia can give rise to ventricular ectopic activity (VEA) that, in turn, could incite fatal arrhythmias. As noted in Chapter 5, the controversy has been incited by the findings of higher rates of coronary mortality, mainly sudden death, in three major trials of the therapy of mild hypertension among patients who had abnormal electrocardiograms (ECGs) at entry to the trials and who were given high doses of diuretic. With diuretics, extracellular potassium concentration tends to fall more than intracellular levels do, thereby hyperpolarizing the cell membrane and leading to an increased threshold for excitation. Although this may reduce the likelihood of arrhythmias due to reentrant phenomena, it may lower the threshold for ventricular fibrillation by delaying conduction and prolonging the duration of the action potential (Hohnloser et al., 1986). This may develop most commonly in the presence of QT prolongation, which in turn can be induced by a number of drugs taken by hypertensives such as antiarrhythmics, phenothiazines, and probucol (Singh et al., 1992).

The problem may be greatest for hypertensives who undergo major stress, particularly if they have underlying left ventricular hypertrophy (LVH), which is associated with an increased frequency of complex ventricular arrhythmias (James and Jones, 1991). During stress, beta$_2$-receptor–mediated activation of the Na^+,K^+–ATPase pump causes potassium to enter cells. Blood potassium levels fall significantly within minutes of the infusion of just enough epinephrine to bring the plasma concentration to ''stress levels'' (Struthers et al., 1983) (Fig. 7.9).

Therefore, the presence of prior diuretic-induced hypokalemia will increase the likelihood of more severe hypokalemia appearing after stress or the use of beta$_2$-agonists (Lipworth et al., 1990). Prevention of such beta-receptor–mediated shifts of potassium could explain much of the protection against mortality in patients given nonselective beta blocker drugs after an acute myocardial infarction.

The issue has been examined by simply observing asymptomatic hypertensives before and after they are made hypokalemic with diuretics. The first study (Holland et al., 1981) gave strong evidence for increased VEA with diuretic-induced hypokalemia; subsequent studies have both confirmed (Siegel et al., 1992; Siscovick et al., 1993) and denied (Papademetriou et al., 1988) the association.

The issue is not settled. The arguments for (Singh et al., 1992) and against (Freis, 1990a) an association between diuretic-induced hypokalemia and VEA have been summarized. As Freis (1990a) argues, most of the studies showing an association can be faulted for various reasons. Nonetheless, the evidence, both circumstantial and direct, strongly suggests the need for caution. The prudent course is to prevent significant falls in serum potassium or, failing that, to correct hypokalemia (Nørgaard and Kjeldsen, 1991).

Effect on BP. Hypokalemia can set off various processes that can raise the BP (Linas et al., 1988), including a worsening of insulin resistance (Langford et al., 1990). Dietary potassium depletion has been found to raise the BP (Krishna et al., 1989), whereas the correction of diuretic-induced hypokalemia lowered the mean BP by an average of 5.5 mm Hg in a group of 16 hypertensives on a constant dose of diuretic (Kaplan et al., 1985).

Management of Diuretic-Induced Hypokalemia.

Prevention. Prevention is preferable. By lowering dietary sodium, increasing dietary potassium, and using the least amount of diuretic needed, potassium depletion may be avoided. A lower dietary sodium intake (72 mmol/day) reduced diuretic-induced K^+ loss by half of that observed on a higher sodium intake (195 mmol/day) (Ram et al., 1981). Fresh vegetables may provide a moderate amount of K^+ without excessive calories. A K^+-sparing agent, beta blocker, or ACE inhibitor given with the diuretic will reduce the degree of K^+ loss (Nader et al., 1988)

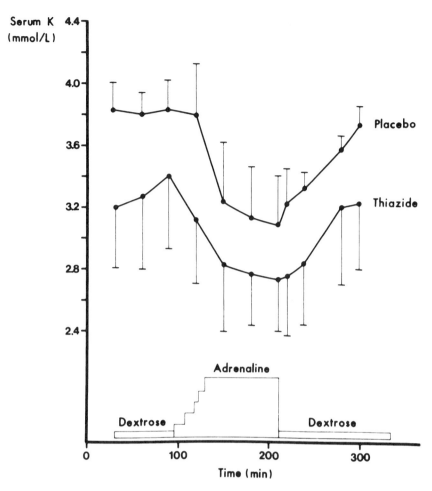

Figure 7.9. Serum potassium (mean ± SD) during infusion of 5% dextrose, 0.06 μg/kg/minute of epinephrine (adrenaline), and 5% dextrose in six healthy subjects after pretreatment with placebo or bendrofluazide (5 mg) for 7 days. (From Struthers AD, Whitesmith R, Reid JL. Prior thiazide diuretic treatment increases adrenaline-induced hypokalemia. *Lancet* 1983;1:1358–1363.)

but may not prevent the development of hypokalemia (Sawyer and Gabriel, 1988).

Repletion. If prevention does not work, the K⁺ deficiency can be replaced with supplemental K⁺, preferably given as the chloride; other anions (as found in most fruits rich in potassium) will not correct the alkalosis or the intracellular K⁺ deficiency as well (Kopyt et al., 1985). However, potassium citrate may be used, particularly in patients given a thiazide to reduce urinary calcium excretion in order to prevent renal stones (Sakhaee et al., 1991). Microencapsulated forms of KCl are more acceptable to patients than the various liquid preparations and have been found to cause fewer upper gastrointestinal mucosal lesions than the wax-matrix form (Hutcheon et al., 1988). The KCl may be given as

a potassium-containing salt substitute; a number are available, and they are less expensive than potassium supplements.

If the patient is continued on the thiazide, 40 mmol/day of supplemental potassium or the addition of a potassium-sparing agent (triamterene) will usually overcome hypokalemia (Schnaper et al., 1989). Concomitant hypomagnesemia will also be corrected with the potassium sparer.

Caution also is advised in giving potassium supplements to patients receiving ACE inhibitors whose aldosterone levels are suppressed and who may be unable to secrete extra potassium. The problem may be compounded in diabetics who may be unable to move potassium rapidly into cells and in those with renal insufficiency who may have a limited ability to excrete potassium.

Hypomagnesemia. Many of the problems attributed to hypokalemia may be caused by hypomagnesemia instead, and potassium repletion may not be possible in the presence of magnesium depletion (Whang et al., 1985).

Incidence. Although loop diuretics tend to cause more urinary magnesium loss than do thiazides, hypomagnesemia and significant cellular depletion may occur with either (Dørup et al., 1993). Hypomagnesemia was rare with doses of thiazide below 100 mg/day but was seen in 12% of patients on that dose (Kroenke et al., 1987).

Clinical Features. The symptoms and signs tend to progress from weakness, nausea, and neuromuscular irritability to tetany, mental changes and convulsions and, finally, to stupor and coma. An important feature is the appearance of ventricular arrhythmias, which are resistant to treatment unless both hypomagnesemia and hypokalemia are corrected (Whang et al., 1985).

Mechanism. The arrhythmias may arise from the inhibiting effect of magnesium deficiency on cell membrane $Na^+, K^+-ATPase$ pump activity, with resultant partial depolarization causing hyperirritability of excitable tissues. Since the impaired pump is less able to transfer extracellular potassium into cells, attempts to correct intracellular potassium depletion by raising blood potassium levels may be unsuccessful. Such pump inhibition may lead not only to cardiac irritability but also, by increasing intracellular free calcium, to increased tone and reactivity of vascular smooth muscle (Altura and Altura, 1984).

Management. Magnesium wastage is lessened by use of smaller doses of diuretics and concomitant use of a potassium-sparing agent (Schnaper et al., 1989). If repletion is needed, oral magnesium oxide, 200 to 400 mg/day (10 to 20 mmol), may be tolerated without gastrointestinal distress.

Hyperuricemia.

Incidence. Plasma uric acid levels are high in as many as 30% of untreated hypertensives (Langford et al., 1987). Thiazide therapy increases the incidence of hyperuricemia and may provoke gout, with an annual incidence of 4.9% at levels above 9 mg/dl (Campion et al., 1987). In the Hypertension Detection and Follow-Up Program, diuretic-induced rises in uric acid were rarely associated with gout (15 episodes over 5 years among 3693 subjects) and

were not associated with loss of renal function or mortality (Langford et al., 1987).

Management. Thiazide-induced hyperuricemia need not be treated until a kidney stone or gout appears (Dykman et al., 1987). If therapy is given, the logical choice is probenecid to increase renal excretion of uric acid. Only in patients who are hyperuricemic from excessive uric acid production, unrelated to diuretic use, should allopurinol be used since it may cause serious toxicity (Dykman et al., 1987).

Calcium Metabolism Alterations. Renal calcium reabsorption also is increased with chronic thiazide therapy, and urinary calcium excretion is decreased by 40% to 50% (Gesek and Friedman, 1992). A slight rise in serum calcium (i.e., 0.1 to 0.2 mg/dl) is usual, and hypercalcemia is often provoked in patients with preexisting hyperparathyroidism or vitamin D-treated hypoparathyroidism. The fact that serum calcium levels do not continue to rise in the face of reduced calcium excretion likely reflects the combination of reduced intestinal absorption of calcium (Sakhaee et al., 1984) and retention of calcium in bone (Giles et al., 1992). The former effect likely reflects a suppression of parathyroid hormone and vitamin D synthesis from the slight hypercalcemia and makes thiazide therapy a practical way to treat patients with renal stones caused by hypercalciuria from increased calcium absorption. The retention of calcium in bone may offer protection from osteoporosis and fractures, giving rise to a call for a proper clinical trial (Cauley et al., 1993).

Hyperlipidemia.

Significance. Although thiazide-induced hypercholesterolemia was reported in 1964 (Schoenfeld and Goldberger, 1964), the problem was not widely recognized until the report by Ames and Hill in 1976 of a rise in serum cholesterol of 12 mg/dl and in serum triglyceride of 26 mg/dl in 32 hypertensives treated for 1 year with chlorthalidone. Since then, multiple reports have documented the adverse effects of various diuretics, raising total serum cholesterol, LDL cholesterol, and triglyceride levels with little effect on high-density lipoprotein (HDL) cholesterol levels (Weidmann et al., 1985; Lardinois and Neuman, 1988; Pollare et al., 1989a; McInnes et al., 1992) (Fig. 7.10).

According to estimates from Framingham data, the adverse lipid changes could largely negate the benefits of the lower BP achieved by diuretic therapy (Ames, 1988). Caution is even more important since hypertension and hyperlip-

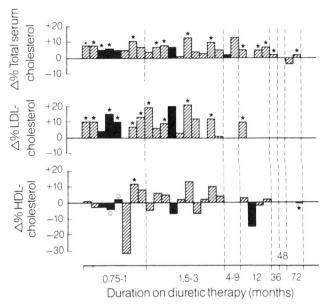

Figure 7.10. Percentage of changes in serum lipoprotein-cholesterol fractions as related to the duration of a monotherapy with thiazide-type (*hatched bars*) or loop diuretics (*solid bars*). The data shown are from published studies with a minimum number of 10 subjects and a minimum duration of 4 weeks. *Asterisks* (*) denote statistically significant changes as compared with pretreatment conditions, p < 0.05. *Open circles* (o) denote measurements by electrophoresis. (From Weidmann P, Uehlinger DE, Gerber A. Antihypertensive treatment of and serum lipoproteins. *J Hypertens* 1985;3:297–306.)

idemia frequently coexist (Bønaa and Thelle, 1991).

Duration. The question has been raised as to the duration of the lipid-altering effects of diuretics (Freis, 1990a). The majority of the studies in Weidmann and associates' survey were of short duration. In two studies, the lipid-raising effect of diuretics appeared to disappear after 1 year (Veterans Administration Cooperative Study Group, 1982) or 2 years (Williams et al., 1986) of continued therapy. On the other hand, persistent hyperlipidemic effects of diuretic therapy have been observed in over 300 patients followed for 5 years (Elliott, 1993) and in the large population of the MRFIT trial (Lasser et al., 1984). In the latter trial, in the presence of diuretic therapy, the fall in plasma cholesterol accomplished with an intensive dietary program was significantly less, as compared with that achieved by the same cholesterol-lowering regimen in the absence of diuretics at the end of 6 years (Lasser et al., 1984).

Mechanism. The mechanism is unknown. The change in cholesterol is correlated with decreases in glucose tolerance that are in turn correlated with falls in serum potassium (Langford et al., 1990), so hypokalemia is shown to be responsible in Figure 7.8, even though the

mechanism has not been established. It can occur with as little as 12.5 mg of HCTZ a day (McKenney et al., 1986) and in the absence of a significant fall in serum potassium (Ames, 1989).

Management. Regardless of how it comes about and even if it is only transient, adverse lipid changes can occur with diuretic use. Lipid levels should be monitored, a diet low in saturated fat should be encouraged and, if dyslipidemia persists, other types of antihypertensive drugs should be considered.

Glucose Intolerance and Insulin Resistance. Insulin resistance (Pollare et al., 1989a), impairment of glucose tolerance, precipitation of overt diabetes (Bengtsson et al., 1992), and worsening of diabetic control (Goldner et al., 1960) have all been observed in patients taking thiazides. Very rarely, diuretics may precipitate hyperosmolar nonketotic diabetic coma (Fonseca and Phear, 1982).

With resistance to the effects of insulin on peripheral glucose utilization, blood glucose levels rise. The pancreas responds with increased insulin secretion, and hyperinsulinemia maintains glucose homeostasis. However, in a prospective study starting with 137 hypertensives with normal glucose tolerance who were treated with diuretics, a progressive loss of tolerance developed so that after 14 years, the 34 of these patients still being followed had higher glucose levels, both fasting and after an oral glucose load (Murphy et al., 1982). Evidence that this glucose intolerance was diuretic-induced came from the significant improvement that was noted 7 months after withdrawal of thiazide therapy. In other studies, an increased risk of developing diabetes over a 9- to 12-year follow-up was noted in patients taking diuretics alone or with a beta blocker (Skarfors et al., 1989; Bengtsson et al., 1992).

Not all studies report a worsening of glucose tolerance with chronic diuretic therapy: 2.5 mg of bendroflumethiazide given to 37 men for 10 years did not (Berglund et al., 1986). In a large case-control study, no association was found between thiazide diuretic use and the initiation of treatment for diabetes mellitus (Gurwitz et al., 1992).

Significance. Hyperinsulinemia appears to be a factor in the cardiovascular risks associated with upper body obesity and a pressor mechanism in the pathogenesis of primary hypertension (see Chapter 3). Beyond those considerations, a retrospective analysis of 759 diabetics treated at the Joslin Clinic between 1972 and 1979 showed a considerably increased mortality rate in those given thiazide diuretics alone for treatment of hypertension, particularly in those with proteinuria (Warram et al., 1991) (Fig. 7.11). The risk was unrelated to the degree of hypertension, but was associated with the years of treatment with diuretics alone. Others have noted an increased mortality rate (Klein et al., 1989) and progression of diabetic nephropathy (Walker et al., 1987) associated with diuretic use in diabetic patients. Therefore, the use of diuretics in diabetics should be minimized.

Hyponatremia. This occurs less commonly in edema-free hypertensives than in edematous patients given thiazides for diuresis. With chronic diuretic use, the contraction of effective blood volume will decrease the ability of the kidney to excrete water, and slight, asymptomatic falls in serum sodium concentration may be noted (Nader et al., 1988). Rarely, severe, symptomatic hyponatremia develops, usually soon after diuretics are started in elderly female patients who appear to have an expanded fluid volume from increased water intake in the face of a decreased ability to excrete free water (Friedman et al., 1989).

Impotence. Impotence has been reported with diuretic therapy, and it may be more common than with other drugs. In the large randomized MRC trial, impotence was complained about by 22.6% of the men on bendrofluazide, as compared with a rate of 10.1% among those on placebo and 13.2% among those on propranolol (Medical Research Council Working Party, 1981). More thorough QOL assessments confirm the association (Chang et al., 1991), and thiazide-induced sexual dysfunction has been documented in a rodent model (Rockhold, 1992).

Other Side Effects. Fever and chills, blood dyscrasias, cholecystitis, pancreatitis, necrotizing vasculitis, acute interstitial nephritis, and noncardiogenic pulmonary edema have been seen rarely. Allergic skin rashes occur in 0.28% of patients, and about the same percentage develop photosensitivity (Diffey and Langtry, 1989).

Loop Diuretics

These agents primarily block chloride reabsorption by inhibition of the $Na^+/K^+/Cl^-$ cotransport system of the luminal membrane of the thick ascending limb of Henle's loop, the site where 35% to 45% of filtered sodium is reabsorbed (Fig. 7.5). Therefore, the loop diuretics are more potent and have a more rapid onset of action than the thiazides. However, they are no more effective in lowering the BP or less likely to cause side effects if given in equipotent amounts. Their major use is in patients with renal insufficiency, in whom large enough doses can be given to achieve an effective luminal concentration (see Chapter 9). In addition, when given intravenously, they provide rapid antihypertensive effects in addition to their diuretic action (Sechi et al., 1992).

Furosemide (Lasix)

Clinical Use. Although some report good antihypertensive effects from once-daily 40-mg doses of furosemide (Frewin et al., 1987), most find that even twice-daily furosemide is less effective than twice-daily HCTZ (Anderson et al., 1971; Araoye et al., 1978; Holland et al., 1979) or once-daily chlorthalidone (Healy et al., 1970) while producing similar hyperuricemia and hypokalemia. The need to maintain a slightly shrunken body fluid volume that is critical for an antihypertensive action from diuretic therapy is not met by the short duration of furosemide action (less than 6 hours for an oral dose); during the remaining hours, sodium is retained, so that net fluid balance over 24 hours is left

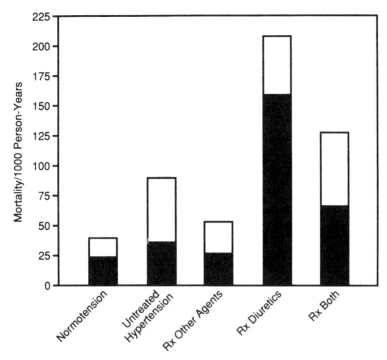

Figure 7.11. Mortality per 1000 person-years in diabetic patients with proteinuria according to hypertension status and type of antihypertensive treatment (℞) during each year of follow-up. *Shaded areas* of bars indicate cardiovascular mortality; *open areas,* other mortality. Mortality during diuretic treatment was significantly higher than with untreated hypertension (p < .025 for cardiovascular mortality; p <.025 for total mortality). Cardiovascular mortality during treatment with both diuretics and other agents was significantly lower than during treatment with diuretics alone (p <.025). Mortality was adjusted by the direct method to the age distribution of all patients receiving antihypertensive treatment. (From Warram JH, et al. Excess mortality associated with diuretic therapy in diabetes mellitus. *Arch Intern Med* 151:1350–1356, 1991.)

unaltered (Wilcox et al., 1983). If furosemide is used twice daily, the first dose should be given early in the morning and the second in the midafternoon, both to provide diuretic action at the time of sodium intake and to avoid nocturia.

One indication for the use of a loop diuretic is in patients on lithium who may have a rise in serum levels when given a thiazide, presumably from enhanced proximal reabsorption of lithium. With furosemide, no increase was seen, perhaps because lithium reabsorption in the loop of Henle was blocked (Jefferson and Kalin, 1979).

Side Effects. Loop diuretics may cause fewer metabolic problems than longer-acting agents because of their shorter duration of action (Nader et al., 1988). With similar durations of action, the side effects are similar, including the hyperlipidemic effect (Fig. 7.10). Pancreatitis (Stenvinkel and Alvestrand, 1988) and allergic reactions (Sullivan, 1991) are two more of the thiazide-associated problems also seen with furosemide.

Bumetanide (Bumex)

This agent, though 40 times more potent and twice more bioavailable than furosemide on a weight basis, is identical in its actions when given in an equivalent dose (Brater et al., 1983).

Ethacrynic Acid (Edecrin)

Though structurally different from furosemide, this drug also works primarily in the ascending limb of Henle and has an equal potency. It is used much less than furosemide, mainly because of its greater propensity to cause permanent hearing loss.

Loop Diuretics Under Investigation

A number of loop diuretics are currently under investigation, including azosemide, etozoline, muzolimine, piretanide, and torasemide (Beermann and Grind, 1987). Muzolimine is considerably longer acting, and piretanide may induce less potassium wastage (Hegbrant et al., 1989). Small, once-daily doses of torasemide have been found to be equipotent to HCTZ and to induce fewer biochemical changes (Baumgart, 1993).

Potassium-Sparing Agents

These drugs act in the distal tubule to prevent potassium loss, one (spironolactone) as an aldosterone antagonist, the others (triamterene and amiloride) as direct inhibitors of potassium secretion (Krishna et al., 1988). All three are effective in reducing diuretic-induced K^+ wastage, but progressive hypokalemia may still occur with their use (Sawyer and Gabriel, 1988). Caution is needed with their use in the presence of renal insufficiency, wherein hyperkalemia may develop because of the decreased ability to excrete potassium.

Spironolactone (Aldactone)

Clinical Use. The similarities in the structure of spironolactone to that of the mineralocorticoid hormones enable this drug, when given in relatively large amounts, to inhibit competitively the binding of those steroids to their intracellular receptors, thereby antagonizing their physiologic effects (Krishna et al., 1988). Three clinical uses for this antagonism are:

—As a diagnostic test and relatively specific therapy for the hypertension associated with primary aldosteronism (see Chapter 13);
—As a diuretic in edematous states such as nephrosis and cirrhosis with ascites, wherein very high levels of aldosterone play a major role;
—As an inhibitor of the aldosterone-mediated exchange of Na^+ and K^+ in the distal tubule to prevent the potassium wastage from thiazide diuretics. When used in combination with HCTZ (as in Aldactazide), 25 mg of spironolactone provided an increase in plasma potassium over 12 hours comparable to that of 32 mmol of potassium chloride (Toner et al., 1990).

The drug will provide a significant antihypertensive effect on its own if given in modest doses. When used alone in average doses of 100 mg once per day, it produced a fall in BP of 18/10 mm Hg over a mean follow-up of 20 months (Jeunemaitre et al., 1988). Aldosterone antagonists may be more widely used if their inhibitions of myocardial fibrosis in experimental animals is seen in humans (Weber et al., 1992).

Side Effects. Impotence and gynecomastia in men and breast tenderness in women are the major side effects. With doses of 25 to 50 mg/day, gynecomastia was seen in 30 of 431 men (Jeunemaitre et al., 1988). The natriuresis induced by spironolactone is antagonized by aspirin (Tweeddale and Ogilvie, 1973).

Triamterene (Dyrenium)

Clinical Use. For many years a combination of HCTZ (25 mg) and triamterene (50 mg), marketed as Dyazide, was the most widely prescribed antihypertensive drug in the United States. A more bioavailable tablet formulation of HCTZ and triamterene (Maxzide) has been marketed and shown to have equal antihypertensive efficacy (Casner and Dillon, 1990).

Though triamterene has less intrinsic antihypertensive action than spironolactone, it acts to inhibit potassium wasting with no hormonal side effects. It enhances the natriuretic effect of thiazides while minimizing their kaliuretic effect (Krishna et al., 1988) and preserves serum and muscle potassium and magnesium levels (Widmann et al., 1988).

Side Effects. Triamterene may be excreted into the urine and may find its way into renal stones (Sörgel et al., 1985). However, no higher frequency of hospitalization for renal stones was found among users of triamterene than among users of HCTZ alone or with other drugs (Jick et al., 1982). The simultaneous use of triamterene and the prostaglandin inhibitor indomethacin has been reported to induce reversible acute renal failure (Sica and Gehr, 1989).

Amiloride (Midamor)

Amiloride is structurally different from both spironolactone and triamterene. It inhibits a number of transport proteins that facilitate the movement of sodium ions either alone or linked with hydrogen or calcium. By blocking the entry of sodium into distal convoluted tubular cells, potassium loss through potassium channels is diminished (Rose, 1991).

Clinical Use. Amiloride has some antihypertensive effect of its own (Katzman et al., 1988) and may therefore potentiate the effect of thiazide diuretic while blunting the renal wastage of potassium. It is largely used in combination with HCTZ as Moduretic, containing 50 mg of HCTZ and 5 mg of amiloride. Other uses than as a potassium-sparer may be developed: by blocking Na-H exchange, it inhibits the rise in intracellular calcium during myocardial ischemia (Murphy et al., 1991). In addition, its action in sodium channels involved in taste may diminish the stimulation of sodium intake that accompanies the use of diuretics (Mattes and Engelman, 1992). Moreover, amiloride blocks the access of lithium to the tubular cells, ameliorating the antidiuretic hormone (ADH)-resistant polyuria often seen with chronic lithium therapy (Battle et al., 1985).

Side Effects. Nausea, flatulence, and skin rash have been the most frequent side effects, and hyperkalemia the most serious. However, a disturbingly large number of cases of hyponatremia in elderly patients have been reported after its use in combination with HCTZ (Mathew et al., 1990).

ADRENERGIC INHIBITING DRUGS

This group of drugs inhibits the sympathetic nervous system, either centrally or peripherally. The effects of the sympathetic nervous system are mediated by the actions of norepinephrine (noradrenaline) released locally from postganglionic nerve endings and epinephrine (adrenaline) released from the adrenal medulla. These actions begin with the binding of the catecholamines to receptors located on the external surface of the effector cell membrane.

Ahlquist (1948) found that the responses to catecholamines in various tissues were mediated through two distinct types of receptors, termed *alpha* and *beta,* based on different degrees of responsiveness to agonists (Fig. 7.12). Subsequently, two subtypes of beta-receptors, termed beta$_1$ and beta$_2$ (Lands et al., 1967), and two subtypes of alpha receptors, termed alpha$_1$ and alpha$_2$, were characterized (Langer, 1974). Since then, at least 11 subtypes of adrenergic receptors have been characterized, but as assessed pharmacologically, they can be subdivided into three major families: beta receptors, which couple to stimulatory G proteins to activate adenylyl cyclase; alpha$_1$ receptors, which couple to a distinct class of G proteins to activate synthesis of the second messengers inositol triphosphate and diacylglycerol; and alpha$_2$ receptors, which couple to inhibitory G proteins to inhibit adenylyl cyclase (Strasser et al., 1992).

Various sympathetic nervous system actions are mediated by different adrenergic receptor types. Some of the alpha and beta effects antagonize one another; others are complementary. A number of drugs act as either *agonists* (i.e., they possess both affinity for and efficacy at receptors) or *antagonists* (i.e., they possess affinity but no efficacy and, therefore, antagonize natural agonists). Weak agonists, termed *partial agonists,* cannot evoke the maximal response of which the cell is capable but have enough affinity for the receptor to antagonize the natural agonists.

The range of actions of some agonists and antagonists on various adrenergic receptors is shown in Figure 7.13 (Strosberg, 1987). Of the agents currently used to treat hypertension, some interfere with the normal release of norepinephrine at the nerve endings and are referred to as peripheral neuronal blocking drugs; others act centrally by stimulating alpha receptors, others block the alpha- or beta-adrenergic receptor sites on the effector cells.

Peripheral Adrenergic Inhibitors

Reserpine

First reported to be an effective antihypertensive in 1942 (Bhatia, 1942), reserpine became

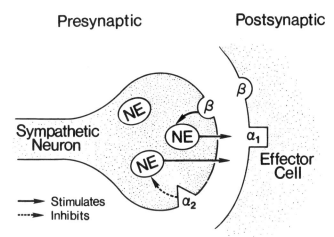

Figure 7.12. Simplified schematic view of the adrenergic nerve ending showing that norepinephrine (*NE*) is released from the storage granules when the nerve is stimulated and enters the synaptic cleft to bind to alpha$_1$ and beta receptors on the effector cell (postsynaptic). In addition, a short feedback loop exists, in which NE binds to alpha$_2$ and beta receptors on the neuron (presynaptic), either to inhibit or to stimulate further release.

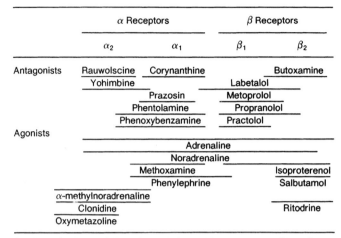

Figure 7.13. Range of actions of adrenergic ligands on alpha and beta receptors. (From Strosberg AD. Molecular and functional properties of beta-adrenergic receptors. *Am J Cardiol* 59:3F–9F, 1987.)

a popular drug in the 1960s and 1970s but has been used less and less since then. The reasons for this reduced use include the following:

—Because it is an inexpensive generic drug, reserpine has no constituency pushing for its use (Lederle et al., 1993);
—Reserpine has become old hat; the advent of every new "miracle" antihypertensive makes it look more and more outdated;
—The scare of cancer tainted reserpine, although the claims have been refuted (Horwitz and Feinstein, 1985);
—The lurking specter of insidious depression.

Pharmacology. Reserpine, one of the many alkaloids of the Indian snakeroot *Rauwolfia serpentina*, has all of the desirable pharmacologic actions of the plant's various preparations. Reserpine is absorbed readily from the gut, is taken up rapidly by lipid-containing tissue, and binds to sites involved with storage of biogenic amines. Its effects start slowly and persist, so only one dose per day is needed.

Mode of Action. Reserpine blocks the transport of norepinephrine into its storage granules so that less of the neurotransmitter is available when the adrenergic nerves are stimulated. The resultant decrease in sympathetic tone results in a decrease in peripheral vascular resistance. Catecholamines also are depleted in the brain, which may account for the sedative and depressant effects of the drug, and in the myocardium, which may decrease cardiac output and induce a slight bradycardia (Cohen et al., 1968).

Efficacy and Dosage. By itself, reserpine has limited antihypertensive potency, resulting in an average decrease of only 3/5 mm Hg;

when combined with a thiazide, the reduction averaged 14/11 mm Hg (VA Cooperative Study, 1962). In a comparison of various regimens in patients with mild hypertension, a combination of *Rauwolfia* and thiazide worked better than a beta blocker plus a thiazide (Veterans Administration Cooperative Study Group, 1977).

With a diuretic, as little as 0.05 mg once daily will provide most of the antihypertensive effect of 0.25 mg and is associated with less lethargy and impotence (Participating VA Centers, 1982).

Side Effects. Side effects are relatively infrequent at appropriately low doses (Prisant et al., 1991). They include:

—Nasal stuffiness;
—Increased gastric acid secretion, which rarely may activate an ulcer;
—Central nervous system depression, which may simply tranquilize an apprehensive patient or may be so severe as to lead to serious depression.

Guanethidine (Ismelin)

Guanethidine at one time was frequently used with many patients with moderate hypertension because it requires only one dose per day and has a steep dose-response relationship, thus producing an effect in almost every patient. As other effective drugs with fewer side effects became available, the use of guanethidine rapidly diminished.

Pharmacology. Guanethidine is one of a group of guanidine compounds that lowers BP. Its absorption from the gut is limited and variable, ranging from 3% to 50% (Woosley and Nies, 1976). The drug is taken into the adrenergic nerves by an active transport mechanism, the same pump that returns extracellular norepinephrine across the nerve membrane. This pump is inhibited by ephedrine, amphetamine, and tricyclic antidepressants, which accounts for their antagonism to the action of guanethidine.

Mode of Action. Once inside the adrenergic nerves, guanethidine initially blocks the exit of norepinephrine; it then causes an active release of norepinephrine from its storage granules, depleting the reserve pool of the neurotransmitter and decreasing the amount released when the nerve is stimulated, thereby reducing peripheral resistance. Myocardial catecholamine stores are partially depleted and cardiac output falls. The drug does not cross the blood-brain barrier, which accounts for the absence of any sedative effect. The BP is reduced somewhat in the supine position, but much more so when the patient is upright since the normal vasoconstrictive response to posture is blunted (Goldberg and Raftery, 1976).

Efficacy and Dosage. Guanethidine is powerful and has a steep dose-response relationship so that the more drug given, the greater the effect. The amount required to lower standing BP to an acceptable and tolerable level varies from 25 to 300 mg daily. The initial dose should be no more than 25 mg, and increments of 10 to 12.5 mg should be made no more often than every 3 to 5 days. The drug need be given only once daily, and the full hypotensive action of a given dose may not become manifest for several days.

Side Effects. Most of the complications are in keeping with the known effects of the drug: postural hypotension, fluid retention, diarrhea, failure of ejaculation. The appearance of minimal postural hypotension may be used as an indication that the therapeutic end-point has been reached.

Others

Guanadrel Sulfate (Hylorel). A close relative of guanethidine, guanadrel sulfate has almost all of the attributes of that drug with a shorter onset and offset of action that diminish the frequency of side effects and make it more tolerable (Owens and Dunn, 1988).

Bethanidine (Tenathan). Another close relative of guanethidine, bethanidine has comparable potency and side effects, except that it produces less diarrhea (VA Cooperative Study, 1977). The main difference is its shorter duration of action, 8 to 12 hours.

Debrisoquin

Debrisoquin undergoes variable metabolic degradation (Silas et al., 1977) and has not been approved for use in the United States.

Central Alpha Agonists

Peripheral adrenergic inhibitors inhibit release of catecholamines, primarily from peripheral adrenergic neurons. We will now examine those that stimulate central alpha$_2$-adrenergic receptors that are involved in depressor sympathoinhibitory mechanisms (van Zwieten, 1992a) (Fig. 7.14). Thus, these drugs have well-defined effects, including:

—A marked decline in sympathetic activity reflected in lower levels of norepinephrine (Bobik et al., 1986);
—A reduction of the ability of the baroreceptor reflex to compensate for a decrease in BP, accounting for the relative bradycardia and enhanced hypotensive action noted upon standing (Jarrott et al., 1987);
—A modest decrease in both peripheral resistance and cardiac output (Bentley, 1987);
—A fall in plasma renin levels (Gavras et al., 1977a);
—Fluid retention, which may not occur with guanabenz (Gehr et al., 1986);
—Maintenance of renal blood flow despite a fall in BP (Lowenstein et al., 1984);
—Common side effects reflecting their central site of action: sedation, decreased alertness, and a dry mouth;
—When abruptly stopped, a rapid rebound and, rarely, an overshoot of the BP may be experienced with or without accompanying features of excess sympathetic nervous activity. This discontinuation syndrome likely represents a sudden surge of catecholamine release, freed from the prior state of inhibition.

Methyldopa (Aldomet)

From the early 1960s to the late 1970s, when beta-blockers became available, methyldopa (Aldomet) was the most popular drug after diuretics used to treat hypertension.

Pharmacology. Methyldopa is the alpha-methylated derivative of dopa, the natural precursor of dopamine and norepinephrine. Originally used to treat hypertension because it inhibited the enzyme dopa decarboxylase (Oates et al., 1960), its mode of action is now thought to involve the formation of methylnorepinephrine and methylepinephrine, which act not as false transmitters but as potent agonists at alpha-adrenergic receptors within the central nervous system, similar to the action of clonidine (van Zwieten et al., 1984) (Fig. 7.14).

Efficacy and Dosage

BP is lowered maximally about 4 hours after an oral dose, and some effect persists for up to

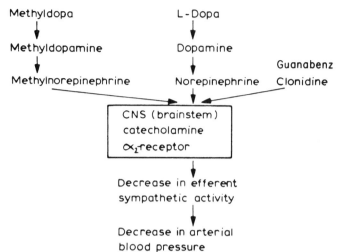

Figure 7.14. Schematic representation of the common mechanism probably underlying the hypotensive actions of methyldopa, L-dopa, clonidine, guanabenz, and guanfacine. (From Henning M. α-Methyldopa and related compounds. In: van Zwieten PA, ed. *Handbook of Hypertension, vol 3, Pharmacology of Antihypertensive Drugs.* Amsterdam: Elsevier, 1984:1564–1593.)

24 hours. For most patients, therapy should be started with 250 mg 2 times per day, and the daily dosage can be increased to a maximum of 3.0 g on a twice-per-day schedule. In patients with renal insufficiency the dosage should be halved. With chronic use, LVH may regress, without apparent relation to changes in BP (Fouad et al., 1982).

Absorption and metabolism of methyldopa may be slowed by concomitant intake of sulfate-containing drugs such as ferrous sulfate with a resultant decrease in its antihypertensive effect (Campbell et al., 1988).

Side Effects.   In addition to the anticipated sedative effects, postural hypotension, and fluid retention, an impairment of reticuloendothelial function (Kelton, 1985) and a variety of ''auto-immune'' side effects, including fever and liver dysfunction, are peculiar to methyldopa. These may reflect an inhibition of suppressor T cells with resultant unregulated autoantibody production by B cells (Kirtland et al., 1980). Liver dysfunction usually disappears when the drug is stopped, but at least 83 cases of serious hepatotoxicity were reported by 1975 (Rodman et al., 1976) with diffuse parenchymal injury similar to that of viral hepatitis (Kaplowitz et al., 1986).

An impairment of psychometric performance (Johnson et al., 1990) and a selective loss of upper airway motor activity (Lahive et al., 1988) may not be obvious until the drug is stopped. Few data are available about lipid changes; in one study, total cholesterol was unchanged, but

HDL cholesterol was reduced by 10% (Leon et al., 1984).

Overall, in large surveys, the number and range of the adverse reactions to methyldopa are impressive (Lawson et al., 1978; Furhoff, 1978). In view of its unique and potentially serious side effects, I believe other central alpha-agonists should be used in place of methyldopa. In the United States, it remains a favored drug only for the treatment of hypertension during pregnancy (see Chapter 11). Fortunately, little of the drug is transferred to the fetus (Jones and Cummings, 1978).

Clonidine (Catapres)

The use of this drug has been limited by concern over a withdrawal syndrome, but its availability as a transdermal preparation has led to an increase in its use.

Pharmacology.   Clonidine is an imidazoline derivative. It is readily absorbed, and plasma levels peak within an hour; the plasma half-life is 6 to 13 hours. It binds to specific sites in the brain, which may be functional receptors that mediate its hypotensive action (van Zwieten, 1992a). In experimental animals, clonidine activates opiate receptors in the brain, and this may play a role in its hypotensive action as well as explain its value for management of opiate withdrawal (van Giersbergen et al., 1989).

Efficacy and Dosage.   When clonidine is taken orally, the BP begins to fall within 30 minutes, with the greatest effect occurring between 2 and 4 hours. The duration of effect is from 12 to 24 hours. The starting dose may be as little as 75 μg twice daily (Clobass Study Group, 1990), with a maximum of 1.2 mg/day. Patients may be given most, and perhaps all, of the daily dose at bedtime to compensate for the sedative effect (Ram et al., 1979). Clonidine has been used to lower markedly elevated BP with an initial 0.1- to 0.2-mg dose followed by hourly 0.05- to 0.1-mg doses (Houston, 1986). Intravenous clonidine is not available in the United States but is used elsewhere (Niarchos and Baksi, 1973).

A transdermal preparation that delivers clonidine continuously over a 7-day interval has been found to be effective and to cause milder side effects than oral therapy (Weber, 1986), but it may cause considerable skin irritation and side effects similar to those seen with the oral drug (Langley and Heel, 1988), including rebound hypertension when discontinued (Metz et al., 1987). It is available in doses of 0.1, 0.2, and 0.3 mg/day.

Clonidine has been used to prevent the reflex sympathetic overactivity that follows direct vasodilator therapy (Mitchell and Pettinger, 1981) and to serve as a screening test for pheochromocytoma (see Chapter 12). It is effective in patients with renal insufficiency, and very little is eliminated during dialysis (Hulter et al., 1979).

Side Effects. Clonidine and methyldopa share the two most common side effects, sedation and dry mouth, though these effects are more common with clonidine (Amery et al., 1970). Rarely, hallucinations and other central nervous system (CNS) effects occur (Brown et al., 1980). Clonidine does not share the "autoimmune" hepatic and hematologic derangements induced by methyldopa.

Rebound and Discontinuation Syndromes. If any antihypertensive therapy is inadvertently stopped abruptly, various "discontinuation syndromes" may occur: (*a*) a rapid asymptomatic return of the BP to pretreatment levels, which occurs in the majority of patients, (*b*) a "rebound" of the BP plus symptoms and signs of sympathetic overactivity, and (*c*) an "overshoot" of the BP above pretreatment levels. In addition, patients who suddenly stop use of beta blockers may experience a different discontinuation syndrome manifested by the sudden appearance of coronary ischemia.

A discontinuation syndrome has been reported with most currently used drugs (Houston, 1981), but most frequently with clonidine (Neusy and Lowenstein, 1989), likely reflecting a rapid return of catecholamine secretion that had been suppressed during therapy (Reid et al., 1977).

Those who take high doses of any antihypertensive drug are vulnerable, particularly if they have underlying severe hypertension and high levels of renin-angiotensin. Those who had been on a combination of a central adrenergic inhibitor (e.g., clonidine) and a beta blocker may be particularly susceptible if the central inhibitor is withdrawn while the beta blocker is continued (Lilja et al., 1982). This leads to a sudden surge in plasma catecholamines in a situation in which peripheral alpha receptors are left unopposed to induce vasoconstriction because the beta receptors are blocked and cannot mediate vasodilation.

If a discontinuation syndrome appears, the previously administered drug should be restarted, and the symptoms will likely recede rapidly. If needed, labetalol will effectively lower a markedly elevated BP (Mehta and Lopez, 1987).

Other Effects. Depression of sinus and atrioventricular (AV) nodal function may be common (Roden et al., 1988), and a few cases of severe bradycardia have been reported (Byrd et al., 1988). This effect may be taken advantage of for the treatment of patients with rapid atrial fibrillation (Roth et al., 1992). Large overdoses will lead to hypertension, presumably by stimulation of peripheral alpha receptors, causing vasoconstriction (Hunyor et al., 1975). The antihypertensive effect of clonidine may be blunted by simultaneous intake of tricyclic antidepressants (Briant et al., 1973) and tranquilizers (van Zwieten, 1977). The drug does not adversely affect lipoproteins or metabolic control in hypertensive diabetics (Nilsson-Ehle et al., 1988).

Other Uses. Clonidine has been reported to be useful in numerous conditions that may accompany hypertension, including:

—Opiate withdrawal (Bond, 1986);
—Menopausal hot flashes (Hammar and Berg, 1985);
—Diarrhea due to diabetic neuropathy (Fedora et al., 1985) or ulcerative colitis (Lechin et al., 1985);
—Sympathetic nervous hyperactivity in patients with alcoholic cirrhosis (Esler et al., 1992).

Guanabenz (Wytensin)

This drug, structurally similar to clonidine, also acts as a central alpha$_2$ agonist, resulting in a decrease of sympathetic outflow from the brain.

However, it has some distinctive features that make it an attractive choice for a centrally acting agent.

Pharmacology. Guanabenz is an aminoguanidine whose absorption is complete, with peak blood levels reached 2 to 5 hours after oral intake (Holmes et al., 1983). It is extensively metabolized, and its mean plasma half-life is 14 hours.

The drug acts centrally in a manner similar to that of clonidine (Holmes et al., 1983). Patients on long-term therapy tend to lose a few pounds in body weight, which is attributed to a natriuresis that in turn may be explained by the drug's effect on chloride reabsorption in the papillary collecting duct (Stein and Osgood, 1984) as well as by its lesser alpha$_1$-mediated vasoconstrictor effect in the kidneys, as compared with that of clonidine (Wolff et al., 1984).

Efficacy and Dosage. Guanabenz lowers BP, as do clonidine and methyldopa, and causes similar side effects; unlike these other agents, it offers the advantages of not causing reactive fluid retention, so it has been approved for initial use as monotherapy. Its use is usually associated with slight lowering of serum cholesterol (Kaplan and Grundy, 1988) and it can be safely used in diabetics (Gutin and Tuck, 1988) and asthmatics (Deitch et al., 1984).

Therapy should begin with 4 mg twice per day, with increments up to a total of 64 mg/day.

Side Effects. The side effects mimic those seen with other central alpha agonists; sedation and dry mouth are the most prominent, being seen in 20% to 30% of patients. Weakness and dizziness each occur in about 6%, whereas gastrointestinal complaints are rare. A withdrawal syndrome may occur if the drug is stopped abruptly (Ram et al., 1979).

Guanfacine (Tenex)

Another clonidine-like drug, guanfacine appears to enter the brain more slowly and to maintain its antihypertensive effect longer (Sorkin and Heel, 1986). These differences translate into a once-per-day dosage and perhaps fewer CNS side effects (Lewin et al., 1990). Withdrawal symptoms are less common than with clonidine (Wilson et al., 1986).

Lofexidine

This is another imidazoline derivative very similar to clonidine in hemodynamics, clinical effectiveness, and side effects (Lopez and Mehta, 1984). It has been effective in managing

withdrawal from both opiates (Washton et al., 1981) and alcohol (Cushman et al., 1985).

Imidazoline Receptor Agonists

A "new generation" of centrally acting drugs is being promoted whose primary site of action is the imidazoline receptor located in the rostral ventrolateral medulla oblongata wherein alpha$_2$ receptors are less abundant (Schäfer et al., 1992). Two of these drugs, *rilmenidine* (Laurent and Safar, 1992) and *moxonidine* (Ollivier et al., 1992), are being investigated with the hope that they will have all of the good effects of the alpha$_2$ agonists but not the sedative effects (Fletcher et al., 1991).

Alpha-Adrenergic Receptor Blockers

Selective alpha$_1$ blockers have had a relatively small share of the overall market for antihypertensive drugs in the United States. Until 1987, prazosin (Minipress) was the only alpha blocker available, but terazosin (Hytrin) and doxazosin (Cardura) are now available. The availability of more of these drugs and the increasing awareness of their special ability to improve lipid levels and insulin sensitivity suggest that their use will expand considerably, as reflected by their inclusion in the drugs recommended for initial monotherapy in the 1993 fifth report of the Joint National Committee on detection, evaluation, and treatment of high blood pressure (JNC-V). In addition, awareness of the influences of alpha-adrenergic mechanisms continues to expand. These include roles in such varied processes as vasoconstriction (Baran et al., 1992), a number of metabolic-hormonal functions (Ruffolo et al., 1991), penile erection (Krane et al., 1989), and vascular hypertrophy (van Kleef et al., 1992). In one area, this expanded potential has already been realized: the relief of the symptoms of urinary tract blockade from prostatic hypertrophy (Guthrie, 1993).

Nonselective Agents

The nonselective alpha blockers, phenoxybenzamine and phentolamine, are used almost exclusively in the medical management of pheochromocytoma, since they are only minimally effective in primary hypertension (see Chapter 12).

Selective Agents

When the two major subtypes of alpha receptors were identified, prazosin, which had been characterized as a nonspecific vasodilator when introduced in 1976, was recognized to act as a competitive antagonist of postsynaptic alpha₁ receptors (van Zwieten, 1988). It remains as the prototype of this class of drugs, but a number of others share this action (Table 7.5).

Mode of Action

These agents block the activation of postsynaptic alpha₁ receptors by circulating or neurally released catecholamines, an activation that normally induces vasoconstriction (Fig. 7.15). This blockade dilates both resistance and capacitance vessels. Peripheral resistance falls without major changes in cardiac output, in part because of a balance between a decrease in venous return (preload) and a slight degree of reflex sympathetic stimulation as a consequence of the vasodilation.

The presynaptic alpha₂ receptors remain open, capable of binding neurotransmitter and thereby inhibiting the release of additional norepineph-

rine (NE) through a direct negative feedback mechanism. This inhibition of NE release explains the lack of tachycardia, increased cardiac output, and rise in renin levels that characterize the response to drugs that block both the presynaptic alpha₂ receptor and the postsynaptic alpha₁ receptor (e.g., phentolamine). Despite this selective blockade, neurally mediated responses to stress and exercise are unaffected, and the baroreceptor reflex remains active. However, the decrease in preload and the blockade of alpha₁ receptors largely prevent the reflex sympathetic activation seen with direct vasodilators (e.g., hydralazine).

Accompanying these desirable attributes, other actions may lessen the usefulness of alpha-adrenergic blockers: they relax the venous bed as well and, at least initially, may affect the visceral vascular bed more than the peripheral vascular bed; the subsequent pooling of blood in the viscera may explain the propensity to first-

Table 7.5. Comparative Characteristics of Alpha₁ Antagonists

Drugs	Duration of Action (hr)	Peak of Action (hr)	Therapeutic Dose (mg)	Frequency of Administration (times/day)
Prazosin	4–6	0.5	1–20	2–3
Terazosin	>18	1–1.7	1–20	1–2
Doxazosin	18–36	6	1–16	1
Trimazosin	3–6	3–7	100–900	2 or 3
Indoramin	>6	2	50–150	2 or 3
Urapidil	6–8	3–5	15–120	1 or 2
Ketanserin	>12	1–2	20–40	1 or 2

From Cubeddu LX. New alpha₁-adrenergic receptor antagonists for the treatment of hypertension: role of vascular alpha receptors in the control of peripheral resistance. *Am Heart J* 1988;116:133–160.

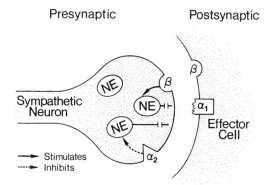

Prazosin Blocks Postsynaptic α₁ Receptor But Not Presynaptic α₂ Receptor

Figure 7.15. Schematic view of the action of prazosin as a postsynaptic alpha blocker. By blocking the alpha₁-adrenergic receptor on the vascular smooth muscle, catecholamine-induced vasoconstriction is inhibited. The alpha₂ receptor on the neuronal membrane is not blocked; therefore inhibition of additional norepinephrine release by the short feedback mechanism is maintained. *NE*, norepinephrine.

dose hypotension (Saxena and Bolt, 1986). Since baroreceptors are active, plasma NE rises after the BP falls, which may limit the antihypertensive potency of these drugs (Izzo et al., 1981). Volume retention is common (Bauer et al., 1984), perhaps because renin and aldosterone levels are less suppressed than they are with other adrenergic-inhibiting drugs (Webb et al., 1987). Moreover, pharmacologic tolerance to the responsiveness to phenylephrine has been observed after 4 weeks of terazosin use in normotensives (Vincent et al., 1992).

Prazosin and other members of this class may also exert some CNS effects that add to their antihypertensive efficacy (Cubeddu, 1988) and side effects. The vascular actions of $alpha_1$ blockers may also involve inhibition of calcium entry (Nichols and Ruffolo, 1988) and angiotensin II–mediated effects on smooth muscle cell growth (van Kleef et al., 1992).

Pharmacology

A quinazoline derivative, prazosin is rapidly absorbed, reaching maximal blood levels at 2 hours and having a plasma half-life of about 3 hours (Schäfers and Reid, 1989). The drug is highly bound to plasma proteins but, in dogs, is rapidly taken into vascular smooth muscle cells. It is metabolized in the liver and excreted largely via bile and feces.

Terazosin and doxazosin are less lipid-soluble and have half or less of the affinity for $alpha_1$ receptors than prazosin does. Therefore, they induce a slower and less profound initial fall in BP, particularly after standing, than does prazosin. This likely translates into a lesser propensity for hypotensive symptoms and certainly provides for a longer duration of action for the second-generation $alpha_1$ blockers.

Individual patients vary in both the degree of fall in BP and the dose required for an effect (Larochelle et al., 1982). In a study of concentration-effect relationships with prazosin, Elliott et al. (1989b) found an attenuation of the antihypertensive response, from 11.5 mm Hg per ng/ml after the first dose of 1 mg to 8.7 mm Hg per ng/ml after 1 week of twice-daily therapy. Thereafter, no further loss of efficacy occurred over 12 weeks.

These agents do not alter plasma renin levels and may be useful in controlling the hypertension of patients who are undergoing dynamic tests of their renin-angiotensin system (Webb et al., 1987).

Efficacy and Dosage

These agents are effective in lowering the BP, equivalent overall to diuretics, beta-blockers, ACE inhibitors, and calcium blockers (Neaton et al., 1993; Carruthers et al., 1993). They work equally well in black and in nonblack patients (Batey et al., 1989) and in the elderly (Cheung et al., 1989) and can be effectively combined with a diuretic, beta-blockers, or calcium entry blockers (Schäfers and Reid, 1989). Prazosin is effective in more severe hypertensives (Ramsay et al., 1987) and in those with chronic renal failure (Lameire and Gordts, 1986). In the presence of renal failure, the hypotensive action is enhanced, so lower doses should be used.

The initial dose should be 1 mg, either at bedtime or on a morning when the patient may be relatively inactive, in case first-dose hypotension occurs. The daily dose should be slowly titrated upward to achieve the desired fall in pressure, with a total daily dose of up to 20 mg sometimes required. No tachyphylaxis to the antihypertensive action has been seen after 5 to 7 years of continual use of prazosin (Kincaid-Smith, 1987) or 3 years of doxazosin (Talseth et al., 1991). However, if reactive fluid retention occurs, the BP may rise, only to fall again with the addition of a small dose of diuretic.

Side Effects

Side effects include headache, drowsiness, fatigue, and weakness—likely nonspecific effects of a lowering of the BP. For most patients, the side effects diminish with continued therapy. Rarely, a first-dose response, with postural hypotension developing in 30 to 90 minutes, is seen, particularly in volume-depleted patients given the shorter-acting prazosin (Stokes et al., 1977). The problem generally can be avoided by initiating therapy with a small dose and making sure the patient is not volume-depleted as a result of diuretic therapy. Even massive overdoses do little harm if the patient remains supine (Rygnestad and Dale, 1983).

Ancillary Effects

Exercise. During isotonic exercise, $alpha_1$ blockers do not reduce performance as do beta blockers but, on the other hand, they will not reduce the exercise-associated rise in systolic pressure, as will beta blockers (Thompson et al., 1989). During isometric exercise, prazosin will suppress the pressor response better than will a beta blocker (Hamada et al., 1987).

Cardiac. In people with coronary disease, alpha$_1$ blockade may be either beneficial or harmful (Feigl, 1987). By limiting the vasoconstriction that is a normal part of the sympathetic activation that occurs during exercise or emotional stress, an alpha$_1$ blocker could improve coronary flow if the vasoconstriction is mainly at the stenotic segment but could worsen coronary flow if the vasoconstriction primarily involves small vessels beyond the stenosis.

Left ventricular hypertrophy has been shown to regress after prazosin therapy (Ram et al., 1989). This is not surprising since alpha$_1$ receptor stimulation is the molecular mediator of cardiac myocyte hypertrophy (Bishopric et al., 1987).

As a balanced arteriolar and venous dilator, prazosin may be a useful drug for treating refractory congestive heart failure (Boman et al., 1989), but tolerance usually develops.

Genital. The nonselective alpha$_1$ and alpha$_2$ blocker phentolamine has been widely used by injection directly into the penis to increase arterial inflow in patients with erectile impotence (Levine et al., 1989). No data are available as to whether oral alpha$_1$ blockers will have any such effect. On the other hand, selective alpha$_1$ blockers have been found to at least temporarily relieve most of the obstructive symptoms of benign prostatic hypertrophy (BPH), apparently by relaxing the tone of prostatic muscle (Guthrie, 1993; Kirby and Barry, 1993).

Lipid Effects. A generally favorable effect of alpha$_1$ blockers on blood lipid levels has been well established; usually observed are a decrease in total and LDL cholesterol and triglycerides and a rise in HDL cholesterol (Pool, 1991) (Fig. 7.16). In a 6-month study comparing prazosin and metoprolol, the mean difference in serum cholesterol at the end of the trial was about 15 mg/dl, or about 9% of the pretreatment value (Lithell et al., 1988). In a parallel study, both captopril and doxazosin induced significant decreases in total cholesterol, but an increase in HDL cholesterol was noted only with doxazosin (Ferrarra et al., 1993). In addition, doxazosin but not atenolol improved the activity of the fibrinolytic system over a 6-month trial (Jansson et al., 1991).

This favorable effect of an alpha$_1$ blocker (doxazosin) versus the detrimental effect of a beta blocker (atenolol) could have a significant impact on overall cardiovascular risk (Carruthers et al., 1993). The mechanisms responsible for these generally favorable effects may include

a decrease in fractional catabolic rate of HDL cholesterol (Sheu et al., 1990), an increase in lipoprotein lipase and lecithin-cholesterol acyltransferase (LCAT) (Rabkin, 1993) activity, and an inhibition of LDL oxidation (Chait and Gilmore, 1993).

Other Metabolic Effects. Alpha$_1$ blockers do not alter glucose tolerance in diabetics (Feher et al., 1990). In obese normoglycemic hypertensives, prazosin improved the disappearance rate of glucose during an intravenous glucose tolerance test and reduced both the peak and the total insulin response (Pollare et al., 1988). Lithell (1991) has reported an improvement in insulin sensitivity with both prazosin and doxazosin. In view of the hyperinsulinemia noted in both obese and nonobese hypertensives described in Chapter 3, this could add to the antihypertensive effect of the drugs.

Other Agents

Trimazosin and Alfuzosin. These drugs, also structurally related to prazosin, may lower the BP by direct arteriolar dilation in addition to alpha$_1$ blockade (Van Kalken et al., 1986; Leto di Priolo et al., 1988).

Indoramin. Also similar in structure and effect to prazosin, indoramin has been introduced for clinical use in numerous places outside the United States. It differs from prazosin in having a direct effect on the heart, reducing contractile force and rate, and it may cause more sedation and other central effects (Holmes and Sorkin, 1986).

Beta-Adrenergic Receptor Blockers

For many years, beta-adrenergic blocking agents were the second most popular antihypertensive drugs after diuretics (Fig. 7.4). Though they are no more effective than other antihypertensive agents and may on occasion induce serious side effects, they are generally well tolerated, and they offer the special advantage of relieving a number of concomitant diseases. In view of their proved ability to provide secondary cardioprotection after an acute myocardial infarction, it was hoped that they would provide special primary protection against initial coronary events as well. As detailed in Chapter 5, this hope remains unfulfilled: when compared with a diuretic in middle-aged patients, no significant difference between the two drugs in protecting against coronary mortality was noted in two large trials (Medical Research Council Working Party, 1985; Wilhelmsen et al., 1987),

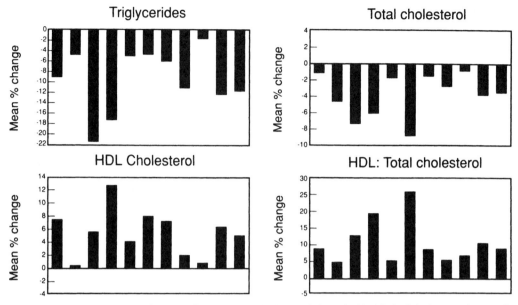

Figure 7.16. Mean percentage of change of lipoproteins with doxazosin in 11 double-blind, clinical comparison studies. (From Pool JL, Taylor AA, Nelson EB. Effects of doxazosin on serum lipids: a review of the clinical data and molecular basis for altered lipid metabolism. *Am J Med* 87[Suppl 2A]:57–61, 1989.)

although half of the patients in the latter trial who received the beta blocker metoprolol did have a lower coronary death rate than did those on a diuretic (Wikstrand et al., 1991). In the MRC trial in the elderly (MRC Working Party, 1992), the beta blocker was significantly less effective than the diuretic in protecting against coronary disease.

Nonetheless, a large number of new beta blockers are being developed with multiple claims of superiority over currently available ones. Although most of these claims remain unproved (Fitzgerald, 1991), they surely will stimulate renewed interest about this class of antihypertensive drugs.

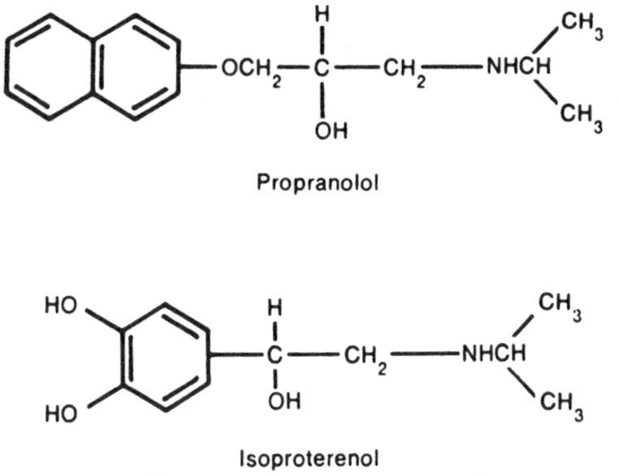

Background

These agents are chemically similar to beta agonists and to each other (Fig. 7.17). Powell and Slater reported in 1958 that the substitution of chlorine for hydroxyl groups on isoproterenol blocked the depressor and vasodilator effects of the beta agonist. Shortly thereafter, Moran and Perkins (1958) showed that dichloroisoproterenol (DCI) blocked adrenergic stimulation of the heart and coined the term "beta-adrenergic blocking drug." DCI also had sympathomimetic effects, so when James Black began his search for drugs that would block only the adrenergic receptors, a series of other compounds were synthesized (Black and Stephenson, 1962). Propran-

Figure 7.17. Structure of propranolol and the beta agonist isoproterenol.

olol was synthesized in 1963, described first in 1964 (Black et al., 1964), shown to be effective in treatment of hypertension that same year (Prichard and Gillam, 1964), and marketed in England in 1965. The time from first animal testing to clinical availability in England took a remarkably short 2 2/3 years.

Since then a large series of similar drugs have been synthesized, about 20 marketed throughout the world (12 in the United States), and another 30 are under investigation (Fitzgerald, 1991). They differ in a number of ways, some having clinical significance, others probably irrelevant. The various beta blockers can be conveniently classified by their relative selectivity for the beta$_1$

receptors (primarily in the heart) and presence of intrinsic sympathomimetic activity (ISA), also referred to as partial agonist activity (PAA) (Fig. 7.18).

Mode of Action

The competitive inhibition of beta blockers on beta-adrenergic activity produces numerous effects on functions that regulate the BP, including a reduction in cardiac output, a diminution of renin release, perhaps a decrease in central sympathetic nervous outflow, a presynaptic blockade that inhibits catecholamine release, and a probable decrease in peripheral vascular resistance.

The traditional view was that the primary effect is a reduction in cardiac output by 15% to 20%, resulting from the blockade of cardiac $beta_1$ receptors, thereby reducing both heart rate and myocardial contractility (Frohlich et al., 1968). This view has been challenged, in part because of studies with a pure $beta_2$ blocking agent (ICI 118551) without $beta_1$ (cardiac) blocking action that produces an antihypertensive effect comparable to propranolol (Vincent et al., 1987). However, others do not find that this agent lowers BP (Robb et al., 1988), so the issue remains unsettled. Moreover, the hemodynamic effects appear to change over time, as documented by two groups of investigators who have examined the acute and chronic effects of multiple beta blockers (Lund-Johansen and Omvik, 1991; van den Meiracker et al., 1988, 1989).

Acute. van den Meiracker et al. examined the hemodynamic changes during the first 24 hours after administration of four beta blockers with disparate characteristics: (*a*) acebutolol:

$beta_1$-selective with moderate ISA, (*b*) atenolol: $beta_1$-selective, no ISA, (*c*) pindolol: nonselective with strong ISA, and (*d*) propranolol: nonselective, no ISA (van den Meiracker et al., 1988). The BP fell quickest after pindolol, which induced no fall in cardiac output (CO) nor any rise in systemic vascular resistance (SVR) (Fig. 7.19). With the other three drugs, the fall in BP was a bit delayed, during which time CO fell and SVR rose. This hemodynamic profile is the one generally provided as the mode of action for the antihypertensive action of beta blockers. Note, however, what followed after 3 to 4 hours with the three agents without strong ISA: CO returned to normal and SVR fell to below normal.

The authors conclude that ''the most important hemodynamic change during the onset of the hypotensive action of β-adrenoceptor antagonists is vasodilation. . . .'' It is the ability of these drugs to interfere with sympathetic vasoconstrictor nerve activity that is likely responsible for their BP-lowering efficacy.

Chronic. Man in't Veld et al. (1988) reviewed the literature on acute and chronic hemodynamic changes with beta blockers, covering 85 studies on 10 drugs in a total of 912 patients, and observed a fairly uniform pattern: cardiac output usually fell acutely (except with high-ISA pindolol) and remained lower chronically; peripheral resistance, on the other hand, usually rose acutely but universally fell toward if not to normal with time (Fig. 7.20). Despite these adaptations, patients on beta blockers have persistently impaired vasodilation in response to exercise or epinephrine (Lenders et al., 1988).

Plasma Catechols. Despite the probable adaptation of peripheral resistance, plasma cate-

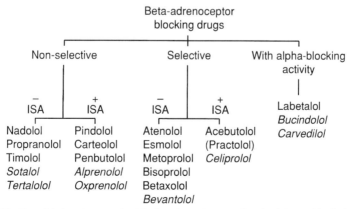

Figure 7.18. Classification of beta-adrenoceptor blockers based on cardioselectivity and intrinsic sympathomimetic activity *(ISA)*. Those not approved for use in the United States are in italics.

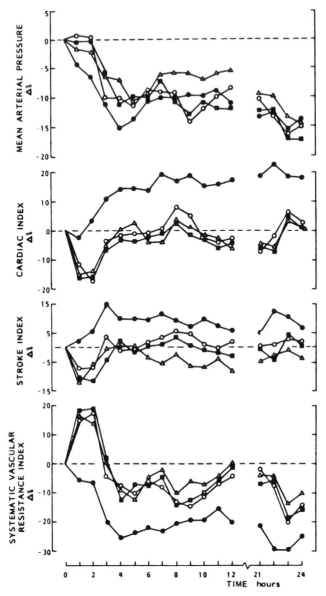

Figure 7.19. Plots of time course of percentage of changes in systemic hemodynamics after the first oral doses of either acebutolol (■), atenolol (Δ), pindolol (●), or propranolol (○). First oral dose was given at time 0. (From van den Meiracker AH et al. Hemodynamic and hormonal adaptations to β-adrenoceptor blockade. A 24-hour study of acebutolol, atenolol, pindolol, and propranolol in hypertensive patients. *Circulation* 78:957, 1988.)

cholamine levels are increased after beta blockade (Rosen et al., 1990); this reflects a reduction in the clearance of both epinephrine and norepinephrine from the circulation during beta blockade (Esler et al., 1981), as well as some baroreflex-mediated activation of the sympathetic nervous system.

Renin Release. Renin levels usually fall promptly after beta blocker therapy, presumably

reflecting the beta₂-receptor mediation of renin release. Some found a close correlation between the falls in renin and BP (Bühler et al., 1972), whereas others did not (Woods et al., 1976).

Pharmacologic Differences

Three major differences have an impact on the clinical use of beta-blockers: lipid solubility, cardioselectivity, and intrinsic sympathomimetic activity (Table 7.6). The first of these helps determines the duration and constancy of action. The latter two help determine the pattern of side effects. In clinical practice, none of these seem to affect antihypertensive efficacy or the side effect profile in a major way (Fitzgerald, 1991).

Lipid Solubility. Beta blockers have varying degrees of lipid solubility. Those that are more lipid-soluble (lipophilic) tend to be taken up and metabolized extensively by the liver (Fig. 7.21). As an example, with oral propranolol and metoprolol, up to 70% is removed on the first pass of portal blood through the liver. The bioavailability of these beta blockers is therefore less after oral than after intravenous administration.

Those such as atenolol and nadolol, which are much less lipid-soluble (lipophobic), escape hepatic metabolism and are mainly excreted by the kidneys, unchanged. As a result, their plasma half-life and duration of action are much longer, and they achieve more stable plasma concentrations. In addition, they enter the brain less and may thereby cause fewer CNS side effects (Yudofsky, 1992).

Cardioselectivity. All currently available beta blockers antagonize cardiac beta$_1$ receptors competitively, but they vary in their degree of beta$_2$-receptor blockade in extracardiac tissues. However, there seems to be little difference in antihypertensive efficacy among those that are more or less cardioselective (Fitzgerald, 1991).

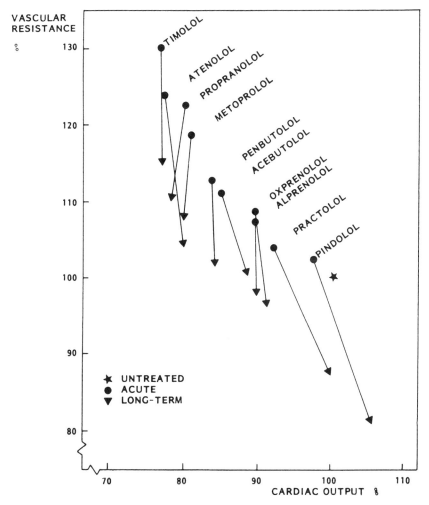

Figure 7.20. Hemodynamic interrelationships during acute (●) and a long-term (▼) beta blockade in hypertension. The *asterisk* indicates the situation before treatment. (From Man in't Veld AJ, Van den Meiracker AH, Schalekamp MA. Do beta-blockers really increase peripheral vascular resistance? Review of the literature and new observations under basal conditions. *Am J Hypertens* 1:91, 1988a.)

Table 7.6. Pharmacologic Properties of Some Beta Blockers

Drug	U.S. Trade Name	Cardio-selectivity	Intrinsic Sympathomimetic Activity	Membrane Stabilizing Activity	Lipid Solubility	Usual Daily Dose (mg)
Acebutolol	Sectral	+	+	+	+ +	200–1200
Alprenolol	Aptin	−	+ +	+	+ + +	400
Atenolol	Tenormin	+	−	−	−	25–100
Betaxolol	Kerlone	+	0	0	−	5–40
Bisoprolol	Zebeta	+	0	0	+ +	5–20
Carteolol	Cartrol	−	+	0	−	2.5–10
Carvedilol	BM 14190	−	0	+ +	+ +	50–100
Celiprolol	Selectol	+	+	0	−	200–400
Esmolol	Brevibloc	+	0	0	−	25–300 μg/kg/min/I.V.
Labetalol	Normodyne, Trandate	−	+	0	+ + +	200–1200
Metoprolol	Lopressor, Toprol	+	−	+	+ + +	50–200
Nadolol	Corgard	−	−	−	−	20–240
Oxprenolol	Trasicor	−	+ +	+	+ + +	60–480
Penbutolol	Levatol	−	+	+	+ + +	20–80
Pindolol	Visken	−	+ + +	+	+ +	10–60
Propranolol	Inderal	−	−	+ +	+ + +	40–240
Sotalol	Betapace	−	−	−	−	160–640
Timolol	Blocadren	−	−	−	+ + +	20–40

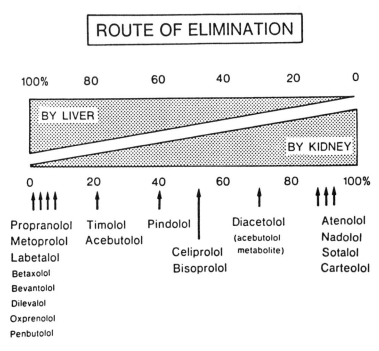

Figure 7.21. Relative degree of clearance by hepatic uptake and metabolism (liver) and renal excretion (kidney) of 10 beta-adrenoceptor-blocking agents. The differences largely reflect differences in lipid solubility, which progressively diminishes from left to right. (From Meier J. β-adrenoreceptor–blocking agents. *Cardiology* 64[Suppl 1]:1–13, 1979 and by permission of S. Karger AG, Basel.)

The major issue revolves around the protection from various side effects that might be anticipated from lesser degrees of beta$_2$-receptor blockade in bronchi, peripheral vessels, and pancreas.

The assumption that an agent with relative cardioselectivity is automatically preferable to one that is less so must be tempered by these considerations:

—No beta blocker is purely cardioselective, particularly in large doses;

—No tissue contains exclusively only one subgroup of receptors: the heart has both, with beta$_1$ predominating; bronchioles have both, with beta$_2$ predominating. Furthermore, the number of cardiac beta$_2$ receptors increases after beta$_1$ blockade (Kaumann, 1991);

—When high endogenous catechol levels are needed, as during an attack of asthma, even minimal degrees of beta$_2$ blockade from a cardioselective drug may cause trouble (Breckenridge, 1983). Similarly, some decrease in respiratory function has been recorded even with bisoprolol, the most cardioselective of beta blockers (Haffner et al., 1992);

—Side effects may reflect not only a beta$_2$ blockade of peripheral vasodilation, but also beta$_1$-mediated falls in cardiac output and limb blood flow.

Nonetheless, cardioselective agents have some advantages. For instance, they have been shown to disturb lipid and carbohydrate metabolism less than nonselective agents, and they will allow diabetics on insulin to raise the blood sugar more rapidly in the event of a hypoglycemic reaction (Clausen-Sjöbom et al., 1987).

On the other hand, in the presence of certain concomitant diseases, such as migraine and tremor, a nonselective beta$_2$ antagonist effect may be preferable. Also, beta$_2$ receptors are involved in stress-induced hypokalemia, so nonselective agents will block this fall in plasma K^+ more than selective ones will (Brown et al., 1983). This could have clinical relevance since stress-induced hypokalemia could cause sudden death.

Intrinsic Sympathomimetic Activity. Of the beta blockers now available in the United States, pindolol and, to a lesser degree, acebutolol have ISA or PAA, implying that even in concentrations that fully occupy the beta receptors, the biologic effect is less than that seen with a full agonist. When background sympathetic activity is low, the partial agonist acts as an agonist; when background activity is high, the partial agonist acts as an antagonist (Cruickshank, 1990).

The presence of intrinsic sympathomimetic activity may be clinically reflected in various beneficial features: less bradycardia, less bronchospasm, less decrease in peripheral blood flow, and less derangement of blood lipids (Fitzgerald, 1991a; Lithell et al., 1992). Moreover, cardiac output is well maintained during exercise with the high-ISA drug pindolol compared with propranolol (Ades et al., 1989). Whereas this could improve exercise performance and achievement of conditioning, it limits the reduction in systolic pressure obtained with non-ISA beta blockers.

Efficacy

Beta blockers have been proposed as initial monotherapy for younger and middle-aged hypertensives, especially white males, and in patients with myocardial ischemia and high levels of stress (Cruickshank, 1992).

Relation to Renin Status. A paradoxic rise in pressure was noted in 11% of low-renin patients given a beta blocker (Drayer et al., 1976), probably reflecting the combination of fluid retention and alpha-adrenergic–mediated peripheral and renal vasoconstriction that occurs in the face of beta$_2$-receptor blockade in the vascular bed. In patients with normal or high renin levels, the inhibition of renin by the beta blocker probably counteracts both of these antagonistic actions.

Claims of lesser response to beta blockers also have been made for two groups of patients who tend to have lower renin levels—blacks and the elderly. The evidence showing a lesser response for blacks is persuasive and uniform (Saunders et al., 1990). However, the claim made by Bühler et al. (1982) that the elderly are less responsive seems to be invalid (Materson et al., 1993).

Dosage

Most beta blockers have a flat dose-response curve, as has been demonstrated for propranolol: the response to 40 mg twice daily was equal to that found with 80, 160, or 240 mg twice daily (Serlin et al., 1980). With atenolol, 25 mg/day was as effective as 50, 75, or 100 mg (Marshall et al., 1979).

A combination of low doses of bisoprolol and 6.25 mg of HCTZ (Ziac) has been approved for first-line therapy with the anticipation of fewer side effects (DeQuattro and Weir, 1993).

In the usual doses prescribed (Table 7.6), various beta blockers have equal antihypertensive efficacy (Davidson et al., 1976; Wilcox, 1978). However, they may not all provide full 24-hour lowering of the BP, which may be particularly critical in protecting against early morning cardiovascular catastrophes. Metoprolol blunted this rapid early morning rise, but atenolol and pindolol did not (Raftery and Carrageta, 1985). Neutel et al. (1990) found a similar lack of 24-hour effect with once-daily atenolol but a sustained effect with acebutolol. Moreover, twice-daily doses of ''cardioselective'' agents may preserve their cardioselectivity better than once-daily large doses (Lipworth et al., 1991).

Lipid-insoluble agents are removed mainly by renal excretion and have relatively longer serum half-lives. In patients with renal insufficiency, higher blood levels are seen with usual doses, so lower doses should be given (McAnish et al., 1980).

Choice of Beta Blocker

In various clinical situations, preference may be given to beta blockers with certain characteristics (Table 7.7). For the majority of patients with uncomplicated hypertension, considering all of these pharmacologic and clinical features, there seems to be some advantage in choosing a relatively cardioselective, lipid-insoluble agent with ISA (such as celiprolol) to provide the certainty of prolonged action and the likelihood of fewer side effects. In the future, beta blockers that also have a vasodilatory effect (e.g., carvedilol or celiprolol) may be especially favored (McAreavey et al., 1991).

Special Uses for Beta Blockers in Hypertensives.

Coexisting Coronary Disease. The antiarrhythmic and antianginal effects of beta blockers make them especially useful in hypertensive patients with coexisting coronary disease (Ardissino et al., 1991). On the other hand, patients with variant angina due to coronary spasm may have their problem made worse with noncardioselective beta blockers, apparently from direct $beta_2$ vascular effects (Hodgson et al., 1989).

A beneficial effect of beta blockers in patients with acute myocardial infarction (MI), both intravenously for acute intervention and orally for chronic use, has been clearly documented (Hampton, 1990). The benefit has been seen with both hydrophilic and lipophilic agents (Lewis, 1992). In a prolonged follow-up of one of the many trials, the benefit of beta blockers after acute MI persisted after 12 months in those who were at high risk for various reasons, but not in those at low risk (Viscoli et al., 1993).

Table 7.7.   Situations Affecting the Choice of Beta Blocker

	Condition	Relative Contraindication	If Used, Type of Beta Blocker Preferred
Cardiac	Left ventricular failure	Almost always	High ISA[a]
	High-degree heart block	Almost always	High ISA
	Severe bradycardia	Often	High ISA
	Variant (Prinzmetal's) angina	Usual	High ISA
	Angina	None	Little ISA
Peripheral vascular	Severe claudication	Almost always	Cardioselective, high ISA (small dose)
Pulmonary	Bronchospasm, asthma	Always	
	Chronic airways disease	Often	Cardioselective (small dose)
Central nervous	Severe depression	Usual	Lipid-insoluble
	Difficult sleep, dreams	Rare	Lipid-insoluble
	Fatigue	Rare	Lipid-insoluble
	Migraine	None	Noncardioselective
Diabetes mellitus	Insulin-requiring	Often	Cardioselective
	Non–insulin-requiring	Rare	Cardioselective
Lipid disorders	High triglycerides Low HDL cholesterol	Often	High ISA
Liver disease		Rare	Lipid-insoluble
Renal disease		Rare	Lipid-soluble

[a]ISA, intrinsic sympathomimetic activity.

Congestive Heart Failure. Although beta blockers have generally been contraindicated in patients with congestive heart failure, those with dilated cardiomyopathy may be helped, particularly by low doses of beta blockers with vasodilatory effects (Persson and Erhardt, 1991).

Patients Needing Antihypertensive Vasodilator Therapy. When used alone, direct vasodilators set off reflex sympathetic stimulation of the heart. The simultaneous use of beta blockers prevents this undesired increase in cardiac output, which not only bothers the patient but also dampens the antihypertensive effect of the vasodilator.

Patients with Hyperkinetic Hypertension. Some hypertensive patients have increased cardiac output that may persist for many years. Beta blockers should be particularly effective in such patients, but a reduction in exercise capacity may restrict their use in young athletes.

Patients with Marked Anxiety and Stress. The somatic manifestations of anxiety—tremor, sweating, and tachycardia—can be reduced with beta blockers, which has been found useful for violin players, surgeons, race-car drivers, and sufferers from phobias and panic attacks (Tyrer, 1988; Ekeberg et al., 1990). This extends to patients with the alcohol withdrawal syndrome (Horwitz et al., 1989) or undergoing day surgery (Mackenzie and Bird, 1989). Atenolol protected patients with acute head injury from stress-induced cardiac damage (Cruickshank et al., 1987).

Other Conditions. Beta blockers may be useful in patients with migraine, intention tremor, or glaucoma.

Side Effects

The side effects of beta blockers reflect the blockade of both $beta_1$ and $beta_2$ receptors. The more cardioselective beta blockers would be expected to induce fewer $beta_2$ effects, and this has been noted (Fodor et al., 1987) (Fig. 7.22). In Fodor et al.'s single-blind study of 52 hypertensive patients who had a past history of side effects with beta blocker therapy, three 8-week courses of beta blocker therapy were given in doses needed to control the BP. The first course was with propranolol (40 to 160 mg twice daily), the second with atenolol (50 to 100 mg once daily), and the third with the previously used dose of propranolol. Most side effects were more common with the nonselective lipid-soluble propranolol, and most recurred with a similar frequency on rechallenge with that drug.

Central Nervous System. As noted in Figure 7.22, CNS side effects—insomnia, nightmares, depressed mood—occur in some patients, though probably less frequently with $beta_1$-selective agents (Dahlöf and Dimenäs, 1990). However, the association between beta blockers and depression has been accounted for by various confounding variables (Bright and Everitt, 1992). In a review of 55 published studies, beta blocker use was found to worsen cognitive function in 17%, improve cognitive function in 16%, and have no significant effect in the rest (Dimsdale et al., 1989).

Carbohydrate Metabolism. Diabetics may have additional problems with beta blockers. The responses to hypoglycemia—both the symptoms and the counter-regulatory hormonal changes that raise the blood sugar—are largely mediated by epinephrine, particularly in those who are insulin-dependent since they usually are also deficient in glucagon. If these patients became hypoglycemic, the beta blockade of epinephrine responses delays the return of the blood sugar. The more cardioselective beta blockers are preferable for those susceptible to hypoglycemia (Clausen-Sjöbom et al., 1987), but all beta blockers may delay recovery. Moreover, hypoglycemia reactions may precipitate a marked rise in BP (Ryan et al., 1985). The only symptom of hypoglycemia may be sweating, which may be enhanced in the presence of a beta blocker (Molnar et al., 1974).

Those diabetics not on insulin may become more hyperglycemic when given a beta blocker, but much more so when they are also given a diuretic (Dornhorst et al., 1985).

The larger population of nondiabetic hypertensives may be at a higher risk for developing diabetes when treated with beta blockers. In 9- to 12-year follow-ups of patients on beta blockers, the relative risk for developing diabetes was 4 to 6 times greater for them than for patients not on antihypertensive drugs (Skarfors et al., 1989; Bengtsson et al., 1992). The effect may reflect insulin resistance: metoprolol and atenolol given for 16 weeks, and pindolol and propranolol given for 6 months, significantly inhibited glucose uptake mediated by insulin; the insulin resistance was accompanied by higher plasma insulin levels (Pollare et al., 1989c; Lithell et al., 1992).

Lipid Metabolism. Beta blockers without ISA raise serum triglycerides and lower HDL cholesterol with little effect on total LDL cholesterol (Lardonis and Neuman, 1988; Vyssoulis et

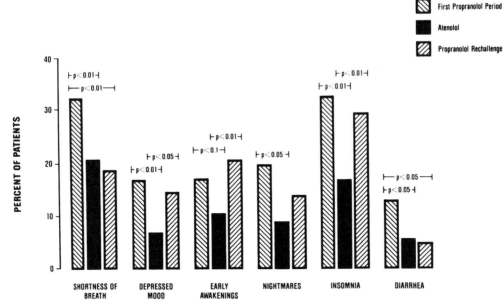

Figure 7.22. Overall incidence rates of side effects during 8 weeks of treatment with propranolol and atenolol (N = 52) (ANOVA). (From Fodor JG, Chockalingam A, Drover A, Fifield F, Pauls CJ. A comparison of the side effects of atenolol and propranolol in the treatment of patients with hypertension. *J Clin Pharmacol* 1987;27:892–901.)

al., 1992). The effects are lessened with cardioselective agents and generally are not seen with agents having ISA activity (e.g., pindolol) or vasodilatory effects (e.g., celiprolol) (Fig. 7.23).

Two mechanisms have been proposed: an effect on hepatic lipoprotein synthesis and interference with lipoprotein catabolism (Lijnen et al., 1992), likely related to reduced lipoprotein lipase activity (Lithell et al., 1992). The problems may arise from a decrease in peripheral blood flow since they are not seen with agents that cause vasodilation. This hypothesis is supported by the finding of increased peripheral production of HDL cholesterol during exercise, interpreted as a reflection of an increased delivery of substrates for lipoprotein lipase through the increased muscle blood flow (Ruys et al., 1989). Peripheral vasoconstriction induced by non-ISA beta blockers could then be reflected in lower peripheral HDL production.

In whatever manner these changes arise, chromium supplements, 200 mg 3 times a day, completely corrected them (Roeback et al., 1991).

Pulmonary. As many as half or more asthmatic patients will develop bronchospasm when given propranolol (Benson et al., 1978). With a cardioselective agent, fewer will get into trouble, and if they do, they can respond better to inhaled beta agonist. Patients with chronic obstructive

pulmonary disease will usually tolerate beta blockers well, but again, a $beta_1$-selective agent is preferred (Lammers et al., 1985).

Renal Function. Although chronic use of propranolol was shown to reduce glomerular filtration rate and renal blood flow, no such falls in renal function were noted in patients given atenolol or nadolol (Bauer, 1985). Renal dysfunction is rarely seen, even in those who have underlying renal insufficiency (Epstein and Oster, 1985).

Potassium. A slight rise in serum potassium may be seen with chronic use of beta blockers (Traub et al., 1980). During exercise, the rise may be even greater (Carlsson et al., 1978). These effects likely reflect blockade of the $beta_2$-mediated epinephrine activation of the Na^+,K^+–ATPase pump that normally transports potassium from extracellular fluid into cells (Rosa et al., 1980). As noted earlier, during stress, plasma K^+ may fall as much as 1.0 mmol/ L; the effect can be blocked by $beta_2$-receptor blockade.

In addition, the beta-blocker suppression of renin release could reduce the secondary aldosteronism seen with diuretic therapy. Despite this, beta-blocking therapy may not protect against diuretic-induced hypokalemia (Steiness, 1984).

Calcium Metabolism. After 6 months on propranolol, patients experienced an increase in plasma-ionized calcium and phosphate levels and a decrease in parathyroid hormone (PTH) levels (Hvarfner et al., 1988). This pattern was attributed to reduced calcium binding to albumin, increasing ionized calcium, which suppresses PTH.

Exercise Capacity. Beta blockers will reduce the ability to perform exercise, in part because of the more rapid onset of the feeling of fatigue and the subjective perception that exercise is harder to perform, which may arise more from central than from peripheral mechanisms (Cooper et al., 1988). In addition, beta$_2$ blockade interferes with circulatory and metabolic responses to exercise (Gullestad et al., 1991). Nonetheless, conditioning can be attained (Chick et al., 1988), probably more easily with cardioselective agents (Ades et al., 1990). High-ISA drugs (e.g., pindolol) allow maintenance of normal cardiac output but do not appear to maintain exercise tolerance any better than non-ISA drugs (e.g., propranolol) (Duncan et al., 1990).

Despite these problems with performance, beta blockers are considered the drugs of choice for suppressing excessive rises in BP during isotonic exercise. They may not do so well in suppressing the rise during isometric exercise (Hamada et al., 1987).

Impotence. Impotence has been noted with beta blockers, as with all antihypertensive agents. In the MRC trial, the frequency of impotence elicited by a questionnaire increased from 10.1% among those on placebo to 13.2% for those on propranolol (Medical Research Council Working Party, 1981).

Peripheral Circulation. Despite reports of vasospastic symptoms in the hand (Eliasson et al., 1984), an analysis of all 11 randomized, controlled trials of beta blockers in patients with peripheral vascular disease found no evidence of worsening of intermittent claudication (Radack and Deck, 1991).

Skin and Connective Tissue. Practolol, the only beta blocker to possess an acetanilide structure, is the only one to cause a serious and progressive oculomucocutaneous syndrome (Wright, 1975).

Despite isolated case reports, there appears to be no causal connection between beta blockers and retroperitoneal fibrosis (Pryor et al., 1983).

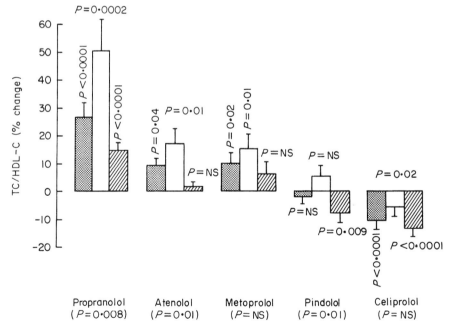

Figure 7.23. Percentage of change in the ratio of total cholesterol to HDL cholesterol after 6 months of beta blocker monotherapy with propranolol, atenolol, metoprolol, pindolol, and celiprolol. Values are given as mean ± SEM. *Stipled bars,* all patients; *white bars,* normolipidemic patients (baseline LDL-C < 160 mg. dl⁻¹); *hatched bars,* dyslipidemic patients (baseline LDL-C ≥ 160 mg. dl⁻¹). (From Vyssoulis GP, et al. Differentiation of β-blocker effects on serum lipids and apolipoproteins in hypertensive patients with normolipidaemic or dyslipidaemic profiles. *Eur Heart J* 13:1506–1513, 1992.)

Psoriasis has been worsened by beta blockers (Savola et al., 1987).

Discontinuation Syndromes. In hypertensives taking beta-adrenergic blockers, abrupt cessation may lead to withdrawal symptoms suggestive of sympathetic overactivity (Houston and Hodge, 1988). However, the more frequent and serious discontinuation syndrome is seen in patients with underlying coronary artery disease who may experience angina, infarction, or sudden death (Psaty et al., 1990). These ischemic episodes likely reflect the phenomenon of supersensitivity: an increased number of beta receptors appear in response to the functional blockade of receptors by the beta blocker; when the beta blocker is discontinued and no longer occupies the receptors, the increased number of receptors are suddenly exposed to endogenous catecholamines, resulting in a greater beta agonist response for a given level of catechols. Hypertensives, with a high frequency of underlying coronary atherosclerosis, may be particularly susceptible to this type of withdrawal syndrome; thus, when the drugs are discontinued, their dosage should be cut by half every 2 or 3 days, and the drugs should be stopped after the third reduction.

Overdose. Massive intoxication of beta blockers may cause profound hypotension, seizures, and coma, which are usually responsive to appropriate beta agonist therapy (Halloran and Phillips, 1981). Membrane stabilizing activity (MSA), a pharmacologic property usually given little attention, may be responsible for the higher rate of deaths from overdoses of drugs that have MSA (e.g., propranolol) than from those that do not (e.g., atenolol) (Henry and Cassidy, 1986).

Drug Interactions (Table 7.8). Most of the interactions listed in Table 7.8 relating to interference with metabolism are of little clinical significance, although smokers have been found to respond less well to beta blockers than to diuretics. Interactions related to beta blockade may be serious, including potentiation of side effects of antiarrhythmic drugs and hypotension with calcium antagonists or alpha blockers. Other interactions lead to pressor reactions: in addition to the reaction noted during hypoglycemia, serious hypertension may occur when exogenous sympathomimetics (diet pills, nose drops) are ingested.

Alpha and Beta-Receptor Blockers

Modification of the conventional beta blocker structure has provided agents with combined

Table 7.8. Selected Drug Interactions with Beta Blockers

Possible situations for decreased antihypertensive effects

NSAIDs may decrease effects of beta blockers

Rifampin, smoking, and phenobarbital decrease serum levels of agents primarily metabolized by liver because of enzyme induction

Possible situations of increased antihypertensive effects

Cimetidine may increase serum levels of beta blockers that are primarily metabolized by liver because of enzyme inhibition

Quinidine may increase risk of hypotension

Effects of beta blockers on other drugs

Combinations of diltiazem or verapamil with beta blockers may have additive sinoatrial and atrioventricular node depressant effects and may also promote negative inotropic effects on failing myocardium

Combination of beta blockers and reserpine may cause marked bradycardia and syncope

Beta blockers may increase serum levels of theophylline, lidocaine, and chlorpromazine because of reduced hepatic clearance

Nonselective beta blockers prolong insulin-induced hypoglycemia and promote rebound hypertension because of unopposed alpha simulation; all beta blockers mask adrenergically mediated symptoms of hypoglycemia and can aggravate diabetes

Beta blockers may make it more difficult to control dyslipidemia

Phenylpropanolamine (which can be obtained over the counter in cold and diet preparations), pseudoephedrine, ephedrine, and epinephrine can cause elevations in blood pressure though unopposed alpha-receptor–induced vasoconstriction

From Joint National Committee. The fifth report of the Joint National Committee on detection, evaluation, and treatment of high blood pressure (JNC V). *Arch Intern Med* 1993;153:154–183.

alpha- and beta-blocking properties. Labetalol is now available; others are being investigated, including carvedilol (Lund-Johansen et al., 1992) and amosulalol (Ando et al., 1992), whereas others that looked promising (medroxalol, dilevalol, prizidilol) have been withdrawn. The following relates only to labetalol.

Pharmacology

Oral labetalol is rapidly absorbed, is lipid-soluble, undergoes first-pass metabolism in the liver, and is about 33% bioavailable (Goa et al., 1989). Bioavailability increases with the patient's age because of decreased clearance of the drug. When administered with food, the bioavailability may be increased by a third, but at the same time absorption is slowed so that the time of maximal drug concentration increases from 1 hour after intake to 3 hours.

Mode of Action

Labetalol is a nonselective beta$_1$- and beta$_2$-receptor blocker and is, like prazosin, highly selective for alpha$_1$ receptors. The ratio of alpha- to beta-blocking action has been estimated as between 1:3 and 1:7. The ratio may fall with increasing plasma concentrations because the upper plateau of the dose-response curve for beta blockade may be reached at lower plasma concentration, whereas maximal alpha blockade may not occur until plasma concentrations are much higher (Goa et al., 1989).

The hemodynamic consequences of the combined alpha and beta blockade are a fall in BP, mainly via a fall in systemic vascular resistance, with little effect on cardiac output (Opie, 1988a) (Fig. 7.24). Note the distinct hemodynamic differences between classic beta blockers and labetalol. Its effect on supine BP is comparable to that of a beta blocker, but its effect on standing BP is greater.

With chronic therapy, renal vascular resistance and forearm resistance are reduced. Coronary blood flow is slightly decreased but less so than with conventional beta blockers. Left ventricular diastolic filling improves more than with beta blockers (Dianzumba et al., 1990).

Acutely, plasma renin activity (PRA) decreases and then rises, whereas norepinephrine levels increase. Chronically, PRA is decreased, plasma aldosterone is unchanged, and catechol levels remain elevated (Weidmann et al., 1978). Weidmann et al. reported increased urinary excretion of catecholamines, but this has subsequently been found to be a chemical interference and not a true increase in excretion. As a result, diagnostic confusion may arise if workup for pheochromocytoma is done while the patient is on labetalol (see Chapter 12).

Efficacy and Dosage

Given orally in doses of 200 to 1200 mg a day, labetalol is effective in patients with mild to severe hypertension; when given twice daily, it maintains good 24-hour control and blunts early morning surges in pressure (DeQuattro et al., 1988). It is more effective than atenolol in black hypertensives (Townsend et al., 1990a) and provides an even greater effect in the elderly than in younger patients because of decreased

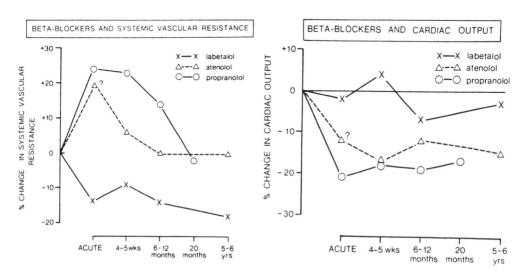

Figure 7.24. *Left,* Systemic vascular resistance (or SVR index) after acute therapy, after approximately 1 month of therapy, after 6 to 12 months, and after 5 to 6 years of therapy with labetalol, atenolol, or propranolol. Data obtained from multiple studies. *Right,* Cardiac output (or cardiac index) for same groups as at left. (From Opie LH. Role of vasodilation in the antihypertensive and antianginal effects of labetalol: implications for therapy of combined hypertension and angina. *Cardiovasc Drugs Ther* 2:369, 1988.)

clearance (Abernethy et al., 1987). During exercise, both heart rate and BP are reduced, so it may be a good choice in patients with concomitant coronary disease (Feit et al., 1991). Although fluid retention may develop when labetalol is used alone, requiring a diuretic (Weidmann et al., 1978), labetalol is effective in patients with chronic renal insufficiency (Innes et al., 1992).

Labetalol has been used both orally and intravenously to treat hypertensive emergencies including postoperative hypertension (Lebel et al., 1985) and acute aortic dissection (Grubb et al., 1987). It has been successfully used to treat hypertension during pregnancy (Pickles et al., 1992).

Side Effects

In a multicenter trial, 22% of 128 patients withdrew from therapy with labetalol because of side effects (New Zealand Hypertension Study Group, 1981). Symptomatic orthostatic hypotension, the most common side effect, is seen most often during initial therapy when large doses are used or during hot weather. A variety of other side effects has been seen including intense scalp itching, ejaculatory failure (Goa et al., 1989), and bronchospasm (George et al., 1985). An increased titer of antinuclear and antimitochondrial antibodies develops in some patients; although a systemic lupus syndrome has not been reported, lichenoid skin eruptions have been (Goa et al., 1989).

Perhaps the most serious side effect is hepatotoxicity: at least three deaths have been reported (Clark et al., 1990). As a result, a warning has been added to its label in the United States, stating: ''Hepatic injury may be slowly progressive despite minimal symptomatology. Appropriate laboratory testing should be done at the first symptom or sign of liver dysfunction.''

In keeping with its alpha-blocking effect, labetalol does not adversely alter blood lipids, as do conventional beta blockers (Lardinois and Neuman, 1988).

VASODILATORS

Direct Vasodilators

Drugs that enter the vascular smooth muscle cell to cause vasodilation are termed *direct* vasodilators. This is in contrast to those that vasodilate in other ways—by inhibiting hormonal vasoconstrictor mechanisms (e.g., ACE inhibitors), by preventing calcium entry into the cells that initiate constriction (e.g., calcium entry

blockers), or by blocking alpha receptor–mediated vasoconstriction (e.g., alpha$_1$-blockers). The various vasodilators differ considerably in their power, mode of action, and relative activities on arteries and veins (Table 7.9).

Hydralazine (Apresoline)

Hydralazine was introduced in the early 1950s (Freis et al., 1953) but was little used because of its activation of the sympathetic nervous system. Its use increased in the 1970s when the rationale for triple therapy—a diuretic, an adrenergic inhibitor, and a direct vasodilator—was demonstrated (Zacest et al., 1972). However, its use receded again with the advent of the newer vasodilating drugs that simultaneously block sympathetic activity. Today, despite its apparent ability to lower lipid levels (Perry and Schroeder, 1955) and to unload the left ventricle (Chatterjee et al., 1980), it is used, as is minoxidil, relatively infrequently, almost always as the third agent in triple therapy of severe hypertension.

Pharmacology. One of several phthalazine derivatives with hypotensive action, hydralazine is the only one approved for use in the United States. Hydralazine is well absorbed from the gut; a maximal blood level is reached in an hour; and the plasma half-life is 2 to 3 hours, although it can persist for up to 24 hours, and it remains even longer within the walls of muscular arteries (Talseth, 1976a). In patients with impaired renal function, the plasma half-life is greatly prolonged, perhaps because of a decrease in both renal clearance and metabolic conversion (Talseth, 1976b).

The inactivation of hydralazine involves acetylation in the liver by the enzyme N-acetyltransferase. The level of this enzyme activity is genetically determined, and rapid acetylators require

Table 7.9. Vasodilator Drugs Used to Treat Hypertension

Drug	Relative Action on Arteries (A) or Veins (V)
Direct	
Hydralazine	A >> V
Minoxidil	A >> V
Nitroprusside	A + V
Diazoxide	A > V
Nitroglycerin	V > A
Calcium entry blockers	A >> V
Angiotensin converting enzyme	
inhibitors	A > V
Alpha blockers	A + V

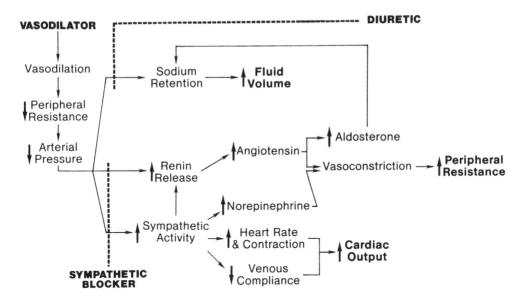

Figure 7.25. Primary and secondary effects of vasodilator therapy in essential hypertension and the manner by which diuretic and beta-adrenergic blocker therapy can overcome the undesirable secondary effects. (From Koch-Weser J. Vasodilator drugs in the treatment of hypertension. *Arch Intern Med* 1974;133:1017–1027, copyright 1974, American Medical Association.)

larger doses to achieve an equivalent effect than do slow acetylators (Ramsay et al., 1984). Perry (1973) showed that patients who develop a lupus-like toxicity tend to be slow acetylators and thus are exposed to the drug longer.

Mode of Action. In a manner that remains uncertain (Vidrio, 1990), the drug acts directly to relax the smooth muscle in the walls of peripheral arterioles, the resistance vessels more so than the capacitance vessels, thereby decreasing peripheral resistance and BP (Saxena and Bolt, 1986).

Compensatory Responses. Coincidental to the peripheral vasodilation, the heart rate, stroke volume, and cardiac output rise, reflecting baroreceptor-mediated reflex increase in sympathetic discharge (Lin et al., 1983) and direct stimulation of the heart (Khatri et al., 1977). In addition, the sympathetic overactivity and the fall in BP increase renin release (Eggertsen and Hansson, 1985), further counteracting the vasodilator's effect and likely adding to the reactive sodium retention that accompanies the fall in pressure (Fig. 7.25).

Efficacy. These compensatory responses sharply limit the use of hydralazine by itself. Furthermore, the average reduction in BP with 200 mg of hydralazine per day plus a thiazide was only 11/12 mm Hg, but when reserpine

(0.25 mg twice daily) was added, the hypotensive effect of the three agents was superior to that of any two, producing an average BP reduction of 23/21 mm Hg (VA Cooperative Study, 1962). More recently, a beta blocker usually is combined with hydralazine and a diuretic in the treatment of more severe hypertension (Eggertsen and Hansson, 1985) (Fig. 7.25).

In older patients, with less responsive baroreceptor reflexes, hydralazine may lower the BP without causing sympathetic overactivity (VA Cooperative Study Group, 1981b).

NSAIDs such as indomethacin attenuate the hypotensive action of hydralazine (Cinquegrani and Liang, 1986).

Dosage. Alone or in combination, hydralazine should usually be started at 25 mg 2 times per day, since the good and bad effects are similar at two doses to what they are for four doses daily (O'Malley et al., 1975). The maximal dose, although often stated as 400 mg, should probably be limited to 200 mg per day for two reasons: to lessen the likelihood of a lupus-like syndrome, and because higher doses seldom provide additional benefit. In one study, when hydralazine was added to therapy with a diuretic and a beta blocker, 50 mg twice daily gave as much antihypertensive effect as did 100 or 200 mg twice daily (Vandenburg et al., 1982).

Side Effects. Three kinds of side effects are seen: those due to reflex sympathetic activation, those due to a lupus-like reaction, and nonspecific problems. Headaches, flushing, and tachycardia should be anticipated and prevented by concomitant use of adrenergic inhibitors. The drug should be given with caution to patients with coronary artery disease and should be avoided in patients with a dissecting aortic aneurysm or recent cerebral hemorrhage, in view of its propensity to increase cardiac output and CBF (Schroeder and Sillesen, 1987).

Lupus-Like Reaction. The reaction has been described by Perry (1973), reviewing his experience with 371 patients given the drug for as long as 20 years. An early, febrile reaction resembling serum sickness was seen in 11 patients; late toxicity developed in 44 (with serious symptoms in 14), resembling systemic lupus erythematosus or rheumatoid arthritis. These symptoms almost invariably went away when therapy was stopped or the dosage was lowered. This late toxicity occurred only among the half of the population who were slow acetylators of the drug. Though Perry noted that remissions of serious hypertension may occur more frequently and overall survival may be better among patients who develop toxicity (Perry et al., 1977), rapidly progressive renal damage has been reported (Sturman et al., 1988).

The syndrome is clearly dose-dependent. In a prospective study of 281 patients, the syndrome did not occur in those taking 50 mg daily, whereas it occurred in 5.4% taking 100 mg daily and in 10.4% taking 200 mg daily (Cameron and Ramsay, 1984). The incidence was fourfold higher in women than in men, and 19.4% of women taking 200 mg daily developed the syndrome. The incidence of a positive antinuclear antibody titer of 1:20 or higher was even greater, found in 50% of patients taking hydralazine, of whom only 3% developed the lupus syndrome (Mansilla-Tinoco et al., 1982).

Other Side Effects. These include anorexia, nausea, vomiting, diarrhea and, less commonly, paresthesias, tremor, and muscle cramps. An additional potential disadvantage of hydralazine and other direct vasodilators is their failure when given alone to regress left ventricular hypertrophy, presumably because of their marked stimulation of sympathetic nervous activity (Leenen et al., 1987).

Despite these multiple problems, in routine clinical use, serious morbidity and mortality were no more common in patients taking hydralazine than in patients taking methyldopa (Franks et al., 1991).

Lipid Effects. One seldom-considered advantage of hydralazine is that it usually *lowers* serum cholesterol, as noted in 1955 (Perry and Schroeder, 1955) and later reconfirmed (Lopez et al., 1983). These authors noted a fall in LDL and a rise in HDL cholesterol levels with hydralazine. The same beneficial lipid effects have been noted with minoxidil (Johnson et al., 1986).

Minoxidil (Loniten)

More potent than hydralazine, minoxidil has become a mainstay in the therapy of severe hypertension associated with renal insufficiency (see Chapter 9). Its propensity to grow hair precludes its use in many women, but this effect has led to its use as a topical ointment for male pattern baldness. Some of the topical drug is absorbed: slight but significant increases in left ventricular (LV) end-diastolic volume, cardiac output, and LV mass have been recorded after use of topical minoxidil for 6 months (Leenen et al., 1988).

Pharmacology. A piperidinopyrimidine derivative, minoxidil is well absorbed, and peak plasma levels are reached within 1 hour (Pettinger, 1980). Though its plasma half-life is only 4 hours, antihypertensive effects persist for about 24 hours, and it can be used once daily (Johnson et al., 1986). It is metabolized in the liver, and the inactive glucuronide is excreted mainly in the urine.

Mode of Action. Minoxidil induces smooth muscle relaxation by modulating potassium channels in vascular smooth muscle, a mechanism apparently unique among vasodilators currently available in the United States but similar to the mode of action of various potassium channel openers (e.g., pinacidil) available elsewhere (Duty and Weston, 1990).

Compensatory Reactions. Since it is both more potent and longer lasting than hydralazine, it is not surprising that minoxidil turns on the various reactions to direct arteriolar vasodilation to an even greater degree. Therefore, large doses of potent loop diuretics and adrenergic blockers will be needed in most patients.

Efficacy and Dosage. Minoxidil is effective when used with diuretics and adrenergic inhibitors, controlling more than 75% of patients previously resistant to multiple drugs (MacKay et al., 1981). However, its propensity for reactive fluid retention often precludes the use of even small doses of minoxidil as a third drug in the treatment of more moderate hypertension (West-wood et al., 1986). It can be given once daily in a range of 2.5 to 80 mg.

Side Effects.   Very rarely, profound hypotension may follow the initial dose (Allon et al., 1986). The most common side effect, seen in about 80% of patients, is hirsutism, beginning with fairly fine hair on the face and then with coarse hair increasing everywhere, including the external ear canal to the extent of causing hearing loss (Toriumi et al., 1988). It is apparently related to the vasodilation of the drug and not to hormonal effects. The hair gradually disappears when the drug is stopped, sometimes leaving less than before the drug was started (Kidwai and George, 1992).

Beyond generalized volume expansion, pericardial effusions appear in about 3% of patients who receive minoxidil (Martin et al., 1980). Since most of these patients had severe renal disease, many of whom were on dialysis, it is difficult to ascribe the effusion specifically to minoxidil.

Two other prior concerns about cardiopulmonary side effects have not been substantiated. Right atrial fibrotic lesions, noted in dogs given massive doses of minoxidil, have not been described in humans (Sobota et al., 1980). Pulmonary hypertension has been reported, but this likely reflects the presence of high pulmonary vascular resistance before minoxidil was administered (Atkins et al., 1977). On the other hand, despite good control of hypertension with triple therapy including minoxidil, left ventricular size often continues to enlarge (Chrysant et al., 1991).

Other Direct Vasodilators

A number of other potassium channel openers are available elsewhere (Duty and Weston, 1990). Of these, pinacidil has been more extensively studied (Friedel and Brogden, 1990). Other direct vasodilators currently under study include flosequinan (Lewis et al., 1989), endralazine (Wu et al., 1986), and cadralazine (McTavish et al., 1990).

Nitrates, both transdermal nitroglycerin (Simon et al., 1986) and oral isosorbide (Pannier et al., 1990), by their vasodilating properties akin to endothelium-derived relaxing factor, can also be used as antihypertensives.

Intravenous direct vasodilators, in particular diazoxide and nitroprusside, are considered in the next chapter.

Calcium Entry Blockers

These drugs, here referred to as calcium entry blockers (CEBs), were called *calcium antagonists* by their leading advocate and developer, the late German physiologist Albrecht Fleckenstein (1990). First reported to lower BP in 1962 (Heidland et al., 1962), they were introduced as antianginal agents in the 1970s and as antihypertensives in the 1980s. Included among the recommended choices for initial monotherapy in the 1988 and 1993 Joint National Committee (JNC-V) reports, they are widely advocated as "first-line" therapy for hypertension (Cummings et al., 1991; Bühler, 1992).

Pharmacology

These agents include some that are related to papaverine (verapamil), others that are dihydropyridines (nifedipine), and others that are benzothiazepines (diltiazem) (Fig. 7.26). In the last few years, a number of other dihydropyridines, most having less inotropic effects than nifedipine, have been introduced. The three major classes of CEBs not only differ in their molecular structure, their sites and modes of action on the slow calcium channel, and their effects on various other cardiovascular functions, but the sensitivities of various vascular tissues to them also differ (Iwanov and Moulds, 1991); there are major pharmacologic differences between the various dihydropyridines as well (Kelly and O'Malley, 1992). Therefore, although all of the CEBs approved for the treatment of hypertension obviously are effective in lowering the BP, they differ in their ancillary effects, duration of action, and side effect profile.

Mode of Action

The CEBs lower the BP by interfering with calcium-dependent contractions of vascular smooth muscle, thereby producing a fall in peripheral vascular resistance (Wysocki et al., 1992). The dihydropyridines are the most powerful in relaxing peripheral vascular smooth muscles and thereby are more likely to activate baroreceptor reflexes that lead to an increase in plasma catecholamines and heart rate (Opie, 1988b). The negative chronotropic effects of verapamil and diltiazem may block this reflex sympathetic stimulation and result in a decreased heart rate (Table 7.10).

Most of the newer dihydropyridines display relative "vasoselectivity"—that is, more peripheral vasodilation and increasingly less cardiac effect on either rate or contractility (Parm-

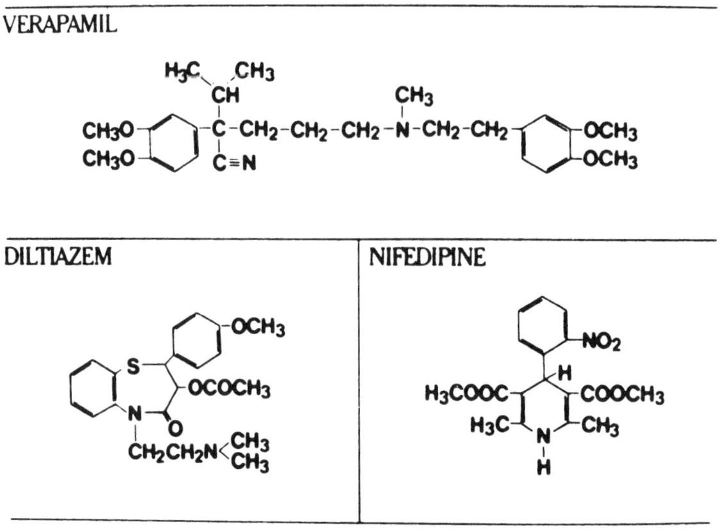

Figure 7.26. Structure of three calcium antagonists.

Table 7.10. Pharmacologic Effects of Calcium Entry Blockers[a]

	Diltiazem	Verapamil	Dihydropyridines
Heart rate	↓	↓	↑ −
Myocardial contractility	↓	↓↓	↓ −
Nodal conduction	↓	↓↓	−
Peripheral vasodilation	↑	↑	↑↑

[a]↓, decrease, ↑, increase, −, no change.

ley, 1990). As a result, unlike other CEBs, amlodipine has been found to improve the exercise capacity of patients with mild-to-moderate congestive failure, likely because it reduced the level of sympathetic activity (Packer et al., 1991).

The blockade of voltage-sensitive slow channels by CEBs may affect multiple vasoconstrictor mechanisms (Nelson et al., 1990). The dihydropyridine nicardipine, but not verapamil or diltiazem, provides functional alpha antagonism, which is demonstrated by blockade of the vasoconstrictor effect of norepinephrine (Pedrinelli et al., 1989; 1991). CEBs decrease vascular (and adrenal) responsiveness to angiotensin II (Donati et al., 1992) and induce a mild natriuresis (Krishna et al., 1991) that may contribute to their antihypertensive action.

Efficacy

The currently available CEBs seem comparable in their antihypertensive potency (Opie, 1988b), although no direct comparisons have been made between them. They have been used alone, in combination with other agents, and

in the treatment of refractory hypertension and hypertensive crisis (Kaplan, 1989b). In patients inadequately controlled on two drugs (i.e., a diuretic and an ACE inhibitor), the addition of a CEB (nifedipine) usually provided satisfactory control (Cummings et al., 1991). Caution is advised against combining either diltiazem or verapamil with a beta blocker because of the potential for arteriovenous conduction problems (Opie, 1987).

Determinants of Efficacy.

Age. Bühler and coworkers (1982) found the response to calcium antagonists used alone to be directly and strongly related to the age and pretreatment renin levels of the patient: the older the patient and the lower the PRA, the better the response, which is opposite the response seen with beta blockers. Whereas CEBs are usually effective in the elderly (Materson et al., 1993), the majority of published reports that compared younger with older patients and that provide actual data on the degree of reduction of BP fail to document a significant difference (Kaplan, 1989a; Zing et al., 1991).

What some have noted as an apparently greater antihypertensive effectiveness of CEBs in the elderly may reflect the characteristically higher BP levels of the elderly and the more pronounced efficacy of CEBs as the level of BP increases (Donnelley et al., 1988). Elderly patients may appear to be more responsive because of pharmacokinetic changes that increase the bioavailability of various CEBs in the elderly, providing more active drug at any given dose than in younger patients (Kelly and O'Malley, 1992).

Race. Most comparisons have shown that blacks respond about as well to CEBs as do nonblacks, and better to CEBs than to ACE inhibitors or to beta blockers (Saunders et al., 1990; Materson et al., 1993).

Duration of Action. Initial experiences with these agents were obtained with formulations requiring two or three doses per day. Longer-lasting formulations are now available, along with other CEBs with inherently longer duration of action, such as amlodipine. The fall in BP, measured by ambulatory monitoring, is maintained throughout the 24 hours with three doses a day of the regular preparations, two doses a day of the sustained-release formulations of verapamil (Calan-SR, Isoptin-SR), and one dose a day of the newer formulations of diltiazem (Cardizem CD), nifedipine (Procardia XL), verapamil (Verelan), and amlodipine (Norvasc).

Additive Effect of Diuretic or Low Sodium Intake. As a corollary to the (unproven) thesis that CEBs are more effective in patients with lower renin levels, a decrease in the antihypertensive efficacy of these drugs has been claimed under two conditions wherein renin levels are raised: dietary sodium restriction (Valdés et al., 1982) and concomitant diuretic therapy (Magagna et al., 1986).

Numerous studies have examined these relationships. In general, the findings support the view that dietary sodium restriction may reduce (but not abolish) the antihypertensive effect of CEBs, whereas high sodium intake may enhance (or not diminish) their efficacy (Nicholson et al., 1987; Luft et al., 1991). Possible explanations for an enhanced antihypertensive action by CEBs with high sodium intake have been provided in studies on hypertensive rats. With sodium loading, the number of dihydropyridine receptors on cell membranes is increased (Garthoff and Bellemann, 1987), and inhibition of sympathetic activity by CEBs increases (Leenen and Yuan, 1992).

On the other hand, most but not all studies have shown an additional antihypertensive effect when diuretics are combined with CEBs. Although a few find no additive effect of the addition of a diuretic to a CEB (Cappuccio et al., 1991; Salvetti et al., 1991), the majority of well-controlled studies show an extra antihypertensive effect from the combination, greater than that seen with either drug alone (Burris et al., 1990; di Somma et al., 1990, Weir et al., 1992). The combination of a diuretic with a CEB has been shown to provide additive effects equal to those seen when a diuretic is added to a beta blocker (Thulin et al., 1991) or to an ACE inhibitor (Elliott et al., 1990).

Natriuretic Effects. Most published data, then, support an additive effect of diuretics when added to a CEB. Nonetheless, there is a rational explanation for a lesser potentiation by diuretics when added to CEBs than to other antihypertensive agents: the CEBs themselves are mildly natriuretic and, having shrunken the vascular volume, thereby would leave less room for additional action from a diuretic. This natriuretic effect has been amply demonstrated for various dihydropyridines (Chellingsworth et al., 1990), perhaps to a greater degree than with diltiazem or verapamil (Krishna et al., 1991). The increased excretion of sodium and water likely reflects the unique ability of CEBs, unlike other vasodilators, to maintain or increase effective renal blood flow, glomerular filtration rate (GFR), and renal vascular resistance (Reams and Bauer, 1990), which, in turn, has been attributed to their selective vasodilatory action on the renal afferent arterioles (Epstein, 1991).

Potential for Good or Bad Renal Effects. On the surface, this preferential vasodilation of afferent arterioles with increases in GFR, renal blood flow, and natriuresis appears to favor the use of CEBs as a way of maintaining good renal function. However, a large body of experimental data suggests that increased renal plasma flow and GFR may accelerate the progression of glomerulosclerosis (see Chapter 9). Increased glomerular perfusion, particularly in the face of systemic hypertension, is viewed as being responsible for the progressive loss of renal function once the process of nephron loss begins in the course of any type of renal disease (Brenner et al., 1988).

The effect of CEBs on renal function remains uncertain, both in experimental animals and in humans. The uncertainty is exemplified by two experimental studies using the same strain of rats who had renal damage produced in the same manner (i.e., by subtotal nephrectomy) and that were followed for 15 weeks on the same CEB, verapamil. Opposing results were found: Harris et al. (1987) found that verapamil provided excellent protection against progression of renal failure; Brunner et al. (1989) noted progressive glomerulosclerosis with verapamil but good protection with the ACE inhibitor enalapril.

The effects of CEBs on renal function in humans also is uncertain. CEBs are useful in protecting against acute ischemic injuries such as radiocontrast-induced acute renal failure and cyclosporine nephrotoxicity (Epstein, 1991). In diabetics with proteinuria, verapamil and diltiazem generally reduce the level of protein excretion, whereas nifedipine increases the level (Bakris, 1991). In hypertensive patients without renal insufficiency, isradapine had little effect on microalbuminuria (Persson et al., 1992). In those with renal insufficiency, nifedipine may induce at least short-term improvements in renal function (Reams et al., 1991), but there are a few reports of acute renal failure developing with CEB therapy (Eicher et al., 1988). Obviously, more information is needed about the long-term effects of CEBs in patients with renal insufficiency.

Cardiac Effects.

Coronary Vasodilation. CEBs were first made available as coronary vasodilators for the treatment of coronary artery disease (CAD) and are widely used for this purpose. Since many hypertensive patients also have CAD, the use of a CEB to treat both diseases is obviously rational and effective. For example, in patients with chronic stable angina, once-daily nifedipine as the extended-release (XL) preparation reduced the number of anginal attacks throughout the 24 hours, including the early morning hours (Parmley et al., 1992).

Cardioprotection. Beyond their unequivocal effects of improving myocardial blood flow while decreasing myocardial oxygen demand, CEBs have other features that suggest that they could protect patients from progression of CAD (i.e., cardioprotection). These include inhibition of endothelial hyperplasia and smooth muscle cell migration, prevention of intracellular calcium overload, and inhibition of platelet aggregation (Oparil and Calhoun, 1991). Moreover, CEBs have been found to be antiatherosclerotic in multiple animal models (van Zwieten, 1993). Studies in humans show that CEBs, particularly dihydropyridines, may inhibit the progression of

coronary atherosclerosis (Lichtlen et al., 1990; Waters et al., 1990). A large prospective study, the Multicenter Isradipine/Diuretic Atherosclerosis Study (MIDAS), may provide more definitive evidence (Furberg et al., 1993).

Despite these favorable features, dihydropyridine CEBs have not been found to be cardioprotective either during or after myocardial infarction (Yusuf et al., 1991). On the other hand, both diltiazem and verapamil have been shown to reduce recurrent episodes, particularly in patients with non–Q wave infarction (Boden, 1992).

There are no data on the effect of CEBs on primary prevention of CAD in patients with hypertension. The potential benefit of CEBs in this regard cannot be excluded even though they do not appear to provide secondary prevention after an acute infarction. Witness the reverse situation with beta blockers: they do provide secondary cardioprotection, but in three of four trials, they have not been shown to provide primary protection (see Chapter 5).

Left Ventricular Hypertrophy. Like most antihypertensive drugs, CEBs have been shown to reduce left ventricular mass and end-diastolic dimension (Dahlöf et al., 1992) without changing diastolic filling indices (Szlachcic et al., 1989).

Exercise. CEBs do not impair the cardiac response to exercise (Harrison et al., 1991) and are clearly superior to beta blockers in maintaining exercise capacity.

Use in Hypertensive Urgencies.

As noted in Chapter 8, liquid nifedipine in capsules has been widely used to quickly reduce BPs deemed to be so high as to need immediate relief (Bertel et al., 1983). Intravenous formulations of nicardipine and felodipine are under investigation, offering more controllable antihypertensive effect while maintaining cerebral blood flow (CBF) (Thulin et al., 1993).

Other Uses for CEBs.

Cerebrovascular Diseases. The dihydropyridine nimodipine (Nimotop) has been approved for relief of vasospasm in patients with subarachnoid hemorrhage (Pickard et al., 1989). Nimodipine was also found to improve neurologic outcome in men after an acute ischemic stroke (Gelmcrs et al., 1988).

Cardiovascular Diseases. Verapamil and, to a lesser degree, diltiazem have been widely used to treat supraventricular tachyarrhythmias, particularly reentrant A-V nodal tachycardias and to control the ventricular rate during atrial fibrillation (Opie, 1988b).

Verapamil improves diastolic filling, decreases gradients, and reduces myocardial oxygen demand in patients with hypertrophic cardiomyopathy (Opie, 1988b).

Other Diseases. Although not officially approved for the other uses listed in Table 7.11, CEBs have proven useful in the management of various conditions, most of them associated with muscular contraction.

Side Effects

Despite all of these real and potential advantages, side effects will preclude the use of these drugs in perhaps 15% of patients. Most side effects—headaches, flushing, local ankle edema—are related to the vasodilation for which the drugs are given. With slow-release and longer-acting formulations, vasodilatory side effects are reduced, but other symptoms may persist (Palmer et al., 1990). It should be no surprise that, in a few patients, the antihypertensive effect may be so marked as to reduce blood flow and induce ischemia of vital organs (O'Mailia et al., 1987). The side effects of the three major classes of CEBs differ considerably (Table 7.12).

Verapamil. Constipation is the most common side effect, and AV block the most serious one. To avoid conduction problems, the drug should generally be avoided in patients with sick sinus syndrome, second- or third-degree AV block, or congestive heart failure. In particular, patients with these conditions who are receiving beta blockers may develop symptomatic bradycardia and heart block if verapamil is added (Carruthers et al., 1989).

Table 7.11. Prospective Uses for Calcium Entry Blockers

Cardiovascular
  Migraine (Andersson and Vinge, 1990)
  Raynaud's phenomenon (Schmidt et al., 1989)
  Nocturnal leg cramps (Baltodano et al., 1988)
  Pulmonary hypertension (Rich et al., 1992)
  High altitude pulmonary edema (Bärtsch et al., 1991)
  Inhibit platelet activation (Addonizio, 1986)

Noncardiovascular
  Esophageal mortality disorders (Konrad-Dalhoff et al., 1991)
  Biliary or renal colic (Bortolotti et al., 1987)
  Epilepsy (Larkin et al., 1988)
  Asthma (Imhof et al., 1991)

Other drug interactions with verapamil include an increase in serum digoxin levels, a reduction in quinidine and cyclosporine clearance, and a decreased bioavailability of verapamil with enzyme-inducing drugs such as rifampin (Kirch et al., 1990).

Diltiazem. The incidence of both gastrointestinal symptoms and conduction problems is less with diltiazem, but this drug is best avoided in patients with the underlying conduction disturbances noted above with verapamil (Waller and Inman, 1989).

Dihydropyridines. Vasodilatory side effects are more common with the dihydropyridines but less so with the second generation of slower-release and longer-acting preparations. For example, headache was no more common with amlodipine than with placebo, and flushing was seen in only 2.4% of patients on the drug (Murdoch and Heel, 1991). On the other hand, dependent edema remains a relatively common problem, related to localized vasodilation and not generalized fluid retention. Interestingly, dependent edema was seen in 14.6% of women who took amlodipine but in only 5.6% of men (versus 5.1% and 1.4%, respectively, on placebo). If this condition bothers the patient, a diuretic will likely not help, and either a nondihydropyridine CEB or a drug from another class should be substituted.

Other Side Effects. Gingival hyperplasia has been noted, most commonly with nifedipine (Ellis et al., 1992). Eye pain, possibly due to ocular vasodilation, has been noted with nifedipine (Coulter et al., 1988). A wide spectrum of adverse cutaneous reactions, some quite serious, have been reported to occur rarely with various CEBs (Stern and Khalsa, 1989).

Overdoses usually are manifested by hypotension and conduction disturbances and can usually be overcome with parenteral calcium and sympathomimetics (Gay et al., 1986).

Other Potential Problems

Since calcium entry is involved in so many cellular functions, concerns have been voiced about other potential adverse effects of CEBs. Calcium metabolism seems little altered (Townsend et al., 1990b). The secretion of various hormones is not affected other than for a reduced adrenal steroid response to both ACTH and angiotensin (Favre et al. 1988; McDermott et al., 1990). Impotence seems rare, but 31 patients reportedly have developed gynecomastia (Tanner and Bosco, 1988).

Table 7.12. Relative Frequency of Side Effects of Calcium Entry Blockers

Effect	Verapamil	Diltiazem	Dihydropyridenes
Cardiovascular system			
Hypotension	+	+	+
Flush	+	−	+ +
Headache	+	+	+ +
Ankle edema	+	+	+ +
Palpitation	−	−	+
Conduction disturbances	+ +	+	−
Heart failure	+	−	(+)
Bradycardia	+ +	+	−
Gastrointestinal tract			
Nausea	+	+	+
Constipation	+ +	(+)	−

CEBs have no unfavorable effects on glucose homeostasis (Trost and Weidmann, 1987; Beer et al., 1993) and do not decrease insulin sensitivity (Pollare et al., 1989b). Unlike the disturbances often seen with diuretics and beta blockers, CEBs tend to have no effects on serum lipids (Lardinois and Neuman, 1988).

Drug Interactions

A problem noted with most other classes of antihypertensive drugs—interference from NSAIDs—may not be seen with CEBs, but only limited data are available (Baez et al., 1987; Morgan and Anderson, 1993).

Another interaction has been noted with the dihydropyridines felodipine and nifedipine: an increased plasma level and duration of action when taken along with grapefruit juice (Bailey et al., 1991). Most other drug interactions with CEBs are of little consequence (Kirch et al., 1990).

Overall Impression

The benefits so greatly outweigh the problems that it is no wonder that these agents have become major drugs for the treatment of various forms of hypertension. They rarely are contraindicated and often are recommended for the treatment of hypertensive patients with a variety of concomitant conditions. With the availability of formulations that are effective on a once or, at most, twice per day schedule, and with the continued publication of glowing reports of efficacy and relative safety of these drugs, their future continues to look promising.

Angiotensin-Converting Enzyme Inhibitors

As detailed in Chapter 3, there are four ways to reduce the activity of the renin-angiotensin system in humans (Fig. 7.27). The first way, the use of beta blockers to reduce renin release from the juxtaglomerular (JG) cells, has been widely used. The second way, the direct inhibition of the activity of renin, is being actively investigated with a variety of renin inhibitors. The third way to block the system is to inhibit the activity of the angiotensin-converting enzyme (ACE), which converts the inactive decapeptide angiotensin I to the potent hormone angiotensin II. These agents, referred to as ACE inhibitors, or ACEIs, are among the fastest-growing drugs used to treat hypertension. The fourth way is to use a competitive antagonist that attaches to angiotensin receptors but does not induce its cellular effects. Such an antagonist, saralasin, was available for a short time as a test for angiotensin-induced hypertension, and others are under investigation for the treatment of hypertension.

This section examines the use of ACEIs. Thereafter, the current status of both renin inhibitors and angiotensin receptor antagonists will be described. Although none are now approved for clinical use, a large number are under investigation (Ménard, 1992).

Pharmacology

After peptides from the venom of the Brazilian viper *Bothrops jararaca* were discovered to inhibit ACE (Ondetti et al., 1971), one, a nonapeptide (teprotide), was found to effectively lower the BP when used intravenously (Gavras et al., 1974). From study of the interaction of ACE and angiotensin, a model of the active site of the zinc-metalloprotein enzyme was developed, and potent, orally effective ACEIs were designed (Fig. 7.28) (Ondetti et al., 1977).

Three chemically different classes of ACEIs have been developed, classified by the ligand of

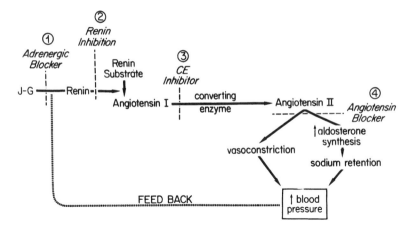

Figure 7.27. Renin-angiotensin system and four sites where its activity may be inhibited.

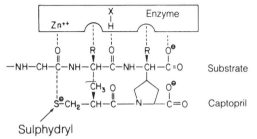

Sulphydryl

Figure 7.28. Hypothetical model of angiotensin-converting enzyme. (From Abrams WB, Davies RO, Gomez HJ. Clinical pharmacology of enalapril. *J Hypertens* 1984;2[Suppl 2]:31–36.)

the zinc ion of ACE: sulfhydryl, carboxyl, and phosphoryl (Table 7.13). Their different structures influence their tissue distribution and routes of elimination (Herman, 1992), differences that could alter their effects on various organ functions beyond their shared ability to lower the BP by blocking the circulating renin-angiotensin mechanism.

Pharmacokinetics. As seen in Table 7.13, most ACEIs are prodrugs, esters of the active compounds that are more lipid-soluble so that they are more quickly and completely absorbed. Captopril, an active drug, reaches a peak blood level within 30 to 60 minutes; enalaprilat, the active metabolite of enalapril, peaks at about 4 hours. Although there are large differences in bioavailability, these seem to make little difference in the clinical effects, likely because of the variable degrees of binding to ACE, tissue penetration, and elimination that contribute to the overall effects (Herman, 1992).

Most ACEIs, except fosinopril and spirapril, are eliminated through the kidneys, having undergone variable degrees of metabolism (Salvetti, 1990). Fosinopril has a balanced route of elimination, with increasingly more of the

Table 7.13. Characteristics of Angiotensin Converting Enzyme Inhibitors

Drug	U.S. Trade Name	Zinc Ligand	Pro-drug	Rate of Elimination	Duration of Action (hr)	Dose Range
Benazepril	Lotensin	Carboxyl	Yes	Renal	24+	10–40
Captopril	Capoten	Sulphydryl	No	Renal	6–10	25–150
Cilazapril	—	Carboxyl	Yes	Renal	24+	2.5–5.0
Enalapril	Vasotec	Carboxyl	Yes	Renal	18–24	5–40
Fosinopril	Monopril	Phosphoryl	Yes	Renal-hepatic	24+	10–40
Lisinopril	Prinivil, Zestril	Carboxyl	No	Renal	18–24	5–40
Perindopril	—	Carboxyl	Yes	Renal	24+	1–16
Quinapril	Accupril	Carboxyl	Yes	Renal	24+	5–80
Ramipril	Altace	Carboxyl	Yes	Renal	24+	1.25–20
Spirapril	—	Carboxyl	Yes	Hepatic	24+	12.5–50

drug removed through the liver as renal function decreases (Hui et al., 1991), so that no decrease in dose should be needed in the presence of renal impairment.

Pharmacodynamics. The pharmacodynamic behavior of ACEIs may be assessed in multiple ways, including changes in the circulating levels of ACE, angiotensin I and II, and renin; hemodynamics changes; and blockade of agonists. The multiple interactions between blood and tissue effects add up to a complicated model to explain the dynamic effects of these drugs (MacFadyen et al., 1991)

Mode of Action

As seen in Figure 7.29, the most obvious manner by which ACEIs lower the BP is to markedly reduce the circulating levels of angiotensin II (van den Meiracker et al., 1992), thereby removing the direct vasoconstriction induced by this peptide. At the same time, the activity of ACE within vessel walls and multiple tissues, including brain and heart, is inhibited, apparently to variable degrees by different ACEIs (Cushman et al., 1989).

Although the presence of the complete renin-angiotensin system within various tissues, including vessel walls, heart, and brain, is certain (Paul et al., 1992), the role of these tissue renin-angiotensin systems in pathophysiology remains uncertain, as does the contribution of inhibition of tissue ACE to the antihypertensive effects of ACEIs.

The reduction by ACEIs of circulating and tissue angiotensin II levels leads to multiple other effects beyond direct vasodilation—effects that likely contribute to their antihypertensive effect. These include:

—A decrease in aldosterone secretion (Gavras et al., 1977b) that may cause natriuresis or at least a lack of reactive renal sodium retention as the BP falls;
—Blunting of the expected increase in sympathetic nervous system activity typically seen after vasodilation (Giannattasio et al., 1992), an effect that may involve both a decrease in sympathetic activity and an increase in parasympathetic activity (Elliott et al., 1989a). As a result, heart rate is not increased and cardiac output does not rise, as is seen with direct vasodilators such as hydralazine.

Effects Other Than on Angiotensin II. ACEIs likely lower BP in ways beyond the inhibition of angiotensin II production. Captopril lowered the pressure in normotensive subjects, but the renin inhibitor Ro 42-5892 did not, despite equal inhibition of the renin-angiotensin system (Kiowski et al., 1992a).

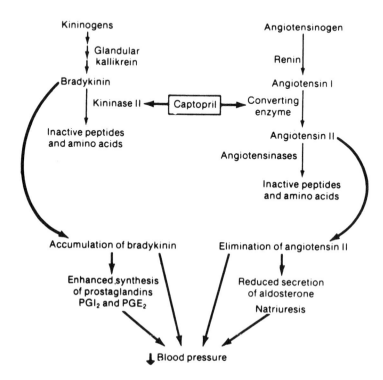

Figure 7.29. Mechanisms by which captopril may lower the blood pressure.

As shown in Figure 7.29, ACE is the same enzyme responsible for the breakdown of bradykinin, a vasodilatory peptide. The role of the presumably elevated levels of active bradykinin after ACEI administration remains uncertain (Gavras, 1992). In experimental models, blockade of endogenous bradykinin by a bradykinin-receptor antagonist blunts the antihypertensive effect of ACEI (Bao et al., 1992). At the least, high levels of bradykinin may be responsible for the frequent cough and rare angioneurotic edema seen with ACEI use.

Figure 7.29 also shows an enhanced synthesis of vasodilatory prostaglandins, presumably via activation by bradykinin of phospholipases that release the precursor arachidonic acid from membrane phospholipids. A role of these prostaglandins in the action of captopril has been suggested by a reduction in its antihypertensive efficacy when prostaglandin synthesis is blocked by the NSAID indomethacin (Quilley et al., 1987).

ACEIs may also lower BP by directly inhibiting vascular hypertrophy (Wang and Prewitt, 1990) and enhancing endothelium-dependent relaxation, as is seen in experimental models (Mombouli et al., 1991; Nakamura et al., 1992). The involvement of EDRF in the response to ACEIs in humans remains uncertain, some finding an improvement in acetylcholine-induced vasodilation after an ACEI (Hirooka et al., 1992), others reporting no effect (Kiowski et al., 1992b).

Ancillary Effects. Regardless of how ACEIs lower the BP, they do so in a manner that tends to protect the function of three vital organs—the heart, the brain, and the kidneys.

Cardiac. As for the heart, ACEIs provide multiple benefits:

—Regression of left ventricular hypertrophy to a greater degree than occurs with other classes of drugs (Dählof et al., 1992);
—Improvement in left ventricular diastolic function beyond that attributable to BP reduction (Zusman et al., 1992);
—Attenuation of sympathetic-mediated coronary vasoconstriction (Perondi et al., 1992) and relief of angina in some patients (van Gilst et al., 1992);
—Prevention of nitrate tolerance both by captopril and enalapril (Katz et al., 1991);
—Attenuation of progressive left ventricular dilatation in patients with low ejection fraction without (Yusuf et al., 1992) or with (Pfeffer et al., 1992) recent acute myocardial infarction accompanied by reductions in cardiac mortality, recurrent MIs, and congestive heart failure;

—Relief of congestive heart failure by altered remodeling and sustained reduction in preload and afterload (Konstam et al., 1992);
—In animal models, inhibition of atherosclerosis (Chobanian et al., 1992) even without affecting BP or plasma lipid levels (Schuh et al., 1993). However, cilazapril did not prevent restenosis after coronary angioplasty (Multicenter European Research Trial, 1992).

Cerebral. Cerebral blood flow is well maintained, and there may be a downward shift in the limits of autoregulation, likely as a result of dilation of large arteries (Torup et al., 1993). This may be responsible for the preservation of cerebral blood flow seen in patients with congestive heart failure given an ACEI (Paulson et al., 1986).

Renal. The kidneys may also be specially protected by the preferential vasodilatation of the efferent arterioles provided by reduction of angiotensin II. Thereby, renal blood flow is increased but, more importantly, intraglomerular pressure is simultaneously reduced. As will be further described in Chapter 9, this action of ACEIs may give them a unique protective effect in patients susceptible to progressive damage from glomerular hypertension, an effect that extends even to normotensive diabetics (Hallab et al., 1993). The amelioration of proteinuria and progressive renal failure by ACEIs almost certainly reflects additional nonhemodynamic effects, including an increased charge selectivity of the glomerular barrier (Erley et al., 1992).

Insulin Sensitivity. Beyond these potential benefits, various ACEIs have been shown to increase sensitivity to insulin and to lower plasma insulin levels (Pollare et al., 1989a; Paolisso et al., 1992). In view of the adverse implications of hyperinsulinemia described in Chapter 3, this could translate into another special advantage of ACEIs.

Differences Among ACEIs. Although some claim that distinct differences in tissue distribution and routes of elimination between various ACEIs may be reflected in different antihypertensive potencies and ancillary properties (Cushman et al., 1989), in most obvious ways all ACEIs seem quite alike. The most widely touted difference—the presence of a sulfhydryl-group in captopril—may be responsible for some additional effects, including scavenging of free radicals (Andreoli, 1993) and attenuating lipid peroxidation (Liu et al., 1992). Although more and more of the presumably unique effects of captopril are being found in ACEIs without a sulfhydryl group (Herman, 1992), in a large 24-week study, various QOL measures were improved with captopril but worsened with enalapril (Testa et al., 1993).

Efficacy

A rather remarkable turnabout has occurred in the few years since captopril was approved "only for use in patients with severe hypertension unresponsive to other agents." ACEIs are now included among the drugs recommended for initial monotherapy of patients with mild and moderate hypertension (Joint National Committee, 1993). This turnabout reflects the use of smaller doses, the recognition of equal efficacy but apparently fewer side effects than seen with other classes, and the potential for some special advantages not provided by other drugs now available.

Monotherapy.   An immediate fall in BP occurs in about 70% of patients given captopril, and the fall is sometimes rather precipitous (Postma et al., 1992). Such a dramatic fall is more likely in those with high renin levels, particularly if they are volume-depleted by prior dietary sodium restriction or diuretic therapy.

Black hypertensives, with lower renin levels as a group, have been found to respond less well to ACEIs than do white hypertensives (Saunders et al., 1990; Materson et al., 1993). On the other hand, elderly patients, who also tend to have lower renin levels, respond as well as do younger patients (Materson et al., 1993).

As expected, patients with high-renin forms of hypertension (i.e., renovascular hypertension) may respond particularly well to ACEIs, but the removal of angiotensin II's support of perfusion to the ischemic kidney may precipitously reduce renal function, particularly in those with bilateral stenoses (Hricik et al., 1993) (see Chapter 10). Patients with hypertension secondary to chronic renal parenchymal disease may also respond well (Opsahl et al., 1990), presumably because they have inappropriately high renin levels and because they retain more of the drug. Sublingual captopril is as effective as sublingual nifedipine in reducing severe hypertension (Angeli et al., 1991).

Combination Therapy.   The addition of a diuretic, even in as low a dose as 6.25 mg of hydrochlorothiazide, will enhance the efficacy of an ACEI (Andrén et al., 1983), normalizing the BP of another 20% to 25% of patients with mild to moderate hypertension more effectively than raising the dose of ACEI would (Townsend

and Holland, 1990). The marked additive effect of a diuretic likely reflects the ACEI blunting of the reactive rise of angiotensin II that usually occurs with diuretic use and that opposes the antihypertensive effect of the diuretic.

Use in Special Patients.   As noted under "Ancillary Effects," ACEIs may provide special benefits to patients with renal damage, either parenchymal or vascular, or various cardiac conditions, including CHF and following an acute myocardial infarction.

Congestive Heart Failure.   ACEIs are particularly useful in the treatment of heart failure, whether caused by hypertension or not, providing not only symptomatic relief but also prolonged survival for patients with CHF (SOLVD Investigators, 1992).

Peripheral Vascular Disease.   ACEIs improve walking distance in hypertensive patients with intermittent claudication (Cosenzi et al., 1992). However, caution in the use of ACEIs is needed in all patients with extensive atherosclerosis because of their higher prevalence of renovascular disease.

Pulmonary Disease.   Even though they may induce a persistent cough, ACEIs are generally safe in patients with asthma (Overlack et al., 1992).

Nonmodulating Hypertensives.   According to the findings described in Chapter 3, almost half of normal-renin hypertensives are not capable of modulating their adrenal and renal responses to volume and angiotensin II in a normal manner. This "nonmodulation" is corrected by an ACEI (Dluhy et al., 1989), suggesting a defect in adrenal and renal receptor or postreceptor responses to angiotensin II.

Dosage

Neither the degree nor the duration of the antihypertensive efficacy of ACEIs can be predicted by their effect on blood ACE or angiotensin II levels. Appropriate dose-response studies reveal that usually recommended initial doses of many may be excessive (Lees, 1992a). Despite careful observations, disagreement remains about the relative effectiveness of different ACEIs. For example, using ambulatory monitors in patients given once-daily doses, Conway et al. (1990) found that 10 mg of lisinopril was more effective than 10 mg of enalapril, but Enström et al. (1992) found equal efficacy from 20-mg doses of the two agents.

Captopril.   Initially, captopril was usually given in doses that are now known to be inordinately high, up to 300 mg 3 times per day. With more experience, doses have come down, particularly in the treatment of mild hypertensives. In the VA Cooperative Study (1984), the response was as good with 12.5 mg 3 times per day as with 25 mg or 50 mg 3 times per day. There is probably no need for using more than 150 mg per day.

The frequency of dosing may also be reduced. In the VA study (1984), 37.5 mg twice per day worked as well as the various doses given 3 times per day. Although some find that 50 to 100 mg of captopril once daily can provide 24-hour BP control, most prefer twice-a-day dosing (Pixley et al., 1989). A starting dose of 25 mg twice a day seems appropriate for most patients. Patients with renal insufficiency or CHF, or who are on prior diuretic therapy, should be started on less, as little as 6.25 mg.

Enalapril. The effect of small doses may not last for the full 24 hours (Pixley et al., 1989), so enalapril should probably be given twice daily. In a controlled study, very little additional response was noted when doses were increased from 10 to 40 mg/day (Salvetti and Arzilli, 1989).

Lisinopril and Others. These agents usually provide full 24-hour effectiveness with one dose per day (Table 7.13).

Side Effects

With large doses of captopril in patients with severe hypertension, many of whom also had renal insufficiency, a high incidence of side effects was reported following the drug's introduction. However, as smaller doses of drug have been used in patients with normal renal function, the incidence of side effects has fallen significantly. For example, the incidence of neutropenia was 7.2% in patients with collagen vascular disease and impaired renal function and 0.4% in patients with renal insufficiency from other causes, but only 0.02% in patients with normal renal function (Warner and Rush, 1988).

The recognized side effects of ACEIs logically can be divided into three types: (*a*) those anticipated from their specific pharmacologic actions, (*b*) those probably related to their chemical structure, and (*c*) nonspecific effects, as seen with any drug that lowers the BP.

The relative incidence of side effects may differ somewhat among the various ACEIs but, in general, they are fairly close. For example, lisinopril shares most, if not all, of the effects of other ACEIs (Cameron and Higgins, 1991).

However, with careful assessment of various QOL measures, equipotent doses of captopril and enalapril had opposite effects—captopril positive, enalapril negative (Testa et al., 1993).

Effects Anticipated from Pharmacologic Actions.

First Dose Hypotension. An immediate fall in mean arterial pressure of more than 30% was seen in 3.3% of 240 hypertensive patients given 25 mg of captopril (Postma et al., 1992).

Elevation of Plasma Potassium. The inhibition of angiotensin II–mediated aldosterone secretion blunts potassium excretion, particularly in patients with underlying renal insufficiency who are given potassium-sparing agents or potassium supplements (Rimmer et al., 1987).

Deterioration of Renal Function. With the very high doses of captopril used initially, an immune-complex glomerulopathy was reported (Hoorntje et al., 1980) but later was shown to reflect preexisting renal damage (Captopril Collaborative Study Group, 1982).

Most subsequent reports of acute loss of renal function concerned patients with renal artery stenoses, either bilateral or in a solitary kidney (Hricik et al., 1983). However, reversible renal insufficiency was noted in 8 of 42 patients without renovascular disease who had relative hypotension after an ACEI (Toto et al., 1991). Moreover, the loss of renal function may be irreversible, leading to acute and persistent renal failure (Devoy et al., 1992). Preexisting volume depletion and extensive atherosclerotic vascular disease potentiate the problem, which may also involve renal artery thrombosis.

Pregnancy. ACEIs are contraindicated in pregnancy because they cause fetal injury and death (Piper et al., 1992).

Blunting of Compensatory Responses to Volume Depletion. An increase in angiotensin II is a major compensatory homeostatic response to volume depletion. Although only isolated cases have been reported (McMurray and Matthews, 1987), the potential for marked hypotension with prerenal azotemia in ACEI-treated patients who experience gastrointestinal fluid loss or other types of volume depletion should be remembered.

Cough. Almost never reported initially, a dry, hacking, nonproductive, and often intolerable cough may be the most frequent side effect of ACEI therapy, reported in 5% to 20% of patients given one of these drugs (Israili and Hall, 1992). It may begin many months after starting any ACEI (Yeo et al., 1991), is more common among women, and may spontaneously disappear (Reisin and Schneeweiss, 1992). It is not accompanied by bronchospasm but may develop more frequently in patients with underlying bronchial hyperreactivity (Overlack et al., 1992). The mechanism for the cough may involve high levels of bradykinin arising from the inhibition of the ACE that is also responsible for the inactivation of kinins. For patients who must continue to take an ACEI, relief may be obtained by switching to fosinopril. If that fails, an NSAID such as indomethacin (Fogari et al., 1992) or sodium cromoglycate (Keogh, 1993) may be helpful.

Angioedema and Anaphylaxis. Angioedema occurs in 0.1% to 0.2% of patients given an ACEI, usually within hours (Israili and Hall, 1992) but sometimes after prolonged use (Chu and Chow, 1993). Anaphylactoid reactions have been seen during dialysis and apheresis in patients on ACEIs, presumably because of an inability to inactivate bradykinin generated by contact of blood with negatively charged surfaces (Olbricht et al., 1992).

Effects Related to Chemical Structure. These may be more common with captopril than with the nonsulfhydryl ACEIs, since most are also seen with other sulfhydryl-containing drugs such as penicillamine (Hammarström et al., 1991). Most, but not all, patients who experience one of these reactions while on captopril can be safely crossed over to enalapril (Jackson et al., 1988).

Taste Disturbance. Although usually of little consequence and self-limited with continued drug intake, taste disturbance may be so bad as to interfere with nutrition. It appears to be related to the binding of zinc by the ACEI (Abu-Hamdan et al., 1988).

Rash. The rash is usually a nonallergic, pruritic maculopapular eruption that appears during the first few weeks of therapy and may disappear despite continuation of the drug. Severe erythema and eczema may appear, possibly as an allergic reaction (Goodfield and Millard, 1985). Onycholysis has also been reported (Borders, 1986).

Leukopenia. This reaction probably occurs exclusively in patients with renal insufficiency (Cooper, 1983), particularly those with underlying immunosuppression either from a disease or from a drug. Though usually reversible, it may be fatal (El Matri et al., 1981).

Nonspecific Side Effects. ACE activity is present in intestinal brush border, and adverse gastrointestinal effects have been reported with ACEI use (Edwards et al., 1992). Other rare effects include pancreatitis (Roush et al., 1991) and cholestatic jaundice (Bellary et al., 1989). Schönlein-Henoch purpura has been reported after use of nonsulfhydryl ACEIs (Disdier et al., 1992).

ACEIs have no major effects on cognitive function (Bulpitt and Fletcher, 1992) and are "lipid neutral" (Lardinois and Neuman, 1988) or "positive" (Keilani et al., 1993), escaping some of the common side effects of other drugs. The improvement in insulin sensitivity observed with some ACEIs may be responsible for rare instances of hypoglycemia (Bell, 1992). Visual hallucinations occurred in two patients given ACEIs (captopril and enalapril) for CHF (Haffner et al., 1993). Headache, dizziness, fatigue, diarrhea, and nausea are listed in reviews but are seldom problems. Sudden withdrawal does not frequently lead to a rebound (Vlasses et al., 1981). Overdose causes hypotension that should be easily managed with fluids and, if needed, dopamine (Augenstein et al., 1988).

Perspective on the Use of ACEIs

Captopril, when first introduced for use in severe hypertensives and in very high doses, got a bad reputation that has quickly been overcome. Because they lead to far fewer side effects with small doses given to patients with good renal function, ACEIs are now recommended for the larger population of milder hypertensives, often for initial monotherapy.

In view of the apparent potential of ACEIs to provide special protection to the kidneys and heart, these drugs clearly will be used more often for the treatment of all degrees of hypertension. Meanwhile, other ways to inhibit the renin-angiotensin system are under investigation as perhaps the most promising of the many drugs for the future.

DRUGS UNDER INVESTIGATION

A large number of new agents are in various phases of study (Van Zwieten, 1992b). The ones that seem most likely to reach clinical use are mentioned briefly.

Other Renin-Angiotensin Blockers

As noted in Figure 7.27, ACE inhibitors are not the only blockers of renin-angiotensin system activity; it can be blocked either near the origin by renin inhibitors or near the final step by angiotensin II–receptor antagonists (Ménard, 1992).

Renin Inhibitors

Inhibitors of the action of renin to cleave the decapeptide angiotensin I from angiotensinogen include some that must be given intravenously, such as enalkiren (A-64662) (Cordero et al., 1991) and CGP 38560A (Chauveau et al., 1992); orally effective agents include Ro 42-5892 (Kobrin et al., 1993) and A-74273 (Verberg et al., 1993). These agents are attractive not only because they can inhibit the production of angiotensin I and II but because they also prevent the reactive rise in renin release that follows the use of ACE inhibitors and angiotensin II–receptor antagonists. Whether any will become available for clinical use remains to be seen.

Angiotensin II–Receptor Antagonists

The first of these agents to reach clinical use, saralasin, was limited by the need for intravenous administration and its pressor effect in low-renin patients resulting from its partial agonist effects (Case et al., 1976). Subsequently, the angiotensin II receptor has been shown to have at least two major subtypes, and agents have been developed that block each (Fig. 7.30).

At this time, the most promising agent that blocks the AT_1 receptor is a nonpeptide imidazole derivative, losartan (DuP 753) (Siegl, 1993), which has been shown to be an orally effective antihypertensive with an additional uricosuric action (Tsunoda et al., 1993). The ability of such an agent to block the pressor and other major actions of angiotensin II without increasing levels of bradykinin (Fig. 7.30) allows patients to escape the cough (Nelson et al., 1993) and other side effects of ACEIs that are attributed to bradykinin.

Neutral Endopeptidase Inhibitors

To provide the vasodilating and natriuretic action of atrial natriuretic peptide (see Chapter 3), inhibitors of the neutral endopeptidase (NEP) that is responsible for its inactivation—EC 34.24.11—have been developed (Richards et al., 1993). Among these, some also inhibit ACE (Dage et al., 1992). They may be particularly useful for patients with hypertension and heart failure.

Serotonin Antagonists

Ketanserin. 5-Hydroxytryptamine (5-HT), or serotonin, is a central and peripheral neuro-

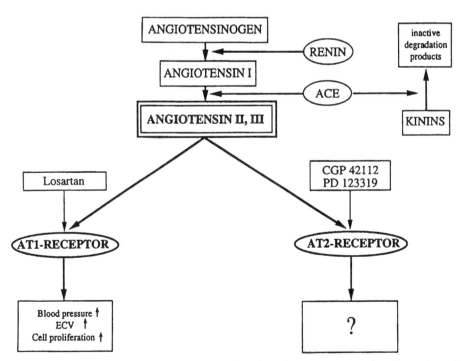

Figure 7.30. Different sites of action of ACE inhibitors and angiotensin receptor antagonists. The renin-angiotensin and kallikrein-kinin systems are linked through ACE. The physiologic responses mediated through angiotensin II by AT_2 receptor stimulation have not yet been described. (From Levens NR, de Gasparo M, Wood JM, Bottari SP. Could the pharmacological differences observed between angiotensin II antagonists and inhibitors of angiotensin converting enzyme be clinically beneficial? *Pharmacol Toxicol* 1992;71:241–249.)

transmitter that is involved in the regulation of BP. Ketanserin is a selective 5-HT$_2$ receptor antagonist with additional alpha$_1$-adrenergic receptor blocking effects that lowers the BP in humans (Robertson, 1990). Ketanserin likely will not be introduced as an antihypertensive in the United States because it prolongs the QT interval in the presence of diuretic-induced hypokalemia, an effect that could predispose to serious ventricular arrhythmias (Prevention of Atherosclerotic Complications with Ketanserin Trial Group, 1989).

Urapidil. This agent is thought to activate 5-HT$_{1A}$ receptors in the CNS, thereby decreasing the firing of serotoninergic neurons and reducing sympathetic nervous activity much like alpha$_1$-adrenergic receptor blockers do (van Zwieten, 1992b).

Dopamine Agonists. Dopamine, the precursor of norepinephrine, induces vasodilation and lowers the BP (Goldberg, 1974). Exogenous dopamine also acts on beta$_1$ receptors to stimulate the heart and on alpha$_1$ and alpha$_2$ receptors to cause vasoconstriction, so that it cannot be used to treat hypertension. Carmoxirole is a selective agonist for presynaptic peripheral DA$_2$-receptors that provides antihypertensive action by inhibition of noradrenaline release from sympathetic nerve endings (Haeusler et al., 1992).

The ergot derivative dihydroergotoxine has a modest antihypertensive effect that may be induced by a dopaminergic mechanism (Mercuro et al., 1992).

Adenosine Receptor Agonists. Adenosine has a direct vasorelaxant effect and inhibits neurotransmitter release. Adenosine agonists are effective in experimental animals, lowering BP while inhibiting renin release and causing a natriuresis (Taylor and Kaplan, 1989).

Potassium Channel Openers. Pinacidil, nicorandil, and cromakalim are representatives of drugs that vasodilate by opening potassium channels and enhancing potassium efflux from vascular smooth muscle cells (Duty and Weston, 1990). Minoxidil and diazoxide work in a similar manner (Nelson, 1993).

Drugs for the Far Future

The drugs described above are under varying stages of clinical investigation. Others are further away, including:

—Neuropeptide Y antagonists (Hedner et al., 1992);
—Endothelin receptor antagonists (Clozel et al., 1993);

—Endothelial protectors, including endothelium-derived relaxing factors (Lüscher, 1993).

Conclusion

The number of drugs under investigation is obviously impressive. Time—and in the United States, the FDA—will tell which of them will become available for clinical use. More drugs will be available, probably in rate-controlled forms, so that a single capsule or a patch may provide smooth control over many days. In the meantime, proper use of what is available will control virtually every hypertensive patient.

CHOICE OF DRUGS: FIRST, SECOND, AND BEYOND

Let us now turn to the practical issue as to which of the many drugs now available (Table 7.14) should be the first, second, or subsequent choices in individual patients. Major changes in these choices are underway: In the United States, a diuretic was chosen as initial therapy up to 90% of the time for patients with mild hypertension in 1983 (Cloher and Whelton, 1986), but the use of diuretics has been declining since then, and ACEIs and CEBs have been growing rapidly in popularity (Fig. 7.4). On the other hand, the 1993 Joint National Committee (JNC) report has recommended that diuretics or beta blockers be the initial choice unless special conditions recommend the use of the newer agents.

In the next few pages, I will attempt to summarize the evidence and provide guidelines for the choices of therapy. Despite my enthusiasm for change, I am well aware that I may be wrong and that the opinions of those who disagree should be respected. Perhaps the best course is to delete "right" and "wrong" because morality is not involved. Since no God-given directions for the treatment of hypertension were included on the tablets brought down by Moses, we should all recognize the frailties of human judgment. We also need to recognize the multiple cultural and conceptual differences that exist in varying parts of the world that lead to major differences in how we treat hypertension (Kaplan, 1991b). We in the United States may think our ways are best, but respect must be given to the opinions of those elsewhere.

Before proceeding into the specifics, we need to recall the overriding issue: to lower the BP in order to maximally reduce cardiovascular risk without decreasing (and perhaps even improving) the enjoyment of life. The preferred qualities of the drugs are fairly obvious, but none

Table 7.14.   Oral Antihypertensive Agents

Type of Drug	Usual Dosage Range (Total mg/day)	Number of Daily Doses	Selected Side Effect[a]
INITIAL ANTIHYPERTENSIVE AGENTS			
Diuretics			
Thiazides and related agents			Hypokalemia, hypomagnesemia,
Bendroflumethiazide (Naturetin)	2.5–5	1	hyponatremia, hyperuricemia,
Benzthiazide (Exna)	12.5–50	1	hypercalcemia, hyperglycemia,
Chlorothiazide (Diuril)	125–500	2	hypercholesterolemia, hypertri-
Chlorthalidone (Hygroton)	12.5–50	1	glyceridemia, sexual dysfunc-
Cyclothiazide (Anhydron)	1–2	1	tion, weakness
Hydrochlorothiazide (Esidrix)	12.5–50	1	
Hydroflumethiazide (Saluron)	12.5–50	1	
Indapamide (Lozol)	2.5–5	1	
Methyclothiazide (Enduron)	2.5–5	1	
Metolazone (Zaroxolyn, Diulo, Mykrox)	0.5–5	1	
Polythiazide (Renese)	1–4	1	
Quinethazone (Hydromox)	25–100	1	
Trichlormethiazide (Naqua)	1–4	1	
Loop diuretics			Same as for thiazides except loop
Bumetanide (Bumex)	0.5–5	2–3	diuretics do not cause hypercal-
Ethacrynic acid (Edecrin)	25–100	2–3	cemia
Furosemide (Lasix)	20–320	2–3	
Potassium-sparing agents			Hyperkalemia, particular in
Amiloride (Midamor)	5–10	1–2	patients with renal failure, in patients treated with an ACE inhibitor or with NSAIDs
Spironolactone (Aldactone)	25–100	2–3	Gynecomastia, mastodynia, menstrual irregularities, diminished libido in males
Triamterene (Dyrenium)	50–150	1–2	Danger of renal calculi
Adrenergic inhibitors			
Beta blockers			Bronchospasm, possible aggrava-
Atenolol (Tenormin)	25–100	1–2	tion of peripheral arterial insuffi-
Betaxolol (Kerlone)	5–40	1	ciency, fatigue, reduced exer-
Bisoprolol (Zebeta)	5–20	1	cise tolerance, insomnia, exacer-
Metoprolol (Lopressor)	50–200	1–2	bation of congestive heart
Metoprolol (Toprol) (extended release)	50–200	1	failure, atrioventricular block in presence of conduction distur-
Nadolol (Corgard)	20–240[b]	1	bances, masking of symptoms
Propranolol (Inderal)	40–240	2	of hypoglycemia, hyperglyceride-
Propranolol (long acting)	60–240	1	mia, decreased high-density
Timolol (Blocarden)	20–40	2	lipoprotein cholesterol (except for those drugs with ISA), exacerbation of angina if abruptly discontinued
Beta blockers with intrinsic sympathomimetic activity (ISA)			Similar to other beta blockers but less bradycardia and lipid changes
Acebutolol (Sectral)	200–12000[b]	2	
Carteolol (Cartrol)	2.5–10†	1	
Penbutolol (Levatol)	20–80†	1	
Pindolol (Visken)	10–60†	2	
Alpha-beta blocker			Similar to other beta blocker, ortho-
Labetalol (Normodyne, Trandate)	200–1200	2	static hypotension, hepatotoxicity
Alpha₁ receptor blockers			Orthostatic hypotension, syncope,
Doxazosin (Cardura)	1–1.6	1	weakness, palpitations, head-
Prazosin (Minipress)	1–20	2–3	ache
Terazosin (Hytrin)	1–20	1–2	

Table 7.14. Oral Antihypertensive Agents, *continued*

Type of Drug	Usual Dosage Range (Total mg/day)	Number of Daily Doses	Selected Side Effect[a]
ACE inhibitors			Cough, rash, angioneurotic
Benazepril (Lotensin)	10–40[b]	1–2	edema, hyperkalemia, dysgeu-
Captopril (Capoten)	12.5–150[b]	2	sia; hypotension with first dose;
Cilazapril	2.5–5.0	1–2	can cause reversible, acute
Enalapril (Vasotec)	2.5–40[b]	1–2	renal failure in patients with bilat-
Fosinopril (Monopril)	10–40	1–2	eral renal arterial stenosis or uni-
Lisinopril (Prinivil, Zestril)	5–40[b]	1–2	lateral stenosis in a solitary kid-
Perindopril	1–16[b]	1–2	ney and in patients with cardiac
Quinapril (Accupril)	5–80[b]	1–2	failure and with volume deple-
Ramipril (Altace)	1.25–20[b]	1–2	tion; rarely can induce neutro-
Spirapril	12.5–50	1–2	penia or proteinuria; absolutely
			contraindicated in second and
			third trimesters of pregnancy
Calcium antagonists			
Diltiazem (Cardizem)	90–360	3	Headache, dizziness, peripheral
Diltiazem (Cardizem SR) (sustained release)	120–360	2	edema, (less common than with dihydropyridines), gingival
Diltiazem (Cardiazem CD, Dilacor) (extended release)	180–360	1	hyperplasia, constipation (especially verapamil), atrioventricular
Verapamil (Calan)	80–480	2–3	block, bradycardia
Verapamil (Calan SR, Isoptin SR, Verelan) (long acting)	120–480	1–2	
Dihydropyridines			Headache, dizziness, peripheral
Amlodipine (Norvasc)	2.5–10	1	edema, tachycardia, gingival
Felodipine (Plendil)	5–20	1	hyperplasia; use with caution in
Isradipine (DynaCirc)	2.5–10	2	patients with congestive heart
Nicardipine (Cardene)	60–120	3	failure and post-MI
Nifedipine (Procardia, Adalat)	30–120	3	
Nifedipine GITS (Procardia XL)	30–90	1	
SUPPLEMENTAL ANTIHYPERTENSIVE AGENTS			
Centrally acting alpha$_2$ agonists			Drowsiness, sedation, dry mouth,
Clonidine (Catapres)	0.1–1.2	2	fatigue, orthostatic dizziness;
Guanabenz (Wytensin)	4–64	2	rebound hypertension with
Guanfacine (Tenex)	1–3	1	abrupt discontinuance
Methyldopa (Aldomet)	250–2000	2	Liver damage, fever, and Coombs-positive hemolytic anemia
Clonidine TTS (patch)	0.1–0.3	once weekly	Same as above; localized skin reaction to the patch
Peripherally acting adrenergic antagonists			
Guanadrel (Hylorel)	10–75	2	Diarrhea, orthostatic and exercise
Guanethidine (Ismelin)	10–100	1	hypotension
Rauwolfia alkaloids			Lethargy, nasal congestion, depression
Rauwolfia (whole root)	50–200	1	
Reserpine (Serpasil)	0.05–0.25	1	Exacerbation of peptic ulcer
Direct vasodilators			Headache, tachycardia, fluid retention; may precipitate angina pectoris in patients with coronary artery disease
Hydralazine (Apresoline)	50–300	2–3	Positive antinuclear antibody test, Lupus syndrome
Minoxidil (Loniten)	2.5–80	1–2	Hypertrichosis, fluid retention

[a]The listing of side effects is not all-inclusive, and clinicians are urged to refer to the package insert for a more detailed listing. Sexual dysfunction, particularly impotence in men, has been reported with the use of all antihypertensive agents. Few data are available on the effect of antihypertensive agents on sexual function in women.

[b]Indicates drugs that are excreted by the kidney and require dosage reduction in the presence of renal impairment (serum creatinine ($\geq$221 μmol/L [2.5 mg/dL]).

now available (or likely to become available) meets all of the criteria for perfection. Nonetheless, currently available choices come close and, used adroitly, can protect almost all patients without much bother.

First Choice

More and more patients with milder and milder hypertension are being treated with drugs. As noted in Chapter 1, that number, in the United States alone, may include 40 million people. These people have two characteristics that must be kept in mind when their hypertension is treated: for the most part, they are asymptomatic; and for the majority, no overt cardiovascular harm would ensue if they were left untreated. I considered the ethics of drug therapy for such patients in Chapter 5.

The choices of therapy, particularly for the first drug, should be made with care. The first drug chosen may be taken for 10, 20, 30, or 40 years. If it successfully lowers the BP by 10 mm Hg, as it will in 50% to 60% of mild hypertensives, no more drugs may be needed. Recall, too, that the tendency of thiazide diuretics, the most commonly used antihypertensive, to raise serum cholesterol levels by 10 to 20 mg/dl was only recognized after they were taken for up to 20 years by millions of people. The need for certainty about long-term safety, in addition to efficacy, should be obvious.

The issue has been nicely portrayed in a review of the impact of predominantly diuretic and beta blocker therapies on the BP and other risk factors in 281 patients treated in a major Australian hypertension center (Jennings and Sudhir, 1990) (Table 7.15). Although hypertension was well controlled, renal function, blood glucose, and cholesterol levels worsened. As summarized in Table 7.14, all drugs may have adverse effects, and precautions are needed in the use of any and all.

Comparative Trials

The only trials that have compared the long-term ability of different drugs to protect patients from overall and cardiovascular morbidity and mortality—the only meaningful criterion—have examined only two classes: diuretics and beta blockers. As described in Chapter 5, three of the five trials directly comparing the two showed no difference between them; the MAPHY portion of the HAPPHY trial found that the beta blocker metoprolol yielded lower coronary mortality rates than did a diuretic, whereas the MRC trial in the elderly found that a diuretic provided better coronary protection than did the beta blocker atenolol.

The issue remains unsettled and, as for now, no one class of drug has been shown to be better in protecting against morbidity or mortality than any other. Unfortunately, no data are available for any agents other than diuretics and beta blockers. Therefore, the decision to change to other drugs must be based on the possibility, or better the probability—but *not* the certainty—that they will be better. Some argue that, in the absence of any such data with other agents, those drugs which have been tested and found to reduce cardiovascular morbidity and mortality—namely, diuretics and beta blockers—should be chosen (Alderman, 1992; Sever et al., 1993).

Joint National Committee Recommendations

This is the position taken in the fifth Joint National Committee Report (1993) (Fig. 7.31): Whereas a diuretic was the sole recommendation for initial therapy in both the 1977 and 1980 reports, less than a full dose of either a thiazide-type diuretic or a beta blocker was recommended in the 1984 report. In the 1988 report, four choices were provided: diuretics, beta blockers, ACEIs, or CEBs. In the 1993 report, six choices are provided, adding alpha and alpha-beta block-

Table 7.15. Effects of Therapy with Diuretics and Beta-blockers in 281 Patients

Values	Before Therapy	After 1 Year
Blood pressure (mm Hg)	160/98	145/88
Weight (kg)	74	74
Potassium level (mmol/L)	4.0	4.1
Creatinine level (mmol/L)	0.08	0.11
Fasting glucose (mmol/L)	5.30	6.33
Total cholesterol (mmol/L)	5.85	6.15

From Jennings GL, Sudhir K. Initial therapy of primary hypertension. Med J Aust 152:198, 1990.

JNC$\underline{V}$ Treatment Algorithm

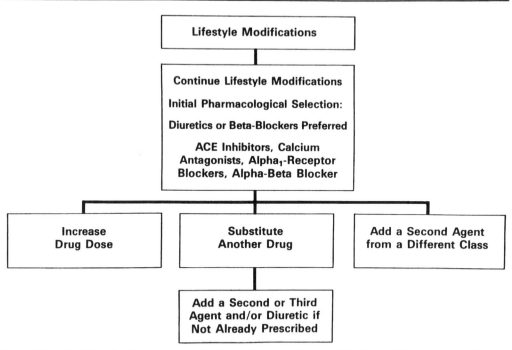

Figure 7.31. Simplified algorithm for treatment of hypertension. (From the Joint National Committee on Detection, Evaluation, and Treatment of High Blood Pressure. The fifth report of the Joint National Committee on Detection, Evaluation, and Treatment of High Blood Pressure [JNC V]. *Arch Intern Med* 1993;153:154–183.)

ers, but preference is given to diuretics and beta blockers. The report states:

Because diuretics and beta blockers have been shown to reduce cardiovascular morbidity and mortality in controlled clinical trials, these two classes of drugs are preferred for initial drug therapy. The alternative drugs—calcium antagonists, angiotensin converting enzyme (ACE) inhibitors, alpha$_1$ receptor blockers, and the alpha-beta blocker—are equally effective in reducing blood pressure (Treatment of Mild Hypertension Research Group, 1991). Although these alternative drugs have potentially important benefits, they have not been used in long-term controlled trials to demonstrate their efficacy in reducing morbidity and mortality and therefore should be reserved for special indications or when diuretics and beta blockers have proved unacceptable or ineffective.

The report immediately proceeds to detail a number of other factors to be considered in selection of drugs: "The cost of medication, metabolic and subjective side effects, and drug-drug interactions . . . [a]lso to be considered in the selection of initial therapy are demographic characteristics, concomitant diseases that may be beneficially or adversely affected by the anti-

hypertensive agent chosen and the use of other drugs that may lead to drug interactions." These additional factors will translate into a continuation of current trends—the use of various classes, the specific drug chosen on the basis of multiple considerations, an approach best described as "individualized."

Individualized Therapy

This approach (Fig. 7.32) is predicated on three major principles:

1. The first choice may be one of a variety of antihypertensives from each class of drugs—diuretics, alpha blockers, beta blockers, ACEIs, or CEBs.
2. The choice can be logically based on the characteristics of the patients, in particular, the presence of concomitant diseases.
3. Rather than proceeding with a second drug if the first does not work well or if side effects ensue, a substitution approach is used—stop the first drug and try another from a different class.

Let us consider further these three principles.

Characteristics of the Drugs (Table 7.16)

Each class of drugs has different features that make its members more or less attractive.

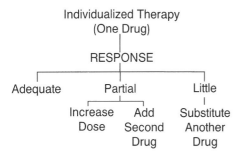

Figure 7.32. Individualized approach to the therapy of hypertension. The choice of initial therapy is based on multiple clinical features.

Diuretics. In the past, diuretics were almost always chosen first, because they were considered free of significant side effects, easy to take, and inexpensive. Moreover, reactive fluid retention with other drugs used without a diuretic often blunted their effect, so the idea of using a diuretic first seemed logical. However, recognition of the "hidden" side effects and costs of diuretics, along with the lesser protection from coronary mortality in the trials wherein they were used, caused many to doubt the wisdom of routine use of diuretics. At the least, these factors have led to the more widespread use of lower doses of diuretics and their combinations with potassium-sparing agents.

Beta-Blockers. Beta blockers then became increasingly popular. However, the need for caution and the contraindications to their use, along with recognition of their potential for altering lipids adversely, dampened their popularity. The failure to find additional protection against coronary disease in trials with a beta blocker, as described in Chapter 5, further weakened the argument for their use.

Indirect Vasodilators. Drugs that act primarily as indirect vasodilators, alpha blockers, ACEIs, and CEBs are being more widely advocated for initial therapy. There seems to be a certain logic in using drugs that induce vasodilation since an elevated peripheral resistance is the hemodynamic fault of established hypertension.

Other Agents. Reserpine works as well as any of these drugs with one dose a day. However, the concern about the subtle onset of depression and the recurrent (but unproved) claims of its carcinogenicity have caused many to stop using it. The other classes of drugs are not recommended in JNC-V (1993) for initial therapy: "The direct-acting smooth muscle vasodilators (e.g., hydralazine, minoxidil) often induce reflex sympathetic stimulation and fluid retention. The [centrally acting] alpha$_2$-agonists and peripherally acting adrenergic antagonists produce annoying side effects in a large number of patients."

Characteristics of the Patients

Demographic Features. Individual patient's characteristics may affect the likelihood of a good response to various classes of drugs (Materson et al., 1993). For example, an elderly, obese black woman will likely respond better to a diuretic than to a beta blocker or an ACEI. A younger, physically active white man would likely respond particularly well to an alpha blocker or an ACEI. In general, black patients tend to do better with a diuretic, less well with a beta blocker or an ACEI, and equally well with a CEB or alpha blocker than do non-black patients. The elderly tend to respond equally well, if not better, to most classes than do younger patients. However, for the individual patient, any drug may work well or poorly, and there is no set formula that can be used to predict certain success without side effects.

Unfortunately, there are very few blinded crossover studies comparing two or more drugs in the same patients to explain what factors are responsible for individual variability. From the few that are available (Brunner et al., 1990; Edmonds et al., 1990; Morgan et al., 1992), it is clear that some patients respond better to one type of drug than to another, but no single factor explains why those who respond do so. The individual patient comparative trial described earlier in this chapter could be used to determine which is the best choice. Practically, if the patient's pressure is well controlled and no bothersome or potentially hazardous adverse effects are present, there is no reason to keep searching for "the best." Rather than searching for perfection, we need simply to weed out the drugs that either produce little good effect or induce significant ill effects.

As noted in JNC-V, demographic features and the presence of concomitant diseases provide a rational approach to the choice of both initial and subsequent therapy (Table 7.17). Table 7.17 differs in a number of specific points from Table 8 of the 1993 JNC-V report, but the general concepts are similar.

Concomitant Conditions. Patients with hypertension, usually being middle-aged or elderly, often have other medical problems, some related to their hypertension, others coincidental (Stewart et al., 1989). As shown in Table

Table 7.16. Choice of Initial Therapy

	Diuretics	Centrally Acting Agents	Alpha-Blockers	Beta-Blockers	ACE Inhibitors	Calcium Antagonists
Hemodynamic effect	Initial volume shrinkage Peripheral vasodilation	Reduce cardiac output	Peripheral vasodilation	Reduce cardiac output	Peripheral vasodilation	Peripheral vasodilation
Side effects						
Overt	Weakness Palpitations	Sedation Dry mouth	Postural dizziness	Bronchospasm Fatigue Prolong hypoglycemia	Cough Taste disturbance Rash	Flushing Local edema Constipation (verapamil)
Hidden	Hypokalemia Hypercholesterolemia Glucose intolerance Hyperuricemia	Withdrawal syndrome Autoimmune syndromes (methyldopa)		Glucose intolerance Hypertriglyceridemia Decrease HDL cholesterol	Leukopenia Proteinuria	AV conduction (verapamil, diltiazem)
Contraindications	Preexisting volume contraction	Orthostatic hypotension Liver disease (methyldopa)	Orthostatic hypotension	Asthma Heartblock	Pregnancy	
Cautions	Diabetes mellitus Gout Digitalis toxicity			Peripheral vascular disease Insulin-requiring diabetes Allergy Coronary spasm Withdrawal angina	Renal insufficiency Renovascular disease	Heart failure
Special advantages	Effective in blacks, elderly Enhance effectiveness of all other agents	No alteration in blood lipids No fluid retention (guanabenz)	No decrease in cardiac output No alteration in blood lipids No sedation Relieves symptoms of prostatic hypertrophy	Reduce recurrences of coronary disease Reduce manifestations of anxiety Coexisting angina, migrane, glaucoma	No CNS side effects Treat CHF Reduce recurrences of coronary disease and development of CHF Probable renal protection	Effective in blacks, elderly No CNS side effects Coronary vasodilation

Table 7.17. Individualized Choices of Therapy

Coexisting Condition	Diuretic	Beta Blocker	Alpha Blocker	Calcium Blocker	ACEI
Older age	+ +	+ / −	+	+	+
Black race	+ +	+ / −	+	+	+ / −
Coronary disease	+ / −	+ +	+	+ +	+
Postmyocardial infarction	+	+ +	+	+ / −	+ +
Congestive failure	+ +	−	+	−	+ +
Cerebrovascular disease	+	+	+ / −	+ +	+
Renal insufficiency	+ +	+ / −	+	+ +	+ +
Diabetes	−	−	+ +	+	+ +
Dyslipidemia	−	−	+ +	+	+
Asthma or chronic obstructive pulmonary disease	+	−	+	+	+

+ + Preferred   + / − Usually not preferred
  + Suitable   − Usually contraindicated

7.17, a hypertensive patient with angina would logically be given a beta blocker or a CEB; a patient with CHF, an ACEI. Alpha blockers, CEBs, and ACEIs are attractive choices for those in whom a diuretic or beta blocker may pose particular problems, such as diabetics or hyperlipidemic patients. In an elderly man with benign prostatic hypertrophy, an alpha blocker would be a logical choice.

Plasma Renin Levels. Laragh and coworkers, as far back as 1972 (Bühler et al., 1972) and persistently since (Devereux and Laragh, 1992), have used the level of plasma renin activity (PRA) to guide the choice of initial therapy. As attractive as the concept is, in practice it often does not work: Donnelley et al. (1992) found that pretreatment PRA accounted for considerably less than 10% of the variability in response to treatment. To be sure, most studies show that patients with lower renin levels respond somewhat better to diuretics, whereas those with higher renin levels respond better to beta blockers and ACEIs (Niutta et al., 1990). The elderly and blacks may respond particularly well to diuretics, perhaps because their renin levels tend to be lower, whereas younger white patients may respond well to beta blockers or ACEIs, perhaps because their renin levels are higher.

Substitution Rather Than Addition

The traditional ''stepped care'' approach meant that if the first drug did not work well, others would be added sequentially. This could mean that the patient is given one, two, or even three drugs, none of which works. The wisdom of substitution rather than addition seems obvious. If the first choice, even if based on all reasonable criteria, does not lower the BP much or is associated with persistent, bothersome side effects, that drug should be stopped and one from another class should be tried. Thereby, the least number of drugs should be needed to achieve the desired fall in BP with the fewest side effects.

Patients with milder hypertension will often need only one drug. Therefore, substitution should work for them. For those with more severe hypertension, the first drug may do all that is expected and still not be enough. Therefore, the addition of a second or, if needed, a third drug added in a stepwise manner is logical.

Cost as a Factor

For some patients, the cost of the medications used to treat hypertension may pose an obstacle to control of their disease (Dustan et al., 1992). The cost per tablet varies between a few cents for a generic hydrochlorothiazide or reserpine to a dollar or more for a brand-name ACEI or CEB. Practitioners concerned about the cost might then choose the least expensive agent.

However, there are additional factors that need to be considered. First, the cost of the tablet may not be the major cost of the medication (Hilleman et al., 1993). If a diuretic causes hypokalemia that must be corrected, potassium supplements may cost a dollar a day or more. Diuretic-induced hyperlipidemia may be an even more serious, albeit less obvious, cost.

Second, more and more agents are available in long-acting formulations so that one tablet a day may provide full coverage. The cost may be reduced further by prescribing larger doses of tablets than can easily be broken in half. Although a dollar or more a day may pose a burden for many, the cost of medication should not interfere with the provision of what is best for most patients. Nonetheless, lacking clear proof that one type of drug is clearly more protective against cardiovascular morbidity and mortality than others, the temptation to go with the least expensive cannot be discounted (Alderman, 1992).

Choice of Second Drug

If a moderate dose of the first choice is well tolerated and effective but not enough to bring the pressure down to the desired level, a second drug can be added or the dose of the first drug can be increased further.

As noted in JNC-V:

Combining antihypertensive drugs with different modes of action will often allow smaller doses of drugs to be used to achieve control, thereby minimizing the potential for dose-dependent side effects. If a diuretic is not chosen as the first drug, it will be useful as a second step agent because its addition usually enhances the effects of other agents.

The wisdom of adding a second drug rather than increasing the dose of the first has been widely accepted but inadequately tested. Nonetheless, there is no question that the addition of two drugs of dissimilar action will usually provide additional effect (Morgan et al., 1992). In patients whose diastolic BP (DBP) remained above 90 mm Hg on isradipine (2.5 mg twice daily) who were randomly assigned to receive more isradipine or to have a diuretic, a beta blocker, or an ACEI added, those given the second agent did better than those given more of the first drug (Lüscher and Waeber, 1993).

The choice of second drug depends largely on the nature of the first. If a diuretic is the first drug, the addition of an adrenergic inhibitor or an ACEI will usually provide significant additional antihypertensive effect. The addition of an alpha blocker will minimize diuretic-induced hyperlipidemia (Black, 1991). If a nondiuretic agent is the first choice, a diuretic can be used as the second choice. However, if a diuretic is to be avoided, combinations of a beta blocker and a CEB or of a CEB and an ACEI will usually provide additive effects (Lüscher and Waeber, 1993).

In the elderly, central alpha agonists may be less attractive because of their tendency to cause sedation, and alpha blockers may cause bothersome postural hypotension. However, all classes of drugs seem to work as well in elderly patients as in younger ones; thus, age per se is probably not an important determinant of the choice of therapy.

Two Drugs as Initial Therapy

Since one-third to one-half of patients will end up on two drugs, some prefer to start with the combination of a diuretic and another agent. That practice is, in general, unwise, for these reasons: (a) even with fairly high BP, many patients will respond adequately to one drug, and there is no certain way to know who will need more than one; (b) if side effects appear, it is preferable to know which drug is responsible; (c) dose-response curves differ with various drugs, so fixed-dose combinations may be inappropriate; and (d) except in those with dangerously high levels of BP, a gradual, gentle reduction in pressure with one drug at a time is easier to tolerate than a sudden, drastic fall from two or more drugs.

Combination Tablets

If the patient ends up on two drugs and the doses match the combinations available, such a combination tablet should be used. Of the combinations available, the addition of a potassium-sparing agent to a diuretic (Dyazide, Maxzide, Moduretic) is eminently sensible. Combinations of a diuretic plus almost every one of the other types of drugs are available; one of these, with only 6.25 mg HCTZ and the beta blocker bisoprolol (Ziac), is approved for initial therapy. Caution is advised in not overdosing the diuretic if larger amounts of other agents are needed.

Choice of Third Drug

Various combinations usually work. In one parallel study, 93 patients uncontrolled on a diuretic and a beta blocker were randomly allocated to either nifedipine, prazosin, or hydralazine (Ramsay et al., 1987). After 6 months, all three drugs lowered BPs significantly, and there were few differences among the three groups other than in the pattern of side effects. In a similar study, captopril, nifedipine, and hydralazine were equally effective, but the ACEI was better tolerated (Bevan et al., 1993). The key, as with two drugs, is to combine agents with different mechanisms of action.

Choice of Fourth Drug

Few patients should need more than three drugs, particularly if the various reasons for resistance to therapy are considered. For those who do, the JNC-V report recommends adding a fourth drug from a different class or having the patient evaluated for the reason behind resistance.

Resistant Hypertension

The reasons for a poor response are numerous (Table 7.18); the most likely is volume overload due to either excessive sodium intake or inade-

Table 7.18. Causes for Lack of Responsiveness to Therapy

Nonadherence to therapy
- Cost of medication
- Instructions unclear and/or not given to the patient in writing
- Inadequate or no patient education
- Lack of involvement of the patient in the treatment plan
- Side effects of medication
- Organic brain syndrome (e.g., memory deficit)
- Inconvenient dosing

Drug-related causes
- Doses too low
- Inappropriate combinations (e.g., two centrally acting adrenergic inhibitors)
- Rapid inactivation (e.g., hydralazine)
- Drug interactions
  Nonsteroidal anti-inflammatory drugs
  Oral contraceptives
  Sympathomimetics
  Antidepressants
  Adrenal steroids
  Nasal decongestants
  Licorice-containing substances (e.g., chewing tobacco)
  Cocaine
  Cyclosporine
  Erythropoietin

Associated conditions
- Increasing obesity
- Alcohol intake more than 1 ounce of ethanol a day

Secondary hypertension
- Renal insufficiency
- Renovascular hypertension
- Pheochromocytoma
- Primary aldosteronism

Volume overload
- Inadequate diuretic therapy
- Excess sodium intake
- Fluid retention from reduction blood pressure
- Progressive renal damage

Pseudohypertension

From Joint National Committee. Fifth report of the Joint National Committee on Detection, Evaluation, and Treatment of High Blood Pressure (JNC V). *Arch Intern Med* 1993;153:154–183.

quate diuretic (Graves et al., 1989). In one series of 91 patients whose pressures remained above 140/90 despite use of three antihypertensive agents, the mechanisms were suboptimal drug regimen (mainly inadequate diuretic) in 43%, intolerance to medications in 22%, noncompliance in 10%, and secondary hypertension in 11% (Yakovlevitch and Black, 1991). In a disadvantaged minority population, uncontrolled hypertension is most closely related to limited access to care, noncompliance with therapy, and alcohol-related problems (Shea et al., 1992).

Before starting work-up for secondary causes and altering drug therapy, BPs should be checked out of the office setting, since as many as half of "resistant" patients turn out to have controlled hypertension (Mejia et al., 1991).

In addition to adequate diuretics, therapy should include an ACEI and a calcium blocker, with minoxidil reserved for those who remain resistant (Pontremoli et al., 1991). Therapy of patients with very severe hypertension in need of immediate reduction will be covered in the next chapter.

Stepping Down or Off Therapy

Once a good response has occurred and has been maintained for a year or longer, medications may be reduced or discontinued. In most studies of patients whose medications were discontinued, the majority have their hypertension reappear in 6 to 12 months; in some studies, however, a significant percentage remain normotensive for 4 years or longer (Schmieder et al., 1991). From their review of all published prospective studies, Schmieder et al. characterize patients who remain normotensive as having mild hypertension with low pretreatment BP, young age, normal body weight, low salt intake, no alcohol consumption, successful therapy with only one drug, and little or no target organ damage. Such paragons may be hard to find, and some of them may be transient or "white coat" hypertensives whose therapy was begun before the diagnosis was established.

Whether it is worth the trouble to stop drug therapy completely is questionable. Withdrawal is certainly worthwhile in elderly patients whose BPs are normal on little therapy and who have no signs of target organ damage (Lernfelt et al., 1990). The more sensible approach in well-controlled patients would be to first decrease the dose of whatever is being used. This approach is feasible, without loss of control, in a significant number of patients who are well controlled on a single drug (Finnerty, 1990). If this succeeds, withdrawal may be attempted with continued surveillance of the BP.

SPECIAL CONSIDERATIONS IN THERAPY

Children are covered in Chapter 16; women who are pregnant or on hormones are covered in Chapter 11.

Women

Partly because of their lesser degree of coronary risk, women have been largely excluded from the large clinical trials, since a difference between placebo and treated subjects should be more obvious in a higher-risk, male population. Therefore, only limited data are available on the ability of therapy to reduce women's risk and on the potential side effects of various therapies in women. Some of the limited data show that white women do not obtain as much benefit from equal degrees of BP reduction as do men or black women (Anastos et al., 1991), but elderly women in the Systolic Hypertension in the Elderly Trial did achieve equal protection (SHEP, 1991).

Blacks and Other Ethnic Groups

As noted in Chapter 4, black hypertensives have many distinguishing characteristics, some that affect their responses to antihypertensive therapy. Poverty and obesity are more prevalent among black hypertensives; both of these conditions may impede the control of hypertension (Shea et al., 1992). When given equal access to the same treatment, blacks respond as whites do and experience an even lower incidence of cardiovascular disease than whites (Ooi et al., 1989). However, they may continue to experience a loss of renal function despite apparently good control of hypertension (Walker et al., 1992).

Blacks respond somewhat less well to beta blockers and ACEIs, perhaps because they tend to have lower renin levels, and equally as well to diuretics, calcium blockers, and alpha blockers (Materson et al., 1993).

Other Ethnic Groups

There is no good evidence that Hispanics, Asians, or other ethnic groups differ in their responses to various antihypertensive agents from Caucasians.

Elderly Patients

Millions of people over age 65 have hypertension; in most such persons, the hypertension is predominantly or purely systolic. As described in Chapter 4, the risks for such patients are significant. As detailed in Chapter 5, the benefits of treating hypertension in the elderly have only recently been documented. Now that such evidence is available, many more elderly hypertensives will be brought into active therapy.

Since the elderly may have sluggish baroreceptor and sympathetic nervous responsiveness, as well as impaired cerebral autoregulation, therapy should be gentle and gradual, avoiding drugs that are likely to cause postural hypotension or to exacerbate other common problems often seen among the elderly (Table 7.19). However, occasional reports of the serious consequences of inappropriate therapy with excessive doses of potent drugs (Jansen et al., 1987) should not deter appropriate therapy of persons with hypertension. On the other hand, caution is advised with the very elderly. Mortality increased significantly over 5 years among some 400 men over age 75 whose diastolic BP was reduced by 5 mm Hg or more while on antihypertensive therapy (Langer et al., 1993).

Lifestyle Modifications

Before we rush into drug therapy, the multiple benefits of nondrug therapies that were described in Chapter 6 need to be reaffirmed. They should be enthusiastically provided and vigorously pursued, preferably before and (one hopes) instead of drug therapy. Fewer trials on these lifestyle modifications have been done on the elderly, but enough data are available to document the efficacy of such measures (Applegate et al., 1992). In particular, dietary sodium should be moderately restricted down to 100 to 120 mmol/day since the pressor effect of sodium excess and the antihypertensive efficacy of sodium restriction progressively increase with age (Weinberger and Fineberg, 1991). However, the elderly may have at least two additional hurdles to overcome in achieving this goal: first, their taste sensitivity may be lessened, so they may ingest more sodium to compensate; second, they may depend more on processed, prepackaged foods that are high in sodium rather than fresh foods that are low in sodium.

Drug Treatment

I can do no better than to paraphrase the recommendations made by a group of British hypertension experts based on their analysis of the data from the six clinical trials of the elderly (Beard et al., 1992):

Table 7.19. Factors That Might Contribute to Increased Risk of Pharmacologic Treatment of Hypertension in the Elderly

Factors	Potential Complications
Diminished baroreceptor activity	Orthostatic hypotension
Impaired cerebral autoregulation	Cerebral ischemia with small falls in systemic pressure
Decreased intravascular volume	Orthostatic hypotension
	Volume depletion, hyponatremia
Sensitivity to hypokalemia	Arrhythmia, muscular weakness
Decreased renal and hepatic function	Drug accumulation
Polypharmacy	Drug interaction
CNS changes	Depression, confusion

—Consider treatment for patients up to age 80 with systolic pressure above 160 mm Hg. (I believe patients at any age who appear to have a reasonable life expectancy should be considered.);

—The goal of therapy should be a BP below 160/90;

—The choice of antihypertensive therapy should be based on the presence of concomitant conditions, individualizing therapy rather than using the stepped care approach. (The table of these researchers on choices is similar to Table 7.17.);

—First-line therapy for those with uncomplicated hypertension should be low doses of a diuretic (e.g., 12.5 mg/day of hydrochlorothiazide, probably with a potassium-sparing agent);

—Beta blockers cannot now be considered the treatment of choice in elderly hypertensive patients, although they may be used in patients with angina or a prior myocardial infarction;

—Even though the newer agents (ACEIs, CEBs, alpha blockers) have not been subjected to controlled trials, "such drugs may be favored on a number of theoretical and practical grounds, particularly when diuretics or beta blockers are contraindicated. They may have a major role in managing patients with coexistent disease, such as heart failure, chronic lung disease, and diabetes" (Beard et al., 1992).

I would add that the number of medications and daily doses should be kept to a minimum, remembering that some elderly patients may have more trouble following complicated dosage schedules, reading the labels, and opening bottles with safety caps. Concerns that treating elderly hypertensives would lead to loss of cognitive function seem not to have been substantiated (Goldstein, 1992), although nifedipine induced subtle impairments of learning and memory in some (Skinner et al., 1992).

Postural Hypotension

As noted in Chapter 4, many elderly patients with systolic hypertension have postural hypotension that may require management before the

hypertension is addressed. Management should begin by correcting precipitating factors and withdrawing offending drugs such as diuretics, vasodilators, tranquilizers, and sedatives. Physical measures should be used, including the following instructions for patients:

—Raise the head of the bed by 15 to 20 degrees;

—Arise slowly, in stages, from supine to seated to standing;

—Engage in dorsiflexion of the feet, handgrip isometric exercise, or mental exercise before standing (Goldstein and Shapiro, 1990);

—Eat small meals to avoid postprandial hypotension;

—Drink one or two cups of strong coffee early in the morning but none thereafter to prevent tolerance to the sympathomimetic effect of caffeine.

—Wear Jobst stockings and, in extreme cases, pressure suits.

If these measures are not adequate, one or another drug may be tried, but none has been particularly successful (Ahmad and Watson, 1990). Drugs should be given in this approximate order:

—Fludrocortisone ± NSAID;

—For "pure" autonomic dysfunction, pindolol;

—For CNS dysfunction, desmopressin;

—If the above fail: ergotamine, yohimbine, alpha-sympathomimetics, dopamine antagonists;

—The somatostatin analogue, octreotide, has been helpful in patients with autonomic neuropathy, presumably by increasing splanchnic vascular resistance and preventing pooling of blood in the gut after eating (Hoeldtke and Davis, 1991).

Patients with Cardiac Disease

Coronary Disease

The presence of angina favors the use of CEBs or beta blockers; beta blockers should be used with caution in those with coronary spasm (Nielsen et al., 1987). Hypertension that persists after an acute myocardial infarction can logically be treated with a beta blocker or, in the presence of a low ejection fraction, an ACEI.

Congestive Failure

For hypertensives with heart failure, diuretics and ACEIs should be used (Groden, 1993). Caution is needed for those elderly hypertensives thought to be in heart failure who have marked hypertrophic cardiomyopathy, since unloaders such as ACEIs may make them hypotensive, whereas beta blockers or CEBs may improve their diastolic dysfunction (Topol et al., 1985).

Left Ventricular Hypertrophy

As noted in Chapter 4, LVH is frequently present on echocardiography, even in patients with mild hypertension. A number of antihypertensive drugs have been shown to reverse LVH, ACEIs perhaps best of all (Dahlöf et al., 1992). Whether such reversal is a desirable goal of therapy remains uncertain, but at the least, regression of LVH does not reduce pump function (Ketelhut et al., 1992) and may protect against potentially serious arrhythmias (Messerli et al., 1989) and cardiovascular events (Koren et al., 1991).

Patients with Cerebrovascular Disease

Immediately after the onset of a stroke, BP may become markedly elevated, only to fall precipitously if potent antihypertensive agents are given (Lisk et al., 1993). Brott and Reed (1989) provide these guidelines for antihypertensive therapy in acute stroke:

—If DBP is above 140 on two readings 5 minutes apart, use intravenous nitroprusside;
—If SBP is over 230 and/or DBP is 121 to 140 on two readings 20 minutes apart, use intravenous labetalol;
—If SBP is 180 to 230 and/or DBP is 105 to 120, defer emergency therapy in the absence of intracranial hemorrhage or left ventricular failure. If the elevation persists over an hour, use oral labetalol, nifedipine, or captopril;
—If SBP is less than 180 and/or DBP is less than 105, antihypertensive therapy is usually not indicated.

Concerns have been expressed over the potential for nitroprusside to induce further rises in intracranial pressure (Garner, 1986). In a study involving measurement of intracranial pressure in patients with hemorrhagic stroke and hypertension, barbiturates were found to be superior to nifedipine, reserpine, or furosemide in reducing both systemic and intracranial pressures (Hayashi et al., 1988). There is a great need for more

such careful study of the treatment of acute stroke. The CEB nimodipine is approved for relief of vasospasm after subarachnoid hemorrhage and, if used early, may provide benefit after acute stroke (Lees, 1992b).

After the acute stages, the BP usually rises (Carlsson and Britton, 1993). For chronic management in those who remain hypertensive, effective antihypertensive treatment has been shown to reduce recurrent strokes (Marshall, 1964; Carter, 1970; Beevers et al., 1973). However, caution is advised: the BP should be lowered gradually and without sudden drops so that cerebral blood flow will not fall (Mori et al., 1993). Elderly patients may have poor cerebral autoregulatory ability (Jansen et al., 1987), and that ability may be further impaired in the presence of cerebrovascular disease. Cerebral blood flow seems least perturbed by ACEIs (Lohmann et al., 1992) and CEBs (Thulin et al., 1993).

Patients with Peripheral Vascular Disease

Hypertensives have more atherosclerotic vascular disease. Beta blockers, including ones with ISA (pindolol), with cardioselectivity (atenolol), and combined with alpha blockade (labetalol), were found to worsen intermittent claudication; an ACEI (captopril), however, did not (Roberts et al., 1987). CEBs and alpha blockers should also provide vasodilation.

Patients with Renal Disease

Since there are so many facets to hypertension in renal disease, Chapter 9 covers that combination in depth.

Hypertension and Diabetes

Both type I and type II diabetics are prone to hypertension and thereby to accelerate the cardiac and renal dysfunctions that are now their leading causes of premature death. About 90% of diabetics have the non–insulin-dependent type II, the end result of obesity-induced insulin resistance. The most critical need for control of both hypertension and diabetes in these patients is weight reduction. If weight can be lost through diet and exercise, marked improvements in insulin resistance can be accomplished (Barnard et al., 1992).

If antihypertensive drugs are needed, they should be chosen carefully, with recognition of their many possible adverse effects (Table 7.20). In particular, diabetic patients at the Joslin Clinic in the late 1970s experienced increased mortality

Table 7.20. Possible Adverse and Beneficial Effects of Antihypertensive Drugs Used in Patients with Diabetes Mellitus

Drug Class	Possible Adverse Effects and Precautions	Possible Benefits
Adrenergic antagonists		Effective in coronary heart disease
Cardioselective beta blockers	Obscure hypoglycemic symptoms: impotence, hypertriglyceridemia, ↓ HDL cholesterol, heart failure, renal excretion (except metoprolol), same as noncardioselective in high doses	
Noncardioselective beta blockers	Same as cardioselective, plus delayed recovery from hypoglycemia, deterioration of glucose control (NIDDM), hyperosmolar coma, hypertension if hypoglycemic, aggravated peripheral vascular disease, ↑ potassium (hypoaldosteronism)	Effective in coronary heart diseases
Combined alpha and beta blockers	Same as noncardioselective blockers	
Peripheral adrenergic inhibitors	Orthostatic hypotension, impotence, sodium retention	
Central adrenergic inhibitors	Same as peripheral inhibitors	
Alpha$_1$-adrenergic inhibitors	Orthostatic hypotension, sodium retention	Rarely cause impotence, no adverse effects on glucose or lipids
Angiotensin-converting enzyme inhibitors	Severe hyperkalemia (hypoaldosteronism); further compromise of renal function in renal failure	Rarely cause impotence, no effect on glucose or lipids, minimize adverse metabolic effects of diuretics, rarely cause orthostatic hypotension, ↓ albuminuria, may reduce rate of renal deterioration
Calcium channel blockers	Orthostatic hypotension (occasionally), glucose intolerance (?)	Rarely cause impotence, no adverse effects on lipids
Direct vasodilators	Aggravate coronary disease, sodium retention	Rarely cause orthostatic hypertension, rarely cause impotence, no effect on glucose or lipids
Diuretics Thiazide	↑ Glucose (NIDDM), impotence, orthostatic hypotension, hypercholesterolemia, ineffective in renal failure, may accelerate renal failure	Minimize sodium retention when used with sodium-retaining drugs
Loop	Same as thiazides (except regarding renal failure)	
Potassium-sparing agents	Severe hyperkalemia (renal failure and hypoaldosteronism), impotence	Effective in real failure, impotence unusual

HDL, high-density lipoprotein; NIDDM, non–insulin-dependent diabetes mellitus.
From Christieb AR. Treatment selection considerations for the hypertensive diabetic patient. *Arch Intern Med* 1990;150:1169–1174.

when diuretics were used (Warram et al., 1991) (Fig. 7.11). For this and various other reasons, Christlieb (1990) and the Canadian Hypertension Society (Dawson et al., 1993) recommend the use of either an ACEI or a CEB for initial therapy for diabetic hypertensives, with a diuretic as a second step. As noted in Chapter 9, ACEIs are proving to be the best choice in the presence of diabetic nephropathy.

Insulin Sensitivity

The differences in insulin sensitivity noted by Lithell (1991) in nondiabetic hypertensives given various antihypertensives for 2 to 3 months (Fig. 7.33) may or may not translate into significant differences in the longterm management of hypertensive diabetics. Significant improvements in insulin sensitivity and glucose tolerance have been observed to persist for 12 months after replacing beta blocker therapy with ACEI therapy (Berntorp et al., 1992). The improvement noted by Lithell with captopril has been observed with other ACEIs as well (Shieh et al., 1992).

Antidiabetic Agents

Outside the United States, metformin is being used to improve insulin sensitivity and help control diabetes. In short-term studies, it also lowers BP (Giugliano et al., 1993). In the future, other agents that improve insulin sensitivity and lower BP in rats (e.g., ciglitazone) (Pershadsingh et al., 1993) may be available. In the meantime, care is needed in the use of insulin since it has been found to raise BP by some researchers

(Randeree et al., 1992) but not by others (Jungmann et al., 1993).

Hypertension and Obesity

Obesity is a major contributor to hypertension (see Chapter 3). The value of weight reduction was covered in Chapter 6. There are few important differences between obese and nonobese hypertensives in response to various antihypertensive agents (Reisin and Weed, 1992), but in general, hypertension in obese persons is less well controlled (Vezù et al., 1992) and their insulin resistance may contribute to resistance to antihypertensive therapy (Isaksson et al., 1993).

Care should be taken with the use of appetite suppressants, particularly sympathomimetics (see Chapter 15). A number of new therapies for obesity that do not adversely affect BP are under investigation (Bray, 1991).

Hypertension and Dyslipidemia

Hypertensives have a higher prevalence of hyperlipidemia even if they are not on therapy (Bønaa and Thelle, 1991). Hypertension and hyperlipidemia are common to certain conditions including upper body obesity (Kaplan, 1989c), diabetes, and alcohol abuse. Even when these mechanisms are excluded, more hypercholesterolemia is found among hypertensives than among age- and sex-matched normotensives, although this may not apply to elderly patients (Simons et al., 1992).

Hypertensives should be assessed for lipid status before antihypertensive therapy is instituted; if hyperlipidemia is present, appropriate

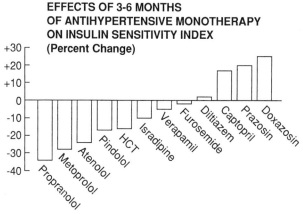

Figure 7.33. The effect on insulin sensitivity of various antihypertensive agents given to groups of hypertensive patients by Lithell and coworkers. (From Lithell HO. Effect of antihypertensive drugs on insulin, glucose, and lipid metabolism. *Diabetes Care* 14:203–209, 1991.)

Table 7.21. Calculated Approximations of the Extent of Drug Effect on Plasma Lipids

	Total Cholesterol	LDL Cholesterol	HDL Cholesterol	Triglycerides
Thiazides	+7%	+10%	+2%	+14%
Beta blockers				
Propranolol	0	−3%	−11%	+16%
Atenolol	0	−2%	−7%	+15%
Pindolol	−1%	−3%	−2%	+7%
Alpha$_1$ blockers	−4%	−13%	+5%	−8%
Central alpha$_2$ agonists	−7%	—	—	—
Calcium entry blockers	0	0	0	0
ACE inhibitors	0	0	0	0

Modified from Johnson BF, Danylchuk MA. The relevance of plasma lipid changes with cardiovascular drug therapy. *Med Clin North Am* 1989;73:449–473.

diet and drug therapy should be provided to control the lipid problem. Unfortunately, the two most widely used antihypertensive agents, diuretics and beta blockers, may induce dyslipidemia, as described in the coverage of these drugs earlier in this chapter and as summarized elsewhere (Lardinois and Neuman, 1988; Johnson and Danylchuk, 1989; Henkin et al., 1992) (Table 7.21). The percentages given in Table 7.21 are based on a thorough but not weighted analysis of published data. Even though these effects may not persist in all patients, in some they last for 5 years or longer (Elliott, 1993). Some discount these negative changes as being inadequate to explain the shortfall in the impact of antihypertensive therapy on coronary disease (Swales, 1991), but they are almost as large as the percentage of positive changes noted in most trials of lipid-lowering drugs that have shown protection from coronary disease.

If either a diuretic or a non-ISA beta blocker is used, the total and HDL cholesterol levels should be rechecked after 2 to 3 months. If a significant alteration has occurred, another drug should be considered or an appropriate lipid-lowering regimen should be instituted. Chromium supplements may raise HDL levels in patients taking beta blockers (Roeback et al., 1991). Fortunately, the other classes of drugs either are lipid-neutral or may actually improve the lipid status (Table 7.21).

Miscellaneous Diseases

Asthma and Chronic Obstructive Pulmonary Disease

Patients with bronchospasm should not be given beta blockers unless there is a powerful indication. ACEIs may cause a cough, perhaps most commonly in people who have underlying bronchial hyperreactivity (Overlack et al., 1992). Some drugs used to treat pulmonary diseases may aggravate hypertension, including sympathomimetic decongestants such as phenylpropanolamine, adrenal steroids, theophylline, and inhaled beta agonists.

Gout

Thiazide-induced hyperuricemia is best neglected, but thiazides should not be given to patients who have gout unless their disease is well controlled with a uricosuric agent. Spironolactone can be used safely.

Impotence and Other Sexual Dysfunction

Impotence, defined as the inability to obtain or maintain an erection, is seen in as many as 10% to 20% of middle-aged men and 35% of men over age 65 (Diokno et al., 1990). The prevalence likely is even greater among hypertensives, even when they are on no treatment (Bansal, 1988). Numerous mechanisms may be involved including psychogenic factors (common), neurogenic causes (less common except among diabetics), hormonal deficiency (rare), and hemodynamic alterations (common, particularly in those with other atherosclerotic risk factors such as smoking and hypercholesterolemia) (Virag et al., 1985). Erection requires relaxation of the smooth muscle of the corpora cavernosa, and this is mediated by release of nitric oxide (Burnett et al., 1992). Diabetic men with impotence have impaired endothelium-dependent mechanisms (Saenz de Tejada et al., 1989).

Before starting any antihypertensive drug therapy, the patient should be asked about sexual dysfunction and, if it is significant, evaluated as completely as is feasible. The evaluation should include a careful history and examination for evidence of neurogenic, hormonal, or hemodynamic problems, often including a study of nocturnal penile tumescence and duplex sonography (Knispel and Huland, 1992). Various therapies may then be provided (Gregoire, 1992), including oral yohimbine, topical application of nitroglycerin or minoxidil (Cavallini, 1991), intracavernosal injections of vasoactive drugs including nitric oxide from donors (Stief et al., 1992), vascular surgery, or penile prosthetic implants. For many patients, an external suction device (EricAid, Osbon Medical Systems, P.O. Box 1478, Augusta, Georgia 30903) works very well (Cookson and Nadig, 1993).

Effects of Antihypertensive Drugs. Antihypertensive drugs are considered to be among the most common causes of impotence. In addition, some drugs may cause retarded ejaculation (guanethidine), gynecomastia (spironolactone), and reduced desire for sex (spironolactone). Most drug-induced problems of sexual dysfunction have been recognized in men. As many as 10% of women aged 35 to 59 have significant sexual dysfunction (Osborn et al., 1988), but there are no data on the effects of antihypertensive drugs on sexual function among women.

Men may lose erectile potency whenever their BP is lowered since much of the problem is due to the vascular insufficiency of the penile artery from atherosclerosis that accompanies their hypertension. Beyond this nonspecific effect, which applies to all antihypertensives, impotence has been reported more frequently after the use of diuretics (Chang et al., 1991) and beta blockers (Croog et al., 1988). In Croog et al.'s study, captopril was less likely to be associated with impotence than other drugs. However, there are few controlled comparative studies to document the relative frequency of the problem with the various classes of drugs (Neaton et al., 1993).

If the problem develops or is made significantly worse after starting any antihypertensive drug, that drug should be stopped. If the patient's hypertension is fairly mild, therapy should be withheld until return of pretreatment potency. When it returns, a very small dose of a drug from another class should be started in an attempt to lower the BP very slowly and gently. Some patients will become impotent whenever the systemic pressure is lowered very much; for them, medical or surgical management of the impotence may be required if the hypertension is to be controlled.

Patients Who Are Pilots

The United States Federal Aviation Administration (FAA) has changed the regulations considerably as to the limits of BP and the types of antihypertensive medications that can be taken by people who wish to be certified as a pilot. These are given in the Guide for Aviation Medical Examiners, United States Department of Transportation, June 1992, pp 86–89. The maximum permitted supine BP for 30- to 39-year-old people is 145/92 or, if cardiac and renal function are normal, 155/98. The permissible levels increase with age. Most antihypertensive drugs can be used with the exceptions of those which may interfere with alertness or performance, including reserpine, guanethidine, guanadrel, and central alpha agonists (methyldopa, clonidine, and guanabenz).

Anesthesia and Surgery

Hypertension, in the absence of significant coronary or myocardial dysfunction, does not add significantly to the cardiovascular risks of noncardiac surgery (Estafanous, 1989). On the other hand, in the presence of preexisting disease, hypertension increases the risk of myocardial ischemia during anesthesia, and the prior administration of antihypertensive therapy reduces that risk (Wolfsthal, 1993). Myocardial ischemia was detected in 11 of 39 untreated hypertensives but in none of 44 receiving atenolol either chronically or with a single dose 2 hours before induction (Stone et al., 1988). Therefore, patients on antihypertensive medications should continue on these drugs, as long as the anesthesiologist is aware of their use and takes reasonable precautions to prevent wide swings in pressure (Charlson et al., 1990).

If hypertension needs to be treated during surgery, intravenous labetalol, nitroprusside, or nicardipine (Sugai et al., 1992) can be used.

Preoperative Precautions

The following precautions seem advisable in handling hypertensive patients before surgery:

—If the BP is uncontrolled and there is time, therapy should be used to bring the pressure down;
—If the patient is uncontrolled and must undergo an operation, special care should be taken to prevent a marked pressor response during intubation by preoperative reassurance and the use of the short-acting beta blocker esmolol (Zsigmond et al., 1988), sublingual nifedipine (Puri and Batra, 1988), or captopril (McCarthy et al., 1990);
—If the patient is potassium-depleted, increased sensitivity to muscle relaxants and, as noted earlier in this chapter, cardiac arrhythmias may occur. A short infusion of 40 mmol of potassium, although it will raise plasma K^+ levels, may do little to

correct longstanding intracellular potassium depletion, and more prolonged replacement therapy should be given. Caution is also needed with the use of local anesthetics with epinephrine, which may further reduce serum potassium levels (Meechan and Rawlins, 1992);

—In patients on adrenergic inhibitors, the pressor response to various sympathomimetic agents may be decreased, so larger doses may be needed to counteract hypotension.

Postoperative Precautions

When any antihypertensive drug is stopped before surgery, life-threatening hypertension may suddenly appear in the immediate postoperative period. This may be a particular problem with short-acting agents, especially clonidine.

For those in need of postoperative BP reduction, successful use of various parenteral forms of various agents has been reported including the short-acting beta blocker esmolol, labetalol, and nicardipine (Halpern et al., 1992). On the other hand, significant lowering of pressure may occur as a nonspecific response to surgery and may persist for months (Volini and Flaxman, 1939). Do not be deceived by what appears to be an improvement in the patient's hypertension: anticipate a gradual return to preoperative levels.

Special problems in postoperative patients after coronary bypass surgery, trauma, and burns

are covered in Chapter 15. Anesthetic considerations in patients with pheochromocytoma are covered in Chapter 12.

Paroxysmal Hypertension and Hypovolemia

Rarely, patients who are severely hypertensive when first seen rapidly go into peripheral vascular collapse when treated with antihypertensive agents (Cohn, 1966). These patients were hypovolemic and hemoconcentrated, and their initial hypertension was at least partly a reflection of compensatory sympathetic nervous system overactivity and, very likely, an activated renin-angiotensin system. When their compensatory support was removed, profound hypotension quickly followed. Similar patients have been observed to have a fall in BP as their shrunken fluid volume is replaced, quieting their activated sympathetic nervous and renin-angiotensin systems (Bissler et al., 1991).

CONCLUSION

The large numbers of drugs now available can be used to successfully treat virtually every hypertensive patient under most any circumstance. Even those at highest risk—the few who develop a hypertensive emergency—can be effectively treated, as is shown in the next chapter.

References

Abernethy DR, Schwartz JB, Plachetka JR, Todd EL, Egan JM. Comparison in young and elderly patients of pharmacodynamics and disposition of labetalol in systemic hypertension. *Am J Cardiol* 1987; 60:697–702.

Abu-Hamdan DK, Desai H, Sondheimer J, Felicetta J, Mahajan S, McDonald F. Taste acuity and zinc metabolism in captopril-treated hypertensive male patients. *Am J Hypertens* 1988;1:303S–308S.

Addonizio VP Jr, Fisher CA, Strauss JF III, Wachtfogel YT, Colman RW, Josephson ME. Effects of verapamil and diltiazem on human platelet function. *Am J Physiol* 1986;250:H366–H371.

Ades PA, Gunther PGS, Meyer WL, Gibson TC, Maddalena J, Orfeo T. Cardiac and skeletal muscle adaptations to training in systemic hypertension and effect of beta blockade (metoprolol or propranolol). *Am J Cardiol* 1990;66:591–596.

Ades PA, Wolfel EE, Hiatt WR, Fee C, Rolfs R, Brammell HL, Horwitz LD. Exercise haemodynamic effects of beta-blockade and intrinsic sympathomimetic activity. *Eur J Clin Pharmacol* 1989;36:5–10.

Ahlquist RP. A study of the adrenotropic receptors. *Am J Physiol* 1948; 153:586–600.

Ahmad RAS, Watson RDS. Treatment of postural hypotension. A review. *Drugs* 1990;39:74–85.

Alderman MH. Which antihypertensive drugs first—and why! *JAMA* 1992; 267:2786–2787.

Allon M, Hall WD, Macon EJ. Prolonged hypotension after initial minoxidil dose. *Arch Intern Med* 1986;146:2075–2076.

Altura BM, Altura BT. Magnesium, electrolyte transport and coronary vascular tone. *Drugs* 1984;28:120–142.

Amery A, Verstraete M, Bossaert H, Verstreken G. Hypotensive action and side effects of clonidine-chlorthalidone and methyldopa-chlorthalidone in treatment of hypertension. *Br Med J* 1970;4:392–395.

Ames R. Effects of diuretic drugs on the lipid profile. *Drugs* 1988;36:33–40.

Ames RP. Thiazide-induced hyperlipidemia is not caused by hypokalemia [Abstract]. *Am J Hypertens* 1989;2:98.

Ames RP, Hill P. Increase in serum lipids during treatment of hypertension with chlorthalidone. *Lancet* 1976;2:721–723.

Anastos K, Charney P, Charon RA, Cohen E, Jones CY, Marte C, Swiderski DM, Wheater ME, Williams S. Hypertension in women: what is really known? *Ann Intern Med* 1991;115:287–293.

Anderson J, Godfrey BE, Hill DM, Munro-Faure AD, Sheldon J. A comparison of the effects of hydrochlorothiazide and of furosemide in the treatment of hypertensive patients. *Q J Med* 1971;40:541–560.

Andersson K-E, Vinge E. β-adrenoceptor blockers and calcium antagonists in the prophylaxis and treatment of migraine. *Drugs* 1990;39:355–373.

Ando K, Noda H, Ogata E, Fujita T. Hemodynamic and endocrine changes associated with hypotensive action of amosulalol in essential hypertension. *J Cardiovasc Pharmacol* 1992;20:7–10.

Andrén L, Weiner L, Svensson A, Hansson L. Enalapril with either a "very low" or "low" dose of hydrochlorothiazide is equally effective in essential hypertension. A double-blind trial in 100 hypertensive patients. *J Hypertens* 1983;1:384–386.

Andreoli SP. Captopril scavenges hydrogen peroxide and reduces, but does not eliminate, oxidant-induced cell injury. *Am J Physiol* 1993;264:F120–F127.

Angeli P, Chiesa M, Caregaro L, Merkel C, Sacerdoti D, Rondana M, Gatta A. Comparison of sublingual captopril and nifedipine in immediate treatment of hypertensive emergencies. *Arch Intern Med* 1991;151:678–682.

Applegate WB, Miller ST, Elam JT, Cushman WC, Derwi DE, Brewer A, Graney MJ. Nonpharmacologic intervention to reduce blood pressure in older patients with mild hypertension. *Arch Intern Med* 1992;152:1162–1166.

Araoye MA, Chang MY, Khatri IM, Freis ED. Furosemide compared with hydrochlorothiazide. Long-term treatment of hypertension. *JAMA* 1978;240:1863–1866.

Ardissino D, Savonitto S, Egstrup K, Marraccini P, Slavich G, Rosenfeld M, Feruglio GA, Roncarolo P, Giordano MP, Wahlqvist I, Rehnqvist N, Barberis P, Specchia G, L'Abbate A. Transient myocardial ischemia during daily life in rest and exertional angina pectoris and comparison of effectiveness of metoprolol versus nifedipine. *Am J Cardiol* 1991;67:946–952.

Atkins JM, Mitchell HC, Pettinger WA. Increased pulmonary vascular resistance with systemic hypertension. *Am J Cardiol* 1977;39:802–807.

Aubert I, Djian F, Rouffy J. Beneficial effects of indapamide on lipoproteins and apoproteins in ambulatory hypertensive patients. *Am J Cardiol* 1990;65:77H–80H.

Augenstein WL, Kulig KW, Rumack BH. Captopril overdose resulting in hypotension. *JAMA* 1988;259:3302–3305.

Baez MA, Alvarez CR, Weidler DJ. Effects of the non-steroidal anti-inflammatory drugs, piroxicam or sulindac, on the antihypertensive actions of propranolol and verapamil. *J Hypertens* 1987;5:S563–566.

Bailey DG, Spence JD, Munoz C, Arnold JMO. Interaction of citrus juices with felodipine and nifedipine. *Lancet* 1991;337:268–269.

Baker D, Roberts DE, Newcombe RG, Fox KAA. Evaluation of drug information for cardiology patients. *Br J Clin Pharmacol* 1991;31:525–531.

Bakris GL. The effects of calcium antagonists on renal hemodynamics, urinary protein excretion, and glomerular morphology in diabetic states [Abstract]. *J Am Soc Nephrol* 1991;2:S21–S29.

Baltodano N, Ballo BV, Weidler DJ. Verapamil vs quinine in recumbent nocturnal leg cramps in the elderly. *Arch Intern Med* 1988;148:1969–1970.

Bansal S. Sexual dysfunction in hypertensive men. A critical review of the literature. *Hypertension* 1988;12:1–10.

Bao G, Gohlke P, Qadri F, Unger T. Chronic kinin receptor blockade attenuates the antihypertensive effect of ramipril. *Hypertension* 1992;20:74–79.

Baran KW, Bache RJ, Dai X-Z, Schwartz JS. Effect of alpha-adrenergic blockade with prazosin on large coronary diameter during exercise. *Circulation* 1992;85:1139–1145.

Barnard RJ, Ugianskis EJ, Martin DA, Inkeles SB. Role of diet and exercise in the management of hyperinsulinemia and associated atherosclerotic risk factors. *Am J Cardiol* 1992;69:440–444.

Bärtsch P, Maggiorini M, Ritter M, Noti C, Vock P, Oelz O. Prevention of high-altitude pulmonary edema by nifedipine. *N Engl J Med* 1991;325:1284–1289.

Batey DM, Nicolich MJ, Lasser VI, Jeffrey SS, Lasser NL. Prazosin versus hydrochlorothiazide as initial antihypertensive therapy in black versus white patients. *Am J Med* 1989;86:74–78.

Battle DC, von Riotte AB, Gaviria M, Grupp M. Amelioration of polyuria by amiloride in patients receiving long-term lithium therapy. *N Engl J Med* 1985;312:408–414.

Baumgart P. Torasemide in comparison with thiazides in the treatment of hypertension. *Cardiovasc Drugs Ther* 1993;7:63–68.

Bauer JH. Adrenergic blocking agents and the kidney. *J Clin Hypertens* 1985;3:199–221.

Bauer JH, Jones LB, Gaddy P. Effects of prazosin therapy on blood pressure, renal function, and body fluid composition. *Arch Intern Med* 1984;114:1196–1200.

Beard K, Bulpitt C, Mascie-Taylor H, O'Malley K, Sever P, Webb S. Management of elderly patients with sustained hypertension. *Br Med J* 1992;304:412–416.

Beer NA, Jakubowicz DJ, Beer RM, Arocha IR, Nestler JE. Effects of nitrendipine on glucose tolerance and serum insulin and dehydroepiandrosterone sulfate levels in insulin-resistant obese and hypertensive men. *J Clin Endocrinol Metab* 1993;76:178–183.

Beermann B, Grind M. Clinical pharmacokinetics of some newer diuretics. *Clin Pharmacokinetics* 1987;12:254–266.

Beevers DG, Fairman MJ, Hamilton M, Harpur JE. Antihypertensive treatment and the course of established cerebral vascular disease. *Lancet* 1973;1:1407–1409.

Bell DSH. Hypoglycemia induced by enalapril in patients with insulin resistance and NIDDM. *Diabetes Care* 1992;15:934–936.

Bellary SV, Isaacs PET, Scott AWM. Captopril and the liver. *Lancet* 1989;2:514.

Bengtsson C, Blohmé G, Lapidus L, Lissner L, Lundgren H. Diabetes incidence in users and non-users of antihypertensive drugs in relation to serum insulin, glucose tolerance and degree of adiposity: a 12-year prospective population study of women in Gothenburg, Sweden. *J Int Med* 1992;231:583–588.

Benson MK, Berrill WT, Cruickshank JM, Sterling GS. A comparison of four β-adrenoceptor antagonists in patients with asthma. *Br J Clin Pharmacol* 1978;5:415–419.

Bentley GA. Clonidine, a widow's curse for pharmacologists. *Clin Exp Pharmacol Physiol* 1987;14:465–470.

Berglund G, Andersson O, Widgren B. Low-dose antihypertensive treatment with a thiazide diuretic is not diabetogenic. A 10-year controlled trial with bendroflumethiazide. *Acta Med Scan* 1986;220:419–424.

Berntorp K, Lindgärd F, Mattiasson I. Long-term effects on insulin sensitivity and sodium transport in glucose-intolerant hypertensive subjects when β-blockade is replaced by captopril treatment. *J Hum Hypertens* 1992;6:291–298.

Bertel O, Conen D, Radü EW, Müller J, Lang C, Dubach UC. Nifedipine in hypertensive emergencies. *Br Med J* 1983;286:19–21.

Beto JA, Bansal VK. Quality of life in treatment of hypertension. A metaanalysis of clinical trials. *Am J Hypertens* 1992;5:125–133.

Bevan EG, Pringle SD, Waller PC, Herrick AL, Findlay JG, Murray GD, Carmichael HA, Reid JL, Weir RJ, Lorimer AR, McInnes GT. Comparison of captopril, hydralazine and nifedipine as third drug in hypertensive patients. *J Hum Hypertens* 1993;7:83–88.

Bhatia BB. On the use of rauwolfia serpentina in high blood pressure. *J Ind Med Assoc* 1942;11:262–265.

Bishopric NH, Simpson PC, Ordahl CP. Induction of the skeletal alpha-actin gene in alpha₁-adrenoceptor–mediated hypertrophy of rat cardiac myocytes. *J Clin Invest* 1987;80:1194–1199.

Bissler JJ, Welch TR, Loggie JMH. Paradoxical hypertension in hypovolemic children. *Pediatr Emerg Care* 1991;7:350–352.

Black HR. Metabolic considerations in the choice of therapy for the patient with hypertension. *Am Heart J* 1991;121:707–715.

Black JW, Crowther AF, Shanks RG, Smith LH, Dornhorst AC. A new adrenergic beta-receptor antagonist. *Lancet* 1964;2:1080–1081.

Black JW, Stephenson JS. Pharmacology of a new adrenergic beta-receptor-blocking compound (nethalide). *Lancet* 1962;2:311–314.

Bobik A, Jennings G, Jackman G, Oddie C, Korner P. Evidence for a predominantly central hypotensive effect of alpha-methyldopa in humans. *Hypertension* 1986;8:16–23.

Boden WE. Meta-analysis in clinical trials reporting: has a tool become a weapon? *Am J Cardiol* 1992;69:681–686.

Boman K, Eriksson P, Slunga L. Is addition of prazosin beneficial in chronic heart failure refractory to angiotensin converting enzyme inhibition? *Eur J Clin Pharmacol* 1989;37:431–432.

Bønaa KH, Thelle DS. Association between blood pressure and serum lipids in a population. The Tromsø study. *Circulation* 1991;83:1305–1314.

Bond WS. Psychiatric indications for clonidine: the neuropharmacologic and clinical basis. *J Clin Psychopharmacol* 1986;6:81–87.

Borders JV. Captopril and onycholysis. *Ann Intern Med* 1986;105:305–306.

Borghi C, Boschi S, Costa FV, Bacchelli S, Esposti DD, Ambrosioni E. Effects of different dosages of hydrochlorothiazide on blood pressure and the renin-angiotensin-aldosterone system in mild to moderate essential hypertension. *Curr Ther Res* 1992;51:859–869.

Bortolotti M, Trisolino G, Barbara L. Nifedipine in biliary and renal colic. *JAMA* 1987;258:3516.

Brater DC. Use of diuretics in chronic renal insufficiency and nephrotic syndrome. *Semin Nephrol* 1988;8:333–341.

Brater DC, Chennavasin P, Day B, Burdette A, Anderson S. Bumetanide and furosemide. *Clin Pharm Ther* 1983;34:207–213.

Bray GA. Treatment for obesity: a nutrient balance/nutrient partition approach. *Nutr Rev* 1991;49:33–45.

Breckenridge A. Which beta blocker? *Br Med J* 1983;286:1085–1088.

Brenner BM, Garcia DL, Anderson S. Glomeruli and blood pressure. *Am J Hypertens* 1988;1:335–347.

Breugnot C, Iliou JP, Privat S, Robin F, Vilaine JP, Lenaers A. In vitro and ex vivo inhibition of the modification of low-density lipoprotein by indapamide. *J Cardiovasc Pharm* 1992;20:340–347.

Briant RH, Reid JL, Dollery CT. Interaction between clonidine and desipramine in man. *Br Med J* 1973;1:522–523.

Bright RA, Everitt DE. β-blockers and depression. Evidence against an association. *JAMA* 1992;267:1783–1787.

Brott T, Reed RL. Intensive care for acute stroke in the community hospital setting. The first 24 hours. *Stroke* 1989; 20:694–697.

Brown MJ, Brown DC, Murphy MB. Hypokalemia from beta-receptor stimulation by circulating epinephrine. *N Engl J Med* 1983;309:1414–1419.

Brown MJ, Salmon D, Rendell M. Clonidine hallucinations. *Ann Intern Med* 1980;93:456–457.

Brunner FP, Thiel G, Hermle M, Bock HA, Mihatsch MJ. Long-term enalapril and verapamil in rats with reduced renal mass. *Kidney Int* 1989;36:969–977.

Brunner HR, Ménard J, Waeber B, Burnier M, Biollaz J, Nussberger J, Bellet M. Treating the individual hypertensive patient: considerations on dose, sequential monotherapy and drug combinations. *J Hypertens* 1990;8:3–11.

Bühler FR. The case for calcium antagonists as first-line treatment of hypertension. *J Hypertens* 1992;10:S17–S20.

Bühler FR, Hulthén UL, Kiowski W, Müller FB, Bolli P. The place of the calcium antagonist verapamil in antihypertensive therapy. *J Cardiovasc Pharm* 1982; 4:S350–S357.

Bühler FR, Laragh JH, Baer L, Vaughan ED Jr, Brunner HR. Propranolol inhibition of renin secretion. A specific approach to diagnosis and treatment of renin-dependent hypertensive diseases. *N Engl J Med* 1972;287:1209–1214.

Bulpitt CJ, Fletcher AE. Cognitive function and angiotensin-converting enzyme inhibitors in comparison with other antihypertensive drugs. *J Cardiovasc Pharm* 1992; 19:S100–S104.

Burnett AL, Lowenstein CJ, Bredt DS, Chang TSK, Snyder SH. Nitric oxide: a physiologic mediator of penile erection. *Science* 1992;257:401–403.

Burris JF, Weir MR, Oparil S, Weber M, Cady WJ, Stewart WH. An assessment of diltiazem and hydrochlorothiazide in hypertension. Application of factorial trial design to a multicenter clinical trial of combination therapy. *JAMA* 1990; 263:1507–1512.

Byrd BF III, Collins HW, Primm RK. Risk factors for severe bradycardia during oral clonidine therapy for hypertension. *Arch Intern Med* 1988;148:729–733.

Cameron HA, Higgins TJC. Clinical experience with lisinopril. Observations on safety and tolerability. *J Hum Hypertens* 1989;3:177–186.

Cameron HA, Ramsay LE. The lupus syndrome induced by hydralazine: a common complication with low dose treatment. *Br Med J* 1984;289:410–412.

Campbell DB, Brackman F. Cardiovascular protective properties of indapamide. *Am J Cardiol* 1990;65:11H–27H.

Campbell N, Paddock V, Sundaram R. *Clin Pharmacol Ther* 1988;43:381–386.

Campion EW, Glynn RJ, DeLabry LO. Asymptomatic hyperuricemia. Risks and consequences in the normative aging study. *Am J Med* 1987;82:421–426.

Cappuccio FP, Markandu ND, Singer DRJ, Buckley MG, Miller MA, Sagnella GA, MacGregor GA. A double-blind crossover study of the effect of concomitant diuretic therapy in hypertensive patients treated with amlodipine. *Am J Hypertens* 1991;4:297–302.

Captopril Collaborative Study Group. Does captopril cause renal damage in hypertensive patients? *Lancet* 1982;1:988–990.

Carlsen JE, Køber L, Torp-Pedersen C, Johansen P. Relation between dose of bendrofluazide, antihypertensive effect, and adverse biochemical effects. *Br Med J* 1990;300:975–978.

Carlsson A, Britton M. Blood pressure after stroke. *Stroke* 1993;24:195–199.

Carlsson E, Fellenius E, Lundborg P, Svensson L. β-adrenoceptor blockers, plasmapotassium, and exercise. *Lancet* 1978; 2:424–425.

Carruthers G, Dessain P, Fodor G, Newman C, Palmer W, Sim D. Comparative trial of doxazosin and atenolol on cardiovascular risk reduction in systemic hypertension. *Am J Cardiol* 1993;71:575–581.

Carruthers SG, Freeman DJ, Bailey DG. Synergistic adverse hemodynamic interaction between oral verapamil and propranolol. *Clin Pharmacol Ther* 1989;46:469–77.

Carter AB. Hypotensive therapy in stroke survivors. *Lancet* 1970;1:485–489.

Case DB, Wallace JM, Keim HJ, Sealey JE, Laragh JH. Usefulness and limitations of saralasin, a partial competitive agonist of angiotensin II for evaluating the renin and sodium factors in hypertensive patients. *Am J Med* 1976;60:825–836.

Casner PR, Dillon KR. A comparison of the anti-hypertensive effectiveness of two triamterene/hydrochlorothiazide combinations: maxzide versus dyazide. *J Clin Pharmacol* 1990;30:715–719.

Cauley JA, Cummings SR, Seeley DG, Black D, Browner W, Kuller LH, Nevitt MC. Effects of thiazide diuretic therapy on bone mass, fractures, and falls. *Ann Intern Med* 1993;118:666–673.

Cavallini G. Minoxidil versus nitroglycerin: a prospective double-blind controlled trial in transcutaneous erection facilitation for organic impotence. *J Urol* 1991; 146:50–53.

Chait A, Gilmore M. Inhibition of low density lipoprotein oxidation by the 6- and 7-hydroxymetabolites of doxazosin, an alpha-1 adrenergic blocking antihypertensive agent [Abstract]. *Am J Hypertens* 1993;6:20A.

Chang SW, Fine R, Siegel D, Chesney M, Black D, Hulley SB. The impact of diuretic therapy on reported sexual function. *Arch Intern Med* 1991;151:2402–2408.

Charlson ME, MacKenzie CR, Gold JP, Ales KL, Topkins M, Shires GT. Intraoperative blood pressure. What patterns identify patients at risk for postoperative complications? *Ann Surg* 1990;212:567–580.

Chatterjee K, Ports TA, Brundage BH, Massie B, Holly AN, Parmley WW. Oral hydralazine in chronic heart failure: sustained beneficial hemodynamic effects. *Ann Intern Med* 1980;92:600–604.

Chauveau D, Guyenne TT, Cumin F, Chatellier G, Corvol P, Ménard J. Investigation of the biochemical effects of renin inhibition in normal volunteers treated by an ACE inhibitor. *Br J Clin Pharmacol* 1992;33:253–260.

Chellingsworth MC, Kendall MJ, Lote CJ, Thewles A. Diuresis and natriuresis after dihydropyridines: role of prostaglandin E. *J Hum Hypertens* 1990;4:241–245.

Cheung DG, Hoffman CA, Ricci ST, Weber MA. Mild hypertension in the elderly. A comparison of prazosin and enalapril. *Am J Med* 1989;86:87–90.

Chick TW, Halperin AK, Gacek EM. The effect of antihypertensive medications on exercise performance: a review. *Med Sci Exerc* 1988;20:447–454.

Chobanian AV, Haudenschild CC, Nickerson C, Hope S. Trandolapril inhibits atherosclerosis in the watanabe heritable hyperlipidemic rabbit. *Hypertension* 1992; 20:473–477.

Christlieb RA. Treatment selection considerations for the hypertensive diabetic patient. *Arch Intern Med* 1990;150:1167–1174.

Chrysant SG, Chrysant C, Sadeghi M, Berlin L. Cardiac changes from beta-blocker, diuretic and minoxidil combination in hypertension. *Cardiology* 1991;78:45–52.

Chu TJ, Chow N. Adverse effects of ACE inhibitors. *Ann Intern Med* 1993;118:314.

Cinquegrani MP, Liang C-S. Indomethacin attenuates the hypotensive action of hydralazine. *Clin Pharmacol Ther* 1986; 39:564–570.

Clark JA, Zimmerman HJ, Tanner LA. Labetalol hepatotoxicity. *Ann Intern Med* 1990;113:210–213.

Clausen-Sjöbom N, Lins P-E, Adamson U, Curstedt T, Hamberger B. Effects of metoprolol on the counter-regulation and recognition of prolonged hypoglycemia in insulin-dependent diabetics. *Acta Med Scand* 1987;222:57–63.

Clobass Study Group. Low-dose clonidine administration in the treatment of mild or moderate essential hypertension: results from a double-blind placebo-controlled study (Clobass). *J Hypertens* 1990; 8:539–546.

Cloher TP, Whelton PK. Physician approach to the recognition and initial management of hypertension. *Arch Intern Med* 1986;146:529–533.

Clozel M, Clozel J, Hess P. Endothelin receptor antagonism: a new therapeutic approach in experimental hypertension [Abstract]. *Circulation* 1993;88(Part 2):316.

Cohen SI, Young MW, Lau SH, Haft JI, Damato AN. Effects of reserpine therapy on cardiac output and atrioventricular conduction during rest and controlled heart rates in patients with essential hypertension. *Circulation* 1968;37:738–745.

Cohn JN. Paroxysmal hypertension and hypovolemia. *N Engl J Med* 1966; 275:643–646.

Conway J, Coats AJS, Bird R. Lisinopril and enalapril in hypertension: a comparative study using ambulatory monitoring. *J Hum Hypertens* 1990;4:235–239.

Conway J, Lauwers P. Hemodynamic and hypotensive effects of long-term therapy with chlorothiazide. *Circulation* 1960; 21:21–26.

Cookson MS, Nadig PW. Long-term results with vacuum constriction device. *J Urol* 1993;149:290–294.

Cooper RG, Stokes MJ, Edwards RHT, Stark RD. Absence of excess peripheral muscle fatigue during β-adrenoceptor blockade. *Br J Clin Pharmacol* 1988;25:405–415.

Cooper RA. Captopril-associated neutropenia. Who is at risk? *Arch Intern Med* 1983;143:659–660.

Cordero P, Fisher ND, Moore TJ, Gleason R, Williams GH, Hollenberg NK. Renal and endocrine responses to a renin inhibitor, enalkiren, in normal humans. *Hypertension* 1991;17:510–516.

Cosenzi A, Piemontesi A, Franca G, Morelli D, Sacerdote A, Bocin E, Bellini G. Chronic antihypertensive treatment with lisinopril in hypertensive patients with peripheral occlusive arterial disease. *Curr Ther Res* 1992;51:275–280.

Coulter DM. Eye pain with nifedipine and disturbance of taste with captopril: a mutually controlled study showing a method of postmarketing surveillance. *Br Med J* 1988;296:1086–1088.

Cranston WI, Juel-Jensen BE, Semmence AM, Jones RPCH, Forbes JA, Mutch LMM. Effects of oral diuretics on raised arterial pressure. *Lancet* 1963;2:966–970.

Croog SH, Kong BW, Levine S, Weir MR, Baume RM, Saunders E. Hypertensive Black men and women. Quality of life and effects of antihypertensive medications. *Arch Intern Med* 1990;150:1733–1741.

Croog SH, Levine S, Sudilovsky A, Baume RM, Clive J. Sexual symptoms in hypertensive patients. A clinical trial of antihypertensive medications. *Arch Intern Med* 1988;148:788–794.

Cruickshank JM. Coronary flow reserve and the J curve relation between diastolic blood pressure and myocardial infarction. *Br Med J* 1988;297:1227–1230.

Cruickshank JM. Measurement and cardiovascular relevance of partial agonist activity (PAA) involving β$_1$- and β$_2$-adrenoceptors. *Pharmacol Ther* 1990;46:199–242.

Cruickshank JM. The case for beta-blockers as first-line antihypertensive therapy. *J Hypertens* 1992;10:S21–S27.

Cruickshank JM, Neil-Dwyer G, Degaute JP, Hayes Y, Kuurne T, Kytta J, Vincent JL, Carruthers ME, Patel S. Reduction of stress/catecholamine-induced cardiac necrosis by beta$_1$-selective blockade. *Lancet* 1987;2:585–589.

Cubeddu LX. New alpha$_1$-adrenergic receptor antagonists for the treatment of hypertension: role of vascular alpha receptors in the control of peripheral resistance. *Am Heart J* 1988;116:133–162.

Cummings DM, Amadio P Jr, Nelson L, Fitzgerald JM. The role of calcium channel blockers in the treatment of essential hypertension. *Arch Intern Med* 1991; 151:250–259.

Cushman P Jr, Forbes R, Lerner W, Stewart M. Alcohol withdrawal syndromes: clinical management with lofexidine. *Alcoholism Clin Exp Res* 1985;9:103–107.

Cushman DW, Wang FL, Fung WC, Harvey CM, DeForrest JM. Differentiation of angiotensin-converting enzyme (ACE) inhibitors by their selective inhibition of ACE in physiologically important target organs. *Am J Hypertens* 1989;2:294–306.

Dage RC, Mehdi S, Giroux EL, French JF, Flynn GA. Dual inhibitor of angiotensin I-converting enzyme and neutral endopeptidase [Abstract]. *Circulation* 1992; 86:I–140.

Dahlöf C, Dimenäs E. Side effects of β-blocker treatments as related to the central nervous system. *Am J Med Sci* 1990; 299:236–244.

Dahlöf B, Hansson L, Acosta JH, Bolzano K, Fairhurst G, Ferreira C, Kaarsalo E, Silva MC, Simone A. Controlled trial of enalapril and hydrochlorothiazide in 200 hypertensive patients. *Am J Hypertens* 1988;1:38–41.

Dahlöf B, Pennert K, Hansson L. Reversal of left ventricular hypertrophy in hypertensive patients. A metaanalysis of 109 treatment studies. *Am J Hypertens* 1992; 5:95–110.

Davidson C, Thadani U, Singleton W, Taylor SH. Comparison of antihypertensive activity of beta-blocking drugs during chronic treatment. *Br Med J* 1976;2:7–9.

Davidson KG, McKenzie JK, Ross SA, Chiasson J-L, Hamet P. Report of the Canadian Hypertension Society Consensus Conference: 5. Hypertension and diabetes. *Can Med Assoc J* 1993;149:821–826.

Deitch MW, Littman GS, Pascucci VL. Antihypertensive therapy with guanabenz in patients with chronic obstructive pulmonary diseases. *J Cardiovasc Pharmacol* 1984;6:S818–S822.

DeQuattro V, De-Ping Lee D, Allen J, Sirgo M, Plachetka J. Labetalol blunts morning pressor surge in systolic hypertension. *Hypertension* 1988;11(Suppl 1):198–201.

DeQuattro V, Weir MR. Bisoprolol fumarate/hydrochlorothiazide 6.25 mg: a new low-dose option for first-line antihypertensive therapy. *Adv Ther* 1993;10:197–206.

Devereux RB, Laragh JH. Angiotensin converting enzyme inhibition of renin system activity induces reversal of hypertensive target organ changes. Do these effects predict a reduction in long-term morbidity? *Am J Hypertens* 1992;5:923–926.

Devoy MAB, Tomson CRV, Edmunds ME, Feehally J, Walls J. Deterioration in renal function associated with angiotensin converting enzyme inhibitor therapy is not always reversible. *J Intern Med* 1992; 232:493–498.

di Somma S, Liguori V, Petitto M, Cavallotti G, Savonitto S, de Divitiis O. Hemodynamic interactions between diuretics and calcium antagonists in the treatment of hypertensive patients. *Cardiovasc Drug Ther* 1990;4:1151–1156.

Dianzumba SB, DiPette D, Joyner CR, Cornman C, Townsend R, Mauro K, Weber E, Theobald T. Left ventricular filling in hypertensive blacks and whites following adrenergic blockade. *Am J Hypertens* 1990;3:48–51.

Diffey BL, Langtry J. Phototoxic potential of thiazide diuretics in normal subjects. *Arch Dermatol* 1989;125:1355–1358.

Dimsdale JE. Reflections on the impact of antihypertensive medications on mood, sedation, and neuropsychologic functioning. *Arch Intern Med* 1992;152:35–39.

Dimsdale JE, Newton RP, Joist T. Neuropsychological side effects of β-blockers. *Arch Intern Med* 1989;149:514–525.

Diokno AC, Brown MB, Herzog AR. Sexual function in the elderly. *Arch Intern Med* 1990;150:197–200.

Disdier P, Harlé J-R, Verrot D, Jouglard J, Weiller P-J. Adult schönlein-henoch purpura after lisinopril. *Lancet* 1992;340:985.

Dluhy RG, Smith K, Taylor T, Hollenberg NK, Williams GH. Prolonged converting enzyme inhibition in non-modulating hypertension. *Hypertension* 1989; 13:371–377.

Donati L, Bühler FR, Beretta-Piccoli C, Kusch F, Heinen G. Antihypertensive mechanism of amlodipine in essential hypertension: role of pressor reactivity to norepinephrine and angiotensin II. *Clin Pharmacol Ther* 1992;52:50–59.

Donnelly R, Elliott HL, Meredith PA. Antihypertensive drugs: individualized analysis and clinical relevance of kinetic-dynamic relationships. *Pharmacol Ther* 1992;53:67–79.

Donnelly R, Elliott HL, Meredith PA, Kelman AW, Reid JL. Nifedipine: individual responses and concentration-effect relationships. *Hypertension* 1988;12:443–449.

Dornhorst A, Powell SH, Pensky J. Aggravation by propranolol of hyperglycaemic effect of hydrochlorothiazide in type II diabetics without alteration of insulin secretion. *Lancet* 1985;1:123–126.

Dørup I, Skajaa K, Thybo NK. Oral magnesium supplementation restores the concentrations of magnesium, potassium and sodium-potassium pumps in skeletal muscle of patients receiving diuretic treatment. *J Intern Med* 1993;233:117–123.

Doyle AE. Sir Horace Smirk. Pioneer in drug treatment of hypertension. *Hypertension* 1991;17:247–250.

Drayer JIM, Keim HJ, Weber MA, Case DB, Laragh JH. Unexpected pressor responses to propranolol in essential hypertension. An interaction between renin, aldosterone and sympathetic activity. *Am J Med* 1976;60:897–903.

Duncan JJ, Vaandrager H, Farr JE, Kohl HW, Gordon NF. *Am J Hypertens* 1990; 3:302–306.

Dustan HP, Caplan LR, Curry CL, De Leon AC Jr, Douglas FL, Frishman W, Hill MN, Washington RL, Steigerwalt S, Shulman NB, Taubert KA, Champagne B, Groom A. Report of the task force on the availability of cardiovascular drugs to the medically indigent. *Circulation* 1992;85:849–860.

Duty S, Weston AH. Potassium channel openers. Pharmacological effects and future uses. *Drugs* 1990;40:785–791.

Dykman D, Simon EE, Avioli LV. Hyperuricemia and uric acid nephropathy. *Arch Intern Med* 1987;147:1341–1345.

Edmonds D, Huss R, Jeck T, Mengden T, Schubert M, Vetter W. Individualizing antihypertensive therapy with enalapril versus atenolol: the Zurich experience. *J Hypertens* 1990;8:S49–S52.

Edwards IR, Coulter DM, Macintosh D. Intestinal effects of captopril. *Br Med J* 1992;304:359–360.

Eggertsen R, Hansson L. Vasodilators in hypertension—a review with special emphasis on the combined used of vasodilators and beta-adrenoceptor blockers. *Int J Clin Pharmacol Ther Toxicol* 1985; 23:411–423.

Eicher JC, Morelon P, Chalopin JM, Tanter Y, Louis P, Rifle G. Acute renal failure during nifedipine therapy in a patient with congestive heart failure. *Critical Care Med* 1988;16:1163–1164.

Eisen SA, Miller DK, Woodward RS, Spitznagel E, Przybeck TR. The effect of prescribed daily dose frequency on patient medication compliance. *Arch Intern Med* 1990;150:1881–1884.

Ekeberg Ø, Kjeldsen SE, Eide IK, Greenwood DT, Enger E. Effects of responses to flight phobia stress. *Clin Pharmacol Ther* 1990;47:599–607.

El Matri A, Larabi MS, Kechrid C, Belkahia C, Ayed HB. Fatal bone-marrow suppression associated with captopril. *Br Med J* 1981;283:277–278.

Eliasson K, Danielson M, Hylander B, Lindblad LE. Raynaud's phenomenon caused by β-receptor blocking drugs. Improvement after treatment with a combined alpha- and β-blocker. *Acta Med Scand* 1984;215:333–339.

Elliott HL, Ajayi AA, Ried JL. The influence of cilazapril on indices of autonomic function in normotensives and hypertensives. *Br J Clin Pharmacol* 1989a;27: 3035–3075.

Elliott HL, Donnelly R, Meredith PA, Reid JL. Predictability of antihypertensive responsiveness and alpha-adrenoceptor antagonism during prazosin treatment. *Clin Pharmacol Ther* 1989b;46:576–583.

Elliott WJ. Glucose and cholesterol elevations from diuretic therapy: intention to treat vs. actual on-therapy experience [Abstract]. *Am J Hypertens* 1993;6:9–10.

Elliott WJ, Polascik TB, Murphy MB. Equivalent antihypertensive effects of combination therapy using diuretic + calcium antagonist compared with diuretic + ACE inhibitor. *J Hum Hypertens* 1990;4: 717–723.

Ellis JS, Seymour RA, Monkman SC, Idle JR. Gingival sequestration of nifedipine in nifedipine-induced gingival overgrowth. *Lancet* 1992;339:1382–1383.

Ellison DH. The physiologic basis of diuretic synergism: its role in treating diuretic resistance. *Ann Intern Med* 1991;114:886–894.

Enström I, Thulin T, Lindholm LH. Comparison between enalapril and lisinopril mild-moderate hypertension: a comprehensive model for evaluation of drug efficacy. *Blood Pressure* 1992;1:102–107.

Epstein M. Calcium antagonists and the kidney. Implications for renal protection. *Am J Hypertens* 1991;4:482S–486S.

Epstein M, Oster JR. Beta blockers and renal function: a reappraisal. *J Clin Hypertens* 1985;1:85–99.

Erley CM, Harrer U, Krämer BK, Risler T. Renal hemodynamics and reduction of proteinuria by a vasodilating beta blocker versus an ACE inhibitor. *Kidney Int* 1992;41:1297–1303.

Esler M, Dudley F, Jennings G, Debinski H, Lambert G, Jones P, Crotty B, Colman J, Willett I. Increased sympathetic nervous activity and the effects of its inhibition with clonidine in alcoholic cirrhosis. *Ann Intern Med* 1992;116:446–455.

Esler M, Jackman G, Leonard P, Skews H, Bobik A, Jennings G. Effect of propranolol on noradrenaline kinetics in patients with essential hypertension. *Br J Clin Pharmacol* 1981;12:375–380.

Estafanous FG. Hypertension in the surgical patient: management of blood pressure and anesthesia. *Cleveland Clin J Med* 1989;56:385–393.

Favre L, Riondel A, Vallotton MB. Effect of calcium-channel blockade on the aldosterone response to sodium depletion and potassium loading in man. *Am J Hypertens* 1988;1:245–248.

Fedorak RN, Field M, Chang EB. Treatment of diabetic diarrhea with clonidine. *Ann Intern Med* 1985;102:197–199.

Feher MD, Henderson AD, Wadsworth J, Poulter C, Gelding S, Richmond W, Sever PS, Elkeles RS. Alpha-blocker therapy; a possible advance in the treatment of diabetic hypertension—results of a cross-over study of doxazosin and atenolol monotherapy in hypertensive non-insulin dependent diabetic subjects. *J Hum Hypertens* 1990;4:571–577.

Feigl EO. The paradox of adrenergic coronary vasoconstriction. *Circulation* 1987;76:737–745.

Feit A, Cohen M, Dimino L, El-Sherif N, Holtzman R, Ram CVS, Gaffeny D, Heller J, Kaplan N. The effects of labetalol and prazosin on exercise haemodynamics in hypertensive patients. *J Hum Hypertens* 1991;5:39–43.

Ferrara LA, Di Marino L, Russo O, Marotta T, Mancini M. Doxazosin and captopril in mildly hypercholesterolemic hypertensive patients. The doxazosin-captopril in hypercholesterolemic hypertensives study. *Hypertension* 1993;21:97–104.

Finnerty FA Jr. Stepped-down therapy versus intermittent therapy in systemic hypertension. *Am J Cardiol* 1990;66:1373–1374.

Finnerty FA Jr, Davidov M, Mroczek WJ, Gavrilovich L. Influence of extracellular fluid volume on response to antihypertensive drugs. *Circ Res* 1970;26(Suppl 1):71–80.

Fitzgerald JD. The applied pharmacology of beta-adrenoceptor antagonists (beta blockers) in relation to clinical outcomes. *Cardiovasc Drugs Ther* 1991a;5:561–576.

Fitzgerald JD. Introduction to focused section on new developments in beta blockade. *Cardiovasc Drugs Ther* 1991b;5:545–548.

Fleckenstein A. History and prospects in calcium antagonist research. *J Mol Cell Cardiol* 1990;22:241–251.

Fletcher AE, Beevers DG, Dollery CT, Wilkinson R, Bulpitt CJ. The effects of two centrally-acting anti-hypertensive drugs on the quality of life. *Eur J Clin Pharmacol* 1991;41:397–400.

Fletcher AE, Bulpitt CJ, Chase DM, Collins WCJ, Furberg CD, Goggin TK, Hewett AJ, Neiss AM. Quality of life with three antihypertensive treatments: cilazapril, atenolol, nifedipine. *Hypertension* 1992;19:499–507.

Flynn MA, Nolph GB, Baker AS, Martin WM, Krause G. Total body potassium in aging humans: a longitudinal study. *Am J Clin Nutr* 1989;50:713–717.

Fodor JG, Chockalingam A, Drover A, Fifield F, Pauls CJ. A comparison of the side effects of atenolol and propranolol in the treatment of patients with hypertension. *J Clin Pharmacol* 1987;27:892–901.

Fogari R, Zoppi A, Tettamanti F, Malamani GD, Tinelli C, Salvetti A. Effects of nifedipine and indomethacin on cough induced by angiotensin-converting enzyme inhibitors: a double-blind, randomized, cross-over study. *J Cardiovasc Pharmacol* 1992;19:670–673.

Fonseca V, Phear DN. Hyperosmolar nonketotic diabetic syndrome precipitated by treatment with diuretics. *Br Med J* 1982;284:36–37.

Fouad FM, Nakashima Y, Tarazi RC, Salcedo EE. Reversal of left ventricular hypertrophy in hypertensive patients treated with methyldopa. Lack of association with blood pressure control. *Am J Cardiol* 49:795–801.

Freis ED. The cardiotoxicity of thiazide diuretics: review of the evidence. *J Hypertens* 1990a;8:S23–S32.

Freis ED. Origins and development of antihypertensive treatment. In: Laragh JH, Brenner BM, eds. Hypertension: Pathophysiology, Diagnosis, and Management. New York: Raven Press, 1990b:2093–2105.

Freis ED, Reda DJ, Materson BJ. Volume (weight) loss and blood pressure response following thiazide diuretics. *Hypertension* 1988;12:244–250.

Freis ED, Rose JC, Higgins TF, Finnerty FA, Kelley RT, Partenope EA. The hemodynamic effects of hypotensive drugs in man. IV. 1-hydrazinophthalazine. *Circulation* 1953;8:199.

Frewin DB, Radeski C, Guerin MD. The effects of substituting fursemide for a thiazide diuretic in the drug regimens of patients with essential hypertension. *Eur J Clin Pharmacol* 1987;33:31–34.

Friedel HA, Brogden RN. Pinacidil. A review of its pharmacodynamic and pharmacokinetic properties, and therapeutic potential in the treatment of hypertension. *Drugs* 1990;39:929–967.

Friedman E, Shadel M, Halkin H, Farfel Z. Thiazide-induced hyponatremia. Reproducibility by single dose rechallenge and an analysis of pathogenesis. *Ann Intern Med* 1989;110:24–30.

Frohlich ED, Tarazi RC, Dustan HP, Page IH. The paradox of beta-adrenergic blockade in hypertension. *Circulation* 1968; 37:417–423.

Furberg CD, Borhani NO, Byington RP, Gibbons ME, Sowers JR. Calcium antagonists and atherosclerosis. The multicenter isradipine/diuretic atherosclerosis study. *Am J Hypertens* 1993;6:24S–29S.

Furhoff A-K. Adverse reactions with methyldopa—a decade's reports. *Acta Med Scand* 1978;203:425–428.

Garner L. Sodium nitroprusside treatment in patients with acute strokes. *Arch Intern Med* 1986;146:1454.

Garthoff B, Bellemann P. Effects of salt loading and nitrendipine on dihydropyridine receptors in hypertensive rats. *J Cardiovasc Pharmacol* 1987;10:S36–S38.

Gavras H, Brunner HR, Laragh JH, Sealey JE, Gavras I, Vukovich RA. An angiotensin converting-enzyme inhibitor to identify and treat vasoconstrictor and volume factors in hypertensive patients. *N Engl J Med* 1974;291:817–821.

Gavras H, Gavras I, Brunner HR, Laragh JH. The antihypertensive action of methyldopa in relation to its effect on the renin-aldosterone system. *J Clin Pharmacol* 1977a; 17:372–378.

Gavras H, Gavras I, Textor S, Volicer L, Brunner HR, Rucinska EJ. Effect of angiotensin converting enzyme inhibition on blood pressure, plasma renin activity and plasma aldosterone in essential hypertension. *J Clin Endocrinol Metab* 1977b; 46:220–226.

Gavras I. Bradykinin-mediated effects of ACE inhibition. *Kidney Int* 1992; 42:1020–1029.

Gay R, Algeo S, Lee R, Olajos M, Morkin E, Goldman S. Treatment of verapamil toxicity in intact dogs. *J Clin Invest* 1986;77:1805–1811.

Gehr M, MacCarthy EP, Goldberg M. Guanabenz: a centrally acting, natriuretic antihypertensive drug. *Kidney Int* 1986; 29:1203–1208.

Gelmers HJ, Gorter K, De Weerdt CJ, Wiezer JHA. A controlled trial of nimodipine in acute ischemic stroke. *N Engl J Med* 1988;318:203–207.

George RB, Light RW, Hudson LD, Conrad SA, Chetty K, Manocha K, Burford JG. Comparison of the effects of labetalol and hydrochlorothiazide on the ventilatory function of hypertensive patients with asthma and propranolol sensitivity. *Chest* 1985;88:815–818.

Gesek FA, Friedman PA. Mechanism of calcium transport stimulated by chlorothiazide in mouse distal convoluted tubule cells. *J Clin Invest* 1992;90:429–438.

Giannattasio C, Cattaneo BM, Omboni S, Seravalle G, Bolla G, Turolo L, Morganti A, Grassi G, Zanchetti A, Mancia G. Sympathomoderating influence of benazepril in essential hypertension. *J Hypertens* 1992;10:373–378.

Giles TD, Sander GE, Roffidal LE, Quiroz AC, Mazzu AL. Comparative effects of nitrendipine and hydrochlorothiazide on calciotropic hormones and bone density in hypertensive patients. *Am J Hypertens* 1992;5:875–879.

Giugliano D, Quatraro A, Consoli G, Minei A, Ceriello A, De Rosa N, D'Onofrio F. Metformin for obese, insulin-treated diabetic patients: improvement in glycaemic control and reduction of metabolic risk factors. *Eur J Clin Pharmacol* 1993; 44:107–112.

Goa KL, Benfield P, Sorkin EM. Labetalol. A reappraisal of its pharmacology, pharmacokinetics and therapeutic use in hypertension and ischaemic heart disease. *Drugs* 1989;37:583–627.

Goldberg AD, Raftery EB. Patterns of blood-pressure during chronic administration of postganglionic sympathetic blocking drugs for hypertension. *Lancet* 1976; 2:1052–1054.

Goldberg LI. Dopamine: clinical uses of an endogenous catecholamine. *N Engl J Med* 1974;291:707–710.

Goldner MG, Zarowitz H, Akgun S. Hyperglycemia and glycosuria due to thiazide derivatives administered in diabetes mellitus. *Med Intelligence* 1960;262:403–405.

Goldstein G. Hypertension and cognitive function in the elderly. *Cardiovasc Risk Factors* 1992;2:127–132.

Goodfield MJ, Millard LG. Severe cutaneous reactions to captopril. *Br Med J* 1985; 290:1111.

Graves JW, Bloomfield RL, Buckalew VM Jr. Plasma volume in resistant hypertension: guide to pathophysiology and therapy. *Am J Med Sci* 1989;298:361–365.

Gregoire A. New treatments for erectile impotence. *Br J Psychiatry* 1992; 160:315–326.

Grimm RH Jr, Cohen JD, Smith WM, Falvo-Gerard L, Neaton JD. Hypertension management in the multiple risk factor intervention trial (MRFIT). Six-year intervention results for men in special intervention and usual care groups. *Arch Intern Med* 1991;145:1191–1199.

Groden DL. Vasodilator therapy for congestive heart failure. *Arch Intern Med* 1993;153:445–454.

Grubb BP, Sirio C, Zelis R. Intravenous labetalol in acute aortic dissection. *JAMA* 1987;258:78–79.

Gullestad L, Birkeland K, Nordby G, Larsen S, Kjekshus J. Effects of selective β_2-adrenoceptor blockade on serum potassium and exercise performance in normal men. *Br J Clin Pharmacol* 1991;32:201–207.

Gurwitz JH, Bohn RL, Glynn RJ, Monane M, Mogun H, Avorn J. Antihypertensive drug therapy and the initiation of treatment of diabetes mellitus. *Ann Intern Med* 1992;118:273–278.

Guthrie R. The treatment of concomitant hypertension and prostatic obstructive symptoms with terazosin [Abstract]. *Am J Hypertens* 1993;6:127A.

Gutin M, Tuck ML. Metabolic control during guanabenz antihypertensive therapy in diabetic patients with hypertension. *Curr Ther Res* 1988;43:775–785.

Guyatt GH, Feeny DH, Patrick DL. Measuring health-related quality of life. *Ann Intern Med* 1993;118:622–629.

Guyatt GH, Keller JL, Jaeschke R, Rosenbloom D, Adachi JD, Newhouse MT. The n-of-1 randomized controlled trial: clinical usefulness. Our three-year experience. *Ann Intern Med* 1990;112:293–299.

Haeusler G, Lues I, Minck K-O, Schelling P, Seyfried CA. Pharmacological basis for antihypertensive therapy with a novel dopamine agonist. *Eur Heart J* 1992; 13(Suppl D):129–135.

Haffner CA, Horton RC, Lewis HM, Hughes B, Kendall MJ. A metabolic assessment of the beta$_1$ selectivity of bisoprolol. *J Hum Hypertens* 1992;6:397–400.

Haffner CA, Smith BS, Pepper C. Hallucinations as an adverse effect of angiotensin converting enzyme inhibition. *Postgrad Med J* 1993;69:240–244.

Hallab M, Gallois Y, Chatellier G, Rohmer V, Fressinaud P, Marre M. Comparison of reduction in microalbuminuria by enalapril and hydrochlorothiazide in normotensive patients with insulin dependent diabetes. *Br Med J* 1993;306:175–182.

Halloran TJ, Phillips CE. Propranolol intoxication. A severe case responding to norepinephrine therapy. *Arch Intern Med* 1981;141:810–811.

Halpern NA, Goldberg M, Neely C, Sladen RN, Goldberg JS, Floyd J, Gabrielson G, Greenstein RJ. Postoperative hypertension: a multicenter, prospective, randomized comparison between intravenous nicardipine and sodium nitroprusside. *Crit Care Med* 1992;20:1637–1643.

Hamada M, Kazatani Y, Shigematsu Y, Ito T, Kokubu T, Ishise S. Enhanced blood pressure response to isometric handgrip exercise in patients with essential hypertension: effects of propranolol and prazosin. *J Hypertens* 1987;5:305–309.

Hammar M, Berg G. Clonidine in the treatment of menopausal flushing. A review of clinical studies. *Acta Obstet Gynecol Scand Suppl* 1985;132:29–31.

Hammarström L, Smith CIE, Berg U. Captopril-induced IgA deficiency. *Lancet* 1991;337:436.

Hampton JR. Secondary prevention of acute myocardial infarction with beta-blocking agents and calcium antagonists. *Am J Cardiol* 1990;66:3C–8C.

Harris DCH, Hammond WS, Burke TJ, Schrier RW. Verapamil protects against progression of experimental chronic renal failure. *Kidney Int* 1987;3:41–46.

Harrison MR, Clifton GD, DeMaria AN. Hemodynamic effects of calcium channel and β-receptor antagonists: evaluation by doppler echocardiography. *Am Heart J* 1991;121:126–132.

Hayashi M, Kobayashi H, Kawano H, Handa Y, Hirose S. Treatment of systemic hypertension and intracranial hypertension in cases of brain hemorrhage. *Stroke* 1988;19:314–321.

Haynes RB. The problems of compliance and their (partial) solution. In: Robertson JIS, ed. Handbook of Hypertension, vol. 1: Clinical Aspects of Essential Hypertension. New York: Elsevier Science Publishers, 1983;437–447.

Healy JJ, McKenna TJ, Canning B, Brien TG, Duffy GJ, Muldowney FP. Body composition changes in hypertensive subjects on long-term diuretic therapy. *Br Med J* 1970;1:716–719.

Hebert PR, Moser M, Mayer J, Glynn RJ, Hennekens CH. Recent evidence on drug therapy of mild to moderate hypertension and decreased risk of coronary heart disease. *Arch Intern Med* 1993;153:578–581.

Hedner T, Sun X, Junggren I-L, Petersson A, Edvinsson L. Peptides as targets for antihypertensive drug development. *J Hypertens* 1992;10(Suppl 7):121–132.

Hegbrant J, Skogström K, Månsby J. Comparison of slow-release piretanide and bendroflumethiazide in the treatment of mild to moderate hypertension. *J Int Med Res* 1989;17:426–434.

Heidland VA, Klütsch K, Öbek A. Myogenbedingte vasodilatation bei nierenischämie. *Münch Med Wochenschr* 1962;35:1636–1637.

Henkin Y, Como JA, Oberman A. Secondary dyslipidemia. Inadvertent effects of drugs in clinical practice. *JAMA* 1992; 267:961–968.

Henry JA, Cassidy SL. Membrane stabilizing activity: a major cause of fatal poisoning. *Lancet* 1986;1:1414–1417.

Herman AG. Differences in structure of angiotensin-converting enzyme inhibitors might predict differences in action. *Am J Cardiol* 1992;70:102C–108C.

Herxheimer A. How much drug in the tablet? *Lancet* 1991;337:346–348.

Hilleman E, Mohiuddin SM, Lucas BD. Cost analysis of initial antihypertension therapy [Abstract]. *Circulation* 1993;88(Part 2):263.

Hirooka Y, Imaizumi T, Masaki H, Ando S-I, Harada S, Momohara M, Takeshita A. Captopril improves impaired endothelium-dependent vasodilation in hypertensive patients. *Hypertension* 1992;20:175–180.

Hodgson JM, Cohen MD, Szentpetery S, Thames MD. Effects of regional alpha- and β-blockade on resting and hyperemic coronary blood flow in conscious, unstressed humans. *Circulation* 1989;79:797–809.

Hoeldtke RD, Davis KM. The orthostatic tachycardia syndrome: evaluation of autonomic function and treatment with octreotide and ergot alkaloids. *J Clin Endocrinol Metab* 1991;73:132–139.

Hohnloser SH, Verrier RL, Lown B, Raeder EA. Effect of hypokalemia on susceptibility to ventricular fibrillation in the normal and ischemic canine heart. *Am Heart J* 1986;112:32–35.

Holland OB, Gomez-Sanchez CE, Kuhnert LV, Poindexter C, Pak CYC. Antihypertensive comparison of furosemide with hydrochlorothiazide for black patients. *Arch Intern Med* 1979;139:1015–1021.

Holland OB, Nixon JV, Kuhnert L. Diuretic-induced ventricular ectopic activity. *Am J Med* 1981;70:762–768.

Holmes B, Brogden RN, Heel RC, Speight TM, Avery GS. Guanabenz. A review of its pharmacodynamic properties and therapeutic efficacy in hypertension. *Drugs* 1983;26:212–229.

Holmes B, Sorkin EM. Indoramin. A review of its pharmacodynamic and pharmacokinetic properties, and therapeutic efficacy in hypertension and related vascular, cardiovascular and airway diseases. *Drugs* 1986;31:467–499.

Hoorntje SJ, Kallenberg CGM, Weening JJ, Donker AJM, The TH, Hoedemaeker PJ. Immune-complex glomerulopathy in patients treated with captopril. *Lancet* 1980;1:1212–1214.

Horwitz RI, Feinstein AR. Exclusion bias and the false relationship of reserpine and breast cancer. *Arch Intern Med* 1985;145:1873–1875.

Horwitz RI, Gottlieb LD, Kraus ML. The efficacy of atenolol in the outpatient management of the alcohol withdrawal syndrome. Results of a randomized clinical trial. *Arch Intern Med* 1989; 149:1089–1093.

Houston MC. Abrupt cessation of treatment in hypertension: consideration of clinical features, mechanisms, prevention and management of the discontinuation syndrome. *Am Heart J* 1981;102:415–430.

Houston MC. Treatment of hypertensive emergencies and urgencies with oral clonidine loading and titration. *Arch Intern Med* 1986;146:586–589.

Houston MC, Hodge R. Beta-adrenergic blocker withdrawal syndromes in hypertension and other cardiovascular diseases. *Am Heart J* 1988;116:515–523.

Hricik DE, Browning PJ, Kopelman R, Goorno WE, Madias NE, Dzau VJ. Captopril-induced functional renal insufficiency in patients with bilateral renal-artery stenoses or renal-artery stenosis in a solitary kidney. *N Engl J Med* 1983;308:373–376.

Hui KK, Duchin KL, Kripalani KJ, Chan D, Kramer PK, Yanagawa N. Pharmacokinetics of fosinopril in patients with various degrees of renal function. *Clin Pharmacol Ther* 1991;49:457–467.

Hulter HN, Licht JH, Ilnicki LP, Singh S. Clinical efficacy and pharmacokinetics of clonidine in hemodialysis and renal insufficiency. *J Lab Clin Med* 1979; 94:223–231.

Hunyor SN, Bradstock K, Somerville PJ, Lucas N. Clonidine overdose. *Br Med J* 1975;4:23.

Hutcheon DF, Skinhj A, Andersen FJ. Gastric irritating effect of potassium chloride formulations. An endoscopic study in humans. *Cur Ther Res* 1988;43:55–61.

Hvarfner A, Bergström R, Lithell H, Mörlin C, Wide L, Ljunghall S. Changes in calcium metabolic indices during long-term treatment of patients with essential hypertension. *Clin Sci* 1988;75:543–549.

Imhof E, Elsasser S, Rosmus B, Ha HR, Follath F, Perruchoud AP. Verapamil in the prophylaxis of bronchial asthma. Is the bronchoprotective effect related to the plasma level? *Eur J Clin Pharmacol* 1991;41:317–319.

Innes A, Gemmell HG, Smith FW, Edward N, Catto GRD. The short term effects of oral labetalol in patients with chronic renal disease and hypertension. *J Hum Hypertens* 1992;6:211–214.

Israili ZH, Hall WD. Cough and angioneurotic edema associated with angiotensin-converting enzyme inhibitor therapy. A review of the literature and pathophysiology. *Ann Intern Med* 1992;117:234–242.

Isaksson H, Cederholm T, Jansson E, Nygren A, Östergren J. Therapy-resistant hypertension associated with central obesity, insulin resistance, and large muscle fibre area. *Blood Pressure* 1993;2:46–52.

Iwanov V, Moulds RFW. Differing calcium sensitivities of human cerebral and digital arteries, human metatarsal veins, and rat aorta. *Br J Clin Pharmacol* 1991; 31:47–54.

Izzo JL Jr, Horwitz D, Keiser HR. Physiologic mechanisms opposing the hemodynamic effects of prazosin. *Clin Pharmacol Ther* 1981;29:7–11.

Jackson B, McGrath BP, Maher D, Johnston CI, Matthews PG. Lack of cross sensitivity between captopril and enalapril. *Aust N Z J Med* 1988;18:21–27.

James MA, Jones JV. An interaction between LVH and potassium in hypertension? *J Hum Hypertens* 1991;5:475–478.

Jansen PAF, Gribnau FWJ, Schulte BPM, Poels EFJ. Contribution of inappropriate treatment for hypertension to pathogenesis of stroke in the elderly. *Br Med J* 1986; 293:914–917.

Jansen PAF, Schulte BPM, Gribnau FWJ. Cerebral ischaemia and stroke as side effects of antihypertensive treatment; special danger in the elderly. A review of the cases reported in the literature. *Netherlands J Med* 1987;30:193–201.

Jansson J-H, Johansson B, Boman K, Nilsson TK. Effects of doxazosin and atenolol on the fibrinolytic system in patients with hypertension and elevated serum cholesterol. *Eur J Clin Pharmacol* 1991; 40:321–326.

Jarrott B, Conway EL, Maccarrone C, Lewis SJ. Clonidine: understanding its disposition, sites and mechanism of action. *Clin Exp Pharmacol Physiol* 1987;14:471–479.

Jefferson JW, Kalin NH. Serum lithium levels and long-term diuretic use. *JAMA* 1979;241:1134–1136.

Jennings GL, Sudhir K. Initial therapy of primary hypertension. *Med J Aust* 1990;152:198–203.

Jeunemaitre X, Kreft-Jais C, Chatellier G, Julien J, Degoulet P, Plouin P-F, Ménard J, Corvol P. Long-term experience with spironolactone in essential hypertension. *Kidney Int* 1988;34:S14–S17.

Jick H, Dinan BJ, Hunter JR. Triamterene and renal stones. *J Urol* 1982; 127:224–225.

Johnson B, Hoch K, Errichetti A, Johnson J. Effects of methyldopa on psychometric performance. *J Clin Pharmacol* 1990;30:1102–1105.

Johnson BF, Danylchuk MA. The relevance of plasma lipid changes with cardiovascular drug therapy. *Med Clin North Am* 1989;73:449–473.

Johnson BF, Errichetti A, Urbach D, Hoch K, Johnson J. The effect of once-daily minoxidil on blood pressure and plasma lipids. *J Clin Pharmacol* 1986; 26:534–538.

Johnston GD. Dose-response relationships with antihypertensive drugs. *Pharmacol Ther* 1992;55:53–93.

Johnston GD, Wilson R, McDermott BJ, McVeigh GE, Duffin D, Logan J. Low-dose cyclopenthiazide in the treatment of hypertension: a one-year community-based study. *Q J Med* 1991;78:135–143.

Joint National Committee. The fifth report of the Joint National Committee on detection, evaluation, and treatment of high blood pressure (JNC V). *Arch Intern Med* 1993;153:154–183.

Jones HMR, Cummings AJ. A study of the transfer of alpha-methyldopa to the human foetus and newborn infant. *Br J Clin Pharmacol* 1978;6:432–434.

Jungmann E, Haak T, Carlberg C, Usadel KH, Wolfgang J. Lack of evidence of insulin-induced hypertension in insulin treated patients with type 2 diabetes mellitus [Abstract]. *Am J Hypertens* 1993;6:52–63.

Kaplan NM. Critical comments on recent literature. Age and the response to antihypertensive drugs. *Am J Hypertens* 1989a;2:213–215.

Kaplan NM. Calcium entry blockers in the treatment of hypertension. Current status and future prospects. *JAMA* 1989b; 262:817–823.

Kaplan NM. Cost-effectiveness of antihypertensive drugs. Fact or fancy? *Am J Hypertens* 1991;4:418–480.

Kaplan NM. New approaches to the treatment of hypertension. *Cardiovasc Drugs Ther* 1991;5:973–978.

Kaplan NM. The appropriate goals of antihypertensive therapy: neither too much nor too little. *Ann Intern Med* 1992; 116:686–690.

Kaplan NM, Carnegie A, Raskin P, Heller JA, Simmons M. Potassium supplementation in hypertensive patients with diuretic-induced hypokalemia. *N Engl J Med* 1985;312:746–749.

Kaplan NM, Grundy S. Comparison of the effects of guanabenz and hydrochlorothiazide on plasma lipids. *Clin Pharmacol Ther* 1988;44:297–302.

Kaplowitz N, Aw TY, Simon FR, Stolz A. Drug-induced hepatotoxicity. *Ann Intern Med* 1986;104:826–839.

Katz RJ, Levy WS, Buff L, Wasserman AG. Prevention of nitrate tolerance with angiotension converting enzyme inhibitors. *Circulation* 1991;83:1271–1277.

Katzman PL, Henningsen NC, Hulthén UL. Amiloride compared with nitrendipine in treatment of essential hypertension. *J Hum Hypertens* 1988;2:147–151.

Kau ST, Howe BB, Johnston PA, Li JH-Y, Halterman J, Zuzack JS, Leszczynska K, Yochim CL, Schwartz JA, Giles RE. Renal and antihypertensive effects of a novel eukalemic diuretic, ICI 207,828. *J Pharmacol Exp Ther* 1992;260:450–457.

Kaumann AJ. Some aspects of heart beta adrenoceptor function. *Cardiovasc Drugs Ther* 1991;5:549–560.

Keilani T, Schlueter WA, Levin ML, Batlle DC. Improvement of lipid abnormalities associated with proteinuria using fosinopril, an angiotensin-converting enzyme inhibitor. *Ann Intern Med* 1993; 118:246–254.

Kelly JG, O'Malley K. Clinical pharmacokinetics of calcium antagonists. *Clin Pharmacokinet* 1992;22:416–433.

Kelton JG. Impaired reticuloendothelial function in patients treated with methyldopa. *N Engl J Med* 1985;313:596–600.

Keogh A. Sodium cromoglycate prophylaxis for angiotensin-converting enzyme inhibitor cough. *Lancet* 1993;341:560.

Kerfoot WW, Carson CC. Pharmacologically induced erections among geriatric men. *J Urol* 1991;146:1022–1024.

Kessler DA. Drug promotion and scientific exchange. The role of the clinical investigator. *N Engl J Med* 1991;325:201–203.

Ketelhut R, Franz IW, Behr U, Toennesmann U, Messerli FH. Preserved ventricular pump function after a marked reduction of left ventricular mass. *J Am Coll Cardiol* 1992;20:864–868.

Khatri I, Uemura N, Notargiacomo A, Freis ED. Direct and reflex cardiostimulating effects of hydralazine. *Am J Cardiol* 1977;40:38–42.

Kidwai BJ, George M. Hair loss with minoxidil withdrawal. *Lancet* 1992;340:609–610.

Kincaid-Smith PS. Alpha blockade. An overview of efficacy data. *Am J Med* 1987; 82:21–25.

Kiowski W, Linder L, Kleinbloesem C, van Brummelen P, Bühler FR. Blood pressure control by the renin-angiotensin system in normotensive subjects. Assessment by angiotensin converting enzyme and renin inhibition. *Circulation* 1992a;85:1–8.

Kiowski W, Linder L, Nuesch R, Martina B. Effects of angiotensin converting enzyme inhibition on endothelial function and vascular design in hypertension [Abstract]. *Circulation* 1992b;86:I–560.

Kirby RS, Barry AC. Doxazosin: antihypertensive effect in hypertensive vs. normotensive BPH patients with BPH [Abstract]. *Am J Hypertens* 1993;6(Part 2):94A.

Kirch W, Kleinbloesem, Belz GG. Drug interactions with calcium antagonists. *Pharmacol Ther* 1990;45:109–136.

Kirtland HH, Mohler DN, Horwitz DA. Methyldopa inhibition of suppressor-lymphocyte function. *N Engl J Med* 1980; 302:825–832.

Klein R, Moss SE, Klein BEK, DeMets DL. Relation of ocular and systemic factors to survival in diabetes. *Arch Intern Med* 1989;149:266–272.

Knispel HH, Huland H. Influence of cause on choice of therapy in 174 patients with erectile dysfunction. *J Urol* 1992; 92:1274–1276.

Knochel JP. Diuretic-induced hypokalemia. *Am J Med* 1984;77:18–27.

Kobrin I, Viskoper RJ, Laszt A, Bock J, Weber C, Charlon V. Effects of an orally active renin inhibitor, ro 42-5892, in patients with essential hypertension. *Am J Hypertens* 1993;6:349–356.

Konrad-Dalhoff I, Baunack AR, Rämsch K-D, Ahr G, Kraft H, Schmitz H, Weihrauch TR, Kuhlmann J. Effect of the calcium antagonists nifedipine, nitrendipine, nimodipine and nisoldipine on oesophageal motility in man. *Eur J Clin Pharmacol* 1991;41:313–316.

Konstam MA, Rousseau MF, Kronenberg MW, Udelson JE, Melin J, Stewart D, Dolan N, Edens TR, Ahn S, Kinan D, Howe DM, Kilcoyne L, Metherall J, Benedict C, Yusuf S, Pouleur H. Effects of the angiotensin converting enzyme inhibitor enalapril on the long-term progression of left ventricular dysfunction in patients with heart failure. *Circulation* 1992;86: 431–438.

Kopyt N, Dalal F, Narins RG. Renal retention of potassium in fruit. *N Engl J Med* 1985;313:582–583.

Koren MJ, Ulin RJ, Laragh JH, Devereux RB. Reduction in left ventricular mass during treatment of essential hypertension is associated with improved prognosis [Abstract]. *Am J Hypertens* 1991;4:1–2.

Krane RJ, Goldstein I, Saenz de Tejada I. Impotence. *N Engl J Med* 1989; 321:1648–1659.

Krishna GG, Miller E, Kapor S. Increased blood pressure during potassium depletion in normotensive men. *N Engl J Med* 1989;320:1177–1182.

Krishna GG, Riley LJ Jr, Deuter G, Kapoor SC, Narins RG. Natriuretic effect of calcium-channel blockers in hypertensives. *Am J Kidney Dis* 1991;18:566–572.

Krishna GG, Shulman MD, Narins RG. Clinical use of the potassium-sparing diuretics. *Semin Nephrol* 1988;8:354–364.

Kroenke K, Wood DR, Hanley JF. The value of serum magnesium determination in hypertensive patients receiving diuretics. *Arch Intern Med* 1987:147:1553–1556.

Lacourcière Y, Provencher P. Comparative effects of zofenopril and hydrochlorothiazide on office and ambulatory blood pressures in mild to moderate essential hypertension. *Br J Clin Pharmacol* 1989; 27:371–376.

Lahive KC, Weiss JW, Weinberger SE. Alpha-methyldopa selectively reduces alae nasi activity. *Clin Sci* 1988;74:547–551.

Lake CR, Ziegler MG, Coleman MD, Kopin IJ. Hydrochlorothiazide-induced sympathetic hyperactivity in hypertensive patients. *Clin Pharmacol Ther* 1979;26:428–432.

Lamas GA, Pfeffer MA, Hamm P, Wertheimer J, Rouleau J-L, Braunwald E. Do the results of randomized clinical trials of cardiovascular drugs influence medical practice? *N Engl J Med* 1992; 327:241–247.

Lameire N, Gordts J. A pharmacokinetic study of prazosin in patients with varying degrees of chronic renal failure. *Eur J Clin Pharmacol* 1986;31:333–337.

Lammers JWJ, Folgering HTM, van Herwaarden CLA. Ventilatory effects of long-term treatment with pindolol and metoprolol in hypertensive patients with chronic obstructive lung disease. *Br J Clin Pharmacol* 1985;20:205–210.

Lands AM, Arnold A, McAuliff JP, Luduena FP, Brown TG Jr. Differentiation of receptor systems activated by sympathomimetic amines. *Nature* 1967;214:597–598.

Langer RD, Criqui MH, Barrett-Connor EL, Klauber MR, Ganiats TG. Blood pressure change and survival after age 75. *Hypertension* 1993;22:551–559.

Langer SZ. Presynaptic regulation of catecholamine release. *Biochem Pharmacol* 1974;23:1793–1800.

Langford HG, Blaufox MD, Borhani NO, Curb JD, Molteni A, Schneider KA, Pressel S. Is thiazide-produced uric acid elevation harmful? Analysis of data from the hypertension detection and follow-up program. *Arch Intern Med* 1987; 147:645–649.

Langford HG, Cutter G, Oberman A, Kansal P, Russell G. The effect of thiazide therapy on glucose, insulin and cholesterol metabolism and of glucose on potassium: results of a cross-sectional study in patients from the hypertension detection and follow-up program. *J Hum Hypertens* 1990;4:491–500.

Langley MS, Heel RC. Transdermal clonidine. A preliminary review of its pharmacodynamic properties and therapeutic efficacy. *Drugs* 1988;35:123–142.

Lardinois CK, Neuman SL. The effects of antihypertensive agents on serum lipids and lipoproteins. *Arch Intern Med* 1988;148:1280–1288.

Larkin JG, Butler E, Brodie MJ. Nifedipine for epilepsy? A pilot study. *Br Med J* 1988;296:530–531.

Larochelle P, du Souich P, Hamet P, Larocque P, Armstrong J. Prazosin plasma concentration and blood pressure reduction. *Hypertension* 1982;4:93–101.

Lasser NL, Grandits G, Caggiula AW, Cutler JA, Grimm RH, Kuller LH, Sherwin RW, Stamler J. Effects of antihypertensive therapy on plasma lipids and lipoproteins in the multiple risk factor intervention trial. *Am J Med* 1984;76:52–66.

Laurent S, Safar M. Rilmenidine: a novel approach to first-line treatment of hypertension. *Am J Hypertens* 1992; 5:99S–105S.

Lawson DH, Gloss D, Jick H. Adverse reactions to methyldopa with particular reference to hypotension. *Am Heart J* 1978;96:572–579.

Lebel M, Langlois S, Belleau LJ, Grose JH. Labetalol infusion in hypertensive emergencies. *Clin Pharmacol Ther* 1985; 37:615–618.

Lechin F, van der Dijs B, Insausti CL, Gømez F, Villa S, Lechin AE, Arocha L, Oramas O. Treatment of ulcerative colitis with clonidine. *J Clin Pharmacol* 1985; 25:219–226.

Lederle FA, Applegate WB, Grimm RH Jr. Reserpine and the medical marketplace. *Arch Intern Med* 1993;153:705–706.

Leemhuis MP, van Damme KJ, Strayvenberg A. Effects of chlorthalidone on serum and total body potassium in hypertensive patients. *Acta Med Scand* 1976;200:37–45.

Leenen FHH, Smith DL, Farkas RM, Reeves RA, Marquez-Julio A. Vasodilators and regression of left ventricular hypertrophy. Hydralazine versus prazosin in hypertensive humans. *Am J Med* 1987;82:969–978.

Leenen FHH, Smith DL, Unger WP. Topical minoxidil: cardiac effects in bald man. *Br J Clin Pharmacol* 1988;26:481–485.

Leenen FHH, Yuan B. Dietary sodium and the antihypertensive effect of nifedipine in spontaneously hypertensive rats. *Am J Hypertens* 1992;5:515–519.

Lees KR. The dose-response relationship with angiotensin converting enzyme inhibitors: effects on blood pressure and biochemical parameters. *J Hypertens* 1992a;10:S3–S11.

Lees KR. Therapeutic interventions in acute stroke. *Br J Clin Pharmacol* 1992b; 34:486–493.

Lenders JWM, de Boo T, Lemmens WAJ, Reyenga J, Thien T. Impaired vasodilation during long-term β₁-selective β-blockade in hypertensive patients. *Clin Pharmacol Ther* 1988;44:195–201.

Leon AS, Agre J, McNally C, Bell C, Neibling M, Grim R Jr, Hunninghake B. Blood lipid effects of antihypertensive therapy: a double-blind comparison of the effects of methyldopa and propranolol. *J Clin Pharmacol* 1984;24:209–217.

Lernfelt B, Landahl S, Svanborg A, Wikstrand J. Overtreatment of hypertension in the elderly? *J Hypertens* 1990;8:483–490.

Leto di Priolo S, Priore P, Cocco G, Sfrisi C, Cazor JL. Dose-titration study of alfuzosin, a new alpha₁-adrenoceptor blocker, in essential hypertension. *Eur J Clin Pharmacol* 1988;35:25–30.

Levine SB, Althof SE, Turner LA, Risen CB, Bodner DR, Kursh ED, Resnick MI. Side effects of self-administration of intracavernous papaverine and phentolamine for the treatment of impotence. *J Urol* 1989; 141:54–57.

Lewin A, Alderman MH, Mathur P. Antihypertensive efficacy of guanfacine and prazosin in patients with mild to moderate essential hypertension. *J Clin Pharmacol* 1990;30:1081–1087.

Lewis HM, Kendall MJ, Smith SR, Bratty JR. A comparison of the effects of flosequinan, a new vasodilator, and propranolol on sub-maximal exercise in healthy volunteers. *Br J Clin Pharmacol* 1989; 27:547–552.

Lewis JA. Treatment of hypertension in older adults. *Br Med J* 1992;304:1245.

Lichtlen PR, Hugenholtz PG, Rafflebeul W, Hecker H, Jost S, Deckers JW. Retardation of angiographic progression of coronary artery disease by nifedipine. *Lancet* 1990;335:1109–1113.

Lijnen P. Biochemical mechanisms involved in the β-blocker-induced changes in serum lipoproteins. *Am Heart J* 1992; 124:549–556.

Lilja M, Jounela AJ, Juustila HJ, Paalzow L. Abrupt and gradual change from clonidine to beta blockers in hypertension. *Acta Med Scand* 1982;211:375–380.

Lin M-S, McNay JL, Shepherd AMM, Musgrave GE, Keeton TK. Increased plasma norepinephrine accompanies persistent tachycardia after hydralazine. *Hypertension* 1983;5:257–263.

Linas SL, Marzec-Calvert R, Ullian ME, O'Brien RF. Mechanism of the antihypertensive effect of K depletion in the spontaneously hypertensive rat. *Kidney Int* 1988;34:18–25.

Lipworth BJ, Irvine NA, McDevitt DG. The effects of time and dose on the relative β₁- and β₂-adrenoceptor antagonism of betaxolol and atenolol. *Br J Clin Pharmacol* 1991;31:154–159.

Lipworth BJ, McDevitt DG, Struthers AD. Electrocardiographic changes induced by inhaled salbutamol after treatment with bendrofluazide: effects of replacement therapy with potassium, magnesium and triamterene. *Clin Sci* 1990;78:225–259.

Lisk DR, Grotta JC, Lamki LM, Tran HD, Taylor JW, Molony DA, Barron BJ. Should hypertension be treated after acute stroke? *Arch Neurol* 1993;50:855–862.

Lithell H, Haglund K, Granath F, Östman J. Are effects of antihypertensive treatment on lipoproteins merely "side effects?" A comparison of prazosin and metoprolol. *Acta Med Scand* 1988;223:531–536.

Lithell H, Pollare T, Vessby B. Metabolic effects of pindolol and propranolol in a double-blind cross-over study in hypertensive patients. *Blood Pressure* 1992; 1:92–101.

Lithell HOL. Effect of antihypertensive drugs on insulin, glucose, and lipid metabolism. *Diabetes Care* 1991;14:203–209.

Liu X, Engelman RM, Rousou JA, Cordis GA, Das DK. Attenuation of myocardial reperfusion injury by sulfhydryl-containing angiotensin converting enzyme inhibitors. *Cardiovasc Drugs Ther* 1992; 6:437–443.

Lohmann FH, Lang S, Gotzen R, Herzfeld O, Koppenhagen K. Cerebral blood flow in elderly people under different long-term antihypertensive treatment [Abstract]. *J Hum Hypertens* 1992;6:255.

Lopez LM, Aguila E, Baz R, Mehta JL. Absence of potentially adverse effects of hydralazine and nitrendipine on serum lipids [Abstract]. *Clin Res* 1983;31:844A.

Lopez LM, Mehta JL. Comparative efficacy and safety of lofexidine and clonidine in mild to moderately severe systemic hypertension. *Am J Cardiol* 1984;53:787–790.

Lowenstein I, Alterman L, Zelen R, Bank DE, Bank N. Comparison of long-term renal hemodynamic effects of methyldopa and propranolol in patients with hypertension and renal insufficiency. *J Clin Pharmacol* 1984;24:436–445.

Luft FC, Fineberg NS, Weinberger MH. Long-term effect of nifedipine and hydrochlorothiazide on blood pressure and sodium homeostasis at varying levels of salt intake in mildly hypertensive patients. *Am J Hypertens* 1991;4:752–760.

Lund-Johansen P, Omvik P. Acute and chronic hemodynamic effects of drugs with different actions on adrenergic receptors: a comparison between alpha blockers and different types of beta blockers with and without vasodilating effect. *Cardiovasc Drugs Ther* 1991;5:605–616.

Lund-Johansen P, Omvik P, Nordrehaug JE, White W. Carvedilol in hypertension: effects on hemodynamics and 24-hour blood pressure. *J Cardiovasc Pharmacol* 1992;12:S27–S34.

Lüscher TF. Possibilities and perspectives of pharmacotherapy for endothelial protection. *Nephrol Hypertens* 1993;2:129–136.

Lüscher TF, Waeber B. Efficacy and safety of various combination therapies based on a calcium antagonist in essential hypertension: results of a placebo-controlled randomized trial. *J Cardiovasc Pharmacol* 1993;21:305–309.

MacFadyen RJ, Lees KR, Reid JL. Tissue and plasma angiotensin converting enzyme and the response to ACE inhibitor drugs. *Br J Clin Pharmacol* 1991;31:1–13.

MacGregor GA, Banks RA, Markandu ND, Bayliss J, Roulston J. Lack of effect of beta-blocker on flat dose response to thiazide in hypertension: efficacy of lose dose thiazide combined with beta-blocker. *Br Med J* 1983;286:1535–1538.

Macharia WM, Leon G, Rowe BH, Stephenson BJ, Haynes RB. An overview of interventions to improve compliance with appointment keeping for medical services. *JAMA* 1992;267:1813–1817.

MacKay A, Isles C, Henderson I, Fife R, Kennedy AC. Minoxidil in the management of intractable hypertension. *Q J Med* 1981;50:175–190.

Mackenzie JW, Bird J. Timolol: a non-sedative anxiolytic premedicant for day cases. *Br Med J* 1989;298:363–364.

Magagna A, Abdel-Haq B, Pedrinelli R, Salvetti A. Does chlorthalidone increase the hypotensive effect of nifedipine? *J Hypertens* 1986;4:S519–S521.

Magee PFA, Freis ED. Is low-dose hydrochlorothiazide effective? *Hypertension* 1986;8(Suppl 2):135–139.

Man in't Veld, Van den Meiracker AH, Schalekamp MA. Do beta-blockers really increase peripheral vascular resistance? Review of the literature and new observations under basal conditions. *Am J Hypertens* 1988;1:91–96.

Mancia G. Autonomic modulation of the cardiovascular system during sleep. *N Engl J Med* 1993;328:347–349.

Mansilla-Tinoco R, Harland SJ, Ryan PJ, Bernstein RM, Dollery CT, Hughes GRV, Bulpitt CJ, Morgan A, Jones JM. Hydralazine, antinuclear antibodies, and the lupus syndrome. *Br Med J* 1982;284:936–939.

Marshall AJ, Barritt DW, Heaton S, Harry JD. Dose response for blood pressure and degree of cardiac β-blockade with atenolol. *Postgrad Med J* 1979;55:537–540.

Marshall J. A trial of long-term hypotensive therapy in cerebrovascular disease. *Lancet* 1964;1:10–12.

Martin WB, Spodick DH, Zins GR. Pericardial disorders occurring during open-label study of 1,869 severely hypertensive patients treated with minoxidil. *J Cardiovasc Pharmacol* 1980;2:S217–S227.

Materson BJ, Reda DJ, Cushman WC, Massie BM, Freis ED, Kochar MS, Hamburger RJ, Fye C, Lakshman R, Gottdiener J, Ramirez EA, Henderson WG. Single-drug therapy for hypertension in men. A comparison of six antihypertensive agents with placebo. *N Engl J Med* 1993;328:914–921.

Mathew TH, Boyd IW, Rohan AP. Hyponatraemia due to the combination of hydrochlorothiazide and amiloride (Moduretic): Australian spontaneous reports 1977–1988. *Med J Aust* 1990;152:308–309.

Mattes RD, Engelman K. Effects of combined hydrochlorothiazide and amiloride versus single drug on changes in salt taste and intake. *Am J Cardiol* 1992;70:91–95.

McAinsh J, Holmes BF, Smith S, Hood D, Warren D. Atenolol kinetics in renal failure. *Clin Pharmacol Ther* 1980; 28:302–309.

McAreavey D, Vermeulen R, Robertson JIS. Newer beta blockers and the treatment of hypertension. *Cardiovasc Drugs Ther* 1991;5:577–588.

McCarthy GJ, Hainsworth M, Lindsay K, Wright JM, Brown TA. Pressor responses to trachael intubation after sublingual captopril. A pilot study. *Anaesthesia* 1990;45:243–245.

McClellan WM, Hall WD, Brogan D, Miles C, Wilber JA. Continuity of care in hypertension. An important correlate of blood pressure control among aware hypertensives. *Arch Intern Med* 1988;148:525–528.

McDermott MT, Walden TL, Bornemann M, Sjoberg RJ, Hofeldt FD, Kidd GS. The effects of theophylline and nifedipine on corticotropin-stimulated cortisol secretion. *Clin Pharmacol Ther* 1990;47:435–438.

McInnes GT, Shelton JR, Harrison IR, Perkins RM, Rigby GV. Diuretic induced hypokalaemia: relationship to dosage interval and plasma aldosterone. *Br J Clin Pharmacol* 1982;14:449–452.

McInnes GT, Yeo WW, Ramsay LE, Moser M. Cardiotoxicity and diuretics: much speculation—little substance. *J Hypertens* 1992;10:317–335.

McKenney JM, Goodman RP, Wright JT Jr, Rifai N, Aycock DG, King ME. The effect of low-dose hydrochlorothiazide on blood pressure, serum potassium, and lipoproteins. *Pharmacotherapy* 1986;6:179–184.

McMurray J, Matthews DM. Consequences of fluid loss in patients treated with ACE inhibitors. *Postgrad Med J* 1987; 63:385–387.

McTavish D, Young RA, Clissold SP. Cadralazine. A review of its pharmacodynamic and pharmacokinetic properties, and therapeutic potential in the treatment of hypertension. *Drugs* 1990;40:543–560.

Medical Research Council Working Party. MRC trial of treatment of mild hypertension: principal results. *Br Med J* 1985;291:97–104.

Medical Research Council Working Party. Comparison of the antihypertensive efficacy and adverse reactions to two doses of bendrofluazide and hydrochlorothiazide and the effect of potassium supplementation on the hypotensive action of bendrofluazide: substudies of the Medical Research Council's trials of treatment of mild hypertension. *J Clin Pharmacol* 1987;27:271–277.

Medical Research Council Working Party. Medical Research Council trial of treatment of hypertension in older adults: principal results. *Br Med J* 1992;304:405–412.

Medical Research Council Working Party on Mild Hypertension. Adverse reactions to bendrofluazide and propranolol for the treatment of mild hypertension. *Lancet* 1981;2:539–543.

Meechan JG, Rawlins MD. The effects of two different local anaesthetic solutions administered for oral surgery on plasma potassium levels in patients taking kaliuretic diuretics. *Eur J Clin Pharmacol* 1992;42:155–158.

Mehta JL, Lopez LM. Rebound hypertension following abrupt cessation of clonidine and metoprolol. Treatment with labetalol. *Arch Intern Med* 1987;147:389–390.

Mejia AD, Egan BM, Schork NJ, Zweifler AJ. Artifacts in measurements of blood pressure and lack of target organ involvement in the assessment of patients with treatment-resistant hypertension. *Ann Intern Med* 1990;112:270–277.

Ménard J. Improving hypertension treatment. Where should we put our efforts: new drugs, new concepts, or new management? *Am J Hypertens* 1992;5:252S–258S.

Ménard J, Serrurier D, Bautier P, Plouin P-F, Corvol P. Crossover design to test antihypertensive drugs with self-recorded blood pressure. *Hypertension* 1988; 11:153–159.

Mercuro G, Rivano CA, Ruscazio M, Lai L, Manca R, Rossetti ZL, Cherchi A. Effects of 1-year's therapy with the dopamine$_2$ agonist dihydroergotoxine on blood pressure and plasma noradrenaline levels in essential hypertension. A preliminary study. *Drug Invest* 1992;4:508–514.

Messerli FH, Nunez BD, Nunez MM, Garavaglia GE, Schmieder RE, Ventura HO.

Hypertension and sudden death. Disparate effects of calcium entry blocker and diuretic therapy on cardiac dysrhythmias. *Arch Intern Med* 1989;149:1263–1267.

Metz S, Klein C, Morton N. Rebound hypertension after discontinuation of transdermal clonidine therapy. *Am J Med* 1987; 82:17–19.

Miller RP, Woodworth JR, Graves DA, Locke CS, Steiger BW, Rotenberg KS. Comparison of three formulations of metolazone: bioavailability and pharmacologic effects. *Cur Ther Res* 1988;43:1133–1142.

Mitchell HC, Pettinger WA. Dose-response of clonidine on plasma catecholamines in the hypernoradrenergic state associated with vasodilator β-blocker therapy. *J Cardiovasc Pharmacol* 1981;3:647–654.

Molnar GW, Read RC, Wright FE. Propranolol enhancement of hypoglycemic sweating. *Clin Pharmacol Ther* 1974; 15:490–496.

Mombouli J-V, Nephtali M, Vanhoutte PM. Effects of the converting enzyme inhibitor cilazaprilat on endothelium-dependent responses. *Hypertension* 1991;18(Suppl 2):22–29.

Moran NC, Perkins ME. Adrenergic blockade of the mammalian heart by a dichloro analogue of isoproterenol. *J Pharmacol Exp Ther* 1958;124:223–237.

Morgan DB, Davidson C. Hypokalaemia and diuretics: an analysis of publications. *Br Med J* 1980;280:905–908.

Morgan T, Anderson A. Interaction of indomethacin (I) with felodipine ER (F) or enalapril (E) [Abstract]. *Am J Hypertens* 1993;6:107A.

Morgan TO, Anderson A, Jones E. Comparison and interaction of low dose felodipine and enalapril in the treatment of essential hypertension in elderly subjects. *Am J Hypertens* 1992;5:238–243.

Mori S, Sadoshima S, Fujii K, Ibayashi S, Iino K, Fujishima M. Decrease in cerebral blood flow with blood pressure reductions in patients with chronic stroke. *Stroke* 1993;24:1376–1381.

Multicenter European Research Trial. Does the new angiotensin converting enzyme inhibitor cilazapril prevent restenosis after percutaneous transluminal coronary angioplasty? Results of the MERCATOR Study: a multicenter, randomized, double-blind placebo-controlled trial. *Circulation* 1992;86:100–110.

Murdoch D, Heel RC. Amlodipine. A review of its pharmacodynamic and pharmacokinetic properties, and therapeutic use in cardiovascular disease. *Drugs* 1991; 41:478–505.

Murphy E, Perlman M, London RE, Steenbergen C. Amiloride delays the ischemia-induced rise in cytosolic free calcium. *Circ Res* 1991;68:1250-1258.

Murphy MB, Lewis PJ, Kohner E, Schumer B, Dollery CT. Glucose intolerance in hypertensive patients treated with diuretics; a fourteen-year follow-up. *Lancet* 1982;2:1293–1296.

Nader PC, Thompson JR, Alpern RJ. Complications of diuretic use. *Semin Nephrol* 1988;8:365–387.

Nakamura M, Funakoshi T, Yoshida H, Arakawa N, Suzuki T, Hiramori K. Endothelium-dependent vasodilation is augmented by angiotensin converting enzyme inhibitors in healthy volunteers. *J Cardiovasc Pharmacol* 1992;20:949–954.

Neal WW. Reducing costs and improving compliance. *Am J Cardiol* 1989; 63:17B–20B.

Neaton JD, Grimm RH Jr, Prineas RJ, Stamler J, Grandits GA, Elmer PJ, Cutler JA, Flack JM, Schoenberger JA, McDonald R, Lewis CE, Liebson PR. Treatment of mild hypertension study (TOMHS): final results. *JAMA* 1993;270:713–724.

Nelson DE, Moyse DM, O'Neil JM, Boger RS, Glassman HN, Kleinert HD. Renin inhibitor, Abbott-72517, does not induce characteristic angiotensin converting enzyme inhibitor (ACEI) cough [Abstract]. *Circulation* 1993;88(Part 2):361.

Nelson MT. Ca^{2+}-activated potassium channels and ATP-sensitive potassium channels as modulators of vascular tone. *Trends Cardiovasc Med* 1993;3:54–60.

Nelson MT, Patlak JB, Worley JF, Standen NB. Calcium channels, potassium channels, and voltage dependence of arterial smooth muscle tone. *Am J Physiol* 1990;259:C3–C18.

Neusy A-J, Lowenstien J. Blood pressure and blood pressure variability following withdrawal of propranolol and clonidine. *J Clin Pharmacol* 1989;29:18–24.

Neutel JM, Schnaper H, Cheung DG, Graettinger WF, Weber MA. Antihypertensive effects of β-blockers administered once daily: 24-hour measurements. *Am Heart J* 1990;120:166–171.

Neuvonen PJ, Kivistö KT. The clinical significance of food-drug interactions: a review. *Med J Aust* 1989;150:36–40.

New Zealand Medical Journal. A multicentre study of labetalol in hypertension. *N Z Med J* 1981;93:215–218.

Niarchos AP, Baksi AK. Treatment of severe hypertension and hypertensive emergencies with intravenous clonidine hydrochloride. *Postgrad Med J* 1973;49:908–913.

Niarchos AP, Weinstein DL, Laragh JH. Comparison of the effects of diuretic therapy and low sodium intake in isolated systolic hypertension. *Am J Med* 1984; 77:1061–1068.

Nichols AJ, Ruffolo RR Jr. The relationship of alpha-adrenoceptor reserve and agonist intrinsic efficacy to calcium utilization in the vasculature. *Trends Pharmacol Sci* 1988;9:236–244.

Nicholson JP, Resnick LM, Laragh JH. The antihypertensive effect of verapamil at extremes of dietary sodium intake. *Ann Intern Med* 1987;107:329–324.

Nielsen H, Egeblad H, Mortensen SA, Sande E. Observations on increased susceptibility to coronary artery vasospasm during beta blockade. *Am Heart J* 1987;114:192–194.

Nilsson-Ehle P, Ekberg M, Fridström P, Ursing D, Lins L-E. Lipoproteins and metabolic control in hypertensive type II diabetics treated with clonidine. *Acta Med Scand* 1988;224:131–134.

Niutta E, Cusi D, Colombo R, Pellizzoni M, Cesana B, Barlassina C, Soldati L, Bianchi G. Predicting interindividual variations in antihypertensive therapy: the role of sodium transport systems and renin. *J Hypertens* 1990;8:S53–S58.

Nørgaard A, Kjeldsen K. Interrelation of hypokalaemia and potassium depletion and its implications: a re-evaluation based on studies of the skeletal muscle sodium, potassium-pump. *Clin Sci* 1991;81:449–455.

Oates JA Jr, Gillespie L Jr, Crout JR, Sjoerdsma A. Inhibition of aromatic amino acid decarboxylation in man and associated pharmacological effects [Abstract]. *J Clin Invest* 1960;39:1015.

Ocon J, Mora J. Twenty-four-hour blood pressure monitoring and effects of indapamide. *Am J Cardiol* 1990;65:58H–61H.

O'Connor DT, Preston RA, Mitas JA, Frigon RP, Stone RA. Urinary kallikrein activity and renal vascular resistance in the antihypertensive response to thiazide diuretics. *Hypertension* 1981;3:139–147.

Olbricht CJ, Schaumann D, Fischer D. Anaphylactoid reactions, LDL apheresis with dextran sulphate, and ACE inhibitors. *Lancet* 1992;340:908–909.

Ollivier JP, Christen MO, Schäfer SG. Moxonidine: a second generation of centrally acting drugs. An appraisal of clinical experience. *J Cardiovasc Pharmacol* 1992;20(Suppl 4):31–36.

O'Mailia JJ, Sander GE, Giles TD. Nifedipine-associated myocardial ischemia or infarction in the treatment of hypertensive urgencies. *Ann Intern Med* 1987; 107:185–186.

O'Malley K, Segal JL, Israili ZH, Boles M, McNay JL, Dayton PG. Duration of hydralazine action in hypertension. *Clin Pharmacol Ther* 1975;18:581–586.

Ondetti MA, Rubin B, Cushman DW. Design of specific inhibitors of angiotensin-converting enzyme: new class of orally active antihypertensive agents. *Science* 1977; 196:441–444.

Ondetti MA, Williams NJ, Sabo EF, Pluscec J, Weaver ER, Kocy O. Angiotensin-converting enzyme inhibitors from the venom of *bothrops jararaca*: isolation, elucidation of structure and synthesis. *Biochemistry* 1971;10:4033–4039.

Ooi WL, Budner NS, Cohen H, Madhavan S, Alderman MH. Impact of race on treatment response and cardiovascular disease among hypertensives. *Hypertension* 1989;14:227–234.

Oparil S, Calhoun DA. The calcium antagonists in the 1990s. An overview. *Am J Hypertens* 1991;4:396S–405S.

Opie LH. Calcium channel antagonists part I: fundamental properties: mechanisms, classification, sites of action. *Cardiovasc Drugs Ther* 1987;1:411–430.

Opie LH. Role of vasodilation in the antihypertensive and antianginal effects of labetalol: implications for therapy of combined hypertension and angina. *Cardiovasc Drugs Ther* 1988a;2:369–376.

Opie LH. Calcium channel antagonists part III: use and comparative efficacy in hypertension and supraventricular arrhythmias. Minor indications. *Cardiovasc Drugs Ther* 1988b;1:625–656.

Opsahl JA, Abraham PA, Keane WF. Renal effects of angiotensin converting enzyme inhibitors: nondiabetic chronic renal disease. *Cardiovasc Drugs Ther* 1990; 4:221–228.

Osborn M, Hawton K, Gath D. Sexual dysfunction among middle aged women in the community. *Br Med J* 1988;296:959–962.

Otterstad JE, Froeland G, Michelsen S, Ekeli T. Are there differences in the blood-pressure-lowering effect of atenolol vs. hydrochlorothiazide + amiloride (Moduretic) when assessed by standard clinic recordings vs. 24-h ambulatory monitoring? *J Intern Med* 1992;231:143–144.

Overlack A, Müller B, Schmidt L, Scheid M-L, Müller M, Stumpe KO. Airway responsiveness and cough induced by angiotensin converting enzyme inhibition. *J Hum Hypertens* 1992;6:387–392.

Owens SD, Dunn MI. Efficacy and safety of guanadrel in elderly hypertensive patients. *Arch Intern Med* 1988;148:1515–1518.

Packer M. Potential role of potassium as a determinant of morbidity and mortality in patients with systemic hypertension and congestive heart failure. *Am J Cardiol* 1990;65:45E–51E.

Packer M, Nicod P, Khandheria BR, et al. Randomized, multicenter, double-blind, placebo-controlled evaluation of amlodipine in patients with mild-to-moderate heart failure [Abstract]. *J Am Coll Cardiol* 1991;17:274.

Palmer A, Fletcher A, Hamilton G, Muriss S, Bulpitt C. A comparison of verapamil and nifedipine on quality of life. *Br J Clin Pharmacol* 1990;30:365–370.

Pannier BM, Kando T, Safarian AA, Isnard RN, Diebold BE, Safar ME. Altered hemodynamic response to isosorbide dinitrate in essential hypertension. *J Clin Pharmacol* 1990;30:127–132.

Paolisso G, Gambardella A, Verza M, D'Amore A, Sgambato S, Varricchio M. ACE inhibition improves insulin-sensitivity in aged insulin-resistant hypertensive patients. *J Hum Hypertens* 1992; 6:175–179.

Papademetriou V, Burris JF, Notargiacomo A, Fletcher RD. Thiazide diuretic therapy is not a cause of arrhythmia in patients with systemic hypertension. *Arch Intern Med* 1988;148:1272–1276.

Parmley WW. New calcium antagonists: relevance of vasoselectivity. *Am Heart J* 1990;120:1408–1413.

Parmley WW, Nesto RW, Singh BN, Deanfield J, Gottlieb SO. Attenuation of the circadian patterns of myocardial ischemia with nifedipine GITS in patients with chronic stable angina. *J Am Coll Cardiol* 1992;19:1380–1389.

Participating Veterans Administration Medical Centers. Low doses v standard dose of reserpine. A randomized, double-blind, multiclinic trial in patients taking chlorthalidone. *JAMA* 1982;248:2471–2477.

Paton RR, Kane RE. Long-term diuretic therapy with metolazone of renal failure and the nephrotic syndrome. *J Clin Pharm* 1977;17:243–251.

Paul M, Bachmann J, Ganten D. The tissue renin-angiotensin systems in cardiovascular disease. *Trends Cardiovasc Med* 1992;2:94–99.

Paulson OB, Jarden JO, Vorstrup S, Holm S, Godtfredsen J. Effect of captopril on the cerebral circulation in chronic heart failure. *Eur J Clin Invest* 1986;16:124–132.

Pedrinelli R, Panarace G, Salvetti A. Calcium entry blockade and adrenergic vascular reactivity in hypertensives: differences between nicardipine and diltiazem. *Clin Pharmacol Ther* 1991;49:86–93.

Pedrinelli R, Taddei S, Salvetti A. Calcium entry blockade and alpha-adrenergic vascular reactivity in human beings: differences between nicardipine and verapamil. *Clin Pharmacol Ther* 1989;45:285–290.

Perondi R, Saino A, Tio RA, Pomidossi G, Gregorini L, Alessio P, Morganti A, Zanchetti A, Manci G. ACE inhibition attenuates sympathetic coronary vasoconstriction in patients with coronary artery disease. *Circulation* 1992;85:2004–2013.

Perry HM Jr. Late toxicity to hydralazine resembling systemic lupus erythematosus or rheumatoid arthritis. *Am J Med* 1973;54:58–72.

Perry HM Jr, Camel GH, Carmody SE, Ahmed KS, Perry EF. Survival in hydralazine-treated hypertensive patients with and without late toxicity. *J Chron Dis* 1977;30:519–528.

Perry HM Jr, Schroeder HA. Depression of cholesterol levels in human plasma following ethylenediamine tetracetate and hydralazine. *J Chron Dis* 1955;2:520–533.

Pershadsingh HA, Szollosi J, Benson S, Hyun WC, Feuerstein BG, Kurtz TW. Effects of ciglitazone on blood pressure and intracellular calcium metabolism. *Hypertension* 1993;21:1020–1023.

Persson B, Andersson OK, Wysocki M, Hedner T, Karlberg B. Calcium antagonism in essential hypertension: effect on renal haemodynamics and microalbuminuria. *J Intern Med* 1992;231:247–252.

Persson H, Erhardt L. Beta receptor antagonists in the treatment of heart failure. *Cardiovasc Drugs Ther* 1991;5:589–604.

Pettinger WA. Minoxidil and the treatment of severe hypertension. *N Engl J Med* 1980;303:922–926.

Pfeffer MA, Braunwald E, Moyé LA, Basta L, Brown EJ Jr, Cuddy TE, Davis BR, Geltman EM, Goldman S, Flaker GC, Klein M, Lamas GA, Packer M, Rouleau J, Rouleau JL, Rutherford J, Wertheimer JH, Hawkins CM. Effect of captopril on mortality and morbidity in patients with left ventricular dysfunction after myocardial infarction. Results of the survival and ventricular enlargement trial. *N Engl J Med* 1992;327:669–677.

Pickard JD, Murray JD, Illingworth R, Shaw MD, Teasdale GM, Foy PM, et al. Effect of oral nimodipine on cerebral infarction and outcome after subarachnoid haemorrhage: British aneurysm nimodipine trial. *Br Med J* 1989;298:636–642.

Pickles CJ, Pipkin FB, Symonds EM. A randomised placebo controlled trial of labetalol in the treatment of mild to moderate pregnancy induced hypertension. *Br J Obstet Gynaecol* 1992;99:964–968.

Piper JM, Ray WA, Rosa FW. Pregnancy outcome following exposure to angiotensin-converting enzyme inhibitors. *Obstet Gynecol* 1992;80:429–432.

Pixley JS, Marshall MK, Stanley H, Starich GH, Ferguson RK. Comparison of once-daily captopril or enalapril in mild essential hypertension. *J Clin Pharmacol* 1989;29:118–122.

Polese A, De Cesare N, Montorsi P, Fabbiocchi F, Guazzi M, Loaldi A, Guazzi MD. Upward shift of the lower range of coronary flow autoregulation in hypertensive patients with hypertrophy of the left ventricle. *Circulation* 1991;83:845–853.

Pollare T, Lithell H, Berne C. A comparison of the effects of hydrochlorothiazide and captopril on glucose and lipid metabolism in patients with hypertension. *N Engl J Med* 1989a;321:868–73.

Pollare T, Lithell H, Mörlin C, Präntare H, Hvarfner A, Ljunghall S. Metabolic effects of diltiazem and atenolol: results from a randomized, double-blind study with parallel groups. *J Hypertens* 1989b;7:551–559.

Pollare T, Lithell H, Selinus I, Berne C. Application of prazosin is associated with an increase of insulin sensitivity in obese patients with hypertension. *Diabetologia* 1988;31:415–420.

Pollare T, Lithell H, Selinus I, Berne C. Sensitivity to insulin during treatment with atenolol and metoprolol: a randomized, double blind study of effects on carbohydrate and lipoprotein metabolism in hypertensive patients. *Br Med J* 1989c;298:1152–1157.

Pontremoli R, Robaudo C, Gaiter A, Massarino F, Deferrari G. Long-term minoxidil treatment in refractory hypertension and renal failure. *Clin Nephrol* 1991;35:39–43.

Pool JL. Effects of doxazosin on serum lipids: a review of the clinical data and molecular basis for altered lipid metabolism. *Am Heart J* 1991;121:251–260.

Pope JE, Anderson JJ, Felson DT. A meta-analysis of the effects of nonsteroidal anti-inflammatory drugs on blood pressure. *Arch Intern Med* 1993;153:477–484.

Postma CT, Dennesen PJW, de Boo T, Thien T. First dose hypotension after captopril; can it be predicted? A study of 240 patients. *J Hum Hypertens* 1992;6:205–209.

Powell CE, Slater IH. Blocking of inhibitory adrenergic receptors by a dichloro analog of isoproterenol. *J Pharmacol Exp Ther* 1958;122:480–488.

Prevention of Atherosclerotic Complications with Ketanserin Trial Group. Prevention of atherosclerotic complications: controlled trial of ketanserin. *Br Med J* 1989;298:424–430.

Prichard BNC, Gillam PMS. Use of propranolol (Inderal) in treatment of hypertension. *Br Med J* 1964;2:725–727.

Prisant LM, Spruill WJ, Fincham JE, Wade WE, Carr AA, Adams MA. Depression associated with antihypertensive drugs. *J Fam Pract* 1991;33:481–485.

Pryor JP, Castle WM, Dukes DC, Smith JC, Watson ME, Williams JL. Do beta-adrenoceptor blocking drugs cause retroperitoneal fibrosis? *Br Med J* 1983;287:639–641.

Psaty BM, Koepsell TD, Wagner EH, LoGerfo JP, Inui TS. The relative risk of incident coronary heart disease associated with recently stopping the use of β-blockers. *JAMA* 1990;263:1653–1657.

Pullar T. Compliance with drug therapy. *Br J Clin Pharmacol* 1991;32:535–539.

Puri GD, Batra YK. Effect of nifedipine on cardiovascular responses to laryngoscopy and intubation. *Br J Anaesth* 1988;60:579–581.

Quilley J, Duchin KL, Hudes EM, McGiff JC. The antihypertensive effect of captopril in essential hypertension: relationship to prostaglandins and the kallikrein-kinin system. *J Hypertens* 1987;5:121–128.

Rabkin SW. Mechanisms of action of adrenergic receptor blockers on lipids during antihypertensive drug treatment. *J Clin Pharmacol* 1993;33:286–291.

Radack K, Deck C. β-adrenergic blocker therapy does not worsen intermittent claudication in subjects with peripheral arterial disease. A meta-analysis of randomized controlled trials. *Arch Intern Med* 1991;151:1769–1776.

Raftery EB, Carrageta MO. Hypertension and beta-blockers. Are they all the same? *Int J Cardiol* 1985;7:337–346.

Ram CVS, Garrett BN, Kaplan NM. Moderate sodium restriction and various diuretics in the treatment of hypertension. *Arch Intern Med* 1981;141:1015–1019.

Ram CVS, Gonzalez D, Kulkarni P, Sunerajan P, Corbett J, Taylor A, Zachariah NY, Kaplan NM. Regression of left ventricular hypertrophy in hypertension. Effects of prazosin therapy. *Am J Med* 1989;86:66–69.

Ram CVS, Holland OB, Fairchild C, Gomez-Sanchez CE. Withdrawal syndrome following cessation of guanabenz therapy. *J Clin Pharmacol* 1979;19:148–150.

Ramsay LE, Parnell L, Waller PC. Comparison of nifedipine, prazosin and hydralazine added to treatment of hypertensive patients uncontrolled by thiazide diuretic plus beta-blocker. *Postgrad Med J* 1987;63:99–103.

Ramsay LE, Silas JH, Ollerenshaw JD, Tucker GT, Phillips FC, Freestone S. Should the acetylator phenotype be determined when prescribing hydralazine for hypertension? *Eur J Clin Pharmacol* 1984;26:39–42.

Randeree HA, Omar MAK, Motala AA, Seedat MA. Effect of insulin therapy on blood pressure in NIDDM patients with secondary failure. *Diabetes Care* 1992;15:1258–1263.

Reams GP, Bauer JH. Effects of calcium antagonists on the hypertensive kidney. *Cardiovasc Drugs Ther* 1990;4:1331–1336.

Reams G, Lau A, Knaus V, Bauer JH. The effect of nifedipine GITS on renal function in hypertensive patients with renal insufficiency. *J Clin Pharmacol* 1991;31:468–472.

Reid JL, Wing LMH, Dargie HJ, Hamilton CA, Davies DS, Dollery CT. Clonidine withdrawal in hypertension. Changes in blood-pressure and plasma and urinary noradrenaline. *Lancet* 1977;1:1171–1174.

Reisin E, Weed SG. The treatment of obese hypertensive black women: a comparative study of chlorthalidone versus clonidine. *J Hypertens* 1992;10:489–493.

Reisin L, Schneeweiss A. Spontaneous disappearance of cough induced by angiotensin-converting enzyme inhibitors (captopril or enalapril). *Am J Cardiol* 1992; 70:398–399.

Rich S, Kaufmann E, Levy PS. The effect of high doses of calcium-channel blockers on survival in primary pulmonary hypertension. *N Engl J Med* 1992;327:76–81.

Richards AM, Wittert GA, Crozier IG, Espiner EA, Yandle TG, Ikram H, Frampton C. Chronic inhibition of endopeptidase 24.11 in essential hypertension: evidence for enhanced atrial natriuretic peptide and angiotensin II. *J Hypertens* 1993; 11:407–416.

Rimmer JM, Horn JF, Gennari FJ. Hyperkalemia as a complication of drug therapy. *Arch Intern Med* 1987;147:867–869.

Robb OJ, Webster J, Petrie JC, Harry JD, Young J. Effects of the β_2-adrenoceptor antagonist ICI 118,551 on blood pressure in hypertensive patients known to respond to β_1-adrenoceptor antagonists. *Br J Clin Pharmacol* 1988;25:433–438.

Roberts DH, Tsao Y, McLoughlin GA, Breckenridge A. Placebo-controlled comparison of captopril, atenolol, labetalol, and pindolol in hypertension complicated by intermittent claudication. *Lancet* 1987;2:650–653.

Robertson JIS. Serotonin and vascular disease: a survey. *Cardiovasc Drugs Ther* 1990;4:137–140.

Rockhold RW. Thiazide diuretics and male sexual dysfunction. *Drug Develop Res* 1992;25:85–95.

Roden DM, Nadeau JHJ, Primm RK. Electrophysiologic and hemodynamic effects of chronic oral therapy with the alpha₂-agonists clonidine and tiamenidine in hypertensive volunteers. *Clin Pharmacol Ther* 1988;43:648–654.

Rodman JS, Deutsch DJ, Gutman SI. Methyldopa hepatitis. A report of six cases and review of the literature. *Am J Med* 1976;60:941–948.

Roeback JR Jr, Hla KM, Chambless LE, Fletcher RH. Effects of chromium supplementation on serum high-density lipoprotein cholesterol levels in men taking beta-blockers. A randomized, controlled trial. *Ann Intern Med* 1991;115:917–924.

Rosa RM, Silva P, Young JB, Landsberg L, Brown RS, Rose JW, Epstein FH. Adrenergic modulation of extrarenal potassium disposal. *N Engl J Med* 1980;302:431–434.

Rose BD. Diuretics. *Kidney Int* 1991; 39:336–352.

Rosen SG, Supiano MA, Perry TJ, Linares OA, Hogikyan RV, Smith MJ, Halter JB. β-adrenergic blockade decreases norepinephrine release in humans. *Am J Physiol* 1990;258:E999–E1005.

Roth A, Kaluski E, Felner S, Heller K, Laniado S. Clonidine for patients with rapid atrial fibrillation. *Ann Intern Med* 1992;116:388–390.

Roush MK, McNutt RA, Gray TF. The adverse effect dilemma: quest for accessible information. *Ann Intern Med* 1991;114:298–299.

Rudd P, Ahmed S, Zachary V, Barton C, Bonduelle D. Compliance with medication timing: implications from a medication trial drug development and clinical practice. *J Clin Res Pharmacoepidemiol* 1992;6:15–27.

Ruffolo RR Jr, Nichols AJ, Hieble JP. Metabolic regulation by alpha₁- and alpha₂-adrenoceptors. *Life Sci* 1991;49:171–183.

Ruys T, Sturgess I, Shaikh M, Watts GF, Nordestgaard BG, Lewis B. Effects of exercise and fat ingestion on high density lipoprotein production by peripheral tissues. *Lancet* 1989;2:1119–1121.

Ryan JR, LaCorte W, Jain A, McMahon FG. Hypertension in hypoglycemic diabetics treated with β-adrenergic antagonists. *Hypertension* 1985;7:443–446.

Rygnestad TK, Dale O. Self-poisoning with prazosin. *Acta Med Scand* 1983; 213:157–158.

Saenz de Tejada I, Goldstein I, Azadzoi K, Krane RJ, Cohen RA. Impaired neurogenic and endothelium-mediated relaxation of penile smooth muscle from diabetic men with impotence. *N Engl J Med* 1989;320:1025–1030.

Sakhaee K, Alpern R, Jacobson HR, Pak CYC. Contrasting effects of various potassium salts on renal citrate excretion. *J Clin Endocrinol Metab* 1991;72:396–400.

Sakhaee K, Nicar MJ, Glass K, Zerwekh JE, Pak CYC. Reduction in intestinal calcium absorption by hydrochlorothiazide in postmenopausal osteoporosis. *J Clin Endocrinol Metab* 1984;59:1037–1043.

Salvetti A. Newer ACE inhibitors. A look at the future. *Drugs* 1990;40:800–828.

Salvetti A, Arzilli F. Chronic dose-response curve of enalapril in essential hypertensives. An Italian multicenter study. *Am J Hypertens* 1989;2:352–354.

Salvetti A, Magagna A, Innocenti P, Ponzanelli F, Cagianelli A, Cipriani M, Gandolfi E, Del Prato C, Ballestra AM, Saba P, Giuntoli F, Panebianco G, Amigoni S. The combination of chlorthalidone with nifedipine does not exert an additive antihypertensive effect in essential hypertensives: a crossover multicenter study. *J Cardiovasc Pharmacol* 1991;17:332–335.

Salvetti A, Pedrinelli R, Bartolomei G, Cagianelli MA, Cinotti G, Innocenti P, Loni C, Saba G, Saba P, Papi L, Bichisao E, Motolese M. Plasma renin activity does not predict the antihypertensive efficacy of chlorthalidone. *Eur J Clin Pharmacol* 1987;33:221–226.

Saunders E, Weir MR, Kong BW, Hollifield J, Gray J, Vertes V, Sowers JR, Zemel MB, Curry C, Schoenberger J, Wright JT, Kirkendall W, Conradi EC, Jenkins P, McLean B, Massie B, Berenson G, Flamenbaum W. A comparison of the efficacy and safety of a β-blocker, a calcium channel blocker, and a converting enzyme inhibitor in hypertensive blacks. *Arch Intern Med* 1990;150:1707–1713.

Savola J, Vehviläinen O, Väätäinen NJ. Psoriasis as a side effect of β-blockers. *Br Med J* 1987;295:637.

Sawyer N, Gabriel R. Progressive hypokalaemia in elderly patients taking three thiazide potassium-sparing diuretic combinations for thirty-six months. *Postgrad Med J* 1988;64:434–437.

Saxena PR, Bolt GR. Haemodynamic profiles of vasodilators in experimental hypertension. *Trends Pharmacol Sci* 1986; 7:501–506.

Schäfer SG, Christen MO, Ernsberger PR. The second generation of centrally acting drugs: moxonidine. *J Cardiovasc Pharmacol* 1992;20:vii–viii.

Schäfers RF, Reid JL. Alpha blockers. In: Kaplan NM, Brenner BM, Laragh JH, eds. New Therapeutic Strategies in Hypertension. New York: Raven Press, 1989: 51–69.

Schappert SM. National ambulatory medical care survey: 1991 summary. From vital and health statistics of the centers for disease control and prevention/national center for health statistics. *Advance Data* 1993; 230:1–20.

Schmidt JF, Valentin N, Nielsen SL. The clinical effect of felodipine and nifedipine in Raynaud's phenomenon. *Eur J Clin Pharmacol* 1989;37:191–192.

Schmieder RE, Rockstroh JK, Messerli FH. Antihypertensive therapy. To stop or not to stop? *JAMA* 1991;265:1566–1571.

Schnaper HW, Freis ED, Friedman RG, Garland WT, Hall WD, Hollifield J, Jain AK, Jenkins P, Marks A, McMahon FG, Sambol NC, Williams RL, Winer N. Potassium restoration in hypertensive patients made hypokalemic by hydrochlorothiazide. *Arch Intern Med* 1989;149:2677–2681.

Schoenfeld MR, Goldberger E. Hypercholesterolemia induced by thiazides: a pilot study. *Curr Ther Res* 1964;6:180–184.

Schroeder T, Sillesen H. Dihydralazine induces marked cerebral vasodilation in man. *Eur J Clin Invest* 1987;17:214–217.

Schuh JR, Blehm DJ, Frierdich GE, McMahon EG, Blaine EH. Differential effects of renin-angiotensin system blockade on atherogenesis in cholesterol-fed rabbits. *J Clin Invest* 1993;91:1453–1458.

Sechi LA, Palomba D, Bartoli E. Acute effects of furosemide on blood pressure in functionally anephric, volume-expanded rats [Abstract]. *J Hypertens* 1992;10:S59.

Serlin MJ, Orme ML'E, Baber NS, Sibeon RG, Laws E, Breckenridge A. Propranolol in the control of blood pressure: a dose-response study. *Clin Pharmacol Ther* 1980;27:586–592.

Sever P, Beevers G, Bulpitt C, Lever A, Ramsay L, Reid J, Swales J. Management guidelines in essential hypertension: report of the second working party of the British Hypertension Society. *Br Med J* 1993; 306:983–987.

Shea S, Misra D, Ehrlich MH, Field L, Francis CK. Predisposing factors for severe, uncontrolled hypertension in an inner-city minority population. *N Engl J Med* 1992;327:776–781.

SHEP Cooperative Research Group. Prevention of stroke by antihypertensive drug treatment in older persons with isolated systolic hypertension. Final results of the systolic hypertension in the elderly program (SHEP). *JAMA* 1991; 265:3255–3264.

Sheu WH-H, Swislocki ALM, Hoffman BB, Reaven GM, Chen Y-DI. Effect of prazosin treatment on HDL kinetics in patients with hypertension. *Am J Hypertens* 1990;3:761–768.

Shieh S-M, Sheu WH-H, Shen DD-C, Fuh MM-T, Jeng C-Y, Jeng JR, Chen Y-Di, Reaven GM. Improvement in metabolic risk factors for coronary heart disease associated with cilazapril treatment. *Am J Hypertens* 1992;5:506–510.

Shulman NB, Porter RS, Levinson RM, Owen SL, Dever GEA, Hall WD. Impact of cost problems on morbidity in a hypertensive population. *Am J Prev Med* 1991;7:374–378.

Sica DA, Gehr TWB. Triamterene and the kidney. *Nephron* 1989;51:454–461.

Siegel D, Hulley SB, Black DM, Cheitlin MD, Sebastian A, Seeley DG, Hearst N, Fine R. Diuretics, serum and intracellular electrolyte levels, and ventricular arrhythmias in hypertensive men. *JAMA* 1992;267:1083–1089.

Siegl PKS. Discovery of losartan, the first specific non-peptide angiotensin II receptor antagonist. *J Hypertens* 1993; 11(Suppl 3):19–22.

Silas JH, Lennard MS, Tucker GT, Smith AJ, Malcolm SL, Marten TR. Why hypertensive patients vary in their response to oral debrisoquine. *Br Med J* 1977;1:422–425.

Simon G, Wittig VJ, Cohn JN. Transdermal nitroglycerin as a step 3 antihypertensive drug. *Clin Pharmacol Ther* 1986; 40:42–45.

Simons LA, Simons J, McCallum J, Friedlander Y. Dubbo study of the elderly: hypertension and lipid levels. *Atherosclerosis* 1992;92:59–65.

Singh BN, Hollenberg NK, Poole-Wilson PA, Robertson JIS. Diuretic-induced potassium and magnesium deficiency: relation to drug-induced QT prolongation, cardiac arrhythmias and sudden death. *J Hypertens* 1992;10:301–316.

Siscovick DS, Raghunathan TE, Wicklund KG, Psaty BM, Rautaharju PM, Koepsell TD, Cobb LA, Eisenberg MS, Copass MK, Wagner EH. Diuretic therapy for hypertension and the risk of primary cardiac arrest [Abstract]. *Circulation* 1993;87:2.

Skarfors ET, Lithell HO, Selinus I, Åberg H. Do antihypertensive drugs precipitate diabetes in predisposed men? *Br Med J* 1989;298:1147–1152.

Skinner MH, Futterman A, Morrissette D, Thompson LW, Hoffman BB, Blaschke TF. Atenolol compared with nifedipine: effect on cognitive function and mood in elderly hypertensive patients. *Ann Intern Med* 1992;116:615–623.

Sobota JT, Martin WB, Carlson RG, Feenstra ES. Minoxidil: right atrial cardiac pathology in animals and in man. *Circulation* 1980;62:376–387.

SOLVD Investigators. Effect of enalapril on survival in patients with reduced left ventricular ejection fractions and congestive heart failure. *N Engl J Med* 1991; 325:293–302.

Sörgel F, Ettinger B, Benet LZ. The true composition of kidney stones passed during triamterene therapy. *J Urol* 1985; 134:871–873.

Sorkin EM, Heel RC. Guanfacine. A review of its pharmacodynamic and pharmacokinetic properties, and therapeutic efficacy in the treatment of hypertension. *Drugs* 1986;31:301–336.

Stein J, Osgood R. Delineation of the site of action of guanabenz in the renal tubule. *J Cardiovasc Pharmacol* 1984; 6:S787–S792.

Steiness E. Thiazide-induced potassium loss not prevented by beta blockade. *Clin Pharmacol Ther* 1984;35:788–791.

Stenvinkel P, Alvestrand A. Loop diuretic-induced pancreatitis with rechallenge in a patient with malignant hypertension and renal insufficiency. *Acta Med Scand* 1988;224:89–91.

Stephenson BJ, Rowe BH, Haynes RB, Macharia WM, Leon G. Is this patient taking the treatment as prescribed? *JAMA* 1993;269:2779–2781.

Stern R, Khalsa JH. Cutaneous adverse reactions associated with calcium channel blockers. *Arch Intern Med* 1989; 149:829–832.

Stewart AL, Greenfield S, Hays RD, Wells K, Rogers WH, Berry SD, McGlynn EA, Ware JE Jr. Functional status and well-being of patients with chronic conditions. Results from the medical outcomes study. *JAMA* 1989;262:907–913.

Stief CG, Holmquist F, Djamilian M, Krah H, Andersson K-E, Jonas U. Preliminary results with the nitric oxide donor linsidomine chlorohydrate in the treatment of human erectile dysfunction. *J Urol* 1992;148:1437–1440.

Stokes GS, Graham RM, Gain JM, Davis PR. Influence of dosage and dietary sodium on the first-dose effects of prazosin. *Br Med J* 1977;1:1507–1508.

Stone JG, Foëx P, Sear JW, Johnson LL, Khambatta HJ, Triner L. Myocardial ischemia in untreated hypertensive patients: effect of a single small oral dose of a beta-adrenergic blocking agent. *Anesthesiology* 1988;68:495–500.

Strandgaard S, Haunsø S. Why does antihypertensive treatment prevent stroke but not myocardial infarction? *Lancet* 1987; 2:658–661.

Strandgaard S, Paulson OB. Cerebral blood flow and its pathophysiology in hypertension. *Am J Hypertens* 1989;2:486–492.

Strasser RH, Ihl-Vahl R, Marquetant R. Molecular biology of adrenergic receptors. *J Hypertens* 1992;10:501–506.

Strosberg AD. Molecular and functional properties of betaadrenergic receptors. *Am J Cardiol* 1987;59:3F–9F.

Struthers AD, Whitesmith R, Reid JL. Prior thiazide diuretic treatment increases adrenaline-induced hypokalemia. *Lancet* 1983;1:1358–1363.

Sturman SG, Kumararatne D, Beevers DG. Fatal hydralazine-induced systemic lupus erythematosus. *Lancet* 1988;2:1304.

Sugai N, Amaha K, Fujita M, Yamamura H. Control of hypertension during anesthesia with continuous infusion of nicardipine hydrochloride. *Curr Ther Res* 1992; 51:617–625.

Sullivan TJ. Cross-reactions among furosemide, hydrochlorothiazide, and sulfonamides. *JAMA* 1991;265:120–121.

Swales JD. Antihypertensive drugs and plasma lipids. *Br Heart J* 1991; 66:409–410.

Szlachcic J, Tubau JF, Vollmer C, Massie BM. Effect of diltiazem on left ventricular mass and diastolic filling in mild to moderate hypertension. *Am J Cardiol* 1989; 63:198–201.

Talseth T. Studies on hydralazine. I. Serum concentrations of hydralazine in man after a single dose and at steady-state. *Eur J Clin Pharmacol* 1976a;10:183–187.

Talseth T. Studies on hydralazine. II. Elimination rate and steady-state concentration in patients with impaired renal function. *Eur J Clin Pharmacol* 1976b;10:311–317.

Talseth T, Westlie L, Daae L. Doxazosin and atenolol as monotherapy in mild and moderate hypertension: a randomized, parallel study with a three-year follow-up. *Am Heart J* 1991;121:280–285.

Tanner LA, Bosco LA. Gynecomastia associated with calcium channel blocker therapy. *Arch Intern Med* 1988;148:379–380.

Taylor DG, Kaplan HR. New antihypertensive drugs. In: Kaplan NM, Brenner BM, Laragh JH, eds. New Therapeutic Strategies in Hypertension. New York: Raven Press, 1989:125–139.

Testa MA, Anderson RB, Nackley JF, Hollenberg NK. Quality of life and antihypertensive therapy in men. A comparison of captopril with enalapril. *N Engl J Med* 1993;328:907–913.

Thompson PD, Cullinane EM, Nugent AM, Sady MA, Sady SP. Effect of atenolol or prazosin on maximal exercise performance in hypertensive joggers. *Am J Med* 1989;86:104–109.

Thulin T, Fagher B, Grabowski M, Ryding E, Elmqvist D, Johansson BB. Cerebral blood flow in patients with severe hypertension, and acute and chronic effects of felodipine. *J Hypertens* 1993;11:83–88.

Thulin T, Hedner T, Gustafsson S, Olsson S-O. Diltiazem compared with metoprolol as add-on-therapies to diuretics in hypertension. *J Hum Hypertens* 1991;5:107–114.

Toner JM, Brawn LA, Yeo WW, Ramsay LE. Adequacy of twice daily dosing with potassium chloride and spironolactone in thiazide treated hypertensive patients. *Br J Clin Pharmacol* 1991;31:457–461.

Topol EJ, Traill TA, Fortuin NJ. Hypertensive hypertrophic cardiomyopathy of the elderly. *N Engl J Med* 1985;312:277–283.

Toriumi DM, Konior RJ, Berktold RE. Severe hypertrichosis of the external ear canal during minoxidil therapy. *Arch Otolaryngol Head Neck Surg* 1988; 114:918–919.

Torup M, Waldemar G, Paulson OB. Ceranapril and cerebral blood flow autoregulation. *J Hypertens* 1993;11:399–405.

Toto RD, Mitchell HC, Lee H-C, Milam C, Pettinger WA. Reversible renal insufficiency due to angiotensin converting enzyme inhibitors in hypertensive nephrosclerosis. *Ann Intern Med* 1991; 115:513–519.

Townsend RR, DiPette DJ, Goodman R, Blumfield D, Cronin R, Gradman A, Katz LA, McCarthy EP, Sopko G. Combined α/β-blockade versus β1-selective blockade in essential hypertension in black and white patients. *Clin Pharmacol Ther* 1990a; 48:665–675.

Townsend R, Dipette DJ, Evans RR, Davis WR, Green A, Graham GA, Wallace JM, Holland OB. Effects of calcium channel blockade on calcium homeostasis in mild to moderate essential hypertension. *Am J Med Sci* 1990b;300:133–137.

Townsend RR, Holland OB. Combination of converting enzyme inhibitor with diuretic for the treatment of hypertension. *Arch Intern Med* 1990;150:1175–1183.

Traub YM, Rabinov M, Rosenfeld JB, Treuherz S. Elevation of serum potassium during beta blockade: absence of relationship to the renin-aldosterone system. *Clin Pharmacol Ther* 1980;28:765–768.

Treatment of Mild Hypertension Research Group. The treatment of mild hypertension study. A randomized, placebo-controlled trial of a nutritional-hygienic regimen along with various drug monotherapies. *Arch Intern Med* 1991;151:1413–1423.

Trost BN, Weidmann P. Effects of calcium antagonists on glucose homeostasis and serum lipids in non-diabetic and diabetic subjects: a review. *J Hypertens* 1987; 5:S81–S104.

Tsunoda K, Abe K, Hagino T, Omata K, Misawa S, Imai Y, Yoshinaga K. Hypotensive effect of losartan, a nonpeptide angiotensin II receptor antagonist, in essential hypertension. *Am J Hypertens* 1993; 6:28–32.

Tweeddale MG, Ogilvie RI. Antagonism of spironolactone-induced natriuresis by aspirin in man. *N Engl J Med* 1973; 289:198–200.

Tyrer P. Current status of β-blocking drugs in the treatment of anxiety disorders. *Drugs* 1988;36:773–783.

Uehara Y, Shirahase H, Nagata T, Ishimitsu T, Morishita S, Osumi S, Matsuoka H, Sugimoto T. Radical scavengers of indapamide in prostacyclin synthesis in rat smooth muscle cell. *Hypertension* 1990;15:216–224.

Valdés G, Soto ME, Croxatto HR, Bellolio T, Corbalán R, Casanegra P. Effects of nifedipine during low, normal and high intakes of sodium in patients with essential hypertension. *Clin Sci* 1982; 63:447s–450s.

van Brummelen P, Man in 't Veld AJ, Schalekamp MADH. Hemodynamic changes during long-term thiazide treatment of essential hypertension in responders and nonresponders. *Clin Pharmacol Ther* 1980;27:328–336.

van den Meiracker AH, Man in 't Veld AJ, Admiraal PJJ, Ritsema van Eck HJ, Boomsma F, Derkx FHM, Schalekamp MADH. Partial escape of angiotensin converting enzyme (ACE) inhibition during prolonged ACE inhibitor treatment: does it exist and does it affect the antihypertensive response? *J Hypertens* 1992;10:803–812.

van den Meiracker AH, Man in 't Veld AJ, Boomsma F, Fischberg DJ, Molinoff PB, Schalekamp MADH. Hemodynamic and β-adrenergic receptor adaptations during long-term β-adrenoceptor blockade. Studies with acebutolol, atenolol, pindolol, and propranolol in hypertensive patients. *Circulation* 1989;80:903–914.

van den Meiracker AH, Man in't Veld AJ, Ritsema van Eck HJ, Boomsma F, Schalekamp MADH. Hemodynamic and hormonal adaptations to β-adrenoceptor blockade. A 24-hour study of acebutolol, atenolol, pindolol, and propranolol in

hypertensive patients. *Circulation* 1988;78:957–968.

van Giersbergen PLM, Tierney SAV, Wiegant VM, de Jong, W. Possible involvement of brain opioid peptides in clonidine-induced hypotension in spontaneously hypertensive rats. *Hypertension* 1989;13:83–90.

van Gilst WH, Tio RA, van Wijngaarden J, de Graeff PA, Wesseling H. Effects of converting enzyme inhibitors on coronary flow and myocardial ischemia. *J Cardiovasc Pharmacol* 1992;19:S134–S139.

van Kalken CK, van der Meulen J, Oe PL, Vriesendorp R, Donker AJM. Pharmacokinetics of trimazosin and its effects on blood pressure, renal function and proteinuria during short-term therapy of patients with impaired renal function and hypertension. *Eur J Clin Pharmacol* 1986;31:63–68.

van Kleef EM, Smits JFM, De Mey JGR, Cleutjens JPM, Lombardi DM, Schwartz SM, Daemen MJAP. α₁-adrenoreceptor blockade reduces the angiotensin II-induced vascular smooth muscle cell DNA synthesis in the rat thoracic aorta and carotid artery. *Circ Res* 1992; 79:1122–1127.

van Schaik BAM, Geyskes GG, Mees EJD. The effect of converting enzyme inhibition on the enhanced proximal sodium reabsorption induced by chronic diuretic treatment in patients with essential hypertension. *Nephron* 1987;47:167–172.

van Zwieten PA. The interaction between clonidine and various neuroleptic agents and some benzodiazepine tranquillizers. *J Pharm Pharmacol* 1977;29:229–234.

van Zwieten PA. Basic pharmacology of alpha-adrenoceptor antagonists and hybrid drugs. *J Hypertens* 1988;6:S3–S11.

van Zwieten PA. Different types of centrally acting antihypertensive drugs. *Eur Heart J* 1992a;13:18–21.

van Zwieten PA. Development and trends in the drug treatment of essential hypertension. *J Hypertens* 1992b;10:S1–S12.

van Zwieten PA. Protective effects of calcium antagonists in different organs and tissues. *Am Heart J* 1993;125:566–571.

van Zwieten PA, Thoolen MJMC, Timmermans PBMWM. The hypotensive activity and side effects of methyldopa, clonidine, and guanfacine. *Hypertension* 1984; 6(Suppl 2):28–33.

Vandenburg MJ, Wright P, Holmes J, Rogers HJ, Ahmad RA. *Br J Clin Pharmacol* 1982;13:747–750.

Vardan S, Mehrotra KG, Mookherjee S, Willsey GA, Gens JD, Green DE. Efficacy and reduced metabolic side effects of a 15-mg chlorthalidone formulation in the treatment of mild hypertension. A multicenter study. *JAMA* 1987;258:484–488.

Verburg KM, Polakowski JS, Kovar PJ, Klinghofer V, Barlow JL, Stein HH, Mantei RA, Fung AKL, Boyd SA, Baker WA, Kleinert HD. Effects of high doses of a-74273, a novel nonpeptidic and orally bioavailable renin inhibitor. *J Cardiovasc Pharmacol* 1993;21:149–155.

Veterans Administration Cooperative Study on Antihypertensive Agents. Double blind control study of antihypertensive agents, II: Further report on the comparative effec-

tiveness of reserpine, reserpine and hydralazine, and three ganglion blocking agents, chlorisondamine, mecamylamine, and pentolinium tartrate. *Arch Intern Med* 1962;110:222–229.

Veterans Administration Cooperative Study on Antihypertensive Agents. Multiclinic controlled trial of bethanidine and guanethidine in severe hypertension. *Circulation* 1977;55:519–525.

Veterans Administration Cooperative Study on Antihypertensive Agents. Comparison of propranolol and hydrochlorothiazide for the initial treatment of hypertension, II: Results of long-term therapy. *JAMA* 1982;248:2004–2011.

Veterans Administration Cooperative Study Group on Antihypertensive Agents. Low-dose captopril for the treatment of mild to moderate hypertension. I. Results of a 14-week trial. *Arch Intern Med* 1984; 144:1947–1953.

Vezù L, La Vecchia L, Vincenzi M. Hypertension, obesity and response to antihypertensive treatment: results of a community survey. *J Hum Hypertens* 1992;6:215–220.

Vidrio H. Interaction with pyridoxal as a possible mechanism of hydralazine hypotension. *J Cardiovasc Pharmacol* 1990; 15:150–156.

Vincent HH, Man in 't Veld AJ, Boomsma F, Derkx FHM, Schalekamp MADH. Is β₁-antagonism essential for the antihypertensive action of β-blockers? *Hypertension* 1987;9:198–203.

Vincent J, Dachman W, Blaschke TF, Hoffman BB. Pharmacological tolerance to α₁-adrenergic receptor antagonism mediated by terazosin in humans. *J Clin Invest* 1992;90:1763–1768.

Virag R, Bouilly P, Frydman D. Is impotence an arterial disorder? A study of arterial risk factors in 440 impotent men. *Lancet* 1985;1:181–184.

Viscoli CM, Horwitz RI, Singer BH. Beta-blockers after myocardial infarction: influence of first-year clinical course on long-term effectiveness. *Ann Intern Med* 1993;118:99–105.

Vlasses PH, Koffer H, Ferguson RK, Green PJ, McElwain GE. Captopril withdrawal after chronic therapy. *Clin Exp Hypertens* 1981;3:929–937.

Volini IF, Flaxman N. The effect of nonspecific operations on essential hypertension. *JAMA* 1939;112:2126–2128.

Vyssoulis GP, Karpanou EA, Pitsavos CE, Skoumas JN, Paleologos AA, Toutouzas PK. Differentiation of β-blocker effects on serum lipids and apolipoproteins in hypertensive patients with normolipidaemic or dyslipidaemic profiles. *Eur Heart J* 1992;13:1506–1513.

Walker WG, Hermann J, Yin D-P, Murphy RP, Patz A. Diuretics accelerate diabetic nephropathy in hypertensive insulin-dependent and non-insulin-dependent subjects. *Trans Assoc Am Phys* 1987; 100:305–315.

Walker WG, Neaton JD, Cutler JA, Neuwirth R, Cohen JD. Renal function change in hypertensive members of the multiple risk factor intervention trial. Racial and treatment effects. *JAMA* 1992;268:3085–3091.

Waller PC, Inman WHW. Diltiazem and heart block. *Lancet* 1989;1:617.

Wang D-H, Prewitt RL. Captopril reduces aortic and microvascular growth in hypertensive and normotensive rats. *Hypertension* 1990;15:68–77.

Warner NJ, Rush JE. Safety profiles of the angiotensin-converting enzyme inhibitors. *Drugs* 1988;35:89–97.

Warram JH, Laffel LMB, Valsania P, Christlieb AR, Krolewski AS. Excess mortality associated with diuretic therapy in diabetes mellitus. *Arch Intern Med* 1991; 151:1350–1356.

Washton AM, Resnick RB, Perzel JF Jr, Garwood J. Lofexidine, a clonidine analogue effective in opiate withdrawal. *Lancet* 1981;1:991–992.

Waters D, Lespérance J, Francetich M, Causey D, Théroux P, Chiang Y-K, Hudon G, Lemarbre L, Reitman M, Joyal M, Gosselin G, Dyrda I, Macer J, Havel RJ. A controlled clinical trial to assess the effect of a calcium channel blocker on the progression of coronary atherosclerosis. *Circulation* 1990;82:1940–1953.

Webb DJ, Fulton JD, Leckie BJ, Malatino LS, McAreavey D, Morton JJ, Murray GD, Robertson JIS. The effect of chronic prazosin therapy on the response of the renin-angiotensin system in patients with essential hypertension. *J Hum Hypertens* 1987;1:195–200.

Weber KT, Brilla CG, Campbell SE, Reddy HK. Myocardial fibrosis and the concepts of cardioprotection and cardioreparation. *J Hypertens* 1992;10:S87–S94.

Weber MA. Transdermal antihypertensive therapy: clinical and metabolic considerations. *Am Heart J* 1986;112:906–912.

Weber MA, Drayer JIM, Rev A, Laragh JH. Disparate patterns of aldosterone response during diuretic treatment of hypertension. *Ann Intern Med* 1977;87:558–563.

Weidmann P, de Châtel R, Ziegler WH, Flammer J, Reubi F. Alpha and beta adrenergic blockade with orally administered labetalol in hypertension. Studies on blood volume, plasma renin and aldosterone and catecholamine excretion. *Am J Cardiol* 1978;41:570–576.

Weidmann P, Uehlinger DE, Gerber A. Antihypertensive treatment and serum lipoproteins. *J Hypertens* 1985;3:297–306.

Weinberger MH, Fineberg NS. Sodium and volume sensitivity of blood pressure. Age and pressure change over time. *Hypertension* 1991;18:67–71.

Weir MR, Weber MA, Punzi HA, Serfer HM, Rosenblatt S, Cady WJ. A dose escalation trial comparing the combination of diltiazem SR and hydrochlorothiazide with the monotherapies in patients with essential hypertension. *J Hum Hypertens* 1992; 6:133–138.

Weisser B, Ripka O. Long-term diuretic therapy: effects of dose reduction on antihypertensive efficacy and counterregulatory systems. *J Cardiovasc Pharmacol* 1992; 19:361–366.

Westwood BE, Wilson M, Heath WC, Hammond JJ, Mashford ML. The unsuitability of minoxidil for the treatment of moderate hypertension. *Med J Aust* 1986; 145:151–152.

Whang R, Flink EB, Dyckner T, Wester PO, Aikawa JK, Ryan MP. Magnesium depletion as a cause of refractory potassium repletion. *Arch Intern Med* 1985; 145:1686–1689.

White WB. Methods of blood pressure determination to assess antihypertensive agents: are casual measurements enough? *Clin Pharmacol Ther* 1989;45:581–586.

Widmann L, Dyckner T, Wester P-O. Effects of triamterene on serum and skeletal muscle electrolytes in diuretic-treated patients. *Eur J Clin Pharmacol* 1988;33:577–579.

Wikstrand J, Warnold I, Tuomilehto J, Olsson G, Barber HJ, Eliasson K, Elmfeldt D, Jastrup B, Karatzas NB, Leer J, Marchetta F, Ragnarsson J, Robitaille N-M, Valkova L, Wesseling H, Berglund G. Metoprolol versus thiazide diuretics in hypertension. Morbidity results from the MAPHY study. *Hypertension* 1991;17:579–588.

Wilcox CS, Mitch WE, Kelly RA, Skorecki K, Meyer TW, Friedman PA, Souney PF. Response of the kidney to furosemide, I: effects of salt intake and renal compensation. *J Lab Clin Med* 1983;102:450–458.

Wilcox RG. Randomised study of six beta-blockers and a thiazide diuretic in essential hypertension. *Br Med J* 1978;2:383–385.

Wilhelmsen L, Berglund G, Elmfeldt D, Fitzsimmons T, Holzgreve H, Hosie J, Hörnkvist P-E, Pennert K, Tuomilehto J, Wedel H. Beta-blockers versus diuretics in hypertensive men: main results from the HAPPHY trial. *J Hypertens* 1987;5:561–572.

Williams WR, Schneider KA, Borhani NO, Schnaper HW, Slotkoff LM, Ellefson RD. The relationship between diuretics and serum cholesterol in hypertension detection and follow-up program participants. *Am J Prev Med* 1986;2:248–255.

Wilson IM, Freis ED. Relationship between plasma and extracellular fluid volume depletion and the antihypertensive effect of chlorothiazide. *Circulation* 1959;20: 1028–1036.

Wilson MF, Haring O, Lewin A, Bedsole G, Stepansky W, Fillingim J, Hall D, Roginsky M, McMahon FG, Jagger P, Strauss M. Comparison of guanfacine versus clonidine for efficacy, safety and occurrence of withdrawal syndrome in step-2 treatment of mild to moderate essential hypertension. *Am J Cardiol* 1986;57:43E–49E.

Wilson TW. The antihypertensive action of hydrochlorothiazide and renal prostacyclin. *Clin Pharmacol Ther* 1986; 39:94–101.

Winer BM. The antihypertensive mechanisms of salt depletion induced by hydrochlorothiazide. *Circulation* 1961; 24:788–796.

Wolff DW, Buckalew VM Jr, Strandhoy JW. Renal α_1- and α_2-adrenoceptor mediated vasoconstriction in dogs: comparison of phenylephrine, clonidine, and guanabenz. *J Cardiovasc Pharmacol* 1984; 6:S793–S798.

Wolfsthal SD. Is blood pressure control necessary before surgery? *Med Clin North Am* 1993;77:349–363.

Woods JW, Pittman AW, Pulliam CC, Werk EE Jr, Waider W, Allen CA. Renin profiling in hypertension and its use in treatment with propranolol and chlorthalidone. *N Engl J Med* 1976;294:1137–1143.

Woosley RL, Nies AS. Guanethidine. *N Engl J Med* 1976;295:1053–1058.

Wright FS. Renal potassium handling. *Semin Nephrol* 1987;7:174–184.

Wright P. Untoward effects associated with practolol administration: oculomucocutaneous syndrome. *Br Med J* 1975; 1:595–598.

Wu, R, Spence JD, Carruthers SG. Evaluation of once daily endralazine in hypertension. *Eur J Clin Pharmacol* 1986;30:553–557.

Wyndham RN, Gimenez L, Walker WG, Whelton PK, Russell RP. Influence of renin levels on the treatment of essential hypertension with thiazide diuretics. *Arch Intern Med* 1987;147:1021–1025.

Wysocki M, Persson B, Bagge U, Andersson OK. Flow resistance and its components in hypertensive men treated with the calcium antagonist isradipine. *Eur J Clin Pharmacol* 1992;43:463–468.

Yakovlevitch M, Black HR. Resistant hypertension in a tertiary care clinic. *Arch Intern Med* 1991;151:1786–1792.

Yeo WW, Maclean D, Richardson PJ, Ramsay LE. Cough and enalapril: assessment by spontaneous reporting and visual analogue scale under double-blind conditions. *Br J Clin Pharmacol* 1991;31:356–359.

Yudofsky SC. β-blockers and depression. The clinician's dilemma. *JAMA* 1992;267:1826–1827.

Yusuf S, Held P, Furberg C. Update of effects of calcium antagonists in myocardial infarction or angina in light of the second Danish verapamil infarction trail (DAVIT-II) and other recent studies. *Am J Cardiol* 1991;67:1295–1297.

Yusuf S, Pepine CJ, Garces C, Pouleur H, Salem D, Kostis J, Benedict C, Rousseau M, Bourassa M, Pitt B. Effect of enalapril on myocardial infarction and unstable angina in patients with low ejection fractions. *Lancet* 1992;340:1173–1178.

Zacest R, Gilmore E, Koch-Weser J. Treatment of essential hypertension with combined vasodilation and beta-adrenergic blockade. *N Engl J Med* 1972; 286:617–622.

Zing W, Ferguson RK, Vlasses PH. Calcium antagonists in elderly and Black hypertensive patients. *Arch Intern Med* 1991; 151:2154–2162.

Zsigmond EK, Barabas E, Korenaga GM. Esmolol attenuates tachycardia caused by tracheal intubation: a double-blind study. *Int J Clin Pharmacol Ther Toxicol* 1988;26:225–231.

Zusman RM, Christensen DM, Higgins J, Boucher CA. Effects of fosinopril on cardiac function in patients with hypertension. Radionuclide assessment of left ventricular systolic and diastolic performance. *Am J Hypertens* 1992;5:219–223.

8 Hypertensive Crises

Life-threatening hypertension may appear in a variety of circumstances (Table 8.1). Hypertensive encephalopathy and accelerated-malignant hypertension may appear on the background of any form of hypertension. These conditions develop in fewer than 1% of patients with primary hypertension, but because 90% or more of hypertension is of unknown cause (i.e., primary), this is the most common setting in which these syndromes appear. Encephalopathy is more common in previously normotensive individuals whose pressures rise suddenly, such as during pregnancy when preeclampsia appears; the accelerated-malignant course often appears without encephalopathy in persons with more chronic hypertension whose pressures progressively rise.

Although the incidence of accelerated-malignant hypertension may be diminishing, and mortality from it is definitely falling (Webster et al., 1993), the syndrome remains all too common, particularly among men in the United States who are young, poor, and black or Hispanic (Shea et al., 1992), as well as among underserved patients everywhere (Clough et al., 1990; Kadiri and Olutade, 1991; Sugiyama and Sesoko, 1992).

Life-threatening hypertension may appear at any age: as congenital renal artery hypoplasia in neonates, as acute glomerulonephritis in children, as eclampsia in young women and as renovascular hypertension in older patients. Clinicians must remain alert to the appearance of such hypertension and manage it aggressively.

DEFINITIONS

The following definitions are generally accepted:

Hypertensive Emergencies. Situations wherein immediate reduction of blood pressure (BP) within minutes is needed, usually with parenteral therapy.

Hypertensive Urgencies. Situations wherein reduction of BP is needed within a period of hours, usually with oral agents.

Accelerated-Malignant Hypertension. Until recently, the term "malignant" hypertension was used for the presence of papilledema (Grade 4 Keith-Wagener [K-W] retinopathy), whereas "accelerated" was used for the presence of hemorrhages and exudates (Grade 3 K-W retinopathy), both with markedly high BP, the diastolic BP usually above 140 mm Hg. The funduscopic differences do not connote different clinical features or prognosis, so the term "accelerated-malignant" hypertension is recommended and will be used (Ahmed et al., 1986).

Hypertensive Encephalopathy. Sudden and usually marked elevation of BP with severe headache and various alterations in consciousness, reversible by reduction of BP.

ACCELERATED-MALIGNANT HYPERTENSION

Mechanisms

When BP reaches some critical level, in experimental animals at a mean arterial pressure of 150 mm Hg, lesions appear in arterial walls, and the syndrome of accelerated-malignant hypertension begins (Fig. 8.1). This may be provoked by one or more vasoactive factors (Möhring, 1977), but the accelerated-malignant phase is likely to be a nonspecific consequence of very

Table 8.1. Circumstances Requiring Rapid Treatment of Hypertension

Hypertensive emergencies
Cerebrovascular
  Hypertensive encephalopathy
  Intracerebral hemorrhage
  Subarachnoid hemorrhage
Cardiac
  Acute aortic dissection
  Acute left ventricular failure
  Acute or impending myocardial infarction
  After coronary bypass surgery
Excessive circulating catecholamines
  Pheochromocytoma crisis
  Food or drug interactions with MAO
    inhibitors
  Sympathomimetic drug abuse (cocaine)
Eclampsia
Head injury
*Postoperative bleeding from vascular suture
  lines*
Severe epistaxis
Hypertensive urgencies
Accelerated-malignant hypertension
*Atherothrombotic brain infarction with severe
  hypertension*
*Rebound hypertension after sudden
  cessation of antihypertensive drugs*
Surgical
  Severe hypertension in patients requiring
    immediate surgery
  Postoperative hypertension
  Severe hypertension after kidney
    transplantation
Severe body burns

high BP (Beilin and Goldby, 1977). Any form of hypertension may progress to the accelerated-malignant phase, some without activation of the renin-angiotensin or other humoral mechanisms (Gavras et al., 1975a). Among the more common causes beyond progression of primary hypertension are renal vascular and certain renal parenchymal diseases such as immunoglobulin A (IgA) nephropathy (Kincaid-Smith, 1991) and reflux nephropathy (Robinson et al., 1992).

Structural Changes

In animal models, the level of the arterial pressure correlates closely with the development of fibrinoid necrosis, the experimental hallmark of accelerated-malignant hypertension (Byrom, 1974). In humans, fibrinoid necrosis is rare, perhaps because those who die from an acute attack have not had time to develop the lesion, and those who live with therapy are able to repair it. The typical lesions, best seen in the kidney,

are hyperplastic arteriosclerosis and accelerated glomerular obsolescence (Jones, 1974). In blacks, myointimal hyperplasia appears to be the typical renal lesion (Pitcock et al., 1976).

Humoral Factors

There is support, however, for the involvement of factors other than the level of the BP in setting off the accelerated-malignant phase, particularly since the range of pressures in patients with severe "benign" hypertension and accelerated-malignant hypertension may overlap (Kincaid-Smith, 1991). As shown on the right side of Figure 8.1, in both rats (Gross et al., 1975) and dogs (Dzau et al., 1981) with unilateral renal artery stenosis, the accelerated-malignant phase was preceded by natriuresis that markedly activated the renin-angiotensin system. The progression was delayed by giving saline loads after the natriuresis.

Whether these animal models involving a major insult to renal blood flow are applicable to all human accelerated-malignant hypertension is uncertain; however, renal artery stenosis is a common cause of accelerated-malignant hypertension in humans, having been found in 35% of 123 patients at Vanderbilt with accelerated-malignant hypertension (Davis et al., 1979).

Evidence for the pathway shown in Figure 8.1 (left) comes from studies on cats made acutely and severely hypertensive, wherein the vascular damage could be inhibited by prior treatment with inhibitors of the cyclooxygenase enzyme involved in prostaglandin synthesis or by topical application of scavengers of free oxygen radicals (Kontos, 1985). More significant abnormalities in the cellular transport mechanisms described in Chapter 3 have been measured in both rats (Touyz et al., 1991) and people (Herlitz et al., 1990) with malignant hypertension. In addition to activation of pressor mechanisms, suppression of vasodepressor mechanisms may be involved, as reflected in decreased urinary kallikrein excretion (Hilme et al., 1993).

In humans, in addition to the presence of renal artery stenosis, the development of accelerated-malignant hypertension has been observed to be more common in association with cigarette smoking (Isles et al., 1979), likely a consequence of the repetitive pressor action of nicotine (Groppelli et al., 1992). High levels of serum immunoglobulins commonly are found, likely as a consequence to vascular damage, but possibly as a primary immunologic disturbance (Hilme et al., 1993).

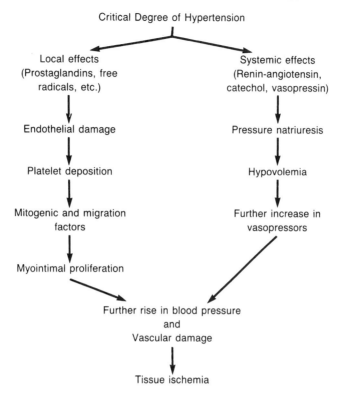

Figure 8.1. Scheme for initiation and progression of accelerated-malignant hypertension.

Clinical Features

Accelerated-malignant hypertension may be accompanied by various symptoms and signs (Table 8.2). However, it is not uncommon to see patients, particularly young black men, who deny any prior symptoms when seen in the end stages of the hypertensive process with their kidneys destroyed, heart failing, and brain function markedly impaired.

Rarely, enough fibrinoid necrosis occurs within abdominal arteries to produce major gut infarction with an ''acute abdomen'' as the presenting feature of malignant hypertension (Padfield, 1975). Rapidly progressive necrotizing vasculitis may present as a hypertensive emergency (O'Connell et al., 1985). An increased association between acute pancreatitis and malignant hypertension has also been noted (Mathur and Warren, 1989).

Table 8.2. Clinical Characteristics of Accelerated-Malignant Hypertension

Blood pressure: usually > 140 mm Hg diastolic
Funduscopic findings: hemorrhages, exudates, papilledema
Neurologic status: headache, confusion, somnolence, stupor, visual loss, focal deficits, seizures, coma
Cardiac findings: prominent apical impulse, cardiac enlargement, congestive failure
Renal: oliguria, azotemia
Gastrointestinal: nausea, vomiting

Funduscopic Findings

The effects of the markedly elevated BP are displayed in the optic fundi, as demonstrated in monkeys with induced accelerated-malignant hypertension (Hayreh et al., 1985a, 1985b, 1986). Beyond the chronic arteriolar sclerosis and hypertrophy, acute changes may include arteriolar spasm, either segmental or diffuse; retinal edema, with a sheen or ripples; retinal hemorrhages, either superficial and flame-shaped, or deep and dot-shaped; retinal exudates, either hard and waxy from resorption of edema or having a cotton-wool appearance, soft from ischemia; and papilledema and engorged retinal veins. In the monkeys, pinpoint, round periarteriolar transudates were particularly common, representing leakage from dilated arterioles

(Hayreh et al., 1985b). These animals had optic neuropathy that was caused by ischemia of the nerve, leading Hayreh et al. (1986) to caution against a precipitous reduction in pressure that could (and has) caused permanent blindness (Cove et al., 1979).

Similar retinopathy with hemorrhages and even papilledema rarely occurs in severe anemia, collagen diseases, and subacute bacterial endocarditis. Some patients have pseudopapilledema associated with congenital anomalies, hyaline bodies (Drusen) in the disk, or severe farsightedness. Fluorescein fundus photography will distinguish between the true and the pseudo states. In addition, benign intracranial hypertension may produce real papilledema but is usually a minimally symptomatic and self-limited process (Jain et al., 1992).

Evaluation

In addition to an adequate history and physical examination, a few laboratory tests should be done immediately to assess the patient's status (Table 8.3).

Laboratory Findings

Hematology and Urine Analysis. Microangiopathic hemolytic anemia with red cell

Table 8.3. Initial Evaluation of Patients with Accelerated-Malignant Hypertension

History
  Prior diagnosis and treatment of
    hypertension
  Intake of pressor agents: street drugs,
    sympathomimetics
  Symptoms of cerebral, cardiac, and visual
    dysfunction
Physical examination
  Blood pressure
  Funduscopic examination
  Neurologic examination
  Cardiopulmonary status
  Body fluid volume assessment
Laboratory evaluation
  Hematocrit and blood smear
  Urine analysis
  Automated chemistry: creatinine, glucose,
    electrolytes
  Plasma renin and aldosterone (some cases)
    (Repeat plasma renin 1 hour after 25 mg
    captopril if renovascular hypertension is
    being considered)
  Spot urine for metanephrine if
    pheochromocytoma is being considered
  Chest radiograph
  Electrocardiogram

fragmentation and intravascular coagulation may occur in accelerated-malignant hypertension, possibly originating from the fibrinoid necrotic arterial lesions (Gavras et al., 1975b).

The urine contains protein and red cells. In a few patients, acute oliguric renal failure may be the presenting manifestation (Meyrier et al., 1984).

Blood Chemistry. Various features of renal insufficiency may be present, including metabolic acidosis, marked azotemia, and hypocalcemia. Hypokalemia is present in about half of patients with accelerated-malignant hypertension, reflecting secondary aldosteronism. The serum sodium level is usually lower than normal, unlike the hypernatremia found in primary aldosteronism.

Renin-Aldosterone. Plasma renin activity (PRA) is usually increased, often to very high levels, in response to intrarenal ischemia (Kawazoe et al., 1987). Aldosterone secretion and excretion are usually increased and return to normal with control of the hypertension (Laragh et al., 1960).

Cardiography. The electrocardiogram (ECG) usually displays evidence of left ventricular hypertrophy, strain, and lateral ischemia. Echocardiography may show incoordinate contractions with impaired diastolic function and delayed mitral valve opening (Shapiro and Beevers, 1983).

Evaluation for Secondary Causes

Once causes for the presenting picture other than severe hypertension are excluded and necessary immediate therapy is provided, an appropriate evaluation for secondary causes of the hypertension should be performed as quickly as possible. It is far easier to obtain necessary blood and urine samples for required laboratory studies before institution of therapies that may markedly complicate subsequent evaluation. None of these procedures should delay effective therapy.

Renovascular Hypertension. Renovascular hypertension is by far the most likely secondary cause and unfortunately the one that may be least obvious by history, physical examination, and routine laboratory tests.

As described in Chapter 10, a single-dose captopril challenge test, measuring plasma renin activity before and 1 hour after administration of 25 mg of captopril, can be performed when the patient presents, since the captopril will almost certainly lower the BP during the subsequent hour, protecting the patient while helping to rule out (or in) renovascular hypertension.

Pheochromocytoma. A spot urine sample should be collected for metanephrine assay since pheochromocytoma is another possible cause and catechol measurements may be invalidated by labetalol and other antihypertensive drugs (see Chapter 12).

Primary Aldosteronism. If significant hypokalemia is noted on the initial blood test, a plasma renin and aldosterone measurement should be obtained to rule out primary aldosteronism (see Chapter 13).

Prognosis

If untreated, most patients with accelerated-malignant hypertension will die within 6 months. The 1-year survival rate was only 10% to 20% without therapy (Dustan et al., 1958). With current therapy, 5-year survival rates of 50% (Clough et al., 1990), 60% (Kawazoe et al., 1988), and 80% (Sugiyama and Sesoko, 1992; Webster et al., 1993) are seen, which clearly shows the major protection provided by antihypertensive therapy.

Importance of Renal Damage

Many patients when first seen with accelerated-malignant hypertension have significant renal damage, which markedly worsens their prognosis. In one series of 100 consecutive patients with malignant hypertension (Bing et al., 1986), the 5-year survival rate of those without renal impairment (serum creatinine less than 1.5 mg/dl) was 96%, no different from that of the general population. However, among those with renal impairment, 5-year survival fell to 65%. When vigorous antihypertensive therapy is begun, renal function often worsens transiently, but those who will eventually improve usually begin to do so within 2 weeks (Lawton, 1982). Marked and sustained improvement of renal function may occur after aggressive therapy when patients present with acute renal failure (Isles et al., 1984), therapy that may need to include dialysis (Bakir et al., 1986).

Causes of Death

Therapy used over the past 35 years has dramatically reduced immediate deaths from acute renal failure, hemorrhagic strokes, and congestive heart failure. With longer survival, death from an acute myocardial infarction is more likely (Webster et al., 1993).

HYPERTENSIVE ENCEPHALOPATHY

With or without the structural defects of accelerated-malignant hypertension, progressively higher BP can lead to hypertensive encephalopathy.

Mechanisms

Breakthrough Vasodilation

With changes in BP, cerebral vessels dilate or constrict to maintain a relatively constant level of cerebral blood flow (CBF), the process of autoregulation that is regulated by sympathetic nervous activity (Tuor, 1992). Direct measurements taken in cats show progressive dilation as pressures are lowered and progressive constriction as pressures rise (MacKenzie et al., 1976) (Fig 8.2). Note, however, that when mean arterial pressures reach a critical level, around 180 mm Hg, the previously constricted vessels, unable to withstand such high pressures, are stretched and dilated—first in areas with less muscular tone, producing irregular sausage-string patterns, and later diffusely, producing generalized vasodilation. This vasodilation allows a breakthrough of CBF, hyperperfusing the brain under high pressure, with leakage of fluid into the perivascular tissue leading to cerebral edema and the clinical syndrome of hypertensive encephalopathy (Strandgaard and Paulson, 1989).

In experimental animals, breakthrough is facilitated by arterial baroreflexes and the release of nitric oxide. When either of these are inhibited, breakthrough is delayed, and the critical level is higher (Talman et al., 1993).

The "breakthrough" vasodilation that leads to hypertensive encephalopathy has also been demonstrated in humans (Strandgaard et al., 1973). By measuring CBF repetitively while arterial BP is lowered by vasodilators or raised by vasoconstrictors, curves of autoregulation have been constructed. Figure 8.3 demonstrates that CBF is constant between mean arterial pressures of 60 and 120 mm Hg in normotensive subjects, the lower six curves. However, as shown in the curves for the upper two normotensive subjects whose pressure was raised beyond the limit of autoregulation, breakthrough hyperperfusion occurs.

Pressures such as these are handled without obvious trouble in chronic hypertensives, whose blood vessels adapt to the chronically elevated BP with structural thickening, presumably mediated by sympathetic nerves (Tuor, 1992).

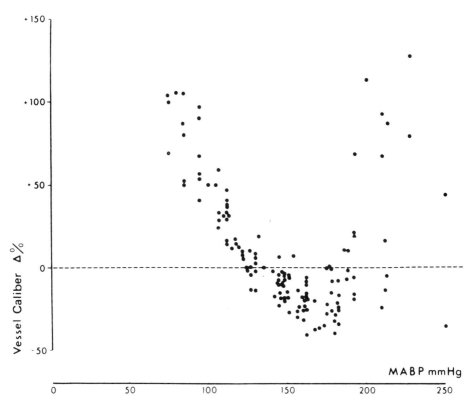

Figure 8.2. Observed change in the caliber of pial arterioles with a caliber less than 50 μm in eight cats, calculated as a percentage of change from the caliber at a mean arterial blood pressure (MABP) of 135 mm Hg. The blood pressure was raised by intravenous infusion of angiotensin II. (From MacKenzie ET, Strandgaard S, Graham DI, et al. Effects of acutely induced hypertension in cats on pial arteriolar caliber, local cerebral blood flow, and the blood-brain barrier. *Circ Res* 39:33, 1976, by permission of the American Heart Association, Inc.)

Thereby the entire curve of autoregulation is shifted to the right, as shown in the upper eight cases in Figure 8.3. Even with this shift, breakthrough will occur if pressures are raised very high, to levels of 170 to 180 mm Hg, as shown in the upper five cases.

These findings explain a number of clinical observations. At the upper portion of the autoregulatory curve, previously normotensive people who suddenly become hypertensive may develop encephalopathy at relatively low levels of hypertension. These include children with acute glomerulonephritis and young women with eclampsia. On the other hand, chronically hypertensive patients less commonly develop encephalopathy, and only at much higher pressures.

At the lower portion of the curve, when the BP is lowered by antihypertensive drugs too quickly, chronic hypertensives often are unable to tolerate the reduction without experiencing cerebral hypoperfusion, manifested by weakness

and dizziness. These symptoms may appear at levels of BP that are still above the upper limit of normal and that are well tolerated by normotensives. The reason is that the entire curve of autoregulation shifts, so that the lower end also is moved, with a fall-off of CBF at levels of 100 to 120 mm Hg mean arterial pressure (Fig. 8.3). Fortunately, as detailed in Chapter 7, if the BP is lowered gradually, the curve can shift back toward the normal so that greater reductions in pressure can eventually be tolerated. Unfortunately, chronic hypertensives may lose their ability to autoregulate, increasing their risk of brain damage when BP is lowered acutely (Jansen et al., 1987).

Maneuvers that increase CBF further and thereby increase intracranial pressure, such as CO_2 inhalation or cerebral vasodilators (e.g., hydralazine and nitroprusside), may be harmful in patients with encephalopathy. In experimentally infarcted brain tissue, autoregulation is lost; therefore, with high BP, perfusion would be accentuated through the damaged tissue, leading to edema and compression of normal brain (Meyer et al., 1972). This provides experimental evidence for the clinical importance of carefully reducing the BP in hypertensive stroke patients.

Thus, hypertensive encephalopathy is the consequence of progressively rising arterial pressures that break through the protection of the blood-brain barrier and the autoregulation of CBF. The underlying causes of encephalopathy

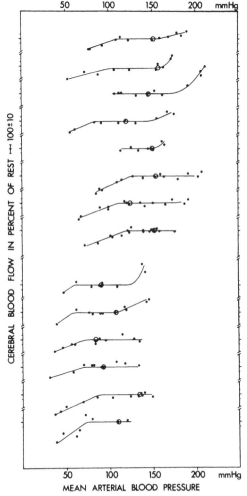

Figure 8.3. Curves of cerebral blood flow with varying levels of blood pressure in 14 people, the top 8 hypertensive, the bottom 6 normotensive. Each patient's habitual pressure is indicated by an *open circle*. The curves reflect autoregulation, with a shift to the right in the hypertensives. Both the lower and the upper limits of autoregulation are shown. Note the breakthrough of CBF when the upper limit is exceeded. (From Johansson B, Strandgaard S, Lassen NA. The hypertensive "breakthrough" of autoregulation of cerebral blood flow with forced vasodilatation, flow increase, and blood-brain-barrier damage. *Circ Res* 1974;34-35[Suppl 1]:167–174.)

are usually conditions involving a sudden rise in pressure, as with sympathomimetic drug abuse (Lake et al., 1990) or preeclampsia-eclampsia (see Chapter 11).

Central Nervous System

Encephalopathic patients have many of the same laboratory findings seen in patients with malignant hypertension, but they also have more central nervous system manifestations. The cerebrospinal fluid is clear but usually under increased pressure. The electroencephalogram (EEG) may show varied, transient, focal, or bilateral disturbances. Computed tomography (CT) scans have revealed widespread areas of diminished density in the white matter representing focal collections of edema that resolve after therapy (Jespersen et al., 1989). Magnetic resonance imaging (MRI) shows more extensive, multifocal areas of extravasation (Hauser et al., 1988).

OTHER HYPERTENSIVE EMERGENCIES

In addition to the two specific presentations of accelerated-malignant hypertension and hypertensive encephalopathy, hypertension may be life-threatening when it accompanies cerebral, cardiac, and other acute conditions wherein a markedly elevated BP contributes to the ongoing tissue damage (Table 8.1). The role of hypertension in most of these conditions was covered in Chapter 4, and some of the other specific circumstances (e.g., pheochromocytoma crises and eclampsia) are covered in their respective chapters. More about some of these specific conditions also is provided later in this chapter under "Therapy for Hypertensive Emergencies."

Differential Diagnosis

Management of the patient with a hypertensive emergency usually does not require knowledge of the specific etiology since the first concern is to lower the BP. However, the choice of therapy may differ with the diagnosis. A less aggressive approach may be indicated in patients with suggestive features, particularly neurologic ones, that represent other diagnoses (Table 8.4).

Differentiating most of the conditions in Table 8.4 from a hypertensive emergency usually is rather easy on clinical grounds. However, aggressive lowering of the BP obviously should be avoided in some of the conditions, particularly after a cerebrovascular accident (CVA), when rapid decrease of cerebral blood flow may

Table 8.4. Diseases That May Mimic a Hypertensive Emergency

Acute left ventricular failure
Uremia from any cause, particularly with
   volume overload
Cerebral vascular accident
Subarachnoid hemorrhage
Brain tumor
Head injury
Epilepsy (postictal)
Collagen diseases, particularly lupus, with
   cerebral vasculitis
Encephalitis
Acute anxiety with hyperventilation syndrome
Drug ingestion: sympathomimetics (cocaine),
   phenyclidine
Acute intermittent porphyria
Hypercalcemia

extend the lesion (Brott and Reed, 1989). The presentation of a CVA is usually abrupt, whereas hypertensive encephalopathy develops more slowly, over days.

THERAPY FOR HYPERTENSIVE EMERGENCIES

The majority of patients with the conditions shown in Table 8.1 will not require immediate reduction in BP. Some patients, such as those with hypertensive encephalopathy, must be treated quickly. If the pressure is not reduced, cerebral edema will worsen, and the lack of autoregulation in ischemic brain tissue may result in further increases in the volume of the ischemic tissue, which may cause either acute herniation or more gradual compression of normal brain (Meyer et al., 1972). Moreover, with increased intracranial pressure, the Cushing reflex may cause the systemic pressure to rise further in an attempt to maintain cerebral blood flow (Jones, 1989).

Initiating Therapy

With encephalopathy or evidence of a progressive stroke or myocardial ischemia, no more than a very few minutes should be taken to admit a patient to an intensive care unit, set up intravenous access and, if possible, place an intra-arterial line for continuous monitoring of the BP. The initial blood and urine samples should be obtained, and antihypertensive therapy should begin immediately thereafter.

Monitoring Therapy

Abrupt falls in pressure should be avoided, and the goal of immediate therapy should be to

lower the diastolic pressure only to about 110 mm Hg. The reductions may need to be even less if signs of tissue ischemia develop as the pressure is lowered. Most of the catastrophes seen with treatment of hypertensive emergencies were related to overly aggressive reduction of the BP (Jansen et al., 1987).

The dilemma is portrayed in two studies appearing within 6 weeks of each other: in one, three children with severe untreated hypertension suffered permanent neurologic damage; blindness resulted in all three, and paraplegia resulted in one (Hulse et al., 1979). In the other study, blindness occurred in two young women soon after successful (and, in one case, quite gradual) treatment of malignant hypertension (Cove et al., 1979).

Particular care should be taken in elderly patients and in patients with known cerebrovascular disease, who are even more vulnerable to sudden falls in systemic BP (Jansen et al., 1987). As described in Chapter 7, patients with acute stroke should have their BP brought down only if it is extremely high and contributing to the neurologic damage, as in the presence of intracranial hemorrhage (Brott and Reed, 1989).

If the neurologic status worsens as treatment proceeds, intracranial pressure may be markedly elevated, most likely from the cerebral edema associated with the hypertensive emergency but also possibly by the further increase in CBF invoked by antihypertensive drugs such as hydralazine (Schroeder and Sillesen, 1987) or nitroprusside (Cottrell et al., 1978b), which dilate cerebral vessels. In this situation, intracranial pressure should be measured and, if markedly elevated, reduced by appropriate therapies such as barbiturates, steroids, or osmotic agents (Lyons and Meyer, 1990).

Adaptation of Cerebral Blood Flow During Therapy

The brain is relatively protected by a large degree of adaptability (Strandgaard and Paulson, 1989). Although the autoregulatory curve is shifted to the right in chronic hypertension, pressures can be lowered about 25% before reaching the lower limit, and symptoms may not occur until pressures are lowered another 25%. Moreover, the brain, unlike the heart, can maintain metabolic functions despite a lower perfusion pressure by extracting more oxygen from the blood. Whereas coronary venous blood is usually only about 30% saturated (near the lower limit of oxygen removal), cerebral venous blood is usually about 60% to 70% saturated, so that considerably more oxygen can be extracted. Over time, as pressures are lowered, the structural changes responsible for the rightward shift in autoregulation recede and the curve returns towards normal, thereby improving the tolerance to a lower pressure. Another factor likely responsible for the relative rarity of cerebral ischemia during therapy is the leftward shift of the lower limit of autoregulation induced by the action of certain antihypertensive drugs on the cerebral vessels. These include alpha blockers and ACE inhibitors, which in different ways both dilate large cerebral arteries and increase downstream pressure, causing smaller-resistance vessels to constrict; thus, during a fall in pressure, these vessels provide a greater autoregulatory dilatory capacity than normal (Barry, 1989). Calcium entry blockers also have been shown to preserve CBF (Thulin et al., 1993).

Cardiac Changes

Benign electrocardiographic changes, mainly T-wave inversions, commonly accompany rapid reduction of BP; this likely may be seen with any drug. These changes, observed during infusions of nitroprusside (Gretler et al., 1992) and after oral nifedipine (Phillips et al., 1991), usually are not accompanied by signs of myocardial ischemia such as left ventricular wall motion abnormalities. Myocardial ischemia is rare because myocardial work is greatly reduced by the reduction in BP.

Parenteral Drugs (Table 8.5)

Need for a Diuretic

In addition to an antihypertensive agent, a potent diuretic, usually furosemide or bumetanide, is usually given intravenously. In one controlled trial involving 64 patients with hypertensive encephalopathy and diastolic pressure above 135 mm Hg, 40 mg of IV furosemide alone brought the pressure down from an average of 225/144 mm Hg to 166/102 mm Hg over 5 hours in 12 patients (McNair et al., 1986). The remaining 52 patients still had a diastolic pressure above 125 mm Hg 1 hour after the furosemide; they were given additional therapy.

Even if not given initially, a diuretic will likely be needed after other antihypertensives are used, since reactive renal sodium retention usually accompanies a fall in pressure and may blunt the efficacy of nondiuretic agents.

On the other hand, if the patient is volume-depleted from pressure-induced natriuresis and

prior nausea and vomiting, additional diuresis could be dangerous. In a few documented instances, volume expansion with intravenous saline has been shown to lower the BP (Kincaid-Smith, 1973; Baer et al., 1977). Most of the patients whose BP improved with salt repletion have had chronic renal disease; it is likely that they start off with salt-wasting interstitial nephritis, as seen with analgesic nephropathy.

Nitroprusside

Clinical Use. The BP always falls when this drug is given, though it occasionally takes much more than the usual starting dose of 0.25 μg/kg/minute for a response (Elliott et al., 1990). The antihypertensive effect disappears within minutes after the drug is stopped. Obviously, the drug should only be used in an intensive care unit, with constant monitoring of the BP. A computer-controlled regulator of the rate of infusion has been described (Martin et al., 1992), and a commercially available unit (Titrator Model 10K, IVAC Corporation, San Diego, CA) has been found to markedly improve the management of postoperative hypertension in a controlled trial (Chitwood et al., 1992).

Mechanism of Action. This exogenous nitrate apparently acts in the same manner as the endogenous vasodilator nitric oxide, the endothelium-derived relaxing factor. The drug is a direct arteriolar and venous dilator and has no effects—good or bad—on the autonomic or central nervous system (Shepherd and Irvine, 1986). The venous dilation reduces return to the heart, causing a fall in cardiac output and stroke volume despite an increase in heart rate, while the arteriolar dilation prevents any rise in peripheral resistance, as would be expected when cardiac output falls (Brush et al., 1989). Nitroprusside may cause redistribution of blood flow away from ischemic areas and could increase the extent of myocardial damage in patients with coronary disease (Mann et al., 1978).

Metabolism and Toxicity. Nitroprusside is metabolized to cyanide by sulfhydryl groups in red cells, and the cyanide is rapidly metabolized to thiocyanate in the liver (Schulz, 1984). If high levels of thiocyanate (above 10 mg/100 ml) remain for days, toxicity may be manifested with fatigue, nausea, disorientation, and psychosis. If cyanide toxicity is suspected because of metabolic acidosis and venous hyperoxemia, nitroprusside should be discontinued, and 4 to 6 mg of a 3% solution of sodium nitrite should be given intravenously over 2 to 4 minutes, fol-

Table 8.5. Parenteral Drugs for Treatment of Hypertensive Emergency (in Order of Rapidity of Action)

Drug	Dosage	Onset of Action	Duration of Action	Adverse Effects
Vasodilators				
Nitroprusside (Nipride, Nitropress)	0.25–10 µg/kg/min as IV infusion	Instantaneous	1–2 min	Nausea, vomiting, muscle twitching, sweating, thiocyanate and cyanide intoxication
Nitroglycerin	5–100 µg/min as IV infusion	2–5 min	3–5 min	Headache, vomiting, methemoglobinemia, tolerance with prolonged use
Diazoxide (Hyperstat)	50–100 m/IV bolus repeated, or 15–30 mg/min by IV infusion	2–4 min	6–12 hr	Nausea, hypotension, flushing, tachycardia, chest pain
Hydralazine (Apresoline)	10–20 mg IV 10–50 mg IM	10–20 min 20–30 min	3–8 hr	Tachycardia, flushing, headache, vomiting, aggravation of angina
Enalaprilat (Vasotec IV)	1.25–5 mg q 6 hr	15 min	6 hr	Precipitous fall in BP in high renin states; response variable
Nicardipine[a]	2–8 mg/hr IV	5–10 min	30–60 min	Tachycardia, headache, flushing, local phlebitis
Adrenergic inhibitors				
Phentolamine (Regitine)	5–15 mg IV	1–2 min	3–10 min	Tachycardia, flushing
Trimethaphan (Arfonad)	0.5–5 mg/min as IV infusion	1–5 min	10 min	Paresis of bowel and bladder, orthostatic hypotension, blurred vision, dry mouth
Esmolol (Brevibloc)	200–500 µg/kg/min for 4 min, then 50–300 µg/kg/min IV	1–2 min	10–20 min	Hypotension, nausea
Labetalol (Normodyne, Trandate)	20–80 mg IV bolus every 10 min 2 mg/min IV infusion	5–10 min	3–6 hr	Vomiting, scalp tingling, burning in throat, postural hypotension, dizziness, nausea

IV, intravenous; IM, intramuscular.
[a]Not approved by Food and Drug Administration.

lowed by an infusion of 50 ml of a 25% solution of sodium thiosulfate (Gifford, 1991). Cyanide toxicity has been prevented by concomitant administration of hydroxocobalamin (Cottrell et al., 1978a). Although nitroprusside may increase intracranial pressure (Cottrell et al., 1978b), most authorities continue to advocate it as the best therapy for hypertensive encephalopathy (Calhoun and Oparil, 1990; Gifford, 1991).

Nitroglycerin

Intravenous nitroglycerin is being used increasingly for coronary vasodilation in patients with myocardial ischemia with or without severe hypertension. Like nitroprusside, it causes cerebral vasodilation and can increase intracranial pressure (Dahl et al., 1989). Methemoglobin is formed during the administration of all organic nitrates, but its mean concentration in patients receiving nitroglycerin for 48 hours or longer averaged only 1.5%, with no clinical symptoms (Kaplan et al., 1985).

Diazoxide

Mechanism of Action.   A congener of the thiazide diuretics, diazoxide dilates the resistance arteries but not the capacitance veins. The compensatory increase in cardiac output and heart rate can be blocked by concomitant beta blocker therapy (Huysmans et al., 1982). Since it does not cross the blood-brain barrier, diazoxide has no direct effects on the cerebral circulation, but of course cerebral blood flow will fall if systemic pressure is reduced below the lower limit of autoregulation (Barry et al., 1983).

Clinical Use.   Diazoxide was initially given as a 300-mg bolus within 10 to 30 seconds to enhance its antihypertensive effect, but the immediate, rather precipitous 30% or greater fall in BP induced some episodes of cerebral and myocardial ischemia (Kanada et al., 1976). The safer course is to give the drug either by slow infusion over 15 to 30 minutes (Garrett and Kaplan, 1982) or by smaller bolus doses, 75 to 100 mg intravenously, every 5 to 10 minutes (Ram and Kaplan, 1979).

Side Effects and Cautions.   These include fluid retention, nausea, flushing, dizziness, and a propensity, with repeated doses, to hyperglycemia, which reflects a direct suppression of insulin secretion (Bergsten et al., 1988).

Hydralazine

The major advantage of this direct vasodilator as a parenteral drug is for the physician, since it can be given by repeated intramuscular injections as well as intravenously with a fairly slow onset and prolonged duration of action. Significant compensatory increases in cardiac output preclude its use as a sole agent except in very young patients (e.g., preeclampsia), who can handle the increased output without inducing ischemia, or very old patients who may not experience the reflex sympathetic discharge and consequent rise in cardiac output because of diminished baroreceptor activity. Parenteral hydralazine has been withdrawn from the U.S. market, so it may no longer be an option.

Trimethaphan

This agent has been popular with anesthesiologists, but, in addition to the problems of generalized autonomic nervous system blockade, it may rarely cause respiratory paralysis (Dale and Schroeder, 1976). Trimethaphan may be the drug of choice with dissecting aneurysms of the aorta (Gifford, 1991).

Labetalol

The combined alpha-beta blocker labetalol has been found to be both safe and effective when given intravenously either by repeated bolus (Huey et al., 1988) or by continuous infusion (Leslie et al., 1987). It starts acting within 5 minutes and lasts for 3 to 6 hours. The oral form can then be used to provide long-term control. Labetalol can likely be used in almost any situation requiring parenteral antihypertensive therapy except when left ventricular dysfunction could be worsened by the predominant beta blockade. Caution is needed to avoid postural hypotension if patients are allowed out of bed. Nausea, itching, tingling of the skin, and beta blocker side effects may be noted.

Esmolol

This relatively cardioselective beta blocker is rapidly metabolized by blood esterases, thereby providing a very short (about 9-minute) half-life and total duration of action (about 30 minutes). Its effects begin almost immediately, and it has found particular use during anesthesia to prevent postintubation hemodynamic perturbations (Oxorn et al., 1990).

Enalaprilat

This intravenous preparation of the active, free form of the prodrug enalapril may be used for treatment of hypertensive emergencies wherein ACE inhibition is thought to offer special advantages, such as severe congestive heart failure (Varriale et al., 1993). Apparently unique effects of ACE inhibitors on cerebral autoregulation, resetting the autoregulatory curve to a lower pressure level, could protect against cerebral ischemia if pressure is lowered abruptly and markedly (Barry, 1989).

Nicardipine and Nimodipine

When given by continuous infusion, the intravenous formulation of these dihydropyridine calcium entry blockers (CEBs) produces a steady, progressive fall in BP with little change in heart rate and a small increase in cardiac output (Lambert et al., 1993). Other IV CEBs also are effective, including verapamil (Brush et al., 1989). One CEB with an apparently greater selectivity for cerebral vessels, nimodipine, has been approved for use in relieving the vasospasm that accompanies subarachnoid hemorrhage (Wong and Haley, 1990).

Other Drugs

Parenteral reserpine and methyldopa have few advantages and many side effects. The alpha blocker phentolamine is specifically indicated for pheochromocytoma or tyramine-induced catecholamine crisis.

Fenoldopam, a dopamine-1 receptor agonist, induces direct vasodilation and BP reduction equal to those of nitroprusside and better effects on renal function (Shusterman et al., 1993). It is not approved for use in the United States.

Criteria for Drug Selection

Since no clinical comparisons of the various agents' eventual outcomes are available, the choice of therapy is based on rapidity of action, ease of administration, and propensity for side effects. There are few data on the effects of these various agents on CBF and autoregulation, intracranial pressure, and most importantly both immediate and eventual outcome.

The data that are available, mostly from animal studies, show that different drugs have different effects on the cerebral circulation (Barry, 1989; Strandgaard and Paulson, 1989). With current techniques to measure global and segmental CBF in humans, such data are becoming available to provide more solid guidelines for the choice of an antihypertensive agent in the treatment of different types of hypertensive emergencies (Thulin et al., 1993).

Although nitroprusside has been most widely used and continues to be preferred for most

hypertensive emergencies by some authors (Calhoun and Oparil, 1990; Gifford, 1991), the recognition of its propensity to increase intracranial pressure and the availability of additional effective parenteral agents have led me to downplay its use. Similarly, diazoxide seems to have outlived its usefulness and should be discarded along with intramuscular reserpine and intravenous methyldopa (because of their sedative effects). Both nitroprusside and diazoxide obviously work and, in thousands of patients, they have overcome hypertensive emergencies. Nonetheless, equally effective and likely safer agents are now available for the relatively few patients who need parenteral therapy.

Specific Hypertensive Emergencies

Unfortunately, there are no comparative studies to suggest the relative order of the choices listed in Table 8.6. Additional agents (e.g., the dopamine-1 receptor agonist fenoldopam) likely soon will be available along with more intravenous alpha blockers, CEBs, and ACE inhibitors.

Cerebrovascular Accidents

Caution is advised in lowering even markedly elevated BP in patients in the immediate post-stroke period. As stated by Lavin (1990): "The protective rise in BP immediately following the stroke is an attempt to maintain adequate perfusion pressure to the ischemic penumbra; thus to artificially lower systemic blood pressure by pharmacological means, except in extreme circumstances, may lead to further neurological damage." Lavin's advice has been amply documented, particularly in studies with agents that raise intracranial pressure as they lower systemic BP (Hayashi et al., 1988).

Although Brott and Reed (1989) have published an algorithm for the treatment of hypertension in acute stroke based on the level of the BP, the advice of Powers (1993) seems best: "In the absence of hypertensive encephalopathy or a systemic cardiovascular emergency requiring immediate BP reduction, the benefits to be derived from acutely lowering BP in patients with acute stroke of any kind remain conjectural and unsupported by good clinical or experimental studies. Designation of any level of elevated BP as too high or prescription of any degree of blood pressure reduction as desirable cannot be supported by existing data." If small-scale studies showing additional benefit with nimodipine in acute ischemic stroke (Gelmers et al., 1988) are confirmed, this agent or others that appear

Table 8.6. Preferred Parenteral Drugs for Specific Hypertensive Emergencies (in Order of Preference)

Emergency	Preferred[a]	Avoid (Reason)
Hypertensive encephalopathy	Labetalol Nicardipine[b] Nitroprusside Trimethaphan	Methyldopa (sedation) Diazoxide (fall in cerebral blood flow) Reserpine (sedation)
Accelerated-malignant hypertension	Labetalol Enalaprilat Nicardipine[b] Nitroprusside	
Stroke or head injury	Labetalol Trimethaphan Nitroprusside Esmolol	Methyldopa (sedation) Reserpine (sedation) Hydralazine (increase cerebral blood flow) Diazoxide (decrease cerebral blood flow)
Left ventricular failure	Enalaprilat Nitroglycerin Nitroprusside	Labetalol, esmolol, and other beta blockers (decrease cardiac output)
Coronary insufficiency	Nitroglycerin Nitroprusside Labetalol Nicardipine[b]	Hydralazine (increase cardiac work) Diazoxide (increase cardiac work)
Dissecting aortic aneurysm	Trimethaphan Nitroprusside Esmolol	Hydralazine (increase cardiac output) Diazoxide (increase cardiac output)
Catecholamine excess	Phentolamine Labetalol	All others (less specific)
Postoperative	Labetalol Nitroglycerin Nicardipine[b] Hydralazine	Trimethaphan (bowel and bladder atony)

[a]A loop diuretic usually will be needed, initially when fluid volume overload is present, or subsequently if reactive fluid retention occurs.
[b]Parenteral form not yet approved in United States.

to reduce tissue damage may be more quickly used. Nimodipine has improved the outcome of patients with aneurysmal subarachnoid hemorrhage (Wong and Haley, 1990).

Cardiac Conditions

Hypertension in patients with acute left ventricular failure from systolic dysfunction should be treated with vasodilators that unload the left ventricle. Whereas nitroprusside and nitroglycerin are preferred for immediate relief, ACE inhibitors will be used more often for more persistent benefit.

Acute coronary insufficiency often precipitates additional hypertension. With or without concomitant hypertension, intravenous parenteral vasodilators, mainly nitroprusside and nitroglycerin, have been tested in 11 trials involving 2170 patients with acute myocardial infarct-

ion and have reduced mortality by a highly significant 43% (Lau et al., 1992).

Acute Aortic Dissection

Hypertension is frequently present in patients who suffer an acute aortic dissection. The usual patient is an elderly man with a long history of hypertension who presents with severe and persistent chest pain. If the event is suspected on clinical grounds, transesophageal echocardiography or CT or MRI scans will usually confirm the diagnosis (Cigarroa et al., 1993).

As described in Chapter 4, the stresses that damage the vessel wall are related not only to the mean pressure but also to the width of the pulse pressure and the maximal rate of rise of the pressure (dp/dt). Drugs that diminish dp/dt, such as trimethaphan or nitroprusside, particularly in combination with a beta blocker, are the best to treat a dissection (Asfoura and Vidt, 1991). Drugs such as direct vasodilators that reflexly stimulate cardiac output and may, thereby, increase the shearing forces that are dissecting the aorta should be avoided.

The choice of definitive therapy of aortic dissection usually is surgery for those with proximal lesions, but chronic medical therapy seems equally as effective for patients with distal lesions confined to the descending aorta (Glower et al., 1990).

Other Specific Circumstances

The management of hypertensive emergencies in a number of special circumstances is considered in specific chapters of theis book, as follows: renal insufficiency (Chapter 9), eclampsia (Chapter 11), pheochromocytoma (Chapter 12), drug abuse (Chapter 15), and in children and adolescents (Chapter 16).

THERAPY FOR HYPERTENSIVE URGENCIES

Hypertensive urgencies (Table 8.1) usually can be managed with oral therapy. This includes most patients with accelerated-malignant hypertension, except for those unable to swallow.

Issue of Need

Hypertensive urgency is seen less often than simple very high BP (i.e., above 200/120 mm Hg). The prudent physician may prefer to ensure the patient's responsiveness to oral therapy before having the patient leave the office or emergency room with a prescription for one or more oral drugs. This holds true even for those patients who have been seen in similar circumstances many times before but who do not adhere to chronic treatment since they, too, may become truly resistant to therapy. Although most such patients could be safely started on one or more oral drugs and sent home to return in 24 or 48 hours for confirmation of their responsiveness, it may be preferable to observe them for a few hours after administration of an antihypertensive drug to ensure responsiveness. A group of such patients was first given 0.2 mg of clonidine and 25 mg chlorthalidone and then randomly assigned either to hourly clonidine until their diastolic BPs were below 105 mm Hg or to placebo (Zeller et al., 1989). When seen 24 hours later, BPs in both groups were equally well controlled, signifying that repeated loading therapy and prolonged observation are likely needed only rarely in asymptomatic patients with severe hypertension.

Oral Agents for Hypertensive Urgencies

Virtually all oral antihypertensive agents have been tried and found to be effective in the treatment of severe hypertension (Opie, 1989). None is clearly better than the rest, and a combination will often be needed for long-term control. Those most widely used are listed in Table 8.7, and complete information about them is provided in Chapter 7.

Nifedipine

This calcium entry blocker has been widely used for the treatment of hypertensive urgencies (Bertel et al., 1983). Liquid nifedipine in a capsule will effectively and usually safely lower BP after a single 5- or 10-mg oral dose (Maharaj and van der Byl, 1992). The drug is effective even more quickly when the capsule is chewed and the contents are swallowed than when it is squirted under the tongue (McAllister, 1986). For a slightly slower and probably safer effect, the sublingual route should be used.

As might be expected with any drug that induces such a significant fall in BP, occasional symptomatic hypotension can occur, but this has been quite rare when the drug is given in no more than a 10-mg initial dose (Opie, 1991).

Captopril

This is the fastest acting of the oral ACE inhibitors now available, and it can also be used sublingually in patients who cannot swallow (Angeli et al., 1991). As noted earlier in this chapter, captopril may be particularly attractive since it shifts the entire curve of cerebral autoregulation to the left, so cerebral blood flow should be well maintained as the systemic pressure falls (Barry, 1989).

Abrupt and marked first dose hypotension has been observed in patients with high renin status given an ACE inhibitor (Postma et al., 1992). Caution is advised in patients who have significant renal insufficiency or who are volume-depleted.

Clonidine

This central alpha agonist has been widely used in repeated hourly doses to safely and effectively reduce very high BP. It works more slowly than nifedipine but eventually brings the pressure down about as well (Jaker et al., 1989).

Significant sedation is the major side effect that contraindicates its use in patients with central nervous system involvement. Since it has a somewhat greater proclivity than other drugs

Table 8.7. Oral Drugs for Hypertensive Urgencies

Drug	Class	Dose	Onset	Duration
Nifedipine (Procardia; Adalat)	Calcium entry blocker	5–10 mg sublingual or swallowed	5–15 min	3–5 hr
Captopril (Capoten)	Angiotensin converting enzyme inhibitor	6.5–50 mg	15 min	4–6 hr
Clonidine (Catapres)	Central alpha agonist	0.2 mg initial then 0.1 mg/hr, up to 0.8 mg total	1/2–2 hr	6–8 hr
Labetalol (Normodyne, Trandate)	Alpha-beta blocker	200–400 mg	1/2–2 hr	8–12 hr

to cause rebound hypertension if it is suddenly discontinued, caution is advised in its use among patients with severe hypertension who have demonstrated poor compliance with therapy.

Labetalol

The alpha-beta blocker labetalol has been given in hourly oral doses ranging from 200 mg to 1200 mg and has markedly reduced elevated pressures as effectively as repeated doses of oral clonidine have (Atkin et al., 1992).

Use of Diuretics

As with the use of parenteral drugs for hypertensive emergencies, diuretics, specifically large intravenous doses of furosemide or bumetanide, often are needed in patients with hypertensive urgencies, both to lower the BP by getting rid of excess volume and to prevent the loss of potency from other antihypertensives because of their tendency to cause fluid retention. However, volume depletion may be overdone, particularly in patients who start off with a shrunken fluid volume. Thereby renin secretion may be further increased, producing more intensive vasoconstriction and worsening the hypertension.

MANAGEMENT AFTER ACUTE THERAPY

Continued Evaluation for Secondary Causes

After the patient is out of danger, a careful search should continue for possible secondary causes, as delineated under the subsection "Evaluation," which is found under the heading "Accelerated-Malignant Hypertension." Secondary causes are much more likely in patients with severe hypertension, in particular renovascular hypertension (Davis et al., 1979).

Chronic Therapy

Most patients will likely require multiple drug therapy. All of the guidelines delineated in Chapter 7 should be followed to ensure adherence to effective therapy.

We will now leave the realm of primary hypertension and look in depth at the various secondary forms of hypertension, starting with the most common: renal parenchymal disease.

References

Ahmed MEK, Walker JM, Beevers DG, Beevers M. Lack of difference between malignant and accelerated hypertension. *Br Med J* 1986;292:235–237.

Angeli P, Chiesa M, Caregaro L, Merkel C, Sacerdoti D, Rondana M, Gatta A. Comparison of sublingual captopril and nifedipine in immediate treatment of hypertensive emergencies. A randomized, single-blind clinical trial. *Arch Intern Med* 1991;151:678–682.

Asfoura JY, Vidt DG. Acute aortic dissection. *Chest* 1991;99:724–729.

Atkin SH, Jaker MA, Beaty P, Quadrel MA, Cuffie C, Soto-Greene ML. Oral labetalol versus oral clonidine in the emergency treatment of severe hypertension. *Am J Med Sci* 1992;303:9–15.

Baer L, Parra-Carrillo JZ, Radichevich I, Williams GS. Detection of renovascular hypertension with angiotensin II blockade. *Ann Intern Med* 1977;86:257–260.

Bakir AA, Bazilinski N, Dunea G. Transient and sustained recovery from renal shutdown in accelerated hypertension. *Am J Med* 1986;80:172–176.

Barry DI. Cerebrovascular aspects of antihypertensive treatment. *Am J Cardiol* 1989; 63:14C–18C.

Barry DI, Strandgaard S, Graham DI, Braendstrup O, Svendsen UG, Bolwig TG. Effect of diazoxide-induced hypotension on cerebral blood flow in hypertensive rats. *Eur J Clin Invest* 1983;13:201–207.

Beilin LJ, Goldby FS. High arterial pressure versus humoral factors in the pathogenesis of the vascular lesions of malignant hypertension. The case of pressure alone. *Clin Sci Mol Med* 1977;52:111–117.

Bergsten P, Gylfe E, Wesslen N, Hellman B. Diazoxide unmasks glucose inhibition of insulin release by counteracting entry of Ca_2+. *Am J Physiol* 1988;255: E422–E427.

Bertel O, Conen D, Radü EW, Müller J, Lang C, Dubach UC. Nifedipine in hypertensive emergencies. *Br Med J* 1983;286:19–21.

Bing BF, Heagerty AM, Russell GI, Swales JD, Thurston H. Prognosis in malignant hypertension. *J Hypertens* 1986;4(Suppl 6):42–44.

Brott T, Reed RL. Intensive care for acute stroke in the community hospital setting. The first 24 hours. *Stroke* 1989;20: 694–697.

Brush JE Jr, Udelson JE, Bacharach SL, Cannon RO III, Leon MB, Rumble TF, Bonow RO. Comparative effects of verapamil and nitroprusside on left ventricular function in patients with hypertension. *J Am Coll Cardiol* 1989;14:515–522.

Byrom FB. The evolution of acute hypertensive arterial disease. *Prog Cardiovasc Dis* 1974;17:31–37.

Calhoun DA, Oparil S. Treatment of hypertensive crisis. *N Engl J Med* 1990;323:1177–1183.

Chitwood WR Jr, Cosgrove DM III, Lust RM, and the Titrator Multicenter Study Group. Multicenter trial of automated nitroprusside infusion for postoperative hypertension. *Ann Thorac Surg* 1992;54:517–522.

Cigarroa JE, Isselbacher EM, DeSanctis RW, Eagle KA. Diagnostic imaging in the evaluation of suspected aortic dissection. *N Engl J Med* 1993;328:35–43.

Clough CG, Beevers DG, Beevers M. The survival of malignant hypertension in blacks, whites and Asians in Britain. *J Hum Hypertens* 1990;4:94–96.

Cottrell JE, Casthely P, Brodie JD, Patel K, Klein A, Turndorf H. Prevention of nitroprusside-induced cyanide toxicity with hydroxocobalamin. *N Engl J Med* 1978a;298:9–11.

Cottrell JE, Patel K, Turndorf H, Ransohoff J. Intracranial pressure changes induced by sodium nitroprusside in patients with intracranial mass lesions. *J Neurosurg* 1978b;48:329–331.

Cove DH, Seddon M, Fletcher RF, Dukes DC. Blindness after treatment for malignant hypertension. *Br Med J* 1979;2:245–246.

Dahl A, Russell D, Nyberg-Hansen R, Rootwelt K. Effect of nitroglycerin on cerebral circulation measured by transcranial Doppler and SPECT. *Stroke* 1989;20:1733–1736.

Dale RC, Schroeder ET. Respiratory paralysis during treatment of hypertension with trimethaphan camsylate. *Arch Intern Med* 1976;136:816–818.

Davis BA, Crook JE, Vestal RE, Oates JA. Prevalence of renovascular hypertension in patients with grade III or IV hypertensive retinopathy. *N Engl J Med* 1979;301:1273–1276.

Dustan HP, Schneckloth RE, Corcoran AC, Page IH. The effectiveness of long-term treatment of malignant hypertension. *Circulation* 1958;18:644–651.

Dzau VJ, Siwek LG, Rosen S, Farhi ER, Mizoguchi H, Barger AC. Sequential renal hemodynamics in experimental benign and malignant hypertension. *Hypertension* 1981;3(Suppl 1):63–68.

Garrett BN, Kaplan NM. Efficacy of slow infusion of diazoxide in the treatment of severe hypertension without organ hypoperfusion. *Am Heart J* 1982;103:390–394.

Gavras H, Brunner HR, Laragh JH, Vaughan ED Jr, Koss M, Cote LJ, Gavras I. Malignant hypertension resulting from deoxycorticosterone acetate and salt excess. *Circ Res* 1975a;36:300–310.

Gavras H, Oliver N, Aitchison J, Begg C, Briggs JD, Brown JJ, Horton PW, Lee F, Lever AF, Prentice C, Robertson JIS. Abnormalities of coagulation and the development of malignant phase hypertension. *Kidney Int* 1975b;8:S252–S261.

Gelmers HJ, Gorter K, de Weerdt CJ, Wiezer HJA. A controlled trial of nimodipine in acute ischemic stroke. *N Engl J Med* 1988;318:203–207.

Gifford RW Jr. Management of hypertensive crises. *JAMA* 1991;266:829–835.

Glower DD, Fann JI, Speier RH, Morrison L, White WD, Smith LR, Rankin JS, Miller DG, Wolfe WG. Comparison of medical and surgical therapy for uncomplicated descending aortic dissection. *Circulation* 1990;82(Suppl 4):39–46.

Gretler DD, Elliott WJ, Moscucci M, Childers RW, Murphy MB. Electrocardiographic changes during acute treatment of hypertensive emergencies with sodium nitroprusside or fenoldopam. *Arch Intern Med* 1992;152:2445–2448.

Groppelli A, Giorgi DMA, Omboni S, Parati G, Mancia G. Persistent blood pressure increase induced by heavy smoking. *J Hypertens* 1992;10:495–499.

Gross F, Dietz R, Mast GJ, Szokol M. Salt loss as a possible mechanism eliciting an acute malignant phase in renal hypertensive rats. *Clin Exp Pharmacol Physiol* 1975;2:323–333.

Hauser RA, Lacey M, Knight R. Hypertensive encephalopathy. Magnetic resonance imaging demonstration of reversible cortical and white matter lesions. *Arch Neurol* 1988;45:1078–1083.

Hayashi M, Kobayashi H, Kawano H, Handa Y, Hirose S. Treatment of systemic hypertension and intracranial hypertension in cases of brian hemorrhage. *Stroke* 1988;19:314–321.

Hayreh SS, Servais GE, Virdi P. Fundus lesions in malignant hypertension. III. Arterial blood pressure, biochemical, and fundus changes. *Ophthalmology* 1985a;92:45–49.

Hayreh SS, Servais GE, Virdi P. Fundus lesions in malignant hypertension. IV. Focal intraretinal periarteriolar transudates. *Ophthalmology* 1985b;92:60–73.

Hayreh SS, Servais GE, Virdi P. Fundus lesions in malignant hypertension. V. Hypertensive optic neuropathy. *Ophthalmology* 1986;93:74–87.

Herlitz H, Hilme E, Jonsson O, Gudbrandsson T, Hansson L. Erythrocyte sodium transport in malignant hypertension. *J Intern Med* 1990;228:133–137.

Hilme E, Hansson L, Sandberg L, Söderström T, Herlitz H. Abnormal immune function in malignant hypertension. *J Hypertens* 1993;11:989–994.

Huey J, Thomas JP, Hendricks DR, Wehmeyer AE, Johns LJ, MacCosbe PE. Clinical evaluation of intravenous labetalol for the treatment of hypertensive urgency. *Am J Hypertens* 1988;1:284S–289S.

Hulse JA, Taylor DSI, Dillion MJ. Blindness and paraplegia in severe childhood hypertension. *Lancet* 1979;2:553–556.

Huysmans FThM, Thien TA, Koene RAP. Combined intravenous administration of diazoxide and beta-blocking agent in acute treatment of severe hypertension or hypertensive crisis. *Am Heart J* 1982;103:395–400.

Isles CG, Brown JJ, Cumming AMM, Lever AF, McAreavey D, Robertson JIS, Hawthorne VM, Stewart GM, Robertson JWK, Wapshaw J. Excess smoking in malignant-phase hypertension. *Br Med J* 1979;1:579–581.

Isles CG, McLay A, Boulton Jones JM. Recovery in malignant hypertension presenting as acute renal failure. *Q J Med* 1984;53:439–452.

Jain N, Rosner F. Idiopathic intracranial hypertension: report of seven cases. *Am J Med* 1992;93:391–395.

Jaker M, Atkin S, Soto M, Schmid G, Brosch F. Oral nifedipine vs oral clonidine in the treatment of urgent hypertension. *Arch Intern Med* 1989;149:260–265.

Jansen PAF, Schulte BPM, Gribnau FWJ. Cerebral ischaemia and stroke as side effects of antihypertensive treatment; special danger in the elderly. A review of the cases reported in the literature. *Neth J Med* 1987;30:193–201.

Jespersen CM, Rasmussen D, Hennild V. Focal intracerebral oedema in hypertensive encephalopathy visualized by computerized tomographic scan. *J Intern Med* 1989;225:349–350.

Johansson B, Strandgaard S, Lassen NA. The hypertensive "breakthrough" of autoregulation of cerebral blood flow with forced vasodilatation, flow increase, and blood-brain-barrier damage. *Circ Res* 1974;34-35(Suppl 1):167–174.

Jones DB. Arterial and glomerular lesions associated with severe hypertension. Light and electron microscopic studies. *Lab Invest* 1974;31:303–313.

Jones JV. Differentiation and investigation of primary versus secondary hypertension (Cushing reflex). *Am J Cardiol* 1989;63:10C–13C.

Kadiri S, Olutade BO. The clinical presentation of malignant hypertension in Nigerians. *J Hum Hypertens* 1991;5:339–343.

Kanada SA, Kanada DJ, Hutchinson RA, Wu D. Angina-like syndrome with diazoxide therapy of hypertensive crisis. *Ann Intern Med* 1976;84:696–699.

Kaplan KJ, Taber M, Teagarden JR, Parker M, Davidson R. Association of methemoglobinemia and intravenous nitroglycerin administration. *Am J Cardiol* 1985;55:181–183.

Kawazoe N, Eto T, Abe I, Takishita S, Ueno M, Kobayashi K, Uezono K, Muratani H, Kimura Y, Tomita Y, Tsuchihashi T, Onoyama K, Kawasaki T, Fukiyama K, Omae T, Fujishima M. Long-term prognosis of malignant hypertension: difference between underlying diseases such as essential hypertension and chronic glomerulonephritis. *Clin Nephrol* 1988;29:53–57.

Kawazoe N, Eto T, Abe I, Takishita S, Ueno M, Kobayashi K, Uezono K, Muratani H, Kimura Y, Tomita Y, Tsuchihashi T, Onoyama K, Kawasaki T, Fukiyama K, Omae T, Fujishima M. Pathophysiology in malignant hypertension: with special reference to the renin-angiotensin system. *Clin Cardiol* 1987;19:513–518.

Kincaid-Smith P. Management of severe hypertension. *Am J Cardiol* 1973;32:575–581.

Kincaid-Smith P. Malignant hypertension. *J Hypertens* 1991;9:893–899.

Kontos HA. Oxygen radicals in cerebral vascular injury. *Circ Res* 1985;57:508–516.

Lake CR, Gallant S, Masson E. Adverse drug effects attributed to phenylpropanolamine:

a review of 142 case reports. *Am J Med* 1990;89:195–208.

Lambert CR, Grady T, Hashimi W, Blakely M, Panayioutou H. Hemodynamic and angiographic comparison of intravenous nitroglycerin and nicardipine mainly in subjects without coronary artery disease. *Am J Cardiol* 1993;71:420–423.

Laragh JH, Ulick S, Januszewicz V, Kelly WG, Lieberman S. Electrolyte metabolism and aldosterone secretion in benign and malignant hypertension. *Ann Intern Med* 1960;53:269–272.

Lau J, Antman EM, Jimenez-Silva J, Kupelnick B, Mosteller F, Chalmers TC. Cumulative meta-analysis of therapeutic trials for myocardial infarction. *N Engl J Med* 1992;327:248–254.

Lavin P. Management of cerebral infarction or transient ischemic attacks. *Arch Intern Med* 1990;150:692–694.

Lawton WJ. The short-term course of renal function in malignant hypertensives with renal insufficiency. *Clin Nephrol* 1982;17:277–283.

Leslie JB, Kalayjian RW, Sirgo MA, Plachetka JR, Watkins WD. Intravenous labetalol for treatment of postoperative hypertension. *Anesthesiology* 1987;67:413–416.

Lyons MK, Meyer FB. Cerebrospinal fluid physiology and the management of increased intracranial pressure. *Mayo Clin Proc* 1990;65:684–707.

MacKenzie ET, Strandgaard S, Graham DI, Jones JV, Harper AM, Farrar JK. Effects of acutely induced hypertension in cats on pial arteriolar caliber, local cerebral blood flow, and the blood-brain barrier. *Circ Res* 1976;39:33–41.

Maharaj B, van der Byl K. A comparison of the acute hypotensive effects of two different doses of nifedipine. *Am Heart J* 1992;124:720–725.

Mann T, Cohn PF, Holman BL, Green LH, Markis JE, Phillips DA. Effect of nitroprusside on regional myocardial blood flow in coronary artery disease. Results in 25 patients and comparison with nitroglycerin. *Circulation* 1978;57:732–737.

Martin JF, Schneider AM, Quinn ML, Smith NT. Improved safety and efficacy in adaptive control of arterial blood pressure through the use of a supervisor. *Trans Biomed Eng* 1992;39:381–388.

Mathur R, Warren JP. Malignant hypertension presenting as acute pancreatitis. *J Hum Hypertens* 1989;3:479–480.

McAllister RG Jr. Kinetics and dynamics in nifedipine after oral and sublingual doses. *Am J Med* 1986;81(Suppl 6A):2–5.

McNair A, Krogsgaard AR, Hilden T, Nielsen PE. Severe hypertension with cerebral symptoms treated with furosemide, fractionated diazoxide or dihydralazine. Danish Multicenter Study. *Acta Med Scand* 1986;220:15–23.

Meyrier A, Laaban JP, Kanfer A. Protracted anuria due to active renal vasoconstriction in malignant hypertension. *Br Med J* 1984;288:1045–1046.

Meyer JS, Teraura T, Marx P, Hashi K, Sakamoto K. Brain swelling due to experimental cerebral infarction. *Brain* 1972; 95:833–852.

Neusy A-J, Lowenstein J. Blood pressure and blood pressure variability following withdrawal of propranolol and clonidine. *J Clin Pharmacol* 1989;29:18–24.

O'Connell MT, Kubrusly DB, Fournier AM. Systemic necrotizing vasculitis seen initially as hypertensive crisis. *Arch Intern Med* 1985;145:265–267.

Opie LH. Treatment of severe hypertension. In: Kaplan NM, Brenner BM, Laragh JH, eds. *New Therapeutic Strategies in Hypertension.* New York: Raven Press, 1989: 183–198.

Opie LH. Sublingual nifedipine. *Lancet* 1991;338:1203.

Oxorn D, Knox JWD, Hill J. Bolus doses of esmolol for the prevention of perioperative hypertension and tachycardia. *Can J Anaesth* 1990;37:206–209.

Padfield PL. Malignant hypertension presenting with an acute abdomen. *Br Med J* 1975;3:353–354.

Phillips RA, Goldman ME, Ardeljan M, Eison HB, Shimabukuro S, Krakoff LR. Isolated T-wave abnormalities and evaluation of left ventricular wall motion after nifedipine for severe hypertension. *Am J Hypertens* 1991;4:432–437.

Pitcock JA, Johnson JG, Hatch FE, Acchiardo S, Muirhead EE, Brown PS. Malignant hypertension in blacks. Malignant intrarenal arterial disease as observed by light and electron microscopy. *Hum Pathol* 1976;7:333–346.

Postma CT, Dennesen PJW, de Boo T, Thien T. First dose hypotension after captopril: can it be predicted? A study of 240 patients. *J Hum Hypertens* 1992;6:205–209.

Powers WJ. Acute hypertension after stroke: the scientific basis for treatment decisions. *Neurology* 1993;43:461–467.

Ram CVS, Kaplan NM. Individual titration of diazoxide dosage in the treatment of severe hypertension. *Am J Cardiol* 1979;43:627–630.

Robinson FO, Johnston SR, Atkinson AB. Accelerated hypertension caused by severe phimosis. *J Hum Hypertens* 1992; 6:165–166.

Rodríguez-Iturbe B, Baggio B, Colina-Chourio J, Favaro S, García R, Sussana F, Castillo L, Borsatti A. Studies on the renin-aldosterone system in the acute nephritic syndrome. *Kidney Int* 1981;19:445–453.

Schroeder T, Sillesen H. Dihydralazine induces marked cerebral vasodilation in man. *Eur J Clin Invest* 1987;17:214–217.

Schulz V. Clinical pharmacokinetics of nitroprusside, cyanide, thiosulphate and thiocyanate. *Clin Pharmacokinet* 1984; 9:239–251.

Shapiro LM, Beevers DG. Malignant hypertension: cardiac structure and function at presentation and during therapy. *Br Heart J* 1983;49:477–484.

Shea S, Misra D, Ehrlich MH, Field L, Francis CK. Predisposing factors for severe, uncontrolled hypertension in an inner-city minority population. *N Engl J Med* 1992;327:776–781.

Shepherd AMM, Irvine NA. Differential hemodynamic and sympathoadrenal effects of sodium nitroprusside and hydralazine in hypertensive subjects. *J Cardiovasc Pharmacol* 1986;8:527–533.

Shusterman NH, Elliott WJ, White WB. Fenoldopam, but not nitroprusside, improves renal function in severely hypertensive patients with impaired renal function. *Am J Med* 1993;95:161–168.

Strandgaard S, Olesen J, Skinhøj, Lassen NA. Autoregulation of brain circulation in severe arterial hypertension. *Br Med J* 1973;1:507–510.

Strandgaard S, Paulson OB. Cerebral blood flow and its pathophysiology in hypertension. *Am J Hypertens* 1989;2:486–492.

Sugiyama K, Sesoko S. Clinical implications of the presence of papilledema in patients with hypertensive retinopathy. *Curr Ther Res* 1992;51:694–703.

Talman WT, Dragon DN, Ohta H. Baroreflexes and nitric oxide contribute to breakthrough of cerebrovascular resistance and cerebral blood flow in hypertension [Abstract]. *Stroke* 1993;24:164.

Thulin T, Fagher B, Grabowski M, Ryding E, Elmqvist D, Johansson BB. Cerebral blood flow in patients with severe hypertension, and acute and chronic effects of felodipine. *J Hypertens* 1993;11:83–88.

Touyz RM, Marshall PR, Milne FJ. Altered cations and muscle membrane ATPase activity in deoxycorticosterone acetate-salt spontaneously hypertensive rats. *J Hypertens* 1991;9:737–750.

Tuor UI. Acute hypertension and sympathetic stimulation: local heterogeneous changes in cerebral blood flow. *Am J Physiol* 1992;263:H511–H518.

Varriale P, David W, Chryssos BE. Hemodynamic response to intravenous enalaprit in patients with severe congestive heart failure and mitral regurgitation. *Clin Cardiol* 1993;16:235–238.

Webster J, Petrie JC, Jeffers TA, Lovell HG. Accelerated hypertension—patterns of mortality and clinical factors affecting outcome in treated patients. *Q J Med* 1993;86:485–493.

Wong MCW, Haley EC Jr. Calcium antagonists: stroke therapy coming of age. *Stroke* 1990;21:494–501.

Zeller KR, Kuhnert LV, Matthews C. Rapid reduction of severe asymptomatic hypertension. A prospective, controlled trial. *Arch Intern Med* 1989;149:2186–2189.

Renal Parenchymal Hypertension

RELATIONSHIP BETWEEN THE KIDNEYS AND HYPERTENSION

The kidney is important in most forms of hypertension. First, as described in Chapter 3, a defect in renal function is almost certainly involved in the pathogenesis of primary hypertension. Second, as noted in Chapter 4, renal damage often develops in the course of primary hypertension. In the United States, hypertension ranks just below diabetes among the causes of end-stage renal disease (ESRD) (Brazy, 1993). In other countries, hypertension is further down the list, considered the cause of about 10% of ESRD (Brown and Whitworth, 1992). The difference between the United States and other countries probably is largely due to the much larger proportion of blacks in the U.S. population and the repeated observation that hypertension is responsible for 4 to 17 times more ESRD in blacks than in nonblacks in the United States (Smith SR et al., 1991). Third, chronic renal disease is the most common cause of secondary hypertension, present in 2% to 5% of all hypertensives or, looked at in another way, responsible for about half of all secondary hypertension. Fourth, hypertension is common in all forms of acquired and congenital forms of renal parenchymal disease. When present, hypertension almost always accelerates the loss of renal function (Perneger et al., 1993) so that control of hypertension in these diseases may be the most important preventative measure available to halt the progressive renal damage.

Thus, it is obvious that some degree of renal damage is common in hypertension and that hypertension is responsible for a large portion of renal failure. The kidney is both the victim and the culprit. Clinically, there is often a vicious cycle: hypertension causes renal damage, which causes more hypertension. One hopes that the cycle can be broken by early and effective antihypertensive therapy, but this is not yet proven.

We will now examine specific varieties of renal disease and how they relate to hypertension, starting from one extreme—the total absence of renal tissue—and going to the other—the presence of only unilateral renal involvement. Renovascular hypertension induced by renal artery stenosis or intrarenal vasculitis and renin-secreting tumors are covered in the next chapter.

HYPERTENSION IN THE ABSENCE OF FUNCTIONING KIDNEYS

Clinical Observations

Using peritoneal dialysis and hemodialysis, it is possible to keep people with nonfunctioning renal tissue alive for years. Since they are unable to excrete sodium and water, their hypertension likely develops in the pattern shown in Figure 9.1: an increase in fluid volume that leads to a rise in cardiac output, followed by a subsequent conversion to an increased peripheral resistance, presumably through whole-body autoregulation (Coleman et al., 1970). Other mechanisms are likely involved (Kim et al., 1980), including the absence of vasodepressors of renal origin (described in Chapter 3). As in patients with ESRD, the accumulation of endogenous inhibitors of nitric oxide synthase may inhibit the vaso-

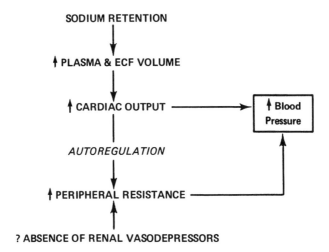

Figure 9.1. Probable mechanism for hypertension in the anephric state.

dilation normally provided by nitric oxide and thereby contribute to the hypertension (Brenner and Yu, 1992).

Effects of Bilateral Nephrectomy

A small number of patients with renal failure and severe hypertension, who are unresponsive to volume control during hemodialysis or drug therapy, may need bilateral nephrectomy before a functioning homotransplant is possible (Sheinfeld et al., 1985). Fortunately, the availability of more effective antihypertensive drugs has diminished the need for this drastic step.

Immediately after bilateral nephrectomy the blood pressure (BP) usually becomes normal, and is controlled predominantly by volume homeostasis. Renin levels are markedly lower after nephrectomy, although some extrarenal renin remains in the circulation and may contribute to inadequate BP control (Campbell et al., 1991). Neither the absence of renal vasodepressors nor the presence of extrarenal renin likely is involved very much.

BLOOD PRESSURE DURING CHRONIC DIALYSIS

The BP is usually variable and rarely maintained within the normal range in patients on chronic dialysis—increasing on the day after dialysis as fluid volume expands, sometimes going even higher at the beginning of dialysis, and often falling to hypotensive levels during the procedure (Cheigh et al., 1992). Hypotension may occur during dialysis for numerous reasons (Daugiradis, 1991; Converse et al., 1992a).

Hypertension between dialyses usually reflects fluid excess, but vasoconstriction from sympathetic nervous system overactivity mediated by an afferent signal arising in the failed kidneys also may be responsible (Converse et al., 1992b).

Continuous ambulatory peritoneal dialysis usually leads to easier control of hypertension, along with reversal of left ventricular hypertrophy (Leenen et al., 1985). This likely reflects the constancy of control of fluid volume, which is not given the chance to reaccumulate as between intermittent dialyses.

Management of Hypertension

Fortunately, the hypertension that is so common before institution of dialysis often disappears with control of fluid volume and various metabolic disturbances. However, as described in Chapter 15, the use of erythropoietin to correct the anemia of renal failure may cause rapid and occasionally severe rises in BP (Fahal et al., 1992).

In patients whose hypertension is not controlled with dialysis, various antihypertensive drugs have been successful, sometimes only on the days between dialysis. The pharmacokinetics of some drugs may be altered both by the absence of renal function and by the variable clearance of dialysis. The review by Bennett (1988) provides data about the effects of various drugs. Angiotensin-converting enzyme (ACE) inhibitors are being used increasingly, not only to control hypertension in patients with increased renin secretion from their native kidneys (Brunner, 1992), but also to ameliorate the marked thirst that drives some dialysis patients to maintain chronic fluid overload (Yamamoto et al., 1986).

HYPERTENSION AFTER KIDNEY TRANSPLANTATION

As more patients are receiving renal transplants and living longer thereafter, hypertension has been recognized as a major complication, one that may, if uncontrolled, quickly destroy the transplant or add to the risk of accelerated atherosclerosis (Raman, 1991).

Epidemiology

Hypertension is noted in more than 50% of the entire postrenal transplant population (Raman, 1991). Among patients who receive a live-related transplant, who undergo bilateral native nephrectomy, who are not taking cyclosporine, and who have excellent graft function, hypertension is unusual. Among patients suffering from chronic rejection while on cyclosporine and high doses of steroids with native kidneys in situ, hypertension is almost always present. If it occurs, hypertension likely reduces graft survival (Laskow and Curtis, 1990).

Hypertension is more likely to occur after transplant in patients who were hypertensive before the transplant. Post-transplant hypertension was noted in 14% of patients who had been normotensive but in 60% of those who had been hypertensive (Rao et al., 1978). On the other hand, receipt of a kidney from a normotensive donor may relieve primary hypertension that preceded (and presumably caused) the renal failure (Curtis et al., 1983).

Causes and Management

Beyond persistence of primary (essential) hypertension, a number of other causes of post-transplant hypertension have been documented (Table 9.1). In addition to those listed, the polycythemia that may follow successful transplantation may induce significant hypertension (Spieker et al., 1992).

Cyclosporine

As described in Chapter 15, cyclosporine can cause both nephrotoxicity and hypertension, and the two may or may not be interrelated. In the overall scheme of management of cyclosporine-induced hypertension described by Laskow and Curtis (1990), the first step is to decrease the dose of cyclosporine. If hypertension persists and renal function is good, antihypertensive drug therapy is advised (see Chapter 15 for details).

Table 9.1. Causes of Posttransplant Hypertension

Immunosuppressive therapy
  Steroids
  Cyclosporine

Allograft failure
  Chronic rejection
  Recurrent disease

Potentially surgically remediable causes
  Allograft renal artery stenosis
  Native kidneys

Speculative cause
  Recurrent essential hypertension:
    As primary cause of ESRD
    From (pre-) hypertensive donor

From Luke RG. Hypertension in renal transplant recipients. *Kidney Int* 1987;31:1024.

Post-Transplant Renal Artery Stenosis

Renal artery stenosis, often at the suture line, is found in about 12% of patients with post-transplant hypertension and may be suspected by appearance of a bruit. Although arteriographic demonstration of narrowing of the lumen greater than 80% is needed to identify an anatomic lesion, the functional significance of the lesion can better be documented by the acute response to a single dose of captopril: a marked rise in plasma renin and a marked fall in glomerular filtration rate (GFR) assessed by renal scintigraphy indicates a functionally significant lesion (Luke, 1987). Doppler ultrasonography may be helpful (Campieri et al., 1988).

If stenosis of the transplant artery is responsible, percutaneous transluminal angioplasty is the treatment of choice. In patients with post-transplant stenosis, caution is needed in the chronic use of ACE inhibitors that may, by removal of the angiotensin II that maintains renal perfusion, lead to rapid loss of graft function (Brunner, 1992).

Native Kidney Hypertension

If graft stenosis is excluded and the hypertension appears to be arising from the host kidneys, percutaneous biopsy and the finding of elevated levels of plasma renin activity (Bresticker et al., 1991) may be needed to recognize chronic allograft rejection. In addition to the use of immunosuppressives, ACE inhibitors may prove useful. If the hypertension persists despite aggressive medical therapy, the native kidneys may have to be removed (Laskow and Curtis, 1990).

Donor Kidney Hypertension

The potential of transference of primary (essential) hypertension from the donor to the recipient is suggested by the finding of more hypertension in recipients of a kidney from hypertensive donors (Guidi et al., 1985), including those who died of a subarachnoid hemorrhage (Strandgaard and Hansen, 1986).

HYPERTENSION WITH CHRONIC RENAL DISEASE

Patients may start at either end of the spectrum: hypertension without overt renal damage on the one end, severe renal insufficiency without hypertension on the other. Eventually, however, both groups move toward the middle—renal insufficiency with hypertension—so that hypertension is found in about 90% of patients with ESRD (Brown and Whitworth, 1992). Despite the reprieves available from dialysis and transplantation, hypertension remains a major risk factor for patients with renal disease. For instance, among 288 patients with biopsy-proven chronic glomerulonephritis, renal function remained normal 5 years later in 92% who were initially normotensive but in only 47% of hypertensive patients (Orofino et al., 1987). Renal insufficiency as a consequence of primary hypertension is described in Chapter 4. This section examines the development of hypertension as a secondary process in the presence of primary renal disease.

As noted earlier in this chapter, recognition of the cause of ESRD may be very difficult clinically. Nonetheless, three points should be remembered: first, hypertension is undoubtedly a major factor in the cardiovascular diseases that are responsible for 30% to 50% of the deaths in patients with ESRD (Rostrand et al., 1991); second, renal insufficiency may develop despite apparently good control of hypertension, particularly among blacks (Smith SR et al., 1991); third, patients whose underlying problem is bilateral renovascular disease may present with refractory hypertension and renal insufficiency (Breyer and Jacobson, 1993). The recognition of their renovascular etiology is critical since revascularization may relieve their hypertension and improve their renal function (Pattison et al., 1992). More about this important group of patients is provided in the next chapter.

Prevalence

Hypertension is common in patients with overt renal insufficiency, as defined by a GFR below 50 ml/minute or a serum creatinine above 1.5 mg/dl. The prevalence of hypertension varies considerably in various forms of renal disease and even within the category of chronic glomerulonephritis, being most common with focal and segmental sclerosis (Brown and Whitworth, 1992). Moreover, within each category of biopsy-proven chronic glomerulonephritis, the prevalence of hypertension varies considerably in different series. For example, hypertension has been reported in as few as 10% and in as many as 52% of patients with mesangial immunoglobulin A (IgA) nephropathy (Berger's disease) (Beaman and Adu, 1988).

In patients with chronic renal disease, BP may remain elevated during sleep, adding further to the cardiovascular burden (Portaluppi et al., 1991).

Significance

Hypertension is associated with a more rapid progression of renal damage regardless of the underlying renal disease. In a series of 86 patients initially seen with an average serum creatinine of 3.8 mg/dl, the rate of subsequent decline of renal function over an average of 33 months was twice as great in those whose diastolic BP (DBP) remained above 90 mm Hg compared with those whose DBP remained below 90 (Brazy et al., 1989).

Most of what follows applies to the most common mechanism for ESRD in the United States—diabetes. However, since diabetic nephropathy has special features, it will be considered separately.

Mechanisms

The mechanism by which hypertension leads to progressive renal damage most likely involves glomerular hypertension, as championed by Brenner and coworkers (Anderson and Brenner, 1989) (Fig. 9.2). Their hypothesis starts with any of a number of factors that increase glomerular capillary plasma flow rate or hydraulic pressure.

As shown in the upper left of Figure 9.2, systemic hypertension is one of these factors. The high systemic pressure may be transmitted into the glomerulus because afferent arteriolar resistance fails to increase adequately (Tolins and Raij, 1991). The higher pressure and/or flow rate, in turn, damages glomerular cells and leads to progressive sclerosis, setting off a vicious cycle. In rats, ischemia of as few as 12% of glomeruli will lead to progressive systemic and glomerular capillary hypertension in the absence

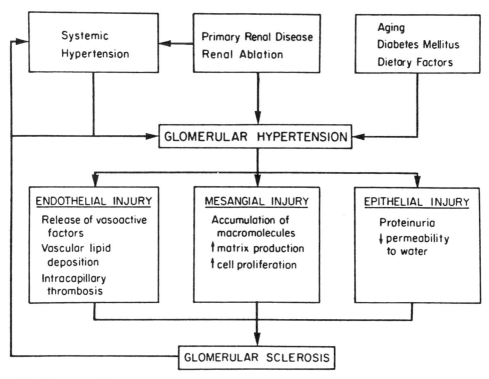

Figure 9.2. Pivotal role of glomerular hypertension in the initiation and progression of structural injury. (From Anderson S, Brenner BM. Progressive renal disease: a disorder of adaptation. *Q J Med* 1989;70:185–189.)

of a measurable reduction in GFR (Miller et al., 1990).

As noted by Jacobson (1991), "We still do not know in molecular or cellular terms how 'haemodynamic damage' occurs." Other factors may be involved beyond glomerular hypertension and hyperfiltration including multiple types of renal injury from angiotensin II (Johnson et al., 1992), glomerular hypertrophy (Yoshida et al., 1989a) and resetting of tubuloglomerular feedback so that glomerular hyperfunction is sustained despite extensive loss of renal function (Salmond and Seney, 1991). The manner by which mechanical forces may induce glomerulosclerosis was demonstrated in rat glomeruli perfused ex vivo, wherein capillary expansion and stretching of mesangial cells by glomerular hypertension provoked increased production of extracellular matrix (Riser et al., 1992).

Secondary Mechanisms

If the progressive sclerosis of glomeruli is responsible for the usual progressive decline in renal function, the manner by which this in turn leads to or aggravates hypertension likely involves an inability of the reduced renal mass to perform a number of its usual functions or the appearance of one or more pressor mechanisms (Table 9.2). Hemodynamically, when renal mass is reduced, the BP rises, first because of volume expansion and an increased cardiac output, later because of elevated peripheral resistance (Ledingham, 1991).

Table 9.2. Mechanisms by Which Renal Damage May Induce Hypertension

Sodium retention and volume expansion
 Increased ouabain-like natriuretic factor
 Increased mineralocorticoid action from nonmetabolized cortisol

Increased production of vasopressors
 Renin-angiotension
 Endothelin

Decreased production of vasodepressors
 Medullipin
 Kinins
 Prostaglandins

Retention of endogenous inhibitors of endothelium-derived relaxing factor (nitric oxide) (e.g., asymmetric dimethylarginine)

The major role played by sodium retention and volume expansion may involve deleterious effects of increased amounts of the endogenous ouabain-like natriuretic factor that inhibits the Na^+,K^+–ATPase pump described in Chapter 3 (Boero et al., 1988). Moreover, the propensity to retain sodium may reflect more than the simple loss of filtering mass: Vierhapper et al. (1991) found that most patients with chronic renal insufficiency had increased ratios of urinary tetrahydrocortisol to tetrahydrocortisone, in keeping with a deficiency of the 11-beta-hydroxysteroid dehydrogenase enzyme, which is needed to convert the usual high levels of mineralocorticoid-acting cortisol to the inactive cortisone, a process more fully described in Chapter 14.

In some patients, secretion of renin from ischemic glomeruli may be excessive. In addition, the damaged kidneys may not produce vasodilatory prostaglandins (Kishimoto et al., 1987) or other renal vasodepressors. And, in keeping with one of the more exciting developments in the pathophysiology of hypertension, Vallance and coworkers (1992) documented the presence of increased levels of an endogenously produced inhibitor of the synthesis of nitric oxide, asymmetric dimethylarginine, in patients with chronic renal failure. As fully described in Chapter 3, inhibition of what appears to be a primary function of endothelial cells to control vascular tone, neurotransmission, and host defense may be involved in many of the clinical problems of renal failure.

Management

Many patients are seen only after significant renal insufficiency has developed, at which time all that can be done is to enter them into dialysis with the hope for transplantation. The total number of ESRD patients on chronic dialysis in the United States will likely reach 250,000 by the year 2000 (National High Blood Pressure Education Program, 1991); this will consume a significant amount of money that could be far more effectively spent on prevention, since the two most common causes of ESRD, nephrosclerosis related to hypertension and diabetic nephropathy, may be largely preventable.

Once renal insufficiency has developed, the goal is to slow its progress by interrupting the vicious cycle shown in Figure 9.2. As of now, the only means known to be effective are control of hypertension and decreasing the intake of dietary protein; however, control of hyperlipid-emia, reduction in the degree of proteinuria, and restriction of phosphorus intake may also be helpful (Klahr, 1991).

Data documenting the ability of antihypertensive therapy to slow the progression of renal insufficiency remain limited, and most of these relate to diabetic nephropathy (Klahr, 1991). The problem may reflect inadequate control of hypertension: in view of the positive correlation between BPs even below 140/90 mm Hg to decreases in renal function (Klahr, 1989), it may take greater reductions of BP or the use of specific agents (e.g., ACE inhibitors) to overcome the glomerular hypertension that is responsible for the progressive loss of renal function (de Jong et al., 1993).

Control of Hypertension

With both diuretics and other antihypertensive agents, transient falls in renal blood flow and glomerular filtration rate may accompany successful reduction of the BP. Unless there is reason to believe that plasma volume is contracted too much or that there is drug-related nephrotoxicity, the best course is to proceed with control of the hypertension despite a rise in the serum creatinine. In the long run, renal function may be preserved by tight control of the hypertension (Pettinger et al., 1989).

The major role of volume excess can be countered by adequate diuretic therapy if renal insufficiency is fairly mild and by removal of fluid via dialysis in overt renal failure.

Diuretics. All diuretics, save spironolactone, must gain entry to the tubular fluid and have access to the luminal side of the nephron to work, reaching the urine by secretion across the proximal tubule by way of organic acid or organic base secretory pathways. ''Their entry to the urinary site of action can be compromised by anything that limits access to the secretory sites (e.g., diminished renal blood flow) or that blocks or competes for the secretory pump (e.g., endogenous organic acids or probenecid for acidic drugs and cimetidine for basic drugs)'' (Brater, 1988).

Patients with chronic renal disease (CRD), then, are resistant to acidic diuretics such as thiazides and the loop diuretics, both because of their reduced renal blood flow and because of the accumulation of organic acid end-products of metabolism. To effect diuresis, enough of the diuretic must be given to deliver adequate amounts of the agent to the tubular sites of action. This translates into a ''sequential doubling of single doses until a ceiling dose is reached'' (Brater, 1988). Once the ceiling dose is reached, that dose should be given as often as needed (usually once a day) as a maintenance dose. In patients with severe renal disease, resistant to conventional diuretic therapy, a continuous, low-dose infusion of a loop diuretic may be more effective and better tolerated (Rudy et al., 1991).

As Brater (1988) points out, thiazides would probably work in many CRD patients if given in high enough doses. "However, such a strategy is still not worth pursuing [because of] the low intrinsic efficacy of these drugs compared to loop diuretics." Most do not try thiazides if the serum creatinine is above 2.0 mg/dl. On the other hand, in severely resistant patients, combining a loop diuretic with a thiazide may effect a response when neither is effective alone (Wollam et al., 1982).

In addition, metolazone may work as well as loop diuretics; furthermore, if control of hypertension requires more persistent volume control than provided by a once-a-day dose of a loop diuretic, metolazone will provide a full 24-hour effect (Bennett and Porter, 1973).

Caution should be taken to avoid excessive diuresis with such potent diuretics on the one hand and interference with diuretic action by nonsteroidal anti-inflammatory drugs (NSAIDs) on the other. Spironolactone, triamterene, and amiloride should be avoided in most patients with severe CRD since hyperkalemia may be induced, particularly in diabetics who cannot secrete extra insulin to enhance transfer of potassium into cells and who may have low renin and aldosterone levels (Perez et al., 1977). Similarly, CRD patients taking beta blockers, who therefore cannot obtain the epinephrine-mediated transfer of potassium across cells, may be susceptible to hyperkalemia (Mitch and Wilcox, 1982).

Sodium Restriction. Patients with CRD may have a narrow range of sodium excretory capacity: if their dietary salt is markedly restricted, these patients may not be able to conserve sodium and will become volume-depleted; if given modest salt loads, they may be unable to excrete enough sodium to prevent volume expansion and hypertension. A very small number have severe salt-losing nephropathy, but few of them are hypertensive (Uribarri et al., 1983). Thus, sodium intake should be carefully monitored.

If $NaHCO_3$ is used to counter the metabolic acidosis, NaCl may have to be more severely restricted. In a practical manner, sodium restriction in the range of 1 to 2 g/day (44 to 88 mEq of sodium per day) is both feasible and necessary to control the hypertension in these patients.

Nondiuretic Antihypertensive Drugs. The ongoing publications by W.M. Bennett (1988) provide the best data about the dosage of antihypertensive and other drugs in patients with varying degrees of CRD (Table 9.3).

Minoxidil. Those with refractory hypertension and renal insufficiency may be successfully treated with minoxidil (Pontremoli et al., 1991). As noted in Chapter 7, minoxidil is a potent vasodilator and must be given with an adrenergic blocker (usually a beta blocker) to prevent reflex cardiac stimulation and with a diuretic (usually furosemide) to prevent fluid retention. The drug need be given only in a single daily dose, as was done in a study of 55 patients with resistant hypertension, 12 of whom had CRD (mean serum creatinine of 2.5 mg/dl) (Spitalewitz et al., 1986).

ACE Inhibitors. In keeping with the hypothesis of Brenner and coworkers (Anderson et al., 1986), ACE inhibitors (ACEIs) have been shown in rat models to provide better control of glomerular hypertension and better preservation of renal function than other drugs that lower the BP equally well (Kakinuma et al., 1992). The observation is in keeping with a greater degree of efferent arteriolar vasodilation provided by blockade of intrarenal angiotensin II. By relieving this efferent constriction to a greater degree than they reduce afferent resistance, ACEIs should reduce both pressure and flow within the glomeruli, thereby providing protection against progressive sclerosis (Tolins and Raij, 1991) (Fig. 9.3). Such is true for some rats but not for others (Yoshida et al., 1989b).

In people, ACEIs clearly lower the BP and reduce proteinuria, and may improve renal function (Apperloo et al., 1991; Brunner, 1992). Preservation of renal function has been amply shown in patients with CRD using various ACEIs (Kamper et al., 1992). In patients with rapidly progressive renal failure from connective tissue disease, an ACEI may provide spectacular effects (Zawada et al., 1981). However, there are no adequate comparisons with other antihypertensive agents to know whether ACEIs are more protective than the others. Moreover, a decrease in proteinuria may not reflect attenuation of renal damage (Remuzzi et al., 1991).

Table 9.3. Guide to Drug Dosage in Renal Failure

Drug	Elimination Half-Life (t$_{1/2}$) (Adults) Normal (hr)	ESRD (hr)	Excreted Unchanged (%)	Normal Dose Interval (hr)	Dose Adjustment for Renal Failure: Creatinine Clearance (ml/min): >50	10–50	<10	Need for Dose Adjustment During Dialysis[a]
Beta-Adrenoceptor Antagonists								
Acebutolol	7–9	7	55	12 or 24	Unchanged	50%	25%	No (H)
Atenolol	6–9	15–35	>90	24	Unchanged	50%	25%	Yes (H) No (P)
Labetalol	3–8	3–8	0–5	12	Unchanged	Unchanged	Unchanged	No (H)
Metoprolol	2.5–4.5	2.5–4.5	5	12	Unchanged	Unchanged	Unchanged	Yes (H)
Nadolol	14–24	45	90	24	Unchanged	50%	25%	Yes (H)
Pindolol	2.5–4	3–4	40	12	Unchanged	Unchanged	Unchanged	?
Propranolol	2–6	1–6	<5	6–12	Unchanged	Unchanged	Unchanged	No (H)
Timolol	2.5–4	4	15	8–12	Unchanged	Unchanged	Unchanged	No (H)
Other Antihypertensive Drugs								
Captopril	1.9	21–32	50–70	12	Unchanged	Unchanged	50%	Yes (H)
Clonidine	6–23	39–42	45	6–8	Unchanged	Unchanged	Unchanged	No (H)
Guanabenz	12–14	?	<5	12	Unchanged	Unchanged	Unchanged	?
Guanethidine	120–240	?	25–50	24	24 hr	24 hr	24–36 hr	?
Hydralazine	2.0–2.5	7–16	25	8–12	8–12 hr	8–12 hr	8–16 hr / 12–24 hr[b]	No (H,P)
Alpha methyldopa	1–1.7	7–16	20–60	6	6 hr	9–18 hr	12–24 hr	Yes (H,P)
Minoxidil	2.8–4.2	2.8–4.2	15–20	8–12	Unchanged	Unchanged	Unchanged	Yes (H)
Nitroprusside sodium	< 10 min	< 10 min	< 10	Constant IV infusion	Unchanged	Unchanged	Unchanged	Yes (H)
Prazosin	1.8–4.6	?	< 5	8–12	Unchanged	Unchanged	Unchanged	No (H,P)
Reserpine	46–168	87–323	< 1	24	Unchanged	Unchanged	Avoid	No (H,P)

[a] H, hemodialysis; P, peritoneal dialysis.
[b] Slow acetylators.
From Bennett WM. Guide to drug dosage in renal failure. *Clin PharmacoKinet* 1988;15:326–354.

As noted in Table 9.3, the excretion of captopril is decreased in ESRD, and a lower dose should be given. The same is true of most other ACEIs except fosinopril, which can be excreted by the liver in the presence of decreased renal function (Murdoch and McTavish, 1992).

Calcium Entry Blockers. These drugs are also effective in controlling the BP and in preserving already impaired renal function, perhaps even better than "standard" therapy (Epstein, 1992). On theoretical grounds, the preferential vasodilation of afferent arterioles that is seen with calcium entry blockers (CEBs) in experimental models would further increase glomerular hyperfiltration (Fig. 9.3). However, in clinical practice, CEBs have not been found to worsen renal function (Tolins and Raij, 1991). The use of a combination of an ACEI and a CEB may be particularly effective (Kloke et al., 1990).

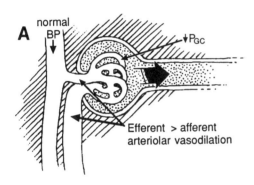

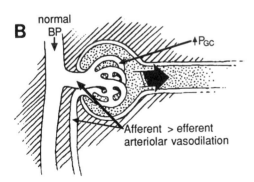

Figure 9.3. Effect of antihypertensive treatment on glomerular hemodynamics as determined by micropuncture studies in the rat. Converting enzyme inhibition results in normalization of blood pressure *(BP)* associated with vasodilatation predominantly of the efferent arteriole, resulting in normalization of intraglomerular capillary pressure (P_{GC}) *(A)*. With calcium channel blockade, reduction of blood pressure is offset by afferent arteriolar vasodilatation, and therefore P_{GC} remains elevated *(B)*. (From Tolins JP, Raij L. Antihypertensive therapy and the progression of chronic renal disease. Are there renoprotective drugs? *Semin Nephrol* 1991;11:538–548.)

Restriction of Dietary Protein

On theoretical and experimental grounds, a reduced protein intake should increase preglomerular resistance by constriction of afferent arterioles, thereby reducing glomerular hyperfiltration and slowing hemodynamically mediated renal disease (de Jong et al., 1993). Such an effect has been observed in clinical trials of patients with renal insufficiency from various causes (Ihle et al., 1989) and from diabetic nephropathy (Zeller et al., 1991). An even larger-scale study of the effect of a diet restricted in protein (and phosphorus) on the progress of CRD is now under way; definitive data should soon be available (Klahr, 1989).

Correction of Anemia

As described further in Chapter 15, the use of recombinant human erythropoietin to correct the anemia of CRD may raise the BP rather markedly (Fahal et al., 1992). This is related to the increase in blood viscosity and volume, so that the anemia should be corrected slowly and with close watch of the BP.

Renin-Dependent Hypertension

A small number of patients with CRD and severe hypertension may have a highly activated renin-angiotensin system—from bilateral renal artery stenosis, one hopes, so that it can be relieved by revascularization (Ying et al., 1984; Rimmer and Gennari, 1993)—but more likely from diffuse intrarenal ischemia that can only be relieved by bilateral nephrectomy (Lazarus et al., 1972). Fortunately, with better control of fluid volume and the use of ACEIs, the need for removal of native kidneys is lessened, but the procedure may relieve hypertension even if the hypertension preceded the renal failure (Curtis et al., 1985).

Sickle Cell Nephropathy

Among 381 patients with sickle cell disease, 26% had proteinuria and 7% had elevated serum creatinine levels (Falk et al., 1992). Proteinuria decreased during therapy with an ACEI, supporting glomerular capillary hypertension as a mechanism for the nephropathy.

Diabetic Nephropathy

The progressive nephropathy seen with diabetes mellitus appears to be another example of the deleterious effects of hyperfiltration and intraglomerular hypertension.

Pathology and Clinical Features

As delineated by Kimmelstiel and Wilson (1936), renal disease occurs among diabetics with a high incidence and with a particular glomerular pathology—nodular intercapillary glomerulosclerosis. The clinical description has been improved very little since their original paper:

The clinical picture appears . . . to be almost as characteristic as the histological one: the patients are relatively old; hypertension is present, usually of the benign type, and the kidneys frequently show signs of decompensation; there is a history of diabetes, usually of long standing; the presenting symptoms may be those of edema of the nephrotic type, renal decompensation or heart failure; the urine contains large amounts of albumin and there is usually impairment of concentrating power with or without nitrogen retention.

The pathologic specificity of the nodular glomerular lesion for diabetes has been upheld. The clinical description should be altered to include younger patients if they have been diabetic over 10 years, to involve hypertension in about 50% to 60% of patients, and to almost always be accompanied by retinal capillary microaneurysms.

Epidemiology

Because more diabetics are living longer, the number of patients with CRD related to diabetic nephropathy continues to increase, with renal failure eventually developing in 30% to 50% of patients afflicted with insulin-dependent diabetes mellitus (IDDM) and in somewhat fewer of those with non–insulin-dependent diabetes mellitus (NIDDM) (Tuttle et al., 1990). The prevalence is more than 3 times higher among blacks with NIDDM, likely explaining the high proportion of ESRD in the U.S. diabetic population (Brancati et al., 1992). There is also a gender difference: among IDDM subjects followed for 30 years, 84% of males and 59% of females developed nephropathy (Orchard et al., 1990).

The mortality rate from coronary and renal disease is 37 times greater in patients with diabetic nephropathy than in the general population, whereas the rate in diabetics without nephropathy is only 4.2 times greater (Borch-Johnsen and Kreiner, 1987). Microalbuminuria is a significant risk marker for future mortality (Mattock et al., 1992).

Diabetic nephropathy occurs in family clusters (Seaquist et al., 1989). Patients with nephropathy have higher sodium-lithium counter-transport activity in red cells than is found in those who do not have nephropathy (Mangili et al., 1988; Krolewski et al., 1988), but Jensen et al. (1990) do not consider this a genetic marker for the development of nephropathy.

Course

The rapidly progressive nature of diabetic nephropathy—usually advancing to renal failure within 10 years after onset of persistent proteinuria (Tuttle et al., 1990) (Fig. 9.4)—reflects features unique to the diabetic state (Mogensen et al., 1992); these features occur in addition to those marking the overall progression of glomerulosclerosis illustrated in Figure 9.2. The primary metabolic abnormality of diabetes—hyperglycemia—is likely responsible for many of the hemodynamic alterations that progressively damage the kidneys (Hostetter, 1992; Pedersen et al., 1992). With increased filtered glucose, the resultant increased tubular reabsorption of glucose carries sodium along; the increased insulin levels (exogenous in Type I, endogenous in Type II) directly stimulate tubular reabsorption of sodium as well (Fujihara et al., 1992). The resultant extracellular fluid volume excess, accentuated by the osmotic pull of hyperglycemia, induces renal hyperfiltration manifested by elevated glomerular filtration rates, which are a hallmark of subsequent nephropathy (Carr et al., 1990). Somewhere in the process, the increased central blood volume activates the release of atrial natriuretic peptide, whose renal vasodilatory action likely contributes to the hyperfiltration (Pedersen et al., 1992).

Other vasoactive control systems may contribute, and glomerular hypertension may be less important than mesangial expansion (Bank, 1991; Mauer et al., 1992). Nonetheless, a cogent argument can be made for the central role of hyperglycemia per se. Once the process starts, the previously inexorable progress of glomerulosclerosis leads to overt nephropathy. Albuminuria is the first recognizable sign: the presence of microalbuminuria almost doubles the prevalence of hypertension, proliferative retinopathy, and neuropathy; the presence of macroalbuminuria doubles them again (Parving, 1991). Microalbuminuria is frequently found even without overt hypertension (Klein et al., 1992), is associated with endothelial dysfunction (Stehouwer et al., 1992), and should be repeatedly monitored in untimed (Nelson et al., 1991) or first-morning (Mogensen, 1992) urine specimens.

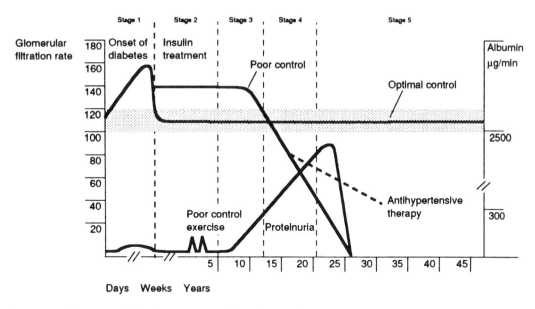

Figure 9.4. The stages of diabetic nephropathy. (From Tuttle KR, Stein JH, DeFronzo RA. The natural history of diabetic nephropathy. *Semin Nephrol* 1990;10:184–193.)

Hypertension is closely correlated with levels of albuminuria and is clearly related to the progress of renal insufficiency. When diabetic nephropathy is responsible for hypertension, patients tend to have albuminuria that is, on average, 100 times more extensive than that of diabetics with coincidental essential hypertension (Christensen et al., 1987). The hypertension is associated with expansion of plasma and extracellular fluid volume with low plasma renin levels that are, nonetheless, inappropriately high for the degree of hypertension and volume expansion (Hommel et al., 1989). High levels of plasma prorenin may predict the development of nephropathy (Luetscher and Kraemer, 1988).

Management

Glycemic Control.   If microalbuminuria is present, tighter glycemic control should be attempted, since hyperglycemia is the cardinal controllable problem. In view of the evidence reviewed in Chapter 3 about the possible deleterious effects of hyperinsulinemia, there may be concern about the use of increased amounts of exogenous insulin to achieve tighter control. Nonetheless, insulin-induced lowering of hyperglycemia will reverse glomerular capillary hypertension in diabetic rats (Scholey and Meyer, 1989), and a number of 1- to 8-year studies in humans have shown a reduction in

albuminuria and in GFR by tighter glycemic control (Tuttle et al., 1991; Feldt-Rasmussen et al., 1991; Diabetes Control and Complications Trial Research Group, 1993).

Antihypertensive Therapy.   The evidence is even stronger for a slowing of the progression of diabetic nephropathy by reduction of elevated BP (Tuttle et al., 1991). The longest protective effect has been reported by Parving et al. (1991), who followed nine insulin-dependent patients for 2 years before and for 10 years after institution of effective antihypertensive therapy. The effects on renal function over the first 6 years (Parving et al., 1987) are similar to those reported over the entire 10 years (Fig. 9.5). Note that this impressive reduction in the rate of decline of renal function was achieved by "traditional" antihypertensive therapy (i.e., without an ACEI). In order to obtain the best protection against the progress of diabetic nephropathy, it may be necessary to lower diastolic BPs to 75 mm Hg or less (Dillon, 1992).

Since Taguma et al. (1985) reported a decrease in heavy proteinuria in 6 of 10 azotemic diabetics with captopril, a large number of studies have documented in humans what has been seen in diabetic rats (Cooper et al., 1992): ACEIs have a special ability to reduce the proteinuria of diabetic nephropathy (Lewis et al., 1993). This has been seen in both normotensive (Stor-

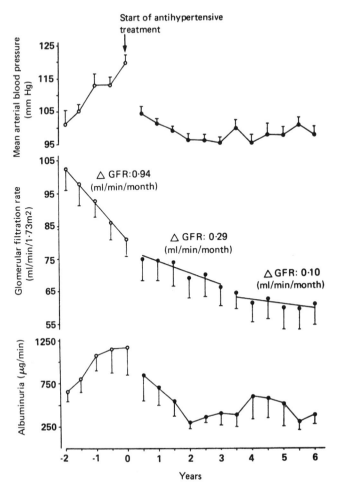

Figure 9.5. Average course of mean arterial blood pressure, glomerular filtration rate, and albuminuria before *(open circles)* and during *(filled circles)* long-term effective antihypertensive treatment of nine insulin-dependent diabetic patients who had nephropathy. Therapy included furosemide, metoprolol, and hydralazine in most patients. (From Parving H-H, Andersen AR, Smidt UM, Hommel E, Mathiesen ER, Svendsen PA. Effect of antihypertensive treatment on kidney function in diabetic nephropathy. *Br Med J* 1987;294:1443–1447.)

nello et al., 1992) and hypertensive (Björck et al., 1992) diabetics with nephropathy using various ACEIs, with a greater effectiveness of ACEIs than of either conventional therapy or calcium antagonists, particularly when little lowering of the BP is accomplished (Lewis et al., 1993; Weidmann et al., 1993) (Fig. 9.6). The fall in proteinuria is usually but not always accompanied by a slowing of the rate of fall in glomerular filtration, the usual index of renal function (Kasiske et al., 1993). As with the effect on proteinuria, ACEIs were uniquely associated with a relative increase in GFR that was independent of effects on BP reduction. Calcium blockers, with the apparent exception of nifedipine, may

be as effective as ACEIs (Bakris, 1992), but subsequent long-term data are not yet available. More controlled long-term studies are being reported (Ravid et al., 1993; Lewis et al., 1993). As a result, earlier ACEI therapy, even in the absence of hypertension, is being advocated (Mogensen, 1992).

Although, as noted in Chapter 7, diuretics may worsen glucose tolerance and insulin sensitivity, they may be needed to control the volume expansion responsible for hypertension (Tuttle et al., 1991). Sodium restriction should also help (Bank et al., 1988).

Low Protein Diet. A diet with only 0.6 g/kg/day of high-biologic-value protein and low in phosphorus given to 20 insulin-dependent diabetics for at least 1 year reduced the rate of renal function decline (Zeller et al., 1991). The mechanism likely involves a decrease in glomerular hyperfiltration by relief from the afferent arteriolar dilation and increased osmotic activity of nitrogenous waste products (de Jong et al., 1993).

Prostaglandin Inhibitors. Indomethacin reduced proteinuria as well as did the ACEI lisinopril, and the two together yielded additive effects but induced a fall in GFR (Heeg et al., 1991), reflecting afferent vasoconstriction by the NSAID and efferent vasodilation by the ACEI (de Jong et al., 1993).

When all else fails, patients who develop ESRD from diabetic nephropathy seem to respond well to the various therapies for renal failure, including continuous ambulatory peritoneal dialysis (Amair et al., 1982) and renal transplantation (Sagalowsky et al., 1983). These patients have a high frequency of low renin hypertension, which may meld into a truly distinctive syndrome seen in CRD—hyporeninemic hypoaldosteronism. Whereas various forms of renal disease may be associated with the syndrome, elderly diabetics are affected more frequently. Such diabetics, unable to mobilize either aldosterone or insulin, which are needed to transfer potassium out of the blood, are partic-

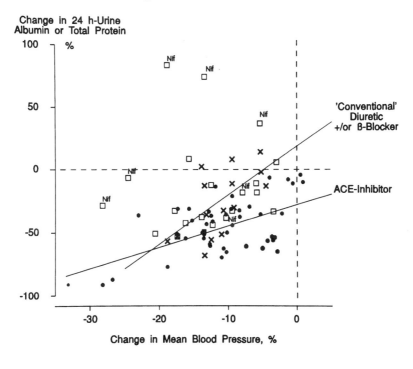

% Changes in Albuminuria - Proteinuria as Related to Blood Pressure Changes in Diabetics on Antihypertensive Drugs

Symbol	Drug	N	r	p <
•	ACE-Inhibitor	45	0.58	0.0001
×	Conventional	14	0.62	0.02
□	Ca-Antagonist	18	0.02	N.S.

Figure 9.6. A meta-analysis of 77 published studies of the percentage in albuminuria or total proteinuria as related to blood pressure changes in diabetic patients with proteinuria on different antihypertensive drug treatments for 4 or more weeks. *Nif,* nifedipine. *N,* number of reported studies. (From Weidmann P, Boehlen LM, de Courten M. Pathogenesis and treatment of hypertension associated with diabetes mellitus. *Am Heart J* 1993;125:1498–1513.)

ularly vulnerable to hyperkalemia (Perez et al., 1977).

HYPERTENSION IN ACUTE RENAL DISEASE

Most acute severe insults to the kidney result in decreased urine formation, retention of salt and water, and hypertension. Acute renal failure with hypertension may result from bilateral renal artery occlusion, either by emboli or thromboses, or by removal of angiotensin II support of blood flow with ACEI therapy in the presence of bilateral renal artery disease (Brunner, 1992). Trauma to the kidney may cause renin-mediated hypertension that is quite variable in onset and severity (Watts and Hoffbrand, 1987). Rarely, a perirenal hematoma may so constrict the kidney as to cause persistent ischemia and hypertension (Hellebusch et al., 1970). Syndromes with a vascular component are discussed further in the next chapter.

Extracorporeal shock wave lithotripsy for kidney stones may be followed by a rise in BP that lasts at least 6 months in 20% to 30% of patients (Hammond et al., 1993). The incidence of persistent hypertension seems quite small (Smith LH et al., 1991), but long-time follow-up is appropriate.

Acute Glomerulonephritis

The classic syndrome is a child with recent streptococcal pharyngitis or impetigo who suddenly passes dark urine and develops facial edema. The renal injury represents the trapping of antibody-antigen complexes within the glomerular capillaries. Although the syndrome has become less common, it still occurs, sometimes in adults past middle age.

Typically, in the acute phase, patients are hypertensive and there is a close temporal relation between oliguria, edema, and hypertension. On occasion, hypertension of a severe, even malignant nature may be the overriding feature.

Mechanism

The hypertension was thought to be secondary to fluid overload with an increased cardiac output, but a careful study of two patients revealed an increased peripheral resistance attributed to an inappropriately high renin level (Birkenhäger et al., 1970).

Treatment and Course

The hypertension should be treated by salt and water restriction and, in mild cases, diuretics and other oral antihypertensives. In keeping with an apparent role of renin, ACEI therapy was very effective in nine patients with acute glomerulonephritis (Parra et al., 1988).

In the classic disease, the patient is free of edema and hypertension within days, of proteinuria within weeks, and of hematuria within months. Hypertension was found in only 3 of 88 children followed for 10 to 17 years (Popovic-Rolovic et al., 1991).

Acute Renal Failure

A rapid decline in renal function may appear from various causes: prerenal (e.g., volume depletion), intrinsic (e.g., glomerulonephritis), or postrenal (e.g., obstructive uropathy) (Diamond and Henrich, 1986). NSAIDs are one of the most common causes of acute renal failure (Shankel et al., 1992), particularly in patients whose renal perfusion depends on prostaglandin-mediated vasodilation (Murray et al., 1990).

Hypertension is rarely a problem, perhaps because peripheral vascular tone often is decreased. Now that dialysis is so readily available, the management of such patients is much less difficult, and virtually complete recovery even after prolonged oliguria is frequent.

Acute Urinary Tract Obstruction

Hypertension may develop after unilateral (Mizuiri et al., 1992) or bilateral (Jones et al., 1987) obstruction to the ureters or urethra (Robinson et al., 1992), an effect in rats that is associated with activation of renin and suppression of kallikrein (El-Dahr et al., 1992). In most patients, the hypertension is fairly mild, but high-pressure chronic retention of urine with hydronephrosis and painless bladder distension from prostatic hypertrophy may be associated with significant hypertension and severe renal insufficiency (Sacks et al., 1989). Catheter drainage of the residual urine may lead to rapid resolution of the hypertension and circulatory overload (Ghose and Harindra, 1989).

HYPERTENSION WITH RENAL PARENCHYMAL DISEASE BUT WITHOUT RENAL INSUFFICIENCY

The hypertension seen with all of the preceding renal diseases seems appropriate to the extensive renal damage, with resultant defects in fluid excretion, renin secretion, or vasodepressor elaboration. Others of a more obvious vascular origin are covered in the next chapter. In some patients, however, hypertension is seen without enough overt renal damage or ischemia to explain the hypertension on any of these bases. This is particularly true in patients with unilateral renal parenchymal disease whose hypertension is relieved by removal of the afflicted kidney.

Renal Donors

In normal humans, the removal of a kidney usually does not result in hypertension, likely because of downward adjustments in renin and aldosterone to maintain normal fluid volume. The issue has been recently explored more thoroughly because of the theoretical possibility— in keeping with the hyperperfusion theory (Fig. 9.2)—that removal of one kidney leads to progressive glomerulosclerosis in the other. This possibility does not seem to have been fully realized: In a long-term follow-up of over 8000 donor nephrectomies, mild, nonprogressive proteinuria was noted in about one-third and a DBP above 90 mm Hg was noted in 25% (Bay and Hebert, 1987). However, both of these findings could also reflect familial renal disease and hypertension. No more hypertension or renal damage was found in 57 living donors than in their siblings after follow-up of 20 years or longer (Najarian et al., 1992). Even after partial removal of a solitary kidney, renal function remains stable, though proteinuria is common (Novick et al., 1991).

It appears that only in the elderly, who have significantly less ability to modulate sodium excretion, might removal of one kidney induce hypertension (Podjarny et al., 1986). Therefore, if unilateral renal disease causes hypertension, something likely is happening in the presumably normal kidney as well.

Chronic Pyelonephritis

Hypertension is found more frequently among patients with radiographic signs of chronic pyelonephritis, even if renal function is well preserved (Jacobson and Lins, 1988) and the pyelonephritis only affects one kidney (Siamopoulos et al., 1983). Hypertensive children are frequently found to have pyelonephritic scarring, usually resulting from vesicoureteric reflux and urinary tract infection. Renal insufficiency and hypertension may not manifest until middle age (Jacobson et al., 1989).

The relationship between the pyelonephritis and the hypertension is uncertain, but an increased level of renin from the pyelonephritic kidney is usually noted in those whose hypertension is relieved by nephrectomy (Siamopoulos et al., 1983).

Drug-Induced Renal Disease

Some patients thought to have chronic pyelonephritis actually have analgesic nephropathy from long-term, regular use of phenacetin (Dubach et al., 1991) or NSAIDs (Sandler et al., 1991), a not uncommon cause of chronic renal failure in the United States but more common in Australia (Kincaid-Smith and Whitworth, 1988). Since renal salt wasting is frequent with this form of interstitial nephritis, hypertension may be somewhat less common, but even malignant hypertension has been seen (Kincaid-Smith and Whitworth, 1988).

A number of other commonly used drugs (e.g., antibiotics, cyclosporine), antineoplastic agents, and diagnostic agents (e.g., contrast media) may cause renal damage (Moore and Porush, 1992). Agents that induce hypertension are covered in Chapter 15.

Polycystic Kidney Disease

Autosomal dominant polycystic kidney disease is the cause of 8% of cases of ESRD. Hypertension is common, even without demonstrable renal insufficiency, and is likely induced by high levels of renin secreted in response to renal ischemia from enlarging cysts (Chapman et al., 1990) or from abnormal expression of renin synthesis in the lining epithelium of the cyst walls (Torres et al., 1992). The hypertension is a risk factor for progression of renal insufficiency (Gabow et al., 1992) but will respond to excision or aspiration of cysts (Bennett et al., 1987) and to ACEIs (Torres et al., 1991).

Renal Tumors

As we shall see in the next chapter, renin-secreting tumors may cause severe hypertension. In addition to those rare tumors, hypertension may be seen with other renal tumors—nephroblastoma (Wilms' tumor), renal cell carcinoma, and hypernephroma (Dahl et al., 1981). Most appear to cause hypertension by activation of the renin system. Radiotherapy for Wilms' tumor may lead to hypertension 10 or more years later (Koskimies, 1982).

Unilateral Renal Disease

In addition to these and other forms of renal disease, hypertension that is not secondary to obvious renal artery stenosis is not infrequently found in patients with a small kidney. After Goldblatt produced hypertension by unilateral renal ischemia, small kidneys were indiscriminately removed from hypertensive patients. Smith (1956) discouraged this practice by calling attention to a cure rate of only 26% in all reports published by 1956.

In most patients cured by unilateral nephrectomy, renovascular disease, not primary parenchymal disease, is probably the cause for both the atrophic kidney and the hypertension, presumably by means of the renin mechanism (Wesson, 1982). Renin levels are increased in the venous blood coming from many of those kidneys whose removal results in relief of hypertension (Gordon et al., 1986). On the other hand, there are reports of cure of hypertension by removal of kidneys thought to be atrophic because of parenchymal disease, usually pyelonephritis, and not because of vascular impairment as reflected by the presence of normal renin levels (Lamberton et al., 1981).

In view of these questions concerning both the frequency and mechanism of unilateral parenchymal disease as a cause of hypertension, caution is advised before nephrectomy is performed in such patients. The cure rate with parenchymal atrophy is probably much less than that with vascular disease. Moreover, nephrectomy should never be done without prior knowledge of the normal functional state of the other kidney. Nephrectomy should probably be reserved for patients with the following conditions:

—Severe hypertension;

—Marked loss of renal function in the afflicted kidney that should be recognizable by renal scintigraphy. In practice, a renal size of less than 8.5 cm usually denotes an inability to salvage the kidney by revascularization;

—Normal renal function in the other kidney.

We will next turn to the disease in which surgical relief and renin are more closely connected, renovascular hypertension.

References

Amair P, Khanna R, Leibel B, Pierratos A, Vas S, Meema E, Blair G, Chisolm L, Vas M, Zingg W, Digenis G, Oreopoulos D. Continuous ambulatory peritoneal dialysis in diabetics with end-stage renal disease. *N Engl J Med* 1982;306:625–630.

Anderson S, Brenner BM. Progressive renal disease: a disorder of adaptation. *Q J Med* 1989;70:185–189.

Anderson S, Rennke HG, Brenner BM. Therapeutic advantage of converting enzyme inhibitors in arresting progressive renal disease associated with systemic hypertension in the rat. *J Clin Invest* 1986;77: 1993–2000.

Apperloo AJ, de Zeeuw D, Sluiter HE, de Jong PE. Differential effects of enalapril and atenolol on proteinuria and renal haemodynamics in non-diabetic renal disease. *Br Med J* 1991;303:821–824.

Bakris G. The antiproteinuric effect of antihypertensive agents in diabetic nephrology. *Arch Intern Med* 1992;152:2137–2139.

Bank N. Mechanisms of diabetic hyperfiltration. *Kidney Int* 1991;40:792–807.

Bank N, Lahorra MAG, Aynedjian HS, Wilkes BM. Sodium restriction corrects hyperfiltration of diabetes. *Am J Physiol* 1988;254:F668–F676.

Bay WH, Hebert LA. The living donor in kidney transplantation. *Ann Intern Med* 1987;106:719–727.

Beaman M, Adu D. Mesangial IgA nephropathy: an autoimmune cause of hypertension? *J Hum Hypertens* 1988;2:139–141.

Bennett WM. Guide to drug dosage in renal failure. *Clin Pharmacokinet* 1988;15: 326–354.

Bennett WM, Elzinga L, Golper TA. Reduction of cyst volume for symptomatic management of polycystic kidney disease. *J Urol* 1987;137:620–622.

Bennett WM, Porter GA. Efficacy and safety of metolazone in renal failure and the nephrotic syndrome. *Clin Pharmacol* 1973;13:357–364.

Birkenhäger WH, Schalekamp MADH, Schalekamp-Kuyken MPA, Kolsters G, Krauss XH. Interrelations between arterial pressure, fluid-volumes, and plasma-renin concentration in the course of acute glomerulonephritis. *Lancet* 1970;1:1086–1087.

Björck S, Mulec H, Johnsen SA, Nordén G, Aurell M. Renal protective effect of enalapril in diabetic nephropathy. *Br Med J* 1992;304:339–343.

Boero R, Guarena C, Berto IM, Forneris G, Borca M, Martina G, Quarello F, Piccoli G. Pathogenesis of arterial hypertension in chronic uraemia: the role of reduced Na,K-ATPase activity. *J Hypertens* 1988; 6(Suppl 4):363–365.

Borch-Johnsen K, Kreiner S. Proteinuria: value as predictor of cardiovascular mortality in insulin dependent diabetes mellitus. *Br Med J* 1987;294:1651–1654.

Brancati FL, Whittle JC, Whelton PK, Seidler AJ, Klag MJ. The excess incidence of diabetic end-stage renal disease among blacks. *JAMA* 1992;268:3079–3084.

Brater DC. Use of diuretics in chronic renal insufficiency and nephrotic syndrome. *Semin Nephrol* 1988;8:333–341.

Brazy PC. Epidemiology and prevention of renal disease. *Curr Opin Nephrol Hypertens* 1993;2:211–215.

Brazy PC, Stead WW, Fitzwilliam JF. Progression of renal insufficiency: role of blood pressure. *Kidney Int* 1989;35: 670–674.

Brenner BM, Yu ASL. Uremic syndrome revisited: a pathogenetic role for retained endogenous inhibitors of nitric oxide synthesis. *Curr Opin Nephrol Hypertens* 1992;1:3–7.

Bresticker M, Nelson J, Wolf J, Anderson B. Plasma renin activity in renal transplant patients with hypertension. *Am J Hypertens* 1991;4:623–626.

Breyer JA, Jacobson HR. Ischemic nephropathy. *Curr Opin Nephrol Hypertens* 1993;2:216–224.

Brown MA, Whitworth JA. Hypertension in human renal disease. *J Hypertens* 1992;10: 701–712.

Brunner HR. ACE inhibitors in renal disease. *Kidney Int* 1992;42:463–479.

Campbell DJ, Kladis A, Skinner SL, Whitworth JA. Characterization of angiotensin peptides in plasma of anephric man. *J Hypertens* 1991;9:265–274.

Campieri C, Mignani R, Prandini R, Terni A, Fatone F, Bonomini V. Doppler ultrasonography in the evaluation of renal graft artery stenosis. *Nephron* 1988;48:341–342.

Carr S, Mbanya J-C, Thomas T, Keavey P, Taylor R, Alberti KGMM, Wilkinson R. Increase in glomerular filtration rate in patients with insulin-dependent diabetes and elevated erythrocyte sodium-lithium countertransport. *N Engl J Med* 1990;322: 500–505.

Chapman AB, Johnson A, Gabow PA, Schrier RW. The renin-angiotensin-aldosterone system and autosomal dominant polycystic kidney disease. *N Engl J Med* 1990; 323:1091–1096.

Cheigh JS, Milite C, Sullivan JF, Rubin AL, Stenzel KH. Hypertension is not adequately controlled in hemodialysis patients. *Am J Kidney Dis* 1992;19:453–459.

Christensen CK, Krusell LR, Mogensen CE. Increased blood pressure in diabetes: essential hypertension or diabetic nephropathy? *Scand J Clin Lab Invest* 1987;47: 363–370.

Coleman TG, Bower JD, Langford HG, Guyton AC. Regulation of arterial pressure in the anephric state. *Circulation* 1970;17: 509–514.

Converse RL Jr, Jacobsen TN, Jost CMT, Toto RD, Grayburn PA, Obregon TM, Fouad-Tarazi F, Victor RG. Paradoxical withdrawal of reflex vasoconstriction as a cause of hemodialysis-induced hypotension. *J Clin Invest* 1992a;90:1657–1665.

Converse RL Jr, Jacobsen TN, Jost CMT, Toto RD, Jost CMT, Cosentino F, Fouad-Tarazi F, Victor RG. Sympathetic overactivity in patients with chronic renal failure. *N Engl J Med* 1992b;327:1912–1918.

Cooper ME, Rumble JR, Allen TJ, O'Brien RC, Jerums G, Doyle AE. Antihypertensive therapy in a model combining spontaneous hypertension with diabetes. *Kidney Int* 1992;41:898–903.

Curtis JJ, Luke RG, Diethelm AG, Whelchel JD, Jones P. Benefits of removal of native kidneys in hypertension after renal transplantation. *Lancet* 1985;2:739–742.

Curtis JJ, Luke GR, Dustan HP, Kashgarian M, Whelchel JD, Jones P, Diethelm AG. Remission of essential hypertension after renal transplantation. *N Engl J Med* 1983; 309:1009–1015.

Daugirdas JT. Dialysis hypotension: a hemodynamic analysis. *Kidney Int* 1991;39: 233–246.

Dahl T, Eide I, Fryjordet A. Hypernephroma and hypertension. *Acta Med Scand* 1981;209:121–124.

de Jong PE, Anderson S, de Zeeuw D. Glomerular preload and afterload reduction as a tool to lower urinary protein leakage: will such treatments also help to improve renal function outcome? *J Am Soc Nephrol* 1993;3:1333–1341.

Diabetes Control and Complications Trial Research Group. The effect of intensive treatment of diabetes on the development and progression of long-term complications in insulin-dependent diabetes mellitus. *N Engl J Med* 1993;329:977–986.

Diamond S, Henrich WL. When acute renal failure complicates severe hypertension. *J Crit Illness* 1986;1:37–50.

Dillon JJ. The relationship between treated blood pressure level and progression of diabetic renal disease [Abstract]. *J Am Soc Nephrol* 1992;3:331.

Dubach UC, Rosner B, Stürmer T. An epidemiologic study of abuse of analgesic drugs. Effects of phenacetin and salicylate on mortality and cardiovascular morbidity (1968 to 1987). *N Engl J Med* 1991;324: 155–160.

El-Dahr SS, Dipp S, Gee J, Hanss B, Vari RC, Chao J. Ureteral obstruction activates renin-angiotensin and suppresses kallikrein-kinin systems [Abstract]. *J Am Soc Nephrol* 1992;3:737.

Epstein M. Calcium antagonists and renal protection. *Arch Intern Med* 1992;152: 1573–1584.

Fahal IH, Yaqoob M, Ahmad R. Phlebotomy for erythropoietin-induced malignant hypertension. *Nephron* 1992;61:214–216.

Falk RJ, Scheinman J, Phillips G, Orringer F, Johnson A, Jennette JC. Prevalence and pathologic features of sickle cell nephropathy and response to inhibition of angiotensin-converting enzyme. *N Engl J Med* 1992; 326:910–915.

Feldt-Rasmussen B, Mathiesen ER, Jensen T, Lauritzen T, Deckert T. Effect of improved metabolic control on loss of kidney function in type 1 (insulin-dependent) diabetic patients: an update of the Steno studies. *Diabetologia* 1991;34:164–170.

Fujihara CK, Padilha RM, Zatz R. Glomerular abnormalities in long-term experimental diabetes. Role of hemodynamic and nonhemodynamic factors and effects of antihypertensive therapy. *Diabetes* 1992;41: 286–293.

Gabow PA, Johnson AM, Kaehny WD, Kimberling WJ, Lezotte DC, Duley IT, Jones RH. Factors affecting the progression of renal disease in autosomal-dominant polycystic kidney disease. *Kidney Int* 1992;41:1311–1319.

Ghose RR, Harindra V. Unrecognised high pressure chronic retention of urine presenting with systemic arterial hypertension. *Br Med J* 1989;298:1626–1628.

Gordon RD, Tunny TJ, Evans EB, Fisher PM, Jackson RV. Unstimulated renal venous renin ratio predicts improvement in hypertension following nephrectomy for unilateral renal disease. *Nephron* 1986;44(Suppl 1): 25–28.

Guidi E, Bianchi G, Rivolta E, Ponticelli C, di Palo FQ, Minetti L, Polli E. Hypertension in man with a kidney transplant: role of familial versus other factors. *Nephron* 1985;41:14–21.

Hammond JJ, Raffaele J, Liddel N, Doyle AE, Costello A, Amerena J. A prospective study to evaluate the effects of extra corporeal shock wave lithotripsy (ESWL) on blood pressure (BP), renal function (RF) and glomerular filtration (GFR) [Abstract]. *J Am Coll Cardiol* 1993;21:257.

Heeg JE, de Jong PE, de Zeeuw D. Additive antiproteinuric effect of angiotensin-converting enzyme inhibition and non-steroidal anti-inflammatory drug therapy: a clue to the mechanism of action. *Clin Sci* 1991; 81:367–372.

Hellebusch AA, Simmons JL, Holland N. Renal ischemia and hypertension from a constrictive perirenal hematoma. *JAMA* 1970;214:757–759.

Hommel E, Mathiesen ER, Giese J, Nielsen MD, Schütten HJ, Parving H-H. On the pathogenesis of arterial blood pressure elevation early in the course of diabetic nephropathy. *Scand J Clin Lab Invest* 1989; 49:537–544.

Hostetter TH. Diabetic nephropathy. Metabolic versus hemodynamic considerations. *Diabetes Care* 1992;15:1205–1215.

Ihle BU, Becker GJ, Whitworth JA, Charlwood RA, Kincaid-Smith PS. The effect of protein restriction on the progression of renal insufficiency. *N Engl J Med* 1989; 321:1773–1777.

Jacobson HR. Chronic renal failure: pathophysiology. *Lancet* 1991;338:419–423.

Jacobson SH, Eklöf O, Eriksson CG, Lins L-E, Tidgren B, Winberg J. Development of hypertension and uraemia after pyelonephritis in childhood: 27 year follow up. *Br Med J* 1989;299:703–706.

Jacobson SH, Lins L-E. Renal hemodynamics and blood pressure control in patients with pyelonephritic renal scarring. *Acta Med Scand* 1988;224:39–45.

Jensen JS, Mathiesen ER, Nrgaard K. Hommel E, Borch-Johnsen K, Funder J, Brahm J, Parving H-H, Deckert T. Increased blood pressure and erythrocyte sodium/lithium countertransport activity are not inherited in diabetic nephropathy. *Diabetologia* 1990;33:619–624.

Johnson RJ, Alpers CE, Yoshimura A, Lombardi D, Pritzl P, Floege J, Schwartz SM. Renal injury from angiotensin II–mediated hypertension. *Hypertension* 1992;19: 464–474.

Jones DA, George NJR, O'Reilly PH, Barnard RJ. Reversible hypertension associated with unrecognised high pressure chronic retention of urine. *Lancet* 1987;1: 1052–1054.

Kakinuma Y, Kawamura T, Bills T, Yoshioka T, Ichikawa I, Fogo A. Blood pressure-independent effect of angiotensin inhibition on vascular lesions of chronic renal failure. *Kidney Int* 1992;42:46–55.

Kamper A-L, Strandgaard S, Leyssac PP. Effect of enalapril on the progression of chronic renal failure. A randomized controlled trial. *Am J Hypertens* 1992;5: 423–430.

Kasiske BL, Kalil RSN, Ma JZ, Liao M, Keane WF. Effect of antihypertensive therapy on the kidney in patients with diabetes: a meta-regression analysis. *Ann Intern Med* 1993;118:129–138.

Kim KE, Onesti G, DelGuercio ET, Greco J, Fernandes M, Eidelson B, Swartz C. Sequential hemodynamic changes in end-stage renal disease and the anephric state during volume expansion. *Hypertension* 1980;2:102–110.

Kimmelstiel P, Wilson C. Intercapillary lesions in the glomeruli of the kidney. *Am J Pathol* 1936;12:83–97.

Kincaid-Smith P, Whitworth JA. Pathogenesis of hypertension in chronic renal disease. *Semin Nephrol* 1988;8:155–162.

Kishimoto T, Terada T, Okahara T, Abe Y, Yamagami S, Maekawa M. Correlation between blood prostaglandins and blood pressure in chronic renal failure. *Nephron* 1987;47:49–55.

Klahr S. The modification of diet in renal disease study. *N Engl J Med* 1989;320: 864–866.

Klahr S. Chronic renal failure: management. *Lancet* 1991;338:423–427.

Klein R, Klein BEK, Linton KLP, Moss SE. Microalbuminuria in a population-based study of diabetes. *Arch Intern Med* 1992; 152:153–158.

Kloke HJ, Wetzels JFM, van Hamersvelt HW, Koene RAP, Kleinbloesem CH, Huysmans FThM. Effects of nitrendipine and cilazapril on renal hemodynamics and albuminuria in hypertensive patients with chronic renal failure. *J Cardiovasc Pharmacol* 1990;16:924–930.

Koskimies O. Arterial hypertension developing 10 years after radiotherapy for Wilm's tumour. *Br Med J* 1982;285:996–998.

Krolewski AS, Canessa M, Warram JH, Laffel LMB, Christlieb AR, Knowler WC, Rand LI. Predisposition to hypertension and susceptibility to renal disease in insulin-dependent diabetes mellitus. *N Engl J Med* 1988;318:140–145.

Lamberton RP, Noth RH, Glickman M. Frequent falsely negative renal vein renin tests in unilateral renal parenchymal disease. *J Urol* 1981;125:477–480.

Laskow DA, Curtis JJ. Post-transplant hypertension. *Am J Hypertens* 1990;3:721–725.

Lazarus JM, Hampers CL, Bennett AH, Vandam LD, Merrill JP. Urgent bilateral nephrectomy for severe hypertension. *Ann Intern Med* 1972;76:733–739.

Ledingham JM. Sodium retention and volume expansion. *Am J Hypertens* 1991;4:534S–540S.

Leenen FHH, Smith DL, Khanna R, Oreopoulos DG. Changes in left ventricular hypertrophy and function in hypertensive patients started on continuous ambulatory peritoneal dialysis. *Am Heart J* 1985;110:102–106.

Lewis EJ, Hunsicker LG, Bain RP, Rohde RD, for the Collaborative Study Group. The effect of angiotensin-converting–enzyme inhibition on diabetic nephropathy. *N Engl J Med* 1993;329:1456–1462.

Luetscher JA, Kraemer FB. Microalbuminuria and increased plasma prorenin. Prevalence in diabetics followed up for four years. *Arch Intern Med* 1988;148:937–941.

Luke RG. Hypertension in renal transplant recipients. *Kidney Int* 1987;31:1024–1037.

Mangili R, Bending JJ, Scott G, Li LK, Gupta A, Viberti GC. Increased sodium-lithium countertransport activity in red cells of patients with insulin-dependent diabetes and nephropathy. *N Engl J Med* 1988;318:146–150.

Mattock MB, Morrish NJ, Viberti G, Keen H, Fitzgerald AP, Jackson G. Prospective study of microalbuminuria as predictor of mortality in NIDDM. *Diabetes* 1992;41:736–741.

Mauer SM, Sutherland DER, Steffes MW. Relationship of systemic blood pressure to nephropathology in insulin-dependent diabetes mellitus. *Kidney Int* 1992;41:736–740.

Miller PL, Rennke HG, Meyer TW. Hypertension and progressive glomerular injury caused by focal glomerular ischemia. *Am J Physiol* 1990;259:F239–F245.

Mitch WE, Wilcox CS. Disorders of body fluids, sodium and potassium in chronic renal failure. *Am J Med* 1982;72:536–550.

Mizuiri S, Amagasaki Y, Hosaka H, Fukasawa K, Nakayama K, Nakamura N, Sakaguchi H. Hypertension in unilateral atrophic kidney secondary to ureteropelvic junction obstruction. *Nephron* 1992;61:217–219.

Mogensen CE. Management of renal disease and hypertension in insulin-dependent diabetes, with an emphasis on early nephropathy. *Curr Opin Nephrol Hypertens* 1992;1:106–115.

Mogensen CE, Petersen MM, Hansen KW, Christensen CK. Micro-albuminuria and the organ-damage concept in antihypertensive therapy for patients with insulin-dependent diabetes mellitus. *J Hypertens* 1992;10(Suppl 1):43–51.

Moore MA, Porush JG. Hypertension and renal insufficiency: recognition and management. *Am Family Phys* 1992;45:1248–1256.

Murdoch D, McTavish D. Fosinopril. A review of its pharmacodynamic and pharmacokinetic properties, and therapeutic potential in essential hypertension. *Drugs* 1992;43:123–140.

Murray MD, Brater DC, Tierney WM, Hui SL, McDonald CJ. Ibuprofen-associated renal impairment in a large general internal medicine practice. *Am J Med Sci* 1990;299:222–229.

Najarian JS, Chavers BM, McHugh LE, Matas AJ. 20 years or more of follow-up on living kidney donors. *Lancet* 1992;340:807–810.

National High Blood Pressure Education Program. National High Blood Pressure Education Program Working Group Report on Hypertension and Chronic Renal Failure. *Arch Intern Med* 1991;151:1280–1287.

Nelson RG, Knowler WC, Pettitt DJ, Saad MF, Charles MA, Bennett PH. Assessment of risk of overt nephropathy in diabetic patients from albumin excretion in untimed urine specimens. *Arch Intern Med* 1991;151:1761–1765.

Novick AC, Gephardt G, Guz B, Steinmuller D, Tubbs RR. Long-term follow-up after partial removal of a solitary kidney. *N Engl J Med* 1991;325:1058–1062.

Orchard TJ, Dorman JS, Maser RE, Becker DJ, Drash AL, Ellis D, LaPorte RE, Kuller LH. Prevalence of complications in IDDM by sex and duration. Pittsburgh Epidemiology of Diabetes Complications Study II. *Diabetes* 1990;39:1116–1124.

Orofino L, Quereda C, Lamas S, Orte L, Gonzalo A, Mampaso F, Ortuno J. Hypertension in primary chronic glomerulonephritis: analysis of 288 biopsied patients. *Nephron* 1987;45:22–26.

Parra G, Rodriguez-Iturbe B, Colina-Chourio J, Garcia R. Short-term treatment with captopril in hypertension due to acute glomerulonephritis. *Clin Nephrol* 1988;29:58–62.

Parving H-H. Impact of blood pressure and antihypertensive treatment on incipient and overt nephropathy, retinopathy, and endothelial permeability in diabetes mellitus. *Diabetes Care* 1991;14:260–269.

Parving H-H, Andersen AR, Smidt UM, Hommel E, Mathiesen ER, Svendsen PA. Effect of antihypertensive treatment on kidney function in diabetic nephropathy. *Br Med J* 1987;294:1443–1447.

Parving H-H, Smidt UM, Mathiesen ER, Hommel E. Ten year's experiences with antihypertensive treatment in diabetic nephropathy [Abstract]. *Diabetologia* 1991;34(Suppl 2):A38.

Pattison JM, Reidy JF, Rafferty MJ, Ogg CS, Cameron JS, Sacks SH, Williams DG. Percutaneous transluminal renal angioplasty in patients with renal failure. *Q J Med* 1992;85:883–888.

Pedersen MM, Christiansen JS, Pedersen EB, Mogensen CE. Determinants of intra-individual variation in kidney function in normoalbuminuric insulin-dependent diabetic patients: importance of atrial natriuretic peptide and glycaemic control. *Clin Sci* 1992;83:445–451.

Perez GO, Lespier L, Knowles R, Oster JR, Vaamonde CA. Potassium homeostasis in chronic diabetes mellitus. *Arch Intern Med* 1977;137:1018–1022.

Perneger TV, Nieto FJ, Whelton PK, Klag MJ, Comstock GW, Szklo M. A prospective study of blood pressure and serum creatinine. *JAMA* 1993;269:488–493.

Pettinger WA, Lee HC, Reisch J, Mitchell HC. Long-term improvement in renal function after short-term strict blood pressure control in hypertensive nephrosclerosis. *Hypertension* 1989;13:766–772.

Podjarny E, Richter S, Magen H, Bachar L, Bernheim J. High incidence of hypertension in older patients after unilateral nephrectomy. *Isr J Med Sci* 1986;22:861–864.

Pontremoli R, Robaudo C, Gaiter A, Massarino F, Deferrari G. Long-term minoxidil treatment in refractory hypertension and renal failure. *Clin Nephrol* 1991;35:39–43.

Popivic-Rolovic M, Kostic M, Antic-Peco A, Jovanovic O, Popovic D. Medium- and long-term prognosis of patients with acute poststreptococcal glomerulonephritis. *Nephron* 1991;58:393–399.

Portaluppi F, Montanari L, Massari M, Di Chiara V, Capanna M. Loss of nocturnal decline of blood pressure in hypertension due to chronic renal failure. *Am J Hypertens* 1991;4:20–26.

Raman GV. Post transplant hypertension. *J Hum Hypertens* 1991;5:1–6.

Rao TKS, Gupta SK, Butt KMH, Kountz SL, Friedman EA. Relationship of renal transplantation to hypertension in end-stage renal failure. *Arch Intern Med* 1978;138:1236–1241.

Ravid M, Savin H, Jutrin I, Bental T, Katz B, Lishner M. Long-term stabilizing effect of angiotensin-converting enzyme inhibition on plasma creatinine and on proteinuria in normotensive type II diabetic patients. *Ann Intern Med* 1993;118:577–581.

Remuzzi A, Perticucci E, Ruggenenti P, Mosconi L, Limonta M, Remuzzi G. Angiotensin converting enzyme inhibition improves glomerular size-selectivity in IgA nephropathy. *Kidney Int* 1991;39:1267–1273.

Rimmer JM, Gennari FJ. Atherosclerotic renovascular disease and progressive renal failure. *Ann Intern Med* 1993;118:712–719.

Riser BL, Cortes P, Zhao X, Bernstein J, Dumler F, Narins RG. Intraglomerular pressure and mesangial stretching stimulate extracellular matrix formation in the rat. *J Clin Invest* 1992;90:1932–1943.

Robinson FO, Johnston SR, Atkinson AB. Accelerated hypertension caused by severe phimosis. *J Hum Hypertens* 1992;6:165–166.

Rostand SG, Brunzell JD, Cannon RO III, Victor RG. Cardiovascular complications in renal failure. *J Am Soc Nephrol* 1991;2:1053–1062.

Rudy DW, Voelker JR, Greene PK, Esparza FA, Brater DC. Loop diuretics for chronic renal insufficiency: a continuous infusion is more efficacious than bolus therapy. *Ann Intern Med* 1991;115:360–366.

Sacks SH, Aparicio SAJR, Bevan A, Oliver DO, Will EJ, Davison AM. Late renal failure due to prostatic outflow obstruction: a preventable disease. *Br Med J* 1989;298:156–159.

Sagalowsky AI, Gailiunas P, Helderman JH, Hull AR, Dickerman RM, Ransler CW, Atkins C, Peters PC. Renal transplantation in diabetic patients: the end result does justify the means. *J Urol* 1983;129: 253–255.

Salmond R, Seney FD Jr. Reset tubuloglomerular feedback permits and sustains glomerular hyperfunction after extensive renal ablation. *Am J Physiol* 1991;260: F395–F401.

Sandler DP, Burr R, Weinberg CR. Nonsteroidal anti-inflammatory drugs and the risk for chronic renal disease. *Ann Intern Med* 1991;115:165–172.

Scholey JW, Meyer TW. Control of glomerular hypertension by insulin administration in diabetic rats. *J Clin Invest* 1989;83: 1384–1389.

Seaquist ER, Goetz FC, Rich S, Barbosa J. Familial clustering of diabetic kidney disease. Evidence for genetic susceptibility to diabetic nephropathy. *N Engl J Med* 1989; 320:1161–1165.

Shankel SW, Johnson DC, Clark PS, Shankel TL, O'Neil WM Jr. Acute renal failure and glomerulopathy caused by nonsteroidal anti-inflammatory drugs. *Arch Intern Med* 1992;152:986–990.

Sheinfeld J, Linke CL, Talley TE, Linke CA. Selective pre-transplant nephrectomy: indications and perioperative management. *J Urol* 1985;133:379–382.

Siamopoulos K, Sellars L, Mishra SC, Essenhigh DM, Robson V, Wilkinson R. Experience in the management of hypertension with unilateral chronic pylonephritis: results of nephrectomy in selected patients. *Q J Med* 1983;52:349–362.

Smith HW. Unilateral nephrectomy in hypertensive disease. *J Urol* 1956;76:685–701.

Smith LH, Drach G, Hall P, Lingeman J, Preminger G. Resnick MI, Segura JW. National High Blood Pressure Education Program (NHBPEP) review paper on complications of shock wave lithotripsy for urinary calculi. *Am J Med* 1991;91:635–641.

Smith SR, Svetkey KP, Dennis VW. Racial differences in the incidence and progression of renal diseases. *Kidney Int* 1991; 40:815–822.

Spieker C, Barenbrock M, Suwelack B, Rahn K-H, Zidek W. Polycythemia-associated hypertension in renal transplantation: efficiency of phlebotomy [Abstract]. *J Hypertens* 1992;10(Suppl 4):107.

Spitalewitz S, Porush JG, Reiser IW. Minoxidil, nadolol, and a diuretic. Once-a-day therapy for resistant hypertension. *Arch Intern Med* 1986;146:882–886.

Stehouwer CDA, Nauta JJP, Zeldenrust GC, Hackeng WHL, Donker AJM, den Ottolander GJH. Urinary albumin excretion, cardiovascular disease, and endothelial dysfunction in non–insulin-dependent diabetes mellitus. *Lancet* 1992;340:319–323.

Stornello M, Valvo EV, Scapellato L. Persistent albuminuria in normotensive non–insulin-dependent (type II) diabetic patients: comparative effects of angiotensin-converting enzyme inhibitors and β-adrenoceptor blockers. *Clin Sci* 1992;82:19–23.

Strandgaard S, Hansen U. Hypertension in renal allograft recipients may be conveyed by cadaveric kidneys from donors with subarachnoid haemorrhage. *Br Med J* 1986;292:1041–1044.

Taguma Y, Kitamoto Y, Futaki G, Ueda H, Monma H, Ishizaki M, Takahashi H, Sekino H, Sasaki Y. Effect of captopril on heavy proteinuria in azotemic diabetics. *N Engl J Med* 1985;313:1617–1620.

Tolins JP, Raij L. Antihypertensive therapy and the progression of chronic renal disease. Are there renoprotective drugs? *Semin Nephrol* 1991;11:538–548.

Torres VE, Donovan KA, Scicli G, Holley KE, Thibodeau SN, Carretero OA, Inagami T, McAteer JA, Johnson CM. Synthesis of renin by tubulocystic epithelium in autosomal-dominant polycystic kidney disease. *Kidney Int* 1992;42:364–373.

Torres VE, Wilson DM, Burnett JC Jr, Johnson CM, Offord KP. Effect of inhibition of converting enzyme on renal hemodynamics and sodium management in polycystic kidney disease. *Mayo Clin Proc* 1991;66:1010–1017.

Tuttle KR, DeFronzo RA, Stein JH. Treatment of diabetic nephropathy: a rational approach based on its pathophysiology. *Semin Nephrol* 1991;11:220–235.

Tuttle KR, Stein JM, DeFronzo RA. The natural history of diabetic nephropathy. *Semin Nephrol* 1990;10:184–193.

Uribarri J, Oh MS, Carroll HJ. Salt-losing nephropathy. Clinical presentation and mechanisms. *Am J Nephrol* 1983; 3:193–198.

Vallance P, Leone A, Calver A, Collier J, Moncada S. Accumulation of an endogenous inhibitor of nitric oxide synthesis in chronic renal failure. *Lancet* 1992;339: 572–575.

Vierhapper H, Derfler K, Nowotny P, Hollenstein U, Waldhäusl W. Impaired conversion of cortisol to cortisone in chronic renal insufficiency—a cause of hypertension or an epiphenomenon? *Acta Endocrinol (Copenh)* 1991;125:160–164.

Watts RA, Hoffbrand BI. Hypertension following renal trauma. *J Hum Hypertens* 1987;1:65–71.

Weidmann P, Boehlen LM, de Courten M. Pathogenesis and treatment of hypertension associated with diabetes mellitus. *Am Heart J* 1993;125:1498–1513.

Wesson LG. Unilateral renal disease and hypertension. *Nephron* 1982;31:1–7.

Wollam GL, Tarazi RC, Bravo EL, Dustan HP. Diuretic potency of combined hydrochlorothiazide and furosemide therapy in patients with azotemia. *Am J Med* 1982; 72:929–937.

Yamamoto T, Shimizu M, Morioka M, Kitano M, Wakabayashi H, Aizawa N. Role of angiotensin II in the pathogenesis of hyperdipsia in chronic renal failure. *JAMA* 1986;256:604–608.

Ying CY, Tifft CP, Gavras H, Chobanian AV. Renal revascularization in the azotemic hypertensive patient resistant to therapy. *N Engl J Med* 1984;311:1070–1075.

Yoshida Y, Fogo A, Ichikawa I. Glomerular hemodynamic changes vs. hypertrophy in experimental glomerular sclerosis. *Kidney Int* 1989a;35:654–660.

Yoshida Y, Kawamura T, Ikoma M, Fogo A, Ichikawa I. Effects of antihypertensive drugs on glomerular morphology. *Kidney Int* 1989b;36:626–635.

Zawada ET Jr, Clements PJ, Furst DA, Bloomer HA, Paulus HE, Maxwell MH. Clinical course of patients with scleroderma renal crisis treated with captopril. *Nephron* 1981;27:74–78.

Zeller K, Whittaker E, Sullivan L, Raskin P, Jacobson HR. Effect of restricting dietary protein on the progression of renal failure in patients with insulin-dependent diabetes mellitus. *N Engl J Med* 1991;324:78–84.

10 Renal Vascular Hypertension

Renovascular disease is one of the more common causes of secondary hypertension; reports of its frequency vary from less than 1% in unselected populations to as many as 20% of patients referred to special centers.

RENOVASCULAR DISEASE VERSUS RENOVASCULAR HYPERTENSION

Renovascular hypertension (RVHT) refers to hypertension caused by renal hypoperfusion. It is important to realize that renovascular disease may or may not cause sufficient hypoperfusion to set off the processes that lead to hypertension. The problem is simply that renovascular disease is much more common than RVHT is. For example, arteriography revealed some degree of renal artery stenosis in 32% of 304 normotensive patients and in 67% of 193 hypertensives with an increasing prevalence with advancing age (Eyler et al., 1962) (Table 10.1). Note that almost half of normotensive patients over 60 had atherosclerotic lesions in their renal vessels.

Before procedures were available to prove the functional significance of stenotic lesions, surgery was frequently performed on hyperten-

sive patients with a unilateral small kidney who did not have reversible RVHT. Homer Smith recognized this as early as 1948 as a misguided application of Goldblatt's experimental model of hypertension induced by clamping the renal artery. Smith found that only 25% of patients were relieved of their hypertension by nephrectomy and warned that only about 2% of all hypertensives probably could be helped by surgery (Smith, 1956).

PREVALENCE

Smith's estimate of the true prevalence of RVHT may be right. The prevalence varies with the nature of the hypertensive population:

—In nonselected patient populations, the prevalence is less than 1%, as noted in Table 1.7;
—Among patients referred for diagnostic studies, 1% to 4% have RVHT (Gifford, 1969; Danielson and Dammström, 1981);
—In patients with suggestive clinical features, the prevalence is higher. Among 490 patients with severe, resistant, or rapidly progressive hypertension, RVHT was found in only 1 of

Table 10.1. Prevalence of Renal Arterial Lesions in Normotensive and Hypertensive Patients[a]

Age (Years)	Normotensive		Hypertensive	
	Normal	Lesion	Normal	Lesion
31–40	7	3	6	10
41–50	26	8	14	22
51–60	99	35	28	50
Over 60	69	56	15	48

[a]Data from Eyler WR, Clark MD, Garman JE, et al. Angiography of the renal areas including a comparative study of renal arterial stenoses in patients with and without hypertension. *Radiology* 1962;78:879.

the 152 below age 40 but in 50 of 338 (15%) of those over age 40, (Horvath et al., 1982);

— Among patients with accelerated or malignant hypertension, the prevalence is even higher. Of 123 adults with diastolic blood pressure (DBP) > 125 mm Hg and grade III or IV retinopathy, 4% of the blacks and 32% of the whites had RVHT (Davis et al., 1979);

— Renovascular disease also is seen more frequently in hypertensive patients with atherosclerotic disease in peripheral, carotid, or coronary arteries (Choudhri et al., 1990; Hurwitz et al., 1990) and in patients with severe hypertension and rapidly progressing renal insufficiency, particularly if it develops after institution of angiotensin-converting enzyme (ACE) inhibitor therapy (Brunner, 1992). On the other hand, RHVT is less common in blacks, found in 9% of blacks versus 18% of whites with suggestive clinical features (Svetkey et al., 1991); RVHT also is less common in diabetics (Munichoodappa et al., 1979), even though they have a higher prevalence of renovascular disease (Sawicki et al., 1991);

— RVHT has been recognized in neonates (Tapper et al., 1987), children (Berkowitz and O'Neill, 1989), and pregnant women (Easterling et al., 1991).

MECHANISMS

Animal Models

A massive body of literature has appeared since Goldblatt and coworkers (1934) first induced hypertension in dogs by partially occluding one renal artery and removing the opposite kidney. Although an increased secretion of renin from the clipped kidney was demonstrated relatively early (Braun-Menendez et al., 1939), it took many more years to reach general agreement that increased renin secretion is responsible for the hypertension caused by renal hypoperfusion (Barger, 1979), whereas renal retention of sodium is the primary mechanism for hypertension resulting from loss of renal tissue (see Chapter 9).

Original Goldblatt Experiment

Goldblatt and coworkers (1934), looking not for RVHT but for a renal cause for essential hypertension, put clamps on both renal arteries of their dogs. Fortunately, the clamps were inserted on separate occasions so that Goldblatt could observe the effect of unilateral obstruction

(Fig. 10.1). However, with the modest degree of constriction that they used, unilateral clamping caused only transient hypertension. For permanent hypertension, both renal arteries had to be clamped, or one clamped and the contralateral kidney removed (Goldblatt, 1975). The sheep and rat have been found to be particularly susceptible to two-kidney, one-clip hypertension, so they are better models than dogs and rabbits for the human (Edmunds et al., 1991).

Two-Kidney, One-Clip Versus One-Kidney, One-Clip

The experimental counterpart to RVHT in the human is unilateral clamping of the renal artery with the contralateral kidney untouched (i.e., "two-kidney, one-clip Goldblatt hypertension"). When one renal artery is clipped and the other kidney is removed (i.e., "one-kidney, one-clip Goldblatt hypertension"), a greater component of sodium retention is introduced, simply by the relative lack of functioning renal mass (de Simone et al., 1992). This then is a model for RVHT plus chronic renal parenchymal dis-

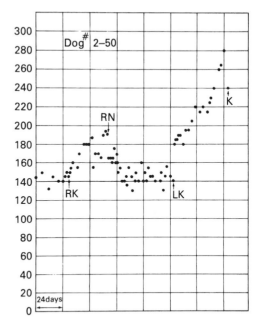

Figure 10.1. One of Goldblatt's original experiments. The graph shows the mean blood pressure of a dog whose right kidney was first moderately constricted (*RK*), with subsequent hypertension that was relieved after right nephrectomy (*RN*). After severe constriction of the left renal artery (*LK*), more severe hypertension occurred and the animal was sacrificed (*K*). (From Hoobler SW. History of experimental renovascular hypertension. In: Stanley JC, Ernst CB, Fry WJ, eds. *Renovascular Hypertension.* Philadelphia: WB Saunders, 1984:12–19.)

ease. In the two-kidney, one-clip model, sodium excretion is increased from the intact contralateral kidney as the pressure rises (i.e., pressure-natriuresis), so there is little sodium retention (Pickering, 1989). Since the two-kidney, one-clip model is more appropriate to RVHT as seen in humans, only this model will be considered further.

After the initial marked rise in renin secretion, renin levels fall but remain inappropriately high and are largely responsible for the hemodynamic changes (Anderson et al., 1990).

Mechanisms Beyond Renin and Volume

Other factors may be involved that interrelate to these primary mechanisms, including the following:

—Activation of the sympathetic nervous system acting through renal nerves (Zimmerman et al., 1987);

—Vasopressin (Ichikawa et al., 1983);

—Endogenous opioid system: administration of an opioid antagonist attenuated development of hypertension in two-kidney, one-clip Goldblatt rats (Chen et al., 1988);

—Increased thromboxane or reduced vasodilatory prostaglandins (Martinez-Maldonado, 1991). A role for renal prostaglandins is supported by the significant fall in BP noted in patients with RVHT who were given aspirin (Imanishi et al., 1989);

—Increased levels of atrial natriuretic factor and kallikrein may attempt to counter the effects of the activated renin-angiotensin system (Martinez-Maldonado, 1991).

Mechanism in Humans

As in the animal models, RVHT in humans is caused by increased renin release from the stenotic kidney (Pickering, 1989). An immediate release of renin has been measured in patients whose renal perfusion pressure was acutely reduced by a balloon-tipped catheter (Fiorentini et al., 1981). The high levels of angiotensin II increase renal vascular resistance, causing a shift in the pressure-natriuresis curve; thus, volume is maintained despite markedly elevated BP (Kimura et al., 1987). Chronically, the stenotic kidney continues to secrete excess renin; fluid volume and peripheral resistance are both elevated (Tarazi and Dustan, 1973). The BP falls when angiotensin antagonists are given and, when the stenosis is relieved, hypertension recedes by a fall in peripheral resistance and fluid volume (Valvo et al., 1987).

As in animal models, humans may enter into a third phase, wherein removal of the stenosis or the entire affected kidney will not relieve the hypertension because of widespread arteriolar damage and glomerulosclerosis in the contralateral kidney by prolonged exposure to high BP and high levels of angiotensin II (Kimura et al., 1991). This phenomenon is clinically relevant: the sooner an arterial lesion that is causing RVHT is removed, the greater the chance of relieving the hypertension. Among 110 patients, corrective surgery for unilateral RVHT was successful in 78% of those with hypertension of less than 5 years' duration but in only 25% of those with a longer duration (Hughes et al., 1981).

Figure 10.2 shows a stepwise scheme for the hemodynamic and hormonal changes that underlie RVHT.

CLASSIFICATION OF RENAL ARTERIAL LESIONS

The majority of renal arterial lesions are atherosclerotic; most of the rest are fibroplastic, but a number of other intrinsic and extrinsic lesions can induce RVHT (Table 10.2). In India, the majority of 205 cases of RVHT seen in one center were caused by progressive aortic arteritis (Takayasu's syndrome) (Chugh et al., 1992). In addition, intrarenal vasculitis can induce hypertension, presumably by producing multiple areas of ischemia.

A classification of the fibrous and fibromuscular stenoses has been established by investigators from the Mayo Clinic (Lüscher et al., 1987) (Fig. 10.3). Of these, medial fibroplasia is the most common (Fig. 10.4). Focal fibroplastic lesions are most common in children (Stanley et al., 1978).

Segmental Disease and Renal Infarction

Stenosis of only a small branch supplying a segment of one kidney may set off RVHT, as was found in 11% of one large series (Bookstein, 1968). Bookstein further recognized the presence of collateral vessels around areas of segmental stenoses with renal infarcts caused by thrombi or emboli. Presumably, if such collaterals are not adequate to relieve the hypoperfusion but the renal tissue remains viable, hypersecretion of renin from the partially infarcted tissue occurs, and hypertension supervenes. After pro-

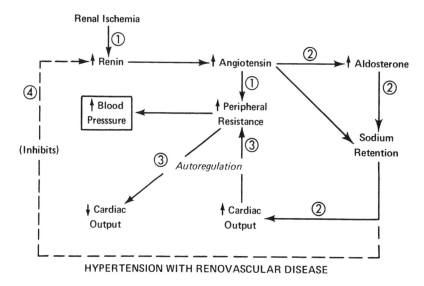

Figure 10.2. Hypertension with renovascular disease. Stepwise hemodynamic changes in the development of renovascular hypertension.

longed medical therapy, the hypertension may remit (Elkik et al., 1984).

CLINICAL FEATURES OF RVHT

General

Clinical features suggestive of renovascular disease as the cause of hypertension are presented in Table 10.3. Some of these features were identified in a cooperative study involving 2442 hypertensive patients, 880 with renovascular disease (Maxwell et al., 1972). Of the 880, 502 had surgery; of these, 60% had atherosclerotic lesions and 35% had fibromuscular disease. Patients with surgically cured renovascular disease were compared with a carefully matched group with essential hypertension (Table 10.4) (Simon et al., 1972).

Abdominal Bruit

Of the features more common in patients with RVHT, only an abdominal bruit was of clear discriminatory value, heard in 46% of those with RVHT but only in 9% of those with essential hypertension. The bruit was heard over the flank in 12% of those with RVHT and only in 1% of those with essential hypertension. Many bruits heard in the epigastrium reflect stenosis within the celiac artery (McLoughlin et al., 1975), but the characteristics of the bruit provide useful information: a bruit that is high-pitched, that is both systolic and diastolic, and that radiates laterally strongly suggests functionally signifi-

cant renal arterial stenosis; a diastolic bruit in a patient with fibrous disease usually indicates a favorable surgical result (Eipper et al., 1976).

Loss of Renal Function with ACEI Therapy

Patients whose renal function rapidly deteriorates after treatment with an ACEI probably have bilateral renovascular disease or a stenosis in the artery to a solitary kidney (Kalra et al., 1990). The loss of renal function reflects a generalized loss of systemic vasoconstriction by angiotensin II that is needed to maintain adequate blood flow beyond the stenosis as well as a specific dilation of renal efferent arterioles that reduces glomerular filtration. This phenomenon may also occur in the stenotic kidney of patients with unilateral renovascular disease and a normal contralateral kidney, but the loss can only be recognized by isotopic renography or other sensitive measures of renal perfusion (Wenting et al., 1984).

Atherosclerotic Versus Fibromuscular Disease

Table 10.5 summarizes the differences between the two major causes of RVHT—atherosclerosis and fibromuscular dysplasia.

Atherosclerotic Lesions

Patients with atherosclerotic renal artery disease are older and have more extensive renal damage, higher systolic pressure, and vascular disease elsewhere (Vidt, 1987). Their disease

Table 10.2. Types of Lesions Associated with Renovascular Hypertension

I. Intrinsic lesions
  A. Atherosclerosis
  B. Fibromuscular dysplasia
    1. Intimal
    2. Medial
      a. Dissection (Edwards et al., 1982)
      b. Segmental infarction (Elkik et al., 1984)
    3. Periarterial or periadventitial
  C. Aneurysm (Nicholas et al., 1992)
  D. Emboli (Preston and Materson, 1992)
  E. Arteritis
    1. Polyarteritis nodosa (Luger et al., 1981)
    2. Takayasu's (Shelhamer et al., 1985)
  F. Arteriovenous malformation or fistula (Ullian and Molitoris, 1987)
  G. Renal artery (Banitt and Clark, 1986) or aortic dissection (Rackson et al., 1990)
  H. Angioma (Farreras-Valenti, 1965)
  I. Neurofibromatosis (Pollard et al., 1989)[a]
  J. Tumor thrombus (Jennings et al., 1964)
  K. Thrombosis after antihypertensive therapy (Shaw and Gopalka, 1982)
  L. Rejection of renal transplant (Raman, 1991)
  M. Injury to the renal artery
    1. Thrombosis after umbilical artery catheterization (Tapper et al., 1987)[a]
    2. Surgical ligation (McCormack et al., 1974)
    3. Trauma (Monstrey et al., 1989)
    4. Radiation (Shapiro et al., 1977)
    5. Lithotripsy (Smith et al., 1991)
  N. Intrarenal cysts (Torres et al., 1991)
  O. Congenital unilateral renal hypoplasia (Ask-Upmark kidney) (Steffens et al., 1991)[a]
  P. Unilateral renal infection (Siamopoulos et al., 1983)
II. Extrinsic lesions
  A. Pheochromocytoma (Brewster et al., 1982)
  B. Congenital fibrous band (Silver and Clements, 1976)[a]
  C. Pressure from diaphragmatic crus (Martin, 1971)[a]
  D. Tumors (Restrick et al., 1992)
  E. Subcapsular or perirenal hematoma (Sterns et al., 1985)
  F. Retroperitoneal fibrosis (Castle, 1973)
  G. Ptosis (Takada et al., 1984)
  H. Ureteral obstruction (Sacks et al., 1989)
  I. Perirenal pseudocyst (Kato et al., 1985)
  J. Stenosis of celiac axis with "steal" of renal blood flow (Alfidi et al., 1972)

[a]More common in children.

tends to progress if the stenoses are not relieved even if the hypertension is controlled. Progression has been noted in about half of 237 such patients followed by multiple investigators for 1 to 15 years (Rimmer and Gennari, 1993).

Medial Fibroplasia

These lesions are usually noted in young women; the process often involves multiple arteries arising from the aorta, including the carotid and celiac vessels (Lüscher et al., 1987). Half of patients with bilateral renal artery medial fibroplasia have extrarenal disease as well, which is rarely symptomatic. Compared with atherosclerotic disease, a progressive course may be somewhat less frequently seen with medial fibroplasia. The following features were found more commonly in 33 patients with fibromuscular dysplasia than in 61 subjects with normal renal arteries: cigarette smoking, HLA-Drw6 antigen, and a family history of cardiovascular disease (Sang et al., 1989). On the other hand, there was no association with oral contraceptive use, abnormal endogenous sex hormone levels, or increased renal mobility.

Other Fibroplasias

Patients with the less common but more sharply localized fibroplastic lesions—intimal,

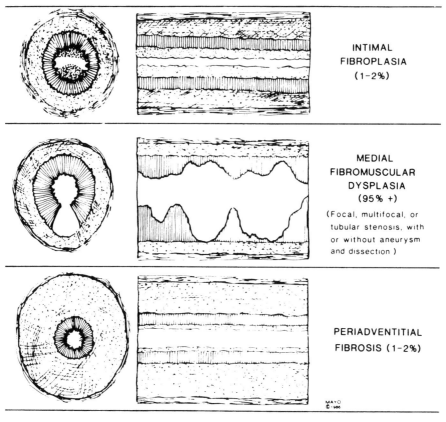

Figure 10.3. Histopathologic classification of arterial fibromuscular dysplasia, based on predominant site of involvement of arterial wall intima (*top*), media (*middle*), and adventitia (*bottom*). (From Lüscher TF, Lie JT, Stanson AW, Houser OW, Hollier LH, Sheps SG. Arterial fibromuscular dysplasia. *Mayo Clin Proc* 1987;62:931–952.)

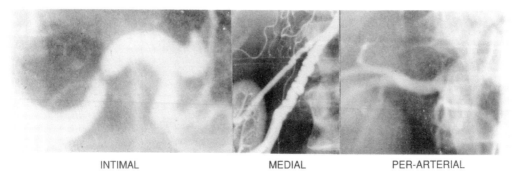

Figure 10.4. Representative radiographs of the three major types of fibromuscular dysplasia. (From Lüscher TF, Lie JT, Stanson AW, Houser OW, Hollier LH, Sheps SG. Arterial fibromuscular dysplasia. *Mayo Clin Proc* 1987;62:931–952.)

perimedial, and periarterial—usually show rapid progression, so severe stenosis and hypertension are frequently observed (Pickering, 1989).

Based on what we have learned about the natural history of the disease and the potential for sometimes acute and often progressive loss of renal function by medical therapy, repair of

any form of functional renovascular disease seems indicated.

Variants

Bilateral Disease with Renal Failure

Renovascular disease, whether atherosclerotic or fibroplastic in origin, was bilateral in 28% of

Table 10.3. Clinical Clues for Renovascular Hypertension

History

Onset of hypertension before age 30 or after age 50
Abrupt onset of hypertension
Severe or resistant hypertension
Symptoms of arteriosclerotic disease elsewhere
Negative family history of hypertension
Smoker
Azotemia with ACE inhibition
Recurrent pulmonary edema

Examination

Abdominal bruits
Other bruits
Advanced fundal changes

Laboratory

Hypokalemia
Proteinuria
High renin concentration

Modified from Pickering TG. The role of laboratory testing in the diagnosis of renovascular hypertension. *Clin Chem* 1991;37:1831.

The possibility of bilateral renovascular disease should be considered in the following groups:

—Young women with severe hypertension, in whom fibroplastic disease is common;

—Older patients with extensive atherosclerotic disease who suddenly have a worsening of renal function (Scoble et al., 1989);

—Azotemic hypertensives who develop multiple episodes of acute pulmonary edema (Pickering et al., 1988; Messina et al., 1992);

—Patients in whom renal function quickly deteriorates after treatment with an ACEI (Rimmer and Gennari, 1993) or other medical therapy;

—Any hypertensive who develops rapidly progressive oliguric renal failure without evidence of obstructive uropathy (O'Donohoe et al., 1990).

Such patients should have arteriography to determine the presence of occlusive disease. Certain features on arteriography suggest viability of the renal tissue, including normal-sized kidneys, a nephrogram, and extensive collateral

Table 10.4. Clinical Characteristics of 131 Patients with Proved Renovascular Hypertension Compared with a Matched Group of Patients with Essential Hypertension

	Essential Hypertension (%)	Renovascular Hypertension (%)
Duration of hypertension < 1 year	12	24
Age of onset after 50	9	15
Family history of hypertension	71	46
Grade 3 or 4 funduscopic changes	7	15
Abdominal bruit	9	46
Blood urea nitrogen > 20 mg/100 ml	8	15
Serum K < 3.4 mEq/L	8	16
Urinary casts	9	20
Proteinuria	32	46

From Simon N, Franklin SS, Bleifer KH, Maxwell MH. Clinical characteristics of renovascular hypertension. *JAMA* 220:1209, 1972, Copyright 1972, American Medical Association.

the patients in the Cooperative Study (Bookstein et al., 1977). Although the disease usually predominates on one side, in some patients it may be sufficiently severe on both sides to induce renal insufficiency (i.e., ischemic renal disease) (Jacobson, 1988). Such patients may be difficult to distinguish from the larger number with essential hypertension or primary renal parenchymal disease who progress into renal failure. The recognition is important since surgical repair or angioplasty may relieve both the hypertension and the renal failure (Ying et al., 1984; Rimmer and Gennari, 1993).

circulation, along with high renin levels from the renal veins.

Hypertension from Contralateral Ischemia

As described previously, hypertension may start with renal stenosis on one side but may persist because of damage to the nonstenotic kidney by the hypertension and high renin (Thal et al., 1963; McAllister et al., 1972). The possibility should be considered if the renal vein renin level is paradoxically high from the nonstenotic kidney. In such cases, if repair of the stenosis does not relieve the hypertension, removal of the nonstenotic kidney should be considered.

Table 10.5. Features of the Two Major Forms of Renal Artery Disease

Renal Artery Disease History	Incidence (%)	Age (yr)	Location of Lesion in Renal Artery	Natural History
Atherosclerosis	65	> 50	Proximal 2 cm; branch disease rare	Progression in 50%, often to total occlusion
Fibromuscular dysplasias				
Intimal	1–2	Children, young adults	Mid-main renal artery and/or branches	Progression in most cases; dissection and/or thrombosis common
Medial	30	25–50	Distal main renal artery and/or branches	Progression in 33%; dissection and/or thrombosis rare
Periarterial	1–2	15–30	Mid to distal main renal artery or branches	Progression in most cases; dissection and/or thrombosis common

Hypertension After Renal Transplantation

As described in Chapter 9, patients who develop severe hypertension after successful renal transplantation should be evaluated for stenosis of the renal artery. These patients have the same propensity for marked loss of renal function if treated with an ACEI as do patients with bilateral renovascular disease.

Hypertension and the Hypoplastic Kidney

As described in Chapter 9, most patients with a small kidney but without a stenotic lesion who respond to nephrectomy have increased plasma renin activity (PRA) from the venous blood draining the diseased kidney, suggesting a renovascular etiology (Mizuiri et al., 1992). In another series, 57 of 174 patients with RVHT had a small, poorly perfused kidney with less than 25% of the total isotopic uptake (Geyskes et al., 1988). The continued secretion of renin into the renal vein is an indication of viability despite the absence of excretory function and the presence of severe tubular atrophy on biopsy. Revascularization, preferably by angioplasty, should always be considered since remarkable return on renal function may follow even when the kidney appears to be nonfunctioning.

Even with a unilateral small kidney, hypertension may arise from renovascular disease in the contralateral kidney. Such was the situation in eight young women with fibroplastic renovascular disease whose hypertension was relieved by relief of the stenosis without surgery on the small kidney (de Jong et al., 1989).

Total absence of one kidney—unilateral renal agenesis—occurs in 1 per 1500 people and should be recognized before evaluation and certainly before surgery on the other kidney. In men, absence of the ipsilateral vas deferens is usually noted in those with renal agenesis (Donohue and Fauver, 1989).

Nephroptosis

Although not observed in the 33 patients seen by Sang and associates (1989), increased mobility of the kidney of 7.5 cm or more as the patient moves from the supine to the upright position (nephroptosis) has been associated with medial fibromuscular dysplasia (de Zeeuw et al., 1977). The possibility that the repeated accordion-like movement of the renal artery results in the fibromuscular disease is an intriguing idea. Patients with hypertension that becomes worse when they stand or who have significant ptosis demonstrated on intravenous pyelography (IVP) should be considered for renin assays and angiography, since nephropexy may relieve the hypertension (Clorius et al., 1981).

Hyperaldosteronism

Patients with RVHT occasionally have profound secondary aldosteronism with hypokalemia due to urinary potassium wasting—all reversed by nephrectomy (Goldberg and McCurdy, 1963).

Nephrotic Syndrome

Proteinuria is common (Zimbler et al., 1987), and a small number of patients with RVHT have the nephrotic syndrome (Kumar and Shapiro, 1980).

Polycythemia

Polycythemia has been seen occasionally in patients with RVHT (Hudgson et al., 1967). Elevated peripheral and renal venous erythropoietin levels without polycythemia are much more common (Grützmacher et al., 1989).

DIAGNOSTIC TESTS

Mann and Pickering (1992) have formulated a sensible guide to the diagnostic work-up for RVHT based on "a selective approach in which only patients with suggestive clinical clues are tested." They provide an Index of Clinical Suspicion (Table 10.6) and then a suggested work-up for patients in the low, moderate, and high categories (Fig. 10.5).

As seen in Figure 10.5, the majority of patients with no suggestive features would get no further work-up. Those with features that indicate a moderate (from 5% to 15%) likelihood of RHVT could be screened with just a peripheral PRA test but more likely with a captopril-augmented PRA test and/or a captopril-augmented renal scan. Although stimulated renal vein renins or duplex ultrasonography are listed as alternative choices, they are less attractive ones because of the discomfort and complexity of the renin ratio and the lack of experience with and variable results of ultrasonography. The relatively few patients with highly suggestive features would most likely have an arteriogram but could be put through the other screening studies first.

The various tests now used to screen and diagnose renovascular disease will be described; they are grouped into those assessing renal perfusion, those measuring renin levels, and those visualizing the renal arteries.

Tests Assessing Renal Perfusion

Intravenous Pyelography

After Maxwell et al. (1964) showed the advantages of the rapid-sequence IVP, this procedure became accepted as the best initial screening test for RVHT, but it subsequently was deemed an unsatisfactory screening test (Mushlin and Thornbury, 1989). Nonetheless, it has been argued that the procedure is the best initial test to screen for both renal parenchymal and vascular causes of hypertension with the recognition that its failure to diagnose about 25% of RVHT cases means that an arteriogram should still be done if it is essential to rule out the disease (Cameron et al., 1992).

Table 10.6.   Testing for Renovascular Hypertension: Clinical Index of Suspicion as a Guide to Selecting Patients for Work-Up

Low (should not be tested)
- Borderline, mild or moderate hypertension, in the absence of clinical clues

Moderate (noninvasive tests recommended)
- Severe hypertension (diastolic blood pressure greater than 120 mm Hg)
- Hypertension refractory to standard therapy
- Abrupt onset of sustained, moderate to severe hypertension at age < 20 or > age 50
- Hypertension with a suggestive abdominal bruit (long, high-pitched, and localized to the region of the renal artery)
- Moderate hypertension (diastolic blood pressure exceeding 105 mm Hg) in a smoker, a patient with evidence of occlusive vascular disease (cerebrovascular, coronary, peripheral vascular), or a patient with unexplained but stable elevation of serum creatinine
- Normalization of blood pressure by an angiotensin-converting enzyme inhibitor in a patient with moderate or severe hypertension (particularly a smoker or a patient with recent onset of hypertension)

High (may consider proceeding directly to arteriography)
- Severe hypertension (diastolic blood pressure greater than 120 mm Hg with either progressive renal insufficiency or refractoriness to aggressive treatment (particularly in a patient who has been a smoker or has other evidence of occlusive arterial disease)
- Accelerated or malignant hypertension (grade III or IV retinopathy)
- Hypertension with recent elevation of serum creatinine, either unexplained or reversibly induced by an angiotensin-converting enzyme inhibitor
- Moderate to severe hypertension with incidentally detected asymmetry of renal size

From Mann SJ, Pickering TG. Detection of renovascular hypertension. State of the art: 1992. *Ann Intern Med* 1992;117:845–853.

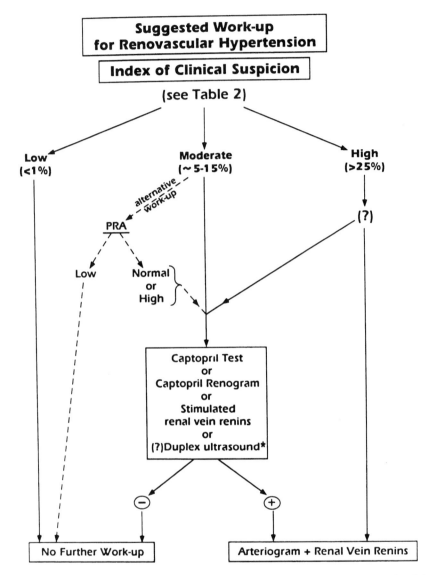

Figure 10.5. Suggested work-up for patients with suspected renovascular hypertension based on the clinical index of suspicion (From Mann SJ, Pickering TG. Detection of renovascular hypertension. State of the art: 1992. *Ann Intern Med* 1992;117:845–853.)

Renal Scan

Technique. Renography may be done with radiolabeled agents that are excreted either by glomerular filtration (technetium-99 diethylene-triamine pentaacetic acid [^{99}Tc-DTPA]) or partially by filtration but mainly by tubular secretion and therefore measure renal blood flow (iodohippurate-131 or ^{99}Tc-mercaptoacetyltriglycine [^{99}Tc-MAG$_3$]).

As described in a consensus statement composed by eight investigators (Nally et al., 1991),

both the scintigraphic images and the time-activity curves should be measured. The time-activity curves are divided into three phases: upslope, maximal activity, and downslope. In addition, the time to maximal activity, the parenchymal transit time, a "split function index" comparing the percentage of uptake in the two kidneys, and the residual cortical activity should be measured. These investigators propose a grading system for the interpretation of renograms and suggest that the probability of functionally significant renal artery stenosis after captopril challenge be defined as "low, indeterminant or high" (Nally et al., 1991).

Captopril-Augmented Renal Scan

When used alone, isotopic renograms provided about 75% sensitivity and specificity for the diagnosis of RVHT, figures similar to those obtained with IVP (Pickering, 1991).

Soon after the observation that renal function in an ischemic kidney could abruptly be reduced further after a single dose of the ACEI captopril (Hricik et al., 1983), the effect of captopril on renal uptake of ^{99}Tc-DTPA was reported (Wenting et al., 1984). As reviewed in a supplement of the *American Journal of Hypertension* (Black and Nally, 1991), either a reduction of the uptake of ^{99}Tc-DTPA or a slowing of the excretion of hippurate or ^{99}Tc-MAG$_3$ can be used to identify the effect of the ACEI in removing the protective actions of the high levels of angiotensin II on the autoregulation of glomerular filtration and the maintenance of renal blood flow, respectively (Fig. 10.6). The use of hippurate or MAG$_3$ with furosemide washout may provide better sensitivity and specificity than ^{99}Tc-DTPA (Erbslöh-Möller et al., 1991).

Postcaptopril renography along with the measurement of peripheral blood renin activity, as will be described later in this chapter, now appears to be the best noninvasive screening test for RVHT (Black and Nally, 1991; Fommei et al., 1992; Elliott et al., 1993). Patients with renal artery stenosis but negative captopril renography results rarely improve after angioplasty, whereas most patients with positive renographic results do (Geyskes and de Bruyn, 1991; Dondi et al., 1992; Elliott et al., 1993). The test may give false-negative results in some patients with very small ischemic kidneys and evidence of unilateral disease when bilateral disease is present (Scoble et al., 1991).

To reduce the cost and time of the work-up, the post-captopril renal scan should be done first. If results are negative (as they will be most of the time), there is no need for a pre-captopril renogram. If they are positive, the procedure should be repeated without captopril to ensure that the differences are related to reversible vascular disease and not parenchymal damage.

Tests Assessing Renin Release

Since hypersecretion of renin from the hypoperfused kidney is the primary event in the pathogenesis of RVHT, it came as no surprise

that increased peripheral PRA levels were found in patients with the disease. However, subsequent experience with PRA assays in peripheral blood showed that many patients with RVHT did not have elevated levels, in keeping with the experimental evidence that secretion of renin from the clipped kidney falls to "normal" soon after RVHT is induced, while renin release from the contralateral kidney is suppressed.

Starting in 1960, reports of PRA assays on renal venous blood appeared, and the presence of an increased concentration of renin coming from the involved kidney was commonly used as a diagnostic and prognostic indicator. More recently, the dynamic effect of the ACEI captopril on renin release has been utilized to enhance the diagnostic accuracy of both peripheral and renal venous PRA assays. More about the control, variability, and measurement of PRA is given in Chapter 3.

Peripheral Blood PRA

Elevated peripheral blood PRA is found in most patients with functionally significant RVHT. However, in the review by Rudnick and Maxwell (1984) of 24 published series, the sensitivity of peripheral PRA in renal vascular hypertension averaged only 57%, the specificity 66%. Of 326 patients with negative tests, 71% were improved by surgery; of 360 with positive tests, 86% were improved.

Captopril-Augmented Peripheral PRA. In view of the discrepancies with peripheral PRA values, various maneuvers have been used to augment PRA release in the hope that patients with curable disease would show a hyperresponsiveness and thereby improve the discriminatory value of peripheral levels. Of these, the response of PRA to captopril has been most widely used after the concept was documented with parenteral ACEIs (Case and Laragh, 1979).

Muller et al. (1986) established criteria for the performance and interpretation of the test (Table 10.7). Using these criteria, Muller et al. found the test to identify all 56 patients in their series with RVHT and to give false-positive results in only 2 of 112 patients with essential hypertension and in 6 with secondary hypertension. They found the test to be neither as sensitive nor as specific in the 46 patients in their series with renal insufficiency.

Although often using different criteria, most researchers have found the test to provide excellent sensitivity but less specificity (Gaul et al., 1989), with overall predictive value of a positive

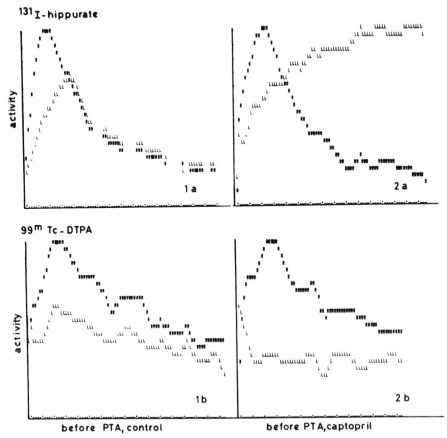

Figure 10.6. Renography in a 42-year-old man with hypertension and stenosis of the left renal artery. *L,* left kidney; *R,* right kidney. After percutaneous transluminal angioplasty (*PTA*), his hypertension was cured. The *upper half* of the figure shows ^{131}I-hippurate (*a*) and the *lower half* shows ^{99m}Tc-diethylenetriamine pentaacetic acid (*DTPA*) (*b*) time-activity curves in two different circumstances: (1) before PTA without any medication (control); (2) before PTA but with 25 mg of captopril taken orally 1 hour before the investigation. Before PTA, captopril slowed down the excretion of ^{131}I-hippurate and reduced the uptake of ^{99m}Tc-DTPA only in the left kidney. After PTA this effect disappeared. (From Geyskes GG, Oei HY, Puylaert CBAJ, et al. Renovascular hypertension identified by captopril-induced changes in the renogram. *Hypertension* 9:451, 1987, and by permission of the American Heart Association, Inc.)

Table 10.7. Criteria for the Captopril-Augmented Peripheral PRA Test

Method
- The patient should maintain a normal salt intake and receive no diuretics.
- If possible, all antihypertensive medications should be withdrawn 3 weeks prior to the test.
- The patient should be seated for at least 30 minutes; a venous blood sample is then drawn for measurement of baseline plasma renin activity.
- Captopril (50 mg diluted in 10 ml of water immediately before the test) is administered orally.
- At 60 minutes, a venous blood sample is drawn for measurement of stimulated plasma renin activity.

Interpretation: A positive test requires:
- Stimulated plasma renin activity of 12 ng/ml/hour or more *and*
- Absolute increase in plasma renin activity of 10 mg/ml/hour or more *and*
- Increase in plasma renin activity of 150% or more, or 400% or more if baseline plasma renin activity is less than 3 ng/ml/hour.

From Muller FB, Sealey JE, Case DB, et al. The captopril test for identifying renovascular disease in hypertensive patients. *Am J Med* 1986;80:633.

test varying between 35% (Gosse et al., 1988) and 92% (Derkx et al., 1985). The number of false-positives is high in patients with high baseline renin levels but quite low in those with low or normal renin levels (Gerber et al., 1992).

Comparison of Renal Vein Renins

Renal Vein Renin Ratio. In view of the poor sensitivity and specificity of measurements of peripheral PRA before the use of captopril challenge, the comparison of renin levels in blood from each renal vein obtained by percutaneous catheterization was used as the most practical and definitive procedure to establish both the diagnosis and surgical curability of this disease. The initial success reported with this technique by Helmer and Judson (1960) has been amply confirmed.

The validity of the procedure was shown in a compilation of the experience of numerous investigators from 1960 to 1983 by Rudnick and Maxwell (1984). In most of these series, a ratio greater than 1.5:1 between the two renal vein PRA levels was considered abnormal or "lateralizing." An abnormal ratio was 92% predictive of curability; the 8% false-positives could represent errors in the renin test, surgical difficulties, or coincidental primary hypertension.

On the other hand, 65% of those whose renal vein PRA level ratio did not lateralize also were improved by surgery. These false-negatives may reflect problems with the technique or pathophysiologic problems, particularly the presence of bilateral disease or the partial relief of ischemia by extensive collateral circulation in the stenotic kidney.

Renal/Systemic Renin Index. To determine the functional significance of bilateral lesions, the renal/systemic renin index can be calculated for each kidney. The index = renal vein renin − systemic (infrarenal vena cava) renin ÷ systemic renin (Fig. 10.7). An index above 0.24 indicates that excess renin is being secreted from the kidney, whereas lower values indicate suppression (Vaughan, 1985). A "pure" unilateral lesion would show an index of zero from the nonischemic side and a ratio between the two renal veins above 1.5:1 (i.e., lateralizing) (Fig. 10.7).

The index or increment of renin for each renal vein over the level in the systemic vein (infrarenal vena cava) was found to be more sensitive and specific than the ratio between the two renal veins (Pickering et al., 1986b). With bilateral but asymmetric disease, the index would be above 0.24 on both sides, and the ratio between the two sides would be below 1.5:1 (i.e., nonlateralizing). However, many patients with incomplete suppression from the contralateral kidney and a nonlateralizing renal vein ratio will improve after repair of the more ischemic kidney. In a series from Michigan (Stanley and Fry, 1977), complete surgical cure was predicted by a high ratio and complete suppression in the contralateral kidney (i.e., index near zero). However, improvement usually occurred in patients with bilateral renin secretion if the more ischemic side was repaired.

Captopril-Augmented Renal Vein Renins. As with peripheral PRA, an ACEI has been used to preferentially stimulate renin release from an ischemic kidney (Re et al., 1978). Although some find that this improves the predictive value of the renal vein renin ratio (Tomoda et al., 1990), Roubidoux et al. (1991) found that it provided only 65% sensitivity in 20 patients with proved renovascular disease and had a 48% false-positive rate in 113 patients without the disease.

Renal Vein Renins with Bilateral and Segmental Disease. Even though lesions are bilateral in 25% of patients with RVHT, one side is usually responsible for the hypertension. Lateralization of renin secretion to one kidney has been found in about two-thirds of the small number of patients with bilateral renal arterial stenosis studied (Rudnick and Maxwell, 1984).

Use of Renal Vein Renins. With the large number of false-negatives, this procedure cannot be used as a screening test. However, it may be useful in confirming the functional significance of a lesion demonstrated by arteriography, particularly if bilateral disease is noted. However, the captopril renogram will serve that purpose in addition to being a more reliable screening test. Therefore, renal vein renin measurements likely will be used less and less, particularly in patients with a significant stenosis and severe hypertension who likely should have either angioplasty or surgery regardless of the results of the renin assay.

Tests Visualizing the Renal Arteries

Renal Arteriography

Rationale. The various tests described in the preceding sections often are recommended before renal arteriography. However, more and more experience seems to confirm the wisdom of a modified Willie Sutton's law: "If you are searching for a lesion, look at the vessel." This

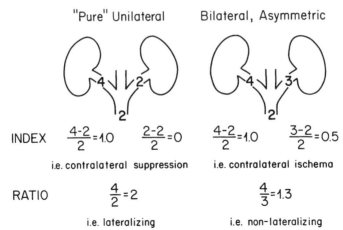

Figure 10.7. Representation of the renal vein renin levels in patients with "pure" unilateral renovascular hypertension (*left*) and bilateral but asymmetric renovascular hypertension (*right*). *Index*, renal vein renin—systemic vein renin ÷ systemic vein renin. *Ratio*, ischemic renal vein renin to contralateral renal vein renin.

seems particularly true for those with highly suggestive clinical features in whom negative screening tests would not be enough to exclude the diagnosis, thus necessitating arteriography regardless of their outcome (Pape et al., 1988).

The reasons for choosing renal arteriography as the initial study in patients with features highly suggestive of RVHT include the following:

—Arteriography provides an immediate answer to the question: Is there renovascular disease that is potentially curable?
—None of the other studies can rule out reversible renovascular disease with certainty. Of course, the finding of a lesion by arteriography usually must be followed by a test proving its functional significance;
—With digital subtraction techniques, small catheters and small quantities of dye are needed so that discomfort and danger for the patient are minimal (Hillman, 1989). Even with conventional arteriography, using either nonionic or ionic contrast agents, the danger of contrast material–induced renal damage is small and can be further minimized by adequate hydration and avoidance of nonsteroidal anti-inflammatory agents (NSAIDs) (Barrett et al., 1992);
—Knowledge of the renal vascular architecture is helpful before collection of renal vein renin samples if these are to be obtained. The recognition of branch or segmental vascular lesions, cysts, and tumors will indicate the need for selective venous sampling, and visualizing extensive collateral flow to a kidney with a major vascular stenosis may indicate

that hypersecretion of renin from the stenotic kidney is diminished so that the renal venous renin ratio no longer lateralizes.

Digital subtraction arteriography is likely to replace conventional arteriography (Hillman, 1989), even though it provides less definition of the renal vasculature. With digital video subtraction angiographic equipment, preexisting images are subtracted from films taken after injection of contrast media; thus, the renal arteries can be visualized with small quantities of diluted (15%) contrast material injected through a small catheter, making the procedure suitable for outpatient use even among children (Tonkin et al., 1988) with excellent safety.

Prognostic Accuracy.   Renal arteriography is almost always successful in diagnosing renal arterial disease. It is of relatively little value, however, in determining surgical curability of renovascular hypertension. In the Cooperative Study, neither the degree of stenosis, nor the presence of poststenotic dilatation, nor the presence of collateral circulation was of significant discriminatory value in predicting success or failure of surgery (Bookstein et al., 1972). In patients with apparently totally occluded main renal arteries, the finding of a markedly delayed and reduced nephrogram is a useful indicator of irreversible renal damage that likely will not respond to revascularization (Feltrin et al., 1986).

The temptation to proceed with transluminal balloon dilation at the time of arteriography will grow. Some are doing so, but most prefer to obtain evidence of functionally significant

RVHT by means of renin studies or renography before or after the arteriogram.

Intravenous Angiography

Digital subtraction intravenous angiography has been recommended for screening (Dunnick et al., 1989). Despite the attractiveness of the ''less invasive'' venous angiographic procedure, arteriography will still be needed to visualize small, intrarenal vessels. In the Cooperative Study of Renovascular Hypertension (Bookstein et al., 1972), stenoses were seen in segmental branches in 6.6% of those with atherosclerotic disease and, in those with fibromuscular disease, the lesions were seen most commonly in the middle and distal third of the renal artery, and in segmental branches in 5% of cases. Therefore, failure to visualize 10% to 20% of renal arteries with intravenous angiography makes arteriography the preferred procedure, although the intravenous procedure can be performed at the time of renal vein renin sampling if that procedure is indicated (Tack and Sos, 1989).

Ultrasonography

Color Doppler imaging and pulsed-Doppler spectral analysis are being increasingly used to visualize the renal arteries (Taylor et al., 1991; Stavros et al., 1992). Although the presence of renal artery stenosis was recognized by ultrasonography in 94% of patients with angiographically demonstrated disease (Bardelli et al., 1992), others report much less diagnostic accuracy (Postma et al., 1992). Even more structural information may be provided by intravascular ultrasonography (Sheikh et al., 1991). As our experience grows, ultrasonography may become a more widely used screening test (Davidson and Wilcox, 1992).

Magnetic Resonance Imaging

Although magnetic resonance imaging (MRI) angiography can visualize most renal arteries, this expensive procedure will likely only be used in patients with markedly impaired renal function in whom neither renal scans nor arteriograms are feasible (Farrugia et al., 1993).

Outdated Procedures

A number of other procedures have been used to diagnose RVHT but they are now outdated. These include:

—Angiotensin infusion test (Kaplan and Silah, 1964);
—Renal biopsy (Vertes et al., 1964);
—Split renal function tests (Schaeffer and Stamey, 1975).

THERAPY

Once a lesion is found and proved to be functionally significant, three choices are available for the treatment of RVHT: medical, surgical, and angioplasty.

No adequately controlled long-term studies comparing the three modalities are available. A nonrandomized study with a mean follow-up of 10.5 years involving 88 patients treated medically and 149 treated nonmedically with either surgery or angioplasty found similar effects on BP and target organ damage but greater total and cardiovascular mortality in those treated medically (Giovannetti et al., 1992). Preliminary data from the first 40 patients enrolled in a randomized study comparing medical and surgical treatment of atherosclerotic renovascular disease with renal impairment noted similar renal function at 12 months but better 18-month event-free survival (74% vs. 44%) in the surgical group (Cairns et al., 1992). In a prospective randomized study, 58 patients with atherosclerotic RVHT have been followed for 2 years after either angioplasty or surgery (Hulthn et al., 1992). Although 6 of the 29 angioplasty patients needed additional intervention to relieve restenosis, the two groups ended up with identical and excellent BP control and renal function at the end of the 2 years.

For each patient, then, the choice must be made individually. For most patients, angioplasty is the first choice. However, surgery is most certain to provide prolonged relief and for a considerable number of patients it is the best choice. Medical therapy, although it has become more effective, often leads to acute decreases in renal perfusion, occasionally to progressive loss of renal structure and function, and rarely to occlusion of stenotic renal arteries (Hannedouche et al., 1991). Therefore, unless the patient is not suited for either surgery or angioplasty, medical therapy is usually given only for short intervals, often to prepare the patient for a reparative procedure. The response to ACEI therapy is usually predictive of the response to angioplasty (Staessen et al., 1988) and to surgery (Von Knorring et al., 1989).

Parenthetically, if patients clearly are not candidates for surgery or angioplasty, there is no reason to subject them to the various procedures needed to make the diagnosis.

In the following description of the results of the three forms of therapy, the terms established by the Cooperative Study (Maxwell et al., 1972) are used: "cure" is a diastolic BP of 90 mm Hg or less without medication; "improved" is a 15% or greater decrease and a diastolic BP between 90 and 110 mm Hg; "failure" is either a less than 15% decrease with a diastolic BP above 90 mm Hg or a diastolic BP greater than 110 mm Hg.

Medical Therapy

The role of antihypertensive drug therapy in the long-term management of RVHT is shrinking because of improving results from surgery and angioplasty and concerns about the adverse long-term effects of medical therapy. However, if hypertension is well controlled and renal function does not deteriorate under careful surveillance, medical therapy may be continued indefinitely.

Renovascular hypertension in the neonate or young child may respond to medical therapy, reducing the need for early nephrectomy (Adelman et al., 1978).

Medical Regimen

Although all classes of antihypertensive drugs have been used to treat RVHT, the most effective therapy is an ACEI (Textor, 1990). In the largest published analysis, captopril was effective for at least 3 months in over 80% of 269 patients with RVHT; progressive renal failure mandating the discontinuation of therapy occurred in only 5% (Hollenberg, 1988).

As noted earlier, the use of an ACEI may markedly decrease blood flow through the stenotic kidney and, if that is the only kidney or if there is bilateral renovascular disease, the result may be rapid though usually reversible renal failure. This is not unique to ACEIs (Textor et al., 1985) but is more likely to occur with their use because of their greater effectiveness, the removal of angiotensin II support of autoregulation, and the preferential dilation of renal efferent vessels that together lead to reduced glomerular filtration and renal perfusion (Rimmer and Gennari, 1993).

Fortunately, return of renal function is usual when the ACEI is stopped (Kalra et al., 1990). Nonetheless, complete occlusions of markedly stenotic renal arteries after ACEI therapy have been seen, particularly if the ACEI is given with a diuretic (Postma et al., 1989; Hannedouche et al., 1991). The recommendation has therefore been made that in patients who are candidates for operation, ACEI "be given for no more than 1 month to allow maximum BP reduction without endangering the stenotic kidney for too long" (Tillman et al., 1984).

Calcium entry blockers such as nifedipine may provide equal control of hypertension and less impairment of renal function than ACEIs (Mimran, 1992). Calcium entry blockers may maintain blood flow better because of their preferential preglomerular vasodilatory effect.

Surgery

The results of published large series from single centers show the expected results from renovascular surgery (Table 10.8). The results with fibromuscular disease are better than with atherosclerotic disease.

Over the past 10 years, surgery has increasingly been performed on sicker and older patients with more extensive atherosclerotic disease, more to preserve renal function than to control hypertension (Libertino et al., 1992). Surgical techniques have expanded, with more aortic replacements and alternate bypass procedures, microvascular and extracorporeal techniques for branch renal artery disease, and renal autotransplantation (Martinez et al., 1990).

Long-Term Follow-Up

Long-term follow-up shows a progressive fall in the number of patients cured or improved, which is not surprising in view of the extensive vascular disease that most have at the time of surgery. In one series, the majority of patients undergoing surgery for fibroplastic disease were alive and normotensive after 15 years, whereas only about half of patients with atherosclerotic disease were alive after 10 years, and only half of them were normotensive (Horvath et al., 1986). In the large series of Lawrie et al. (1989), the best BP responses were seen in those with higher preoperative BP and more severe renal artery stenosis, whereas long-term survival was lower in males, older patients, patients with bilateral renal stenosis, and patients in whom other vascular operations also were needed.

Results in Special Groups

In addition to these overall results, special consideration should be given to special groups and situations.

Children. Renovascular hypertension is second only to coarctation as a surgically remediable form of hypertension among children.

Table 10.8. Results of Surgery for Renovascular Hypertension

	Source				
	Foster et al., 1975	Stanley et al., 1982	Novick et al., 1987	Van Brockel et al., 1988	Lawrie et al., 1989
No. of patients	502	313	345	172	919
Time of study	1961–69	1961–80	1975–84	1959–83	1955–86
Mean follow-up (mo)	12	≈60	38	8	88
Overall benefit (%)	66	89	92	76	82
Fibromuscular disease benefit (%)	63	94	93	79	—
Atherosclerotic disease benefit (%)	71	81	92	74	—
Technical success (%)	≈80	86	96	94	89
Perioperative mortality (%)	6.8	1.9	1.4	6.4	5.5

Modified from Tack C, Sos TA. Radiologic diagnosis of renovascular hypertension and percutaneous transluminal renal angioplasty. *Semin Nucl Med* 1989;19:89.

Results of surgical repair generally have been very good. Cure or improvement was reported in 17 of 17 patients by Berkowitz and O'Neill (1989), and in 27 of 28 treated with surgery from 1978 to 1988 by Martinez et al. (1990).

Elderly Patients. With their predominance of atherosclerotic disease, patients over 65 might be expected to do worse. Nonetheless, in the Cleveland Clinic series, patients over 65 did better with surgery than with medical therapy or angioplasty (Vidt, 1987), and the surgical results were as good in patients over 65 years of age as in patients under 65 (Bedoya et al., 1989). Repair of coexistent significant carotid or coronary vascular disease should be considered before renovascular surgery.

Nonfunctioning Kidneys. Even after complete occlusion of the renal artery, revascularization may be successful, even if delayed for as long as 56 days (Libertino et al., 1980). Patients who suddenly become anuric should be considered for immediate angiography and, if a correctable vascular lesion is identified, revascularization should be performed (Williams et al., 1988).

Renal Insufficiency. Patients with bilateral renovascular disease or disease in the artery to a solitary kidney may present with renal insufficiency (Ying et al., 1984; Rimmer and Gennari, 1993). In a review of four surgical series involving 268 patients with bilateral ischemic renal disease, Jacobson (1988) noted that operative mortality ranged from 2% to 15%, and that the majority of patients showed improved renal function over 2- to 3-year follow-up. Similarly good overall results were noted in 19 patients with a single, ischemic kidney (McCready et al., 1987) and in 18 patients with Takayasu's disease (Lagneau and Michel, 1985).

Arterial Stenosis after Transplantation. As discussed in Chapter 9, this is one of the more common causes of post-transplant hypertension. Operative intervention may be indicated (Dickerman et al., 1980), although angioplasty will usually be the first choice (McMullin et al., 1992).

Transluminal Angioplasty

After the first report of successful treatment of RVHT by percutaneous transluminal dilation (Grüntzig et al., 1978), fairly extensive experience has been reported and the technical aspects have continually improved (Tack and Sos, 1989). However, restenosis occurs within a year in at least one-sixth of patients after a first successful angioplasty, particularly in those with ostial lesions in association with severe aortic atherosclerosis (Plouin et al., 1993).

A careful analysis of all 10 large series reported up to the end of 1987 found that, of 691 angioplasties attempted, 12% were technical failures; the overall BP responses were 24% cured, 43% improved, and 33% failed (Ramsay and Waller, 1990). As with surgery, results with fibromuscular disease were better than with atherosclerotic disease (Table 10.9). Complications were reported in 9%, and 3 of the 691 patients died.

Ramsay and Waller (1990) conclude that "the evidence for the value of angioplasty in treating RVHT has serious limitations. Angioplasty for fibromuscular disease seems to be worthwhile, but for atherosclerotic lesions the benefit appears to be small and its efficacy needs to be compared with medical therapy in randomised trials."

Attempts to predict the outcome of angioplasty identify youth as the most significant

Table 10.9. Summary of Outcome After Angioplasty in 10 Published Series[a]

Type of Disease	Number of Technically Successful Operations	Blood Pressure Response (%)		
		Cured	Improved	Failed
Atheromatous	391	19	52	30
(Range in %)		(9–29)	(29–75)	(10–54)
Fibromuscular	175	50	42	9
(Range in %)		(25–85)	(13–63)	(0–25)

[a]Data from Ramsay and Waller, 1990.

factor; little value is derived from the various screening tests for RVHT described earlier in this chapter (Postma et al., 1991).

Patients with Renal Insufficiency

Improvement in BP and renal function has been noted in one-half or more of these patients (Pickering et al., 1986a; Tykarski et al., 1993) but about 20% develop progressive renal failure (Textor et al., 1992). Even renal arteries that appear to be totally occluded may be dilated successfully (Sniderman and Sos, 1982).

Complications

Complications occur in about 10% of patients; the rate and severity almost always decrease with increasing experience (Hayes et al., 1988). Since the balloon causes cracking and occasional separation of the intima from the media rather than compression of atherosclerotic plaques, it is remarkable that so few complications have been observed. Rupture of the renal artery may occur as long as 9 days after the procedure (Olin and Wholey, 1987), but serious complications are relatively rare. However, the ready availability of surgical backup for possible serious complications is considered mandatory before angioplasty is performed.

Renal Embolization

In a few instances, percutaneous renal embolization by injection of ethanol into the renal artery has been successfully used to treat severe hypertension in patients with RVHT in whom neither surgery nor angioplasty was feasible and in whom medical therapy was unsuccessful (Iaccarino et al., 1989).

Recommendations for Therapy

There are no valid comparisons among the three major forms of therapy, and there likely never will be. For now, balloon angioplasty should be offered as the easiest and safest initial approach, particularly for those with fibromuscular disease and nonostial lesions; surgery should be offered to patients who cannot be approached with angioplasty; and medical therapy should be offered only for patients unwilling to have or too sick for repair.

INTRARENAL VASCULITIS

Hypertension with renal damage is common in various vasculitic syndromes including Wegener's granulomatosis (Woodrow et al., 1990) and systemic lupus erythematosus (Ward and Stadenski, 1992). All of these patients may enter into an acute, severe hypertensive phase, usually associated with markedly elevated plasma renin levels, likely reflecting intrarenal stenoses from multiple arteriolar lesions. The hypertension can sometimes be rather remarkably reversed by ACEI therapy (Coruzzi and Novarini, 1992).

RENIN-SECRETING TUMORS (PRIMARY RENINISM)

Since the recognition of the first case of primary reninism in 1967 (Robertson et al., 1967), more than 30 have been reported, and the syndrome has been well described (McVicar et al., 1993). Most such tumors are relatively small and are composed of juxtaglomerular cells that have been shown to make renin (Fallo et al., 1992). In addition to these juxtaglomerular cell tumors, or *hemangiopericytomas,* hypertension and high renin levels that revert to normal after nephrectomy have been reported in children with Wilms' tumor (Sheth et al., 1978), in patients with adenocarcinoma of the kidney (Steffens et al., 1992), and in tumors of various external sites including lung, ovary (Anderson et al., 1989), liver, pancreas, and sarcomas (Geddy and Main, 1990). Large intrarenal tumors also can produce high renin hypertension by compressing renal vessels. Two patients with apparently unilateral juxtaglomerular cell hyperplasia but no tumor have been described (Kuchel et al., 1993).

Primary reninism is not common, but clinicians should be aware that hypertension with a high renal venous renin level from one kidney may not always represent RVHT. Most of the renin-secreting tumors of renal origin fit a rather typical pattern:

—Severe hypertension in relatively young patients: the oldest reported has been 53 (Corvol et al., 1988), but most are below 25;

—Very high prorenin and renin levels in the peripheral blood and even higher levels from the kidney harboring the tumor;

—Secondary aldosteronism usually manifested by hypokalemia;

—The tumor should be recognizable by computed tomography (CT) scan or by selective angiography;

—The tumor is morphologically a hemangiopericytoma arising from the juxtaglomerular apparatus, and it contains large amounts of renin and prorenin.

Cure should be possible by removal of the tumor; if that is not possible, an ACEI or calcium antagonist should be used.

Now that the renal causes of hypertension have been covered, we will turn to the only other common causes of secondary hypertension, those seen during pregnancy and with the use of oral contraceptives.

References

Adelman RD, Merten D, Vogel J, Goetzman BW, Wennberg RP. Nonsurgical management of renovascular hypertension in the neonate. *Pediatrics* 1978;62:71–76.

Alfidi RJ, Tarar R, Fosmoe RJ, Ferrario C, Boltuch RL, Gifford R W Jr. Renal-splanchnic steal and hypertension. *Radiology* 1972;102:545–549.

Anderson PW, Macaulay L, Do YS, Sherrod A, d'Ablaing G, Koss M, Shinagawa T, Tran B, Montz FJ, Hsueh WA. Extrarenal renin-secreting tumors: insights into hypertension and ovarian renin production. *Medicine* 1989;68:257–268.

Anderson WP, Ramsey DE, Takata M. Development of hypertension from unilateral renal artery stenosis in conscious dogs. *Hypertension* 1990;16:441–451.

Banitt PF, Clark CW. Isolated dissecting aneurysm of the renal artery. *J Urol* 1986; 135:998–999.

Bardelli M, Jensen G, Volkmann R, Aurell M. Non-invasive ultrasound assessment of renal artery stenosis by means of the Gosling pulsatility index. *J Hypertens* 1992; 10:985–989.

Barger AC. The Goldblatt memorial lecture. Part I: experimental renovascular hypertension. *Hypertension* 1979;1:447–455.

Barrett BJ, Parfrey PS, Vavasour HM, McDonald J, Kent G, Hefferton D, O'Dea F, Stone E, Reddy R, McManamon PJ. Contrast nephropathy in patients with impaired renal function: high versus low osmolar media. *Kidney Int* 1992; 41: 1274–1279.

Bedoya L, Ziegelbaum M, Vidt DG, Badhwar K, Novick AC. Gifford FW Jr. Baseline renal function and surgical revascularization in atherosclerotic renal arterial disease in the elderly. *Clev Clin J Med* 1989; 56:415–421.

Berkowitz HD, O'Neill JA Jr. Renovascular hypertension in children. *J Vasc Surg* 1989;9:46–55.

Black HR, Nally JV Jr. Introduction. The role of captopril scintigraphy in the diagnosis and management of renovascular hypertension: a consensus conference. *Am J Hypertens* 1991;4:661S–662S.

Bookstein JJ. Segmental renal artery stenosis in renovascular hypertension. *Radiology* 1968;90:1073–1083.

Bookstein JJ, Abrams HL, Buenger RE, Reiss MD, Lecky JW, Franklin SS, Bleifer KH,

Varady PD, Maxwell MH. Radiologic aspects of renovascular hypertension. Part 3. Appraisal of arteriography. *JAMA* 1972;221:368–374.

Bookstein JJ, Maxwell MH, Abrams HL, Buenger RE, Lecky J, Franklin SS. Cooperative study of radiologic aspects of renovascular hypertension. Bilateral renovascular disease. *JAMA* 1977; 237: 1706–1709.

Braun-Menendez E, Fasciolo JC, Leloir FL, Munoz JM. La substancia hipertensinora de la sangre del rinon isquemiado [Abstract]. *Rev Soc Argent Biol* 1939; 15:420.

Brewster DC, Jensen SR, Novelline RA. Reversible renal artery stenosis associated with pheochromocytoma. *JAMA* 1982; 248:1094–1096.

Brunner HR. ACE inhibitors in renal disease. *Kidney Int* 1992;42:463–479.

Cairns HS. Conference. Atherosclerotic renal artery stenosis. *Lancet* 1992;340:298–299.

Cameron HA, Close CF, Yeo WW, Jackson PR, Ramsay LE. Investigation of selected patients with hypertension by the rapid-sequence intravenous urogram. *Lancet* 1992;339:658–661.

Case DB, Laragh JH. Reactive hyperreninemia in renovascular hypertension after angiotensin blockade with saralasin or converting enzyme inhibitor. *Ann Intern Med* 1979;91:153–160.

Castle CH. Iatrogenic renal hypertension: two unusual complications of surgery for familial pheochromocytoma. *JAMA* 1973; 225:1085–1088.

Chen M, Lee J, Malvin RL, Huang BS. Naloxone attenuates development of hypertension in two-kidney one-clip Goldblatt rats. *Am J Physiol* 1988;255:E839–E842.

Choudhri AH, Cleland JGF, Rowlands PC, Tran TL, McCarty M, Al-Kutoubi MAO. Unsuspected renal artery stenosis in peripheral vascular disease. *Br Med J* 1990;301:1197–1198.

Chugh KS, Jain S, Sakhuja V, Malik N, Gupta A, Gupta A, Sehgal S, Jha V, Gupta KL. Renovascular hypertension due to Takayasu's Arteritis among Indian patients. *Q J Med* 1992;85:833–843.

Clorius JH, Schmidlin P, Raptou E, Huber W, Georgi P. Hypertension associated with massive, bilateral, posture-dependent renal

dysfunction. *Radiology* 1981;140: 231–235.

Coruzzi P, Novarini A. Which antihypertensive treatment in renal vasculitis? *Nephron* 1992;62:372.

Corvol P, Pinet F, Galen FX, Plouin PF, Chatellier G, Pagny JY, Corvol MT, Menard J. Seven lessons from seven renin secreting tumors. *Kidney Int* 1988;34(Suppl 25): 38–44.

Danielson M, Dammström B-G. The prevalence of secondary and curable hypertension. *Acta Med Scand* 1981;209:451–455.

Davidson RA, Wilcox CS. Newer tests for the diagnosis of renovascular disease. *JAMA* 1992;268:3353–3358.

Davis BA, Crook JE, Vestal RE, Oates JA. Prevalence of renovascular hypertension in patients with grade III or IV hypertensive retinopathy. *N Engl J Med* 1979; 301: 1273–1276.

de Jong PE, van Bockel JH, de Zeeuw D. Unilateral renal parenchymal disease with contralateral renal artery stenosis of the fibrodysplasia type. *Ann Intern Med* 1989;110:437–445.

de Simone G, Devereux RB, Camargo MJF, Volpe M, Wallerson DC, Atlas SA, Laragh JH. In vivo left ventricular anatomy in rats with two-kidney, one clip and one-kidney, one clip renovascular hypertension. *J Hypertens* 1992;10:725–732.

de Zeeuw D, Donker AJM, Burema J, van der Hem GK, Mandema E. Nephroptosis and hypertension. *Lancet* 1977;1:213–215.

Derkx FHM, Tan-Tjiong LH, Wenting GJ, Man in't Veld A, Schalekamp MADH. Use of captopril in the diagnostic work-up of renovascular hypertension. *J Hypertens* 1985;3(Suppl 3):287–289.

Dickerman RM, Peters PC, Hull AR, Curry TS, Atkins C, Fry WJ. Surgical correction of posttransplant renovascular hypertension. *Ann Surg* 1980;192:639–644.

Dondi M, Fanti S, De Fabritiis A, Zuccalà A, Gaggi R, Mirelli M, Stella A, Marengo M, Losinno F, Monetti N. Prognostic value of captopril renal scintigraphy in renovascular hypertension. *J Nucl Med* 1992;33:2040–2044.

Donohue RE, Fauver HE. Unilateral absence of the vas deferens. A useful clinical sign. *JAMA* 1989;261:1180–1182.

Dunnick NR, Svetkey LP, Cohan RH, Newman GE, Braun SD, Himmelstein SI, Bollinger RR, McCann RL, Wilkinson RH Jr, Klotman PE. Intravenous digital subtraction renal angiography: use in screening for renovascular hypertension. *Radiology* 1989;171:219–222.

Easterling TR, Brateng D, Goldman ML, Strandness DE, Zaccardi MJ. Renal vascular hypertension during pregnancy. *Obstet Gynecol* 1991;78:921–925.

Edmunds ME, Russell GI, Bing RF. Reversal of experimental renovascular hypertension. *J Hypertens* 1991;9:289–301.

Edwards BS, Stanson AW, Holley KE, Sheps SG. Isolated renal artery dissection. Presentation, evaluation, management, and pathology. *Mayo Clin Proc* 1982; 57: 564–571.

Eipper DR, Gifford RW Jr, Stewart BH, Alfidi RJ, McCormack LJ, Vidt DG. Abdominal bruits in renovascular hypertension. *Am J Cardiol* 1976;37:48–52.

Elkik F, Corvol P, Idatte J-M, Ménard J. Renal segmental infarction: a cause of reversible malignant hypertension. *J Hypertens* 1984;2:149–156.

Elliott WJ, Martin WB, Murphy MB. Comparison of two noninvasive screening tests for renovascular hypertension. *Arch Intern Med* 1993;153:755–764.

Erbslöh-Möller B, Dumas A, Roth D, Sfakianakis GN, Bourgoignie JJ. Fursemide-^{131}I-hippuran renography after angiotensin-converting enzyme inhibition for the diagnosis of renovascular hypertension. *Am J Med* 1991;90:23–29.

Eyler WR, Clark MD, Garman JE, Rian RL, Meininger DE. Angiography of the renal areas including a comparative study of renal arterial stenoses in patients with and without hypertension. *Radiology* 1962; 78:879–892.

Fallo F, D'Agostino D, Armanini D, Caregaro L, Mantero F. Concomitant release of renin, angiotensin I, and angiotensin II during superfusion of human juxtaglomerular cell tumor. *Am J Hypertens* 1992; 5:566–569.

Farreras-Valenti P, Rozman C, Jurado-Grau J, del Rio G, Elizalde C. Grönblad-Strandberg-Touraine syndrome with systemic hypertension due to unilateral renal angioma. *Am J Med* 1965;39:355–360.

Farrugia E, King BF, Larson TS. Magnetic resonance angiography and detection of renal artery stenosis in a patient with impaired renal function. *Mayo Clin Proc* 1993;68:157–160.

Feltrin GP, Rossi G, Talenti E, Pessina AC, Miotto D, Thiene G, Dal Palu C. Prognostic value of nephrography in atherosclerotic occlusion of the renal artery. *Hypertension* 1986;8:962–964.

Fiorentini C, Guazzi MD, Olivari MT, Bartorelli A, Necchi G, Magrini F. Selective reduction of renal perfusion pressure and blood flow in man: humoral and hemodynamic effects. *Circulation* 1981; 63: 973–978.

Fommei E, Ghione S, Hilson AJW, Mezzasalma L, Oei HY, Piepsz A, Volterrani D. European Multicentre Study: captopril radionuclide test in renovascular hypertension [Abstract]. *J Hypertens* 1992; 10 (Suppl 4):83.

Gaul MK, Linn WD, Mulrow CD. Captopril-stimulated renin secretion in the diagnosis of renovascular hypertension. *Am J Hypertens* 1989;2:335–340.

Geddy PM, Main J. Renin-secreting retroperitoneal leiomyosarcoma: an unusual cause of hypertension. *J Hum Hypertens* 1990; 4:57–58.

Gerber LM, Mann SJ, Alderman MH, Pickering TG, Sealey JE, Mueller FB. High specificity of the captopril test in all but high renin patients [Abstract]. *Am J Hypertens* 1992;5:131A.

Geyskes GG, de Bruyn AJG. Captopril renography and the effect of percutaneous transluminal angioplasty on blood pressure in 94 patients with renal artery stenosis. *Am J Hypertens* 1991;4:685S–689S.

Geyskes GG, Oei HY, Klinge J, Kooiker CJ, Puylaert CBAJ, Dourhout Mees EJ. Renovascular hypertension: the small kidney updated. *Q J Med* 1988;66:203–217.

Geyskes GG, Oei HY, Puylaert CBAJ, Dourhout Mees EJ. Renovascular hypertension identified by captopril-induced changes in the renogram. *Hypertension* 1987; 9: 451–458.

Gifford RW Jr. Evaluation of the hypertensive patient with emphasis on detecting curable causes. *Milbank Mem Fund Q* 1969;47:170–199.

Giovannetti R, Arzilli F, Salvetti A. Surgical vs medical treatment in the outcome of renovascular hypertensives [Abstract]. *Am J Hypertens* 1992;5:130.

Goldberg JM, McCurdy DK. Hyperaldosteronism and hypergranularity of the juxtaglomerular cells in renal hypertension. *Ann Intern Med* 1963;59:24–36.

Goldblatt H. Reflections. *Urol Clin North Am* 1975;2:219–221.

Goldblatt H, Lynch J, Hanzal RF, Summerville WW. Studies on experimental hypertension. I. The production of persistent elevation of systolic blood pressure by means of renal ischemia. *J Exp Med* 1934; 59:347–378.

Gosse Ph, Dupas JY, Reynaud P, Jullien E, Dallocchio M. The captopril test in the detection of renovascular hypertension in a population with low prevalence of the disease. A prospective study [Abstract]. *Am J Hypertens* 1988;1:79A.

Grüntzig A, Kuhlmann U, Vetter W, Lütolf U, Meier B, Siegenthaler W. Treatment of renovascular hypertension with percutaneous transluminal dilatation of a renal-artery stenosis. *Lancet* 1978;1:801–802.

Grützmacher P, Radtke HW, Stahl RAK, Rauber K, Schoeppe W. Renal artery stenosis and erythropoietin [Abstract]. *Kidney Int* 1989;35:326.

Hannedouche T, Godin M, Fries D, Fillastre JP. Acute renal thrombosis induced by angiotensin-converting enzyme inhibitors in patients with renovascular hypertension. *Nephron* 1991;57:230–231.

Hayes JM, Risius B, Novick AC, Geisinger M, Zelch M, Gifford RW Jr, Vidt DG, Olin JW. Experience with percutaneous transluminal angioplasty for renal artery stenosis at the Cleveland Clinic. *J Urol* 1988; 139:488–492

Helmer OM, Judson WE. The presence of vasoconstrictor and vasopressor activity in renal vein plasma of patients with arterial hypertension. In: Skelton RF, ed. *Hypertension: Proceedings of the Council for High Blood Pressure Research.* New York: American Heart Association, 1960; 8: 38–52.

Hillman BJ. Imaging advances in the diagnosis of renovascular hypertension. *Am J Radiol* 1989;153:5–14.

Hollenberg NK. Medical therapy for renovascular hypertension. A review. *Am J Hypertens* 1988;1:338S–343S.

Hoobler SW. History of experimental renovascular hypertension. In: Stanley JC, Ernst CB, Fry WJ, eds. *Renovascular Hypertension.* Philadelphia: WB Saunders, 1984:12–19.

Horvath JS, Fischer WE, May J, Waugh RC, Sheil AG, Eyres A, Johnson JR, Duggin GG, Hall BM, Tiller DJ. Surgical management of renovascular hypertension—A comparison between fibromuscular hyperplasia and atherosclerotic lesions: a 20-year study. *J Hypertens* 1986;4(Suppl 6):688–690.

Horvath JS, Waugh RC, Tiller DJ, Duggin GG. The detection of renovascular hypertension: a study of 490 patients by renal angiography. *Q J Med* 1982;51:139–146.

Hricik DE, Browning PJ, Kopelman R, Goorno WE, Madias NE, Dzau VJ. Captopril-induced functional renal insufficiency in patients with bilateral renal-artery stenoses or renal-artery stenosis in a solitary kidney. *N Engl J Med* 1983;308:373–376.

Hudson P, Pearce JMS, Yeates WK. Renal artery stenosis with hypertension and high haematocrit. *Br Med J* 1967;1:18–21.

Hughes JS, Dove HG, Gifford RW Jr, Feinstein AR. Duration of blood pressure elevation in accurately predicting surgical cure of renovascular hypertension. *Am Heart J* 1981;101:408–413.

Hulthén UL, Weibull H, Bergqvist D, Bergentz S-E, Jonsson K, Nöström F, Manhem P. Percutaneous transluminal renal angioplasty versus vascular surgery in atherosclerotic unilateral renal artery stenosis—a prospective, randomized study [Abstract]. *J Hypertens* 1992;10(Suppl 4):112.

Hurwitz GA, Mattar AG, Bhargava R, Powe JE, Driedger AA. Screening for a renovascular etiology in hypertensive patients undergoing myocardial scintigraphy: differential renal thallium-201 uptake. *Can J Cardiol* 1990;6:198–204.

Iaccarino V, Russo D, Niola R, Muto R, Testa A, Andreucci VE, Porta E. Total or partial percutaneous renal ablation in the treatment of renovascular hypertension: radiological and clinical aspects. *Br J Radiol* 1989;62:593–598.

Ichikawa I, Ferrone RA, Duchin DL, Manning M, Dzau VJ, Brenner BM. Relative contribution of vasopressin and angiotensin II to the altered renal microcirculatory dynamics in two-kidney Goldblatt hypertension. *Circ Res* 1983;53:592–602.

Imanishi M, Kawamura M, Akabane S, Matsushima Y, Kuramochi M, Ito K, Ohta M, Kimura K, Takamiya M, Omae T. Aspirin lowers blood pressure in patients with renovascular hypertension. *Hypertension* 1989;14:461–468.

Jacobson HR. Ischemic renal disease: an overlooked clinical entity? *Kidney Int* 1988;34:729–743.

Jennings RC, Shaikh VAR, Allen WMC. Renal ischaemia due to thrombosis of renal artery resulting from metastases from primary carcinoma of bronchus. *Br Med J* 1964;2:1053–1054.

Kalra PA, Mamtora H, Holmes AM, Waldek S. Renovascular disease and renal complications of angiotensin-converting enzyme inhibitor therapy. *Q J Med* 1990; 77: 1013–1018.

Kaplan NM, Silah JG. The angiotensin infusion test. *N Engl J Med* 1964;271:536–541.

Kato K, Takashi M, Narita H, Kondo A. Renal hypertension secondary to perirenal pseudocyst: resolution by percutaneous drainage. *J Urol* 1985;134:942–943.

Kimura G, London GM, Safar ME, Kuramochi M, Omae T. Glomerular hypertension in renovascular hypertensive patients. *Kidney Int* 1991;39:966–972.

Kimura G, Saito F, Kojima S, Yoshimi H, Abe H, Kawano Y, Yoshida K, Ashida T, Kawamura M, Kuramochi M, Ito K, Omae T. Renal function curve in patients with secondary forms of hypertension. *Hypertension* 1987;10:11–15.

Kuchel O, Horky K, Cantin M, Roy P. Unilateral juxtaglomerular hyperplasia, hyperreninism and hypokalaemia relieved by nephrectomy. *J Hum Hypertens* 1993; 7:71–78.

Kumar A, Shapiro AP. Proteinuria and nephrotic syndrome induced by renin in patients with renal artery stenosis. *Arch Intern Med* 1980;140:1631–1634.

Lagneau P, Michel JB. Renovascular hypertension and Takayasu's disease. *J Urol* 1985;134:876–879.

Lawrie GM, Morris GC, Glaeser DH, DeBakey ME. Renovascular reconstruction: factors affecting long-term prognosis in 919 patients followed up to 31 years. *Am J Cardiol* 1989;63:1085–1092.

Libertino JA, Bosco PJ, Ying CY, Breslin DJ, Woods BO'B, Tsapatsaris NP, Swinton NW Jr. Renal revascularization to preserve and restore renal function. *J Urol* 1992;147:1485–1487.

Libertino JA, Zinman L, Breslin DJ, Swinton NW, Legg MA. Renal artery revascularization. *JAMA* 1980;244:1340–1342.

Luger AM, Bauer JH, Neviackas JA, Le HT, Nichols WK. Primary necrotizing arteritis of the main renal artery presenting as accelerated renovascular hypertension. *Am J Nephrol* 1981;1:168–172.

Lüscher TF, Lie JT, Stanson AW, Houser OW, Hollier LH, Sheps SG. Arterial fibromuscular dysplasia. *Mayo Clin Proc* 1987;62:931–952.

Mann SJ, Pickering TG. Detection of renovascular hypertension. State of the art: 1992. *Ann Intern Med* 1992;117:845–853.

Martin DC Jr. Anomaly of right crus of the diaphragm involving the right renal artery. *Am J Surg* 1971;121:351–354.

Martinez A, Novick AC, Cunningham R, Goormastic M. Improved results of vascular reconstruction in pediatric and young adult patients with renovascular hypertension. *J Urol* 1990;144:717–720.

Martinez-Maldonado M. Pathophysiology of renovascular hypertension. *Hypertension* 1991;17:707–719.

Maxwell MH, Bleifer KH, Franklin SS, Varady PD. Demographic analysis of the study. *JAMA* 1972;220:1195–1204.

Maxwell MH, Gonick HC, Wiita R, Kaufman JJ. Use of the rapid-sequence intravenous pyelogram in the diagnosis of renovascular hypertension. *N Engl J Med* 1964; 270: 213–220.

McAllister RG, Michelakis AM, Oates JA, Foster JH. Malignant hypertension due to renal artery stenosis. *JAMA* 1972; 221: 865–868.

McCormack JL, Bain RC, Kenny GM, Tocantins R. Iatrogenic renal hypertension. *Arch Surg* 1974;108:220–222.

McCready RA, Daugherty ME, Nighbert EJ, Hyde GL, Freedman AM, Ernst CB. Renal revascularization in patients with a single functioning ischemic kidney. *J Vasc Surg* 1987;6:185–190.

McLoughlin MJ, Colapinto RF, Hobbs BB. Abdominal bruits. Clinical and angiographic correlation. *JAMA* 1975; 232: 1238–1242.

McMullin ND, Reidy JF, Koffman G, Rigden SPA, Haycock G, Chantler C, Bewick M. The management of renal transplant artery stenosis in children by percutaneous transluminal angioplasty. *Transplantation* 1992;53:559–563.

McVicar M, Carman C, Chandra M, Jumari Abbi R, Teichberg S, Kahn E. Hypertension secondary to renin-secreting juxtaglomerular cell tumor: case report and review of 38 cases. *Pediatr Nephrol* 1993;7:404–412.

Messina LM, Zelenock GB, Yao KA, Stanley JC. Renal revascularization for recurrent pulmonary edema in patients with poorly controlled hypertension and renal insufficiency: a distinct subgroup of patients with arteriosclerotic renal artery occlusive disease. *J Vasc Surg* 1992;15:73–82.

Mimran A. Renal effects of antihypertensive agents in parenchymal renal disease and renovascular hypertension. *J Cardiovasc Pharmacol* 1992;19(Suppl 6):45–50.

Mizuiri S, Amagasaki Y, Hosaka H, Fukasawa K, Nakayama K, Nakamura N, Sakaguchi H. Hypertension in unilateral atrophic kidney secondary to ureteropelvic junction obstruction. *Nephron* 1992; 61:217–219.

Monstrey SJM, Beerthuizen GIJM, vander Werken CHR, Debruyne FMJ, Goris RJA. Renal trauma and hypertension. *J Trauma* 1989;29:65–70.

Muller FB, Sealey JE, Case DB, Atlas SA, Pickering TG, Pecker MS, Preibisz JJ, Laragh JH. The captopril test for identifying renovascular disease in hypertensive patients. *Am J Med* 1986;80:633–644.

Munichoodappa C, D'Elia JA, Libertino JA, Gleason RE, Christlieb AR. Renal artery stenosis in hypertensive diabetics. *J Urol* 1979;121:555–558.

Mushlin AI, Thornbury JR. Intravenous pyelography: the case against its routine use. *Ann Intern Med* 1989;111:58–70.

Nally JV Jr, Chen C, Fine E, Fommei E, Ghione S, Geyskes GG, Hoffer PB, Sfakianakis G. Diagnostic criteria of renovascular hypertension with captopril renography. A consensus statement. *Am J Hypertens* 1991;4:749S–752S.

Nicholas WC, Cranston Pe, Weems WL. Severe hypertension associated with an intrarenal aneurysm. *South Med J* 1992; 85:853–856.

O'Donohoe MK, Donohoe J, Corrigan TP. Acute renal failure of renovascular origin: cure by aortorenal reconstruction after 24 days of anuria. *Nephron* 1990;56:92–93.

Olin JW, Wholey M. Rupture of the renal artery nine days after percutaneous transluminal angioplasty. *JAMA* 1987; 257: 518–520.

Pape JF, Gudmundsen TE, Pedersen HK. Renal angiography may be used primarily in the diagnosis of renovascular hypertension. *Scand J Urol Nephrol* 1988; 22: 41–44.

Pickering TG. Renovascular hypertension: etiology and pathophysiology. *Semin Nucl Med* 1989;19:79–88.

Pickering TG. The role of laboratory testing in the diagnosis of renovascular hypertension. *Clin Chem* 1991;37:1831–1837.

Pickering TG, Herman L, Devereux RB, Sotelo JE, James GD, Sos TA, Silane MF, Laragh JH. Recurrent pulmonary oedema in hypertension due to bilateral renal artery stenosis: treatment by angioplasty or surgical revascularisation. *Lancet* 1988; 2: 551–552.

Pickering TG, Sos TA, Saddekni S, Rozenblit G, James GD, Orenstein A, Helseth G, Laragh JH. Renal angioplasty in patients with azotaemia and renovascular hypertension. *J Hypertens* 1986a;4(Suppl 6): 667–669.

Pickering TG, Sos TA, Vaughan ED Jr, Laragh JH. Differing patterns of renal vein renin secretion in patients with renovascular hypertension, and their role in predicting the response to angioplasty. *Nephron* 1986b;44(Suppl 1):8–11.

Plouin P-F, Darné B, Chatellier G, Pannier I, Battaglia C, Raynaud A, Azizi M. Restenosis after a first percutaneous transluminal renal angioplasty. *Hypertension* 1993;21:89–96.

Pollard SG, Hornick P, Macfarlane R, Calne RY. Renovascular hypertension in neurofibromatosis. *Postgrad Med J* 1989; 65:31–33.

Postma CT, Hoefnagels WHL, Barentsz JO, de Boo T, Thien T. Occlusion of unilateral stenosed renal arteries—relation to medical treatment. *J Hum Hypertens* 1989; 3:185–190.

Postma CT, van Aalen J, de Boo T, Rosenbusch G, Thien T. Doppler ultrasound scanning in the detection of renal artery stenosis in hypertensive patients. *Br J Radiol* 1992;65:857–860.

Postma CT, van Oijen AHAM, Barentsz JO, de Boo T, Hoefnagels WHL, Corstens FHM, Thien T. The value of tests predicting renovascular hypertension in patients with renal artery stenosis treated by angioplasty. *Arch Intern Med* 1991; 151: 1531–1535.

Preston RA, Materson BJ. Renal cholesterol emboli: a cause of hypertension in the elderly. *Cardiovasc Risk Factors* 1992; 2:101–104.

Rackson ME, Lossef SV, Sos TA. Renal artery stenosis in patients with aortic dissection: increased prevalence. *Radiology* 1990;177:555–558.

Raman GV. Post transplant hypertension. *J Hum Hypertens* 1991;5:1–6.

Ramsay LE, Waller PC. Blood pressure response to percutaneous transluminal angioplasty for renovascular hypertension: an overview of published series. *Br Med J* 1990;300:569–572.

Re R, Novelline R, Escourrou M-T, Athanasoulis C, Burton J, Haber E. Inhibition of angiotensin-converting enzyme for diagnosis of renal-artery stenosis. *N Engl J Med* 1978;298:582–586.

Restrick LJ, Ledermann JA, Hoffbrand BI. Primary malignant retroperitoneal germ cell tumour presenting with accelerated hypertension. *J Hum Hypertens* 1992; 6:243–244.

Rimmer JM, Gennari FJ. Atherosclerotic renovascular disease and progressive renal failure. *Ann Intern Med* 1993; 118: 712–719.

Robertson PW, Klidjian A, Harding LK, Walters G, Lee MR, Robb-Smith AHT. Hypertension due to a renin-secreting renal tumour. *Am J Med* 1967;43:963–976.

Rudnick MR, Maxwell MH. Limitations of renin assays. In: Narins RG, ed. *Controversies in Nephrology and Hypertension.* New York: Churchill Livingstone, 1984: 123–160.

Sacks SH, Aparicio SAJR, Bevan A, Oliver DO, Will EJ, Davison A. Late renal failure due to prostatic outflow obstruction: a preventable disease. *Br Med J* 1989; 298:156–159.

Sang CN, Whelton PK, Hamper UM, Connolly M, Kadir S, White RI, Sanders R, Liang K-Y, Bias W. Etiologic factors in renovascular fibromuscular dysplasia. A case-control study. *Hypertension* 1989; 14:472–479.

Sawicki PT, Kaiser S, Heinemann L, Frenzel H, Berger M. Prevalence of renal artery stenosis in diabetes mellitus—an autopsy study. *J Intern Med* 1991;229:489–492.

Schaeffer AJ, Stamey TA. Ureteral catheterization studies. *Urol Clin North Am* 1975;2:327–335.

Scoble JE, McClean A, Stansby G, Hamilton G, Sweny P, Hilson AJW. The use of captopril-DTPA scanning in the diagnosis of atherosclerotic renal artery stenosis in patients with impaired renal function. *Am J Hypertens* 1991;4:721S–723S.

Shapiro AL, Cavallo T, Cooper W, Lapenas D, Bron K, Berg G. Hypertension in radiation nephritis. Report of a patient with unilateral disease, elevated renin activity levels, and reversal after unilateral nephrectomy. *Arch Intern Med* 1977; 137: 848–851.

Shaw AB, Gopalka SK. Renal artery thrombosis caused by antihypertensive treatment. *Br Med J* 1982;285:1617.

Sheikh KH, Davidson CJ, Newman GE, Kisslo KB, Schwab SJ. Intravascular ultrasound assessment of the renal artery. *Ann Intern Med* 1991;115:22–25.

Shelhamer JH, Volkman DJ, Parrillo JE, Lawley TJ, Johnston MR, Fauci AS.

Takayasu's arteritis and its therapy. *Ann Intern Med* 1985;103:121–126.

Sheth KJ, Tang TT, Blaedel ME, Good TA. Polydipsia, polyuria, and hypertension associated with renin-secreting Wilms tumor. *J Pediatr* 1978;92:921–924.

Siamopoulos K, Sellars L, Mishra SC, Essenhigh DM, Robson V, Wilkinson R. Experience in the management of hypertension with unilateral chronic pylonephritis: results of nephrectomy in selected patients. *Q J Med* 1983;52:349–362.

Silver D, Clements JB. Renovascular hypertension from renal artery compression by congenital bands. *Ann Surg* 1976; 183: 161–166.

Simon N, Franklin SS, Bleifer KH, Maxwell MH. Clinical characteristics of renovascular hypertension. *JAMA* 1972; 220: 1209–1218.

Smith HW. Unilateral nephrectomy in hypertensive disease. *J Urol* 1956;76:685–701.

Smith LH, Drach G, Hall P, Lingeman J, Preminger G, Resnick MI, Segura JW. National High Blood Pressure Education Program (NHBPEP) review paper on complications of shock wave lithotripsy for urinary calculi. *Am J Med* 1991;91:635–641.

Sniderman KW, Sos TA. Percutaneous transluminal recanalization and dilatation of totally occluded renal arteries. *Radiology* 1982;142:607–610.

Staessen J, Wilms G, Baert A, Fagard R, Lijnen P, Suy R, Amery A. Blood pressure during long-term converting-enzyme inhibition predicts the curability of renovascular hypertension by angioplasty. *Am J Hypertens* 1988;1:208–214.

Stanley JC, Fry WJ. Surgical treatment of renovascular hypertension. *Arch Surg* 1977;112:1291–1297.

Stanley P, Gyepes MT, Olson DL, Gates GF. Renovascular hypertension in children and adolescents. *Radiology* 1978;129: 123–131.

Stavros AT, Parker SH, Yakes WF, Chantelois AE, Burke BJ, Meyers RR, Schenck JJ. Segmental stenosis of the renal artery: pattern recognition of tardus and parvus abnormalities with duplex sonography. *Radiology* 1992;184:487–492.

Steffens J, Bock R, Braedel HU, Isenberg E, Bührle CP, Ziegler M. Renin-producing renal cell carcinomas—clinical and experimental investigations on a special form of renal hypertension. *Urol Res* 1992; 20: 111–115.

Steffens J, Mast GJ, Braedel HU, Hoffman W, Isenberg E, Püschel W, Bock R, Ziegler M. Segmental renal hypoplasia of vascular origin causing renal hypertension in a 3-year-old girl. *J Urol* 1991;146:826–829.

Sterns RH, Rabinowitz R, Segal AJ, Spitzer RM. ''Page kidney.'' Hypertension caused by chronic subcapsular hematoma. *Arch Intern Med* 1985;145:169–171.

Svetkey LP, Kadir S, Dunnick NR, Smith SR, Dunham DB, Lambert M, Klotman PE. Similar prevalence of renovascular hypertension in selected blacks and whites. *Hypertension* 1991;17:678–683.

Tack C, Sos TA. Radiologic diagnosis of renovascular hypertensin and percutaneous transluminal renal angioplasty. *Semin Nucl Med* 1989;29:89–100.

Takada Y, Shimizu H, Kazatani Y, Azechi H, Hiwada K, Kokubu T. Orthostatic hypertension with nephroptosis and aortitis disease. *Arch Intern Med* 1984; 144: 152–154.

Tapper D, Brand T, Hickman R. Early diagnosis and management of renovascular hypertension. *Am J Surg* 1987; 153: 495–500.

Tarazi RC, Dustan HP. Neurogenic participation in essential and renovascular hypertension assessed by acute ganglionic blockade: correlation with haemodynamic indices and intravascular volume. *Clin Sci* 1973;44:197–212.

Taylor DC. Duplex ultrasound in the assessment of vascular disease in clinical hypertension. *Am J Hypertens* 1991;4:550–556.

Textor SC. ACE inhibitors in renovascular hypertension. *Cardiovasc Drugs Ther* 1990;4:229–235.

Textor SC, Kos P, Schirger A, Taler S, McKusick M, Sheps S. Does angioplasty (PTA) protect renal function in azotemic atherosclerotic (ASO) renovascular disease [Abstract]? *J Am Soc Nephrol* 1992;3:538.

Textor SC, Novick AC, Tarazi RC, Klimas V, Vidt DG, Pohl M. Critical perfusion pressure for renal function in patients with bilateral atherosclerotic renal vascular disease. *Ann Intern Med* 1985;102:308–314.

Thal AP, Grage TB, Vernier RL. Function of the contralateral kidney in renal hypertension due to renal artery stenosis. *Circulation* 1963;27:36–43.

Tillman DM, Malatino LS, Cumming AMM, Hodsman GP, Leckie BJ, Lever AF, Morton JJ, Webb DJ, Robertson JI. Enalapril in hypertension with renal artery stenosis: long-term follow-up and effects on renal function. *J Hypertens* 1984;2(Suppl 2):93–100.

Tomoda F, Takata M, Ohashi S, Ueno H, Ikeda K, Yasumoto K, Iida H, Sasayama S. Captopril-stimulated renal vein renin in hypertensive patients with or without renal artery stenosis. *Am J Hypertens* 1990; 3:918–926.

Tonkin IL, Stapleton FB, Roy S III. Digital subtraction angiography in the evaluation of renal vascular hypertension in children. *Pediatrics* 1988;81:150–158.

Torres VE, Wilson DM, Burnett JC Jr, Johnson CM, Offord KP. Effect of inhibition of converting enzyme on renal hemodynamics and sodium management in polycystic kidney disease. *Mayo Clin Proc* 1991;66:1010–1017.

Tykarski A, Edwards R, Dominiczak AF, Reid JL. Percutaneous transluminal renal angioplasty in the management of hypertension and renal failure in patients with renal artery stenosis. *J Hum Hypertens* 1993;7:491–496.

Ullian ME, Molitoris BA. Bilateral congenital renal arteriovenous fistulas. *Clin Nephrol* 1987;27:293–297.

Valvo E, Bedogna V, Gammaro L, Taddei G, Maso R, Cavaggioni M, Tonon M, Maschio G. Systemic haemodynamics in renovascular hypertension: changes after revascularization with percutaneous transluminal angioplasty. *J Hypertens* 1987;5: 629–632.

Vaughn ED Jr. Renovascular hypertension. *Kidney Int* 1985;27:811–827.

Vertes V, Grauel JA, Goldblatt H. Renal arteriography, separate renal-function studies and renal biopsy in human hypertension. Selection of patients for surgical treatment. *N Engl J Med* 1964;270:656–659.

Vidt DG. Geriatric hypertension of renovascular origin: diagnosis and management. *Geriatrics* 1987;42:59–70.

Von Knorring J, Lepäntalo M, Fyhrquist F. Long-term prognosis of surgical treatment of renovascular hypertension. *J Intern Med* 1989;225:303–309.

Ward MM, Studenski S. Clinical prognostic factors in lupus nephritis. The importance of hypertension and smoking. *Arch Intern Med* 1992;152:2082–2088.

Wenting GJ, Tan-Tjiong H, Derkx FHM, de Bruyn JHB, Man in't Veld AJ, Schalekamp MADH. Split renal function after captopril in unilateral renal artery stenosis. *Br Med J* 1984;288:886–890.

Williams B, Feehally J, Attard A, Bell PRF. Recovery of renal function after delayed revascularisation of acute occlusion of the renal artery. *Br Med J* 1988; 296: 1591–1592.

Woodrow G, Cook JA, Brownjohn AM, Turney JH. Is renal vasculitis increasing in incidence? *Lancet* 1990;336:1583.

Ying CY, Tifft CP, Gavras H, Chobanian AV. Renal revascularization in the azotemic hypertensive patient resistant to therapy. *N Engl J Med* 1984;311:1070–1075.

Zimbler MS, Pickering TG, Sos TA, Laragh JH. Proteinuria in renovascular hypertension and the effects of renal angioplasty. *Am J Cardiol* 1987;59:406–408.

Zimmerman JB, Robertson D, Jackson EK. Angiotensin II—noradrenergic interactions in renovascular hypertensive rats. *J Clin Invest* 1987;80:443–457.

11 Hypertension with Pregnancy and the Pill

Hypertension occurs in well over 5% of all pregnancies and in as many as 5% of women who take oral contraceptives for 5 years. In developed countries, hypertensive disorders of pregnancy are among the leading causes of maternal (Dudley, 1992) and perinatal mortality (Lenox et al., 1990). Hypertension associated with the use of oral contraceptives may rapidly accelerate or more slowly cause vascular damage. Although the causes of neither gestational nor pill-induced hypertension are completely known, if they are recognized early and handled appropriately, the morbidity and mortality they cause can be largely prevented.

TYPES OF HYPERTENSION DURING PREGNANCY

A small percentage of women enter pregnancy with preexisting hypertension; a larger number develop hypertension during pregnancy—as many as 20% of women in their first pregnancy (National High Blood Pressure Education Program Working Group, 1990).

Classification

In the previous edition of this book, Davey and MacGillivray's (1988) classification was followed since it had been approved by the International Society for the Study of Hypertension in Pregnancy. However, experts—individually (Chamberlain, 1991a; Goldberg and Schrier, 1991; Roberts and Redman, 1993) and in groups

(National High Blood Pressure Education Program Working Group, 1990), both in the United States and in England—continue to use the simpler terminology proposed in 1972 by the American College of Obstetricians and Gynecologists (Hughes, 1972). The term "pregnancy-induced hypertension" (PIH) also is being used less and less. Therefore, the following definitions will be used:

—*Chronic hypertension.* Hypertension present before pregnancy or diagnosed before the 20th week of gestation or that persists beyond 6 weeks postpartum;

—*Preeclampsia.* Increased blood pressure (BP) appearing after 20 weeks' gestation, usually accompanied by proteinuria and edema;

—*Eclampsia.* The occurrence of seizures that cannot be attributed to other causes in a patient with preeclampsia;

—*Preeclampsia superimposed on chronic hypertension.* In women with chronic hypertension, increases of BP of 30 mm Hg systolic or 15 mm Hg diastolic together with the appearance of proteinuria or edema;

—*Transient hypertension.* Elevated BP during pregnancy or in the first 24 hours postpartum with no other signs of preeclampsia or preexisting hypertension. This pattern, a manifestation of latent chronic hypertension, usually recurs in subsequent pregnancies and is responsible for most misdiagnoses of preeclampsia in multiparous women.

Problems of Diagnosing Preeclampsia

There are problems inherent in diagnosing a syndrome of unknown cause only on the basis of highly nonspecific signs (Roberts and Redman, 1993). For example, as will be noted, the BP in normal pregnancy usually falls during the first and middle trimester, only to return toward the prepregnant level during the third trimester. Since women with preexisting hypertension have an even greater fall early on, their subsequent "normal" rise may give the appearance of the onset of preeclampsia. In addition, some of those with chronic hypertension may have persistent but previously unrecognized proteinuria as well as nonspecific edema; thus, when they are seen with the full triad, the diagnosis of preeclampsia looks rather certain. On the other hand, some women with preeclampsia may have neither proteinuria nor edema initially (Morgan and Thurnau, 1988), and thereby are thought to have either chronic or transient hypertension.

The distinction between chronic hypertension and preeclampsia is of more than academic interest: in the former, hypertension is the major problem; in the latter, hypertension is "important primarily as a sign of the underlying disorder (of) poor perfusion of many organs" (National High Blood Pressure Education Program Working Group, 1990). The management of both the hypertension and the pregnancy, as well as the prognosis for future pregnancies, varies with the diagnosis. The bottom line, however, is clear: when in doubt, diagnose preeclampsia and institute its treatment, since even mild preeclampsia may rapidly progress; if it is correctly diagnosed and managed, the risks to both mother and baby can be largely overcome.

BLOOD PRESSURE MONITORING DURING PREGNANCY

Techniques of Measurement

The various guidelines described in Chapter 2 should be followed in measuring the BP during pregnancy. However, confusion persists among those who measure BP (Perry et al., 1991). The confusion involves whether to use the Korotkoff phase 4 (muffling) or phase 5 (disappearance) for the diastolic level. Although the British Hypertension Society and the World Health Organization have recommended the use of phase 4, U.S. authorities almost uniformly recommend phase 5 (Cunningham and Lindheimer, 1992), as do more and more English obstetricians (Perry et al., 1990; de Swiet, 1991). The

best course is to use phase 5, reserving phase 4 only for the small number of women whose phase 5 is very low or indeterminate (Johenning and Barron, 1992; Lopez et al., 1992). Lopez et al. (1992) followed 1194 women with frequent BP measurements from week 20 until delivery. They found fewer than 0.5% of readings down to zero, a difference of 6 mm Hg between phases 4 and 5, and evidence that phase 5 provided greater specificity and predictive value for the development of intrauterine growth retardation and preeclampsia.

Home Recording

A logical way to improve both the accuracy and predictive value of BP measurements is to have patients monitor their own BP with the semiautomatic, inexpensive devices described in Chapter 2 (Zuspan and Rayburn, 1991). If there is an urgent need to confirm newly recognized elevated office readings, the home readings can be telemetrically transmitted (Mooney et al., 1990).

Ambulatory Monitoring

With ambulatory devices, 24-hour BPs have now been recorded in large numbers of normal and preeclamptic pregnancies. Relatively stable readings throughout normal pregnancy with lower pressures during sleep have been documented (Cugini et al., 1992; Contard et al., 1993; Halligan et al., 1993). In preeclampsia, the nocturnal fall is blunted very early in the course, many weeks before clinical manifestations appear (Cugini et al., 1992).

Findings in Pregnancy

In most normal pregnancies, BPs are lower during the midportion and gradually return toward nonpregnancy levels during the third trimester (Christianson, 1976). If these low-normal diastolic levels rise to above 84 mm Hg at any gestational age, fetal mortality is increased, even more so if proteinuria accompanies the rise in pressure (Friedman and Neff, 1978). Patients destined to develop preeclampsia often have higher than normal BP well before they become overtly hypertensive (Moutquin et al., 1985) (Fig. 11.1). The systolic level has been largely disregarded, but it is a better guide to fetal outcome than the diastolic value (Anonymous, Lancet, 1991).

CIRCULATION IN NORMAL PREGNANCY

The multiple changes that occur in pregnancy are "adaptations [that] generally move to mini-

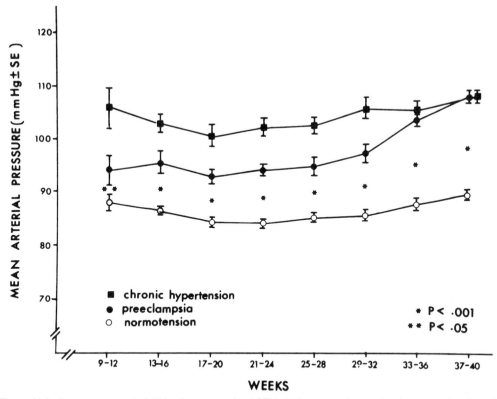

Figure 11.1. Average mean arterial blood pressures (+ 1 SE) in 710 women who remained normotensive throughout pregnancy, in 46 who developed preeclampsia, and in 37 with chronic hypertension. (From Moutquin JM, Rainville C, Giroux L, Raynauld P, Amyot G, Bilodeau R, Pelland N. A prospective study of blood pressure in pregnancy: prediction of preeclampsia. *Am J Obstet Gynecol* 1985;151:191–196.)

mize the stresses imposed and to provide the best environment for the growing fetus'' (Chamberlain, 1991b). Of these adaptations, those affecting the BP and circulation are among the most profound.

Hemodynamic Changes

Normal pregnancy is associated with a progressive increase in plasma and extracellular fluid volume and with a rise in cardiac output (Robson et al., 1989b), which are likely adaptations (via renal sodium retention) to progressive vasodilation induced by the hormonal milieu (Goldberg and Schrier, 1991). A host of causes for vasodilation are present: the placenta imposes an arteriovenous shunt on the maternal circulation, the endothelial cells make more vasodilatory prostaglandins, and high levels of progesterone and estrogen may contribute. As a result of these vasodilatory forces, the pressor response to exogenous angiotensin II becomes progressively lessened (Abdul-Karim and Assali, 1961; Ito et al., 1992). Plasma levels of

atrial natriuretic factor are normal (Lowe et al., 1992), further evidence that despite an increased fluid volume, the central circulation is not overexpanded.

Along with the increased blood volume, peripheral edema is common, but this often arises from interference of venous return by the enlarged uterus (Thomson et al., 1967).

Sodium Transport

As noted in Chapter 3, various measures of sodium transport in blood cells are altered in patients with primary hypertension. Numerous changes have been reported in normotensive pregnancy, including a decrease in erythrocyte sodium concentration and increases in ouabain-sensitive sodium flux, the sodium pump rate constant, and maximum velocity (MacPhail et al., 1992). These various indices of increased sodium transport across cells are accompanied by high plasma levels of a ouabain-like factor that is thought to inhibit the membrane Na^+,K^+–ATPase pump (Delva et al., 1989). The presence of this factor, which may arise in the placenta, could lead to the synthesis of more pump units (ouabain binding sites).

Renal Function

Renal blood flow and glomerular filtration rate are increased by about 50% early in pregnancy, with a gradual return to nonpregnant levels toward the end of gestation and without significant changes in intraglomerular pressure or permeability and normal renal hemodynamic reserve (Davison, 1992).

Renin-Angiotensin-Aldosterone

Plasma renin levels, both active and inactive, and renin substrate are increased in normal pregnancy (Brown et al., 1963). The levels of renin activity and concentration are elevated, in part, as a consequence of the estrogen-induced stimulation of renin substrate, which increases about sixfold (Sealey et al., 1982). Two other factors contribute: first, the various hemodynamic and renal changes described above, which tend to activate the release of renin; and second, the contribution of renin synthesized in the placenta (Lenz et al., 1989).

Prorenin, the biosynthetic precursor of renin, is produced in large amounts early in pregnancy in the ovaries, later in the uteroplacental unit, but its function remains uncertain (Itskovitz et al., 1992).

The probable importance of high levels of active renin and angiotensin II in maintaining BP and uterine blood flow during normal pregnancy is supported by the following finding: when the action of endogenous angiotensin II was blocked by the angiotensin-converting enzyme inhibitor (ACEI) captopril, the mean BP of normal pregnant women fell from 78 to 64 mm Hg (Taufield et al., 1988). In addition, the increased levels of angiotensin II in the maternal circulation increase the secretion of aldosterone and 11-deoxycorticosterone (Dörr et al., 1989).

At the same time, as various forces raise levels of renin-angiotensin-aldosterone, normal pregnancy brings forth numerous mechanisms to protect the circulations of both mother and fetus from the intense vasoconstriction, volume retention, and potassium wastage that high angiotensin II and aldosterone levels would ordinarily engender.

Responsiveness to Angiotensin and Aldosterone

Pregnant women are relatively resistant to the pressor effects of exogenous angiotensin II (Abdul-Karim and Assali, 1961; Ito et al., 1992); this reflects down-regulation of angiotensin II receptors by the high levels of circulating angiotensin II (Baker et al., 1992b) and antagonism by endothelium-derived vasodilating prostacyclin and nitric oxide, which are vasodilatory (Magness et al., 1992). Moreover, the placenta is less responsive to angiotensin II than most nonreproductive tissues, which results in a preferential maintenance of perfusion through the uteroplacental bed (Loquet et al., 1990).

The large amounts of potent mineralocorticoids present during pregnancy would be expected to maintain sodium balance at the cost of progressive renal wastage of potassium, yet pregnant women are normokalemic. This appears to be due to the high level of progesterone, which acts as an aldosterone antagonist (Brown et al., 1986).

Prostaglandin Synthesis

As noted, the resistance to angiotensin likely reflects the increased synthesis of vasodilatory prostanoids reflected by progressively higher plasma levels of prostacyclin and lower levels of thromboxane during normal pregnancy (Wang et al., 1991). When normal pregnant women were given inhibitors of prostaglandin synthesis (indomethacin or aspirin), they lost their refractoriness (Everett et al., 1978), and vasoconstriction developed within the placenta (Broughton-Pipkin et al., 1984).

Overview of the Circulation in Normal Pregnancy

Normal pregnancy, then, is a low-BP state associated with marked vasodilation that reduces peripheral resistance but an expanded fluid volume that increases cardiac output. Renal blood flow is markedly increased, and the renin-aldosterone system is activated (Table 11.1).

PREECLAMPSIA

All of the preceding is a prologue to our understanding of preeclampsia. Almost all of these various hemodynamic, renal, and hormonal changes of normal pregnancy are altered in preeclampsia (Table 11.1).

Hemodynamic Changes

The basic abnormality appears to be "profound vasoconstriction [that] reduces the intravascular capacity even more than blood volume" (Roberts and Redman, 1993). Intense vasospasm often can be seen in the nail beds,

Table 11.1. Changes in Normal Pregnancy and Preeclampsia

	Normal Pregnancy	Changes Occurring with Preeclampsia[a]
Hemodynamics		
Plasma volume	Expanded	Decreased
Extracellular fluid volume	Increased	Unchanged
Cardiac output	Increased	Decreased
Peripheral resistance	Reduced	Increased
Vascular reactivity:		
To norepinephrine	Unchanged	Increased
To angiotensin	Reduced	Increased
Uterine blood flow		Decreased
Renal function		
Blood flow	Increased	Decreased
Glomerular filtration	Increased	Decreased
Plasma uric acid	Decreased	Increased
Excretion of sodium load	Normal	Unchanged
Hormonal changes		
Plasma renin substrate	Increased	Unchanged
Plasma renin activity	Increased	Decreased
Plasma angiotensin II	Increased	Decreased
Angiotensin II receptors	Decreased	Increased
Plasma aldosterone	Increased	Decreased
Mineralocorticoid receptors	Increased	Decreased
Atrial natriuretic factor	Normal	Increased
Endogenous ouabain-like factor	Increased	Increased
Plasma insulin	Increased	Increased
Plasma endothelin	Normal	Increased or unchanged
Prostacyclin synthesis	Increased	Decreased
Thromboxane synthesis	Increased	Increased

[a]These changes are relative, as compared with those seen in normal pregnancy, and are not compared with those seen in nonpregnant women.

retinas, and coronary arteries (Bauer et al., 1982). The hypoxia resulting from the vasospasm is responsible for the various changes in tissue structure and function. Beyond spasm, structural alterations with increased thickness of the media relative to lumen diameter were found in omental resistance vessels from women with preeclampsia (Aalkjaer et al., 1984). Deposition of fibrin products is also widespread and may play a role in the diminution of blood flow.

Most of the data on the hemodynamics of preeclampsia have been obtained from women with severe disease relatively late in its course. In such patients, plasma volume is reduced by 10% to 40%, cardiac output is low, and peripheral resistance is increased (Wallenburg, 1988) (Fig. 11.2). However, in women with less severe preeclampsia, the hemodynamic findings are more heterogeneous: some have high cardiac output and low peripheral resistance (Easterling and Benedetti, 1989).

Pathogenesis

The cause of preeclampsia must explain the following features, as delineated by Chesley (1985):

—It occurs almost exclusively during the first pregnancy: nulliparas are from 6 to 8 times more susceptible than are multiparas;

—It occurs more frequently in the young and in those with multiple fetuses, hydatidiform mole, or diabetes;

—The incidence increases as term approaches; it is unusual before the end of the second trimester;

—The features of the syndrome are hypertension, edema, proteinuria and, when advanced, convulsions and coma;

—There is characteristic renal and hepatic pathology;

—The syndrome has a hereditary tendency. In the families of women who had preeclampsia, the syndrome developed in 25% of their

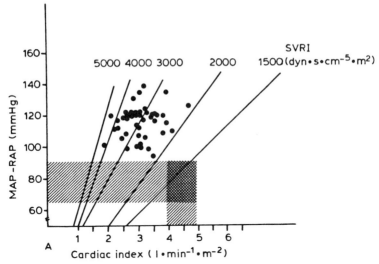

Figure 11.2. Relationship between systemic perfusion pressure *(MAP—RAP)*, cardiac index, and systemic vascular resistance index *(SVRI)* in 44 untreated nulliparous preeclamptic patients. Values for normotensive pregnant women fall within the *crosshatched area*. (From Wallenburg HCS. Hemodynamics in hypertensive pregnancy. In: Rubin PC, ed. *Handbook of Hypertension, Vol 10: Hypertension in Pregnancy.* Amsterdam: Elsevier Science Publishers, 1988:66–101.)

daughters and granddaughters, but only in 6% of their daughters-in-law (Chesley, 1980);
—It rapidly disappears when the pregnancy is terminated.

The risk factors for preeclampsia and its often erratic course have been well studied. Many of the mechanisms for various consequences are known (e.g., increased sensitivity to angiotensin II), and lessened production of vasodilating prostaglandins likely explains the rise in BP. But what remains elusive is the initiating mechanism, the match that sets off the ofttimes explosive course of this strange malady that disturbs up to one in five first pregnancies and hardly ever is seen again.

Deficient Trophoblastic Migration

The mystery may have been solved, as noted by Geoffrey Chamberlain (1991a):

The cause of pregnancy induced hypertension is now almost completely understood, with reasonable educated guesses being possible in unknown cases. The primary defect is failure of the second wave of trophoblastic invasion. Usually the trophoblast invades the entire length of the spiral arteries by 22 weeks of gestation. This leads to an appreciable fall in peripheral resistance and therefore a fall in BP. In addition, as the trophoblast usually removes all the muscle coat of the spiral arteries, blood flows unimpeded into the intervillous space, gushing like a fountain over the villous tree that contains the fetal vessels. This ensures adequate time for exchange of oxygen, nutrients, and the waste products of metabolism [Fig. 11.3].

Support for Chamberlain's construct certainly exists (Redman, 1991b; Roberts and Redman, 1993). Histopathologists have shown absent or aberrant trophoblastic invasion (Pijnenborg et al., 1991; Khong et al., 1992). Not only is trophoblastic invasion limited, but the expression of adhesion molecules from these cells is diminished, leading the investigators to conclude that "the delicate balance of adhesive interactions that normally permit cytotrophoblast invasion is tipped in favor of those which restrain this process, with the net effect of shallow uterine invasion" (Zhou et al., 1993).

Uteroplacental Hypoperfusion

The consequences of deficient trophoblastic migration with retention of musculoelastic media in spiral arteries could explain the major phenomenon that is usually held responsible for the pathophysiology of preeclampsia: uteroplacental hypoperfusion (Fig. 11.4). In addition to the histopathologic evidence noted above, other data support uteroplacental hypoperfusion:

—Some features can be induced by chronic uterine ischemia in various experimental animals (Phippard and Horvath, 1988);
—Uteroplacental blood flow is decreased, as measured by an isotopic accumulation curve (Lunell et al., 1982) and by Doppler ultrasonography (Kevin and Stuart, 1992);
—The clearance of steroid precursors for the synthesis of estrogens by the placenta, used

as an indicator of placental perfusion, is markedly reduced after hypertension develops (Everett et al., 1980).

Uteroplacental hypoperfusion fits with the recognized clinical circumstances wherein preeclampsia is most common: *reduced placental mass relative to need* (first pregnancies in young women, twins, hydatidiform mole) and *compromised uterine vasculature* (diabetes and preexisting hypertension).

Prostaglandin Imbalance

The next step in the scheme shown in Figure 11.4 is decreased fetoplacental production of prostacyclin, as originally suggested by Speroff

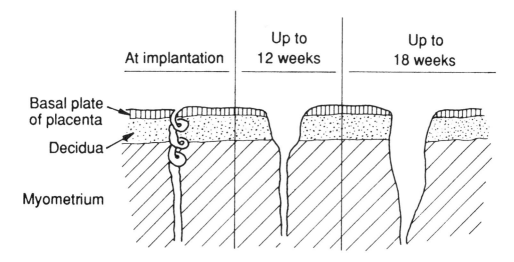

Figure 11.3. The normal invasion of spiral arteries by the trophoblast converts them into deltas and so improves blood flow. This invasion is defective in preeclampsia. (From Chamberlain G. Raised blood pressure in pregnancy. *Br Med J* 1991a;302:1454–1458.)

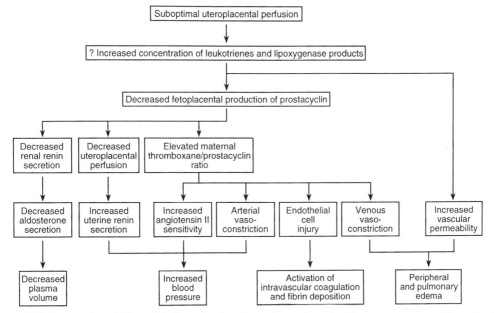

Figure 11.4. Proposed model to explain the pathophysiology of preeclampsia. (The consequences of the activation of intravascular coagulation and fibrin deposition are shown in Fig. 11.6). (From Friedman SA. Preeclampsia: a review of the role of prostaglandins. *Obstet Gynecol* 1988;71:122–137, reprinted with permission from The American College of Obstetricians and Gynecologists.)

in 1973. The evidence continues to mount that preeclampsia represents an imbalance in the placental production of the two major prostaglandins, decreased vasodilatory prostacyclin and increased vasoconstrictor thromboxane, along with increases in toxic lipid peroxides (Wang et al., 1992). These alterations have been shown to precede the onset of preeclampsia and to be related to uteroplacental blood flow (Meagher and Fitzgerald, 1993). On the other hand, the source of the prostaglandin imbalance may be endothelial cells altered by a circulating factor that arises from the hypoperfused placenta (Roberts and Redman, 1993).

Treatment with Low-Dose Aspirin.   The hypothesis that an imbalance between prostacyclin and thromboxane is responsible for preeclampsia suggests that small doses of aspirin (which block platelet synthesis of thromboxane but do not interfere with endothelial synthesis of prostacyclin) would be beneficial.

The evidence accumulated over the past few years suggests that the effectiveness of aspirin may be related to the degree of risk. A meta-analysis of six small controlled trials of low-dose aspirin therapy showed a significant reduction in the incidence of preeclampsia in women at high risk (Imperiale et al., 1991). A multicenter controlled trial studied 1106 women between 16 and 32 weeks of gestation considered to be at intermediate risk for various reasons; the half given 50 mg a day of aspirin had no significant differences from the half given no treatment in multiple end-points, including the frequency of preeclampsia (Italian Study of Aspirin in Pregnancy, 1993). In another multicenter trial involving 2985 women at low risk, 60 mg a day of aspirin was given to half starting from 13 to 27 weeks of gestation (Sibai et al., 1993). The incidence of preeclampsia was reduced from 6.3% in the placebo-treated half to 4.6% (relative risk, 0.7; 95% confidence interval, 0.6–1.0; p = .05). Most of the reduction was seen in patients with initially elevated systolic pressures. However, the frequency of abruptio placenta increased from 0.1% to 0.7% in the aspirin-treated half, and perinatal outcomes were not affected. The investigators concluded as follows: "We do not recommend the routine use of low-dose aspirin therapy in healthy nulliparous women" (Sibai et al., 1993).

These negative results in women at low and intermediate risk do not preclude the potential benefit for low-dose aspirin in women at relatively high risk for preeclampsia (Dekker and Sibai, 1993). In the future, selective inhibitors of thromboxane synthesis or receptors may prove to be safer and more effective (Wilkes et al., 1992).

Endothelial Alterations

Whether arising form the placenta or from the endothelial cells, changes in prostaglandins may have systemic effects that induce the multiple features of preeclampsia (Fig. 11.4). There is evidence for placental release of substances that circulate to alter endothelial cells; either (a) they do not produce vasodilatory autocrine and paracrine factors such as nitric oxide and prostacyclin (McCarthy et al., 1992) or (b) they do produce vasoconstricting factors such as endothelin (Schiff et al., 1992) or platelet-derived growth factor (Roberts et al., 1991, 1992). Whatever the mechanism, endothelium-derived relaxation is impaired in preeclampsia (Pinto et al., 1991). Despite the uncertainty as to the exact mechanism, the potential for treatment with nitric oxide precursors has already been suggested (Giles et al., 1992).

Increased Responsiveness to Angiotensin II

Women who develop preeclampsia have an increased pressor responsiveness to angiotensin II as early as the 22nd week of gestation, often 10 to 15 weeks before hypertension appears (Gant et al., 1973) (Fig. 11.5). This hypersensitivity is thought to reflect an increased vascular responsiveness and not a better-filled vascular bed, since a study showed that volume expansion did not decrease the resistance of normotensive women near term to that seen in women destined to develop preeclampsia (Cunningham et al., 1975). Perhaps as a result of the increased pressor sensitivity to angiotensin II, plasma renin and angiotensin II levels decrease, so that the number and binding affinity of angiotensin II receptors on platelets increase (Baker et al., 1992a).

Other Theories

A host of other theories have been proposed for the pathogenesis of preeclampsia. Although each is supported by various types of evidence, none seems to fulfill all of the requirements needed to explain the syndrome better than the theory of uteroplacental hypoperfusion.

Genetic Susceptibility

Whatever else is responsible, there is clearly a familial factor that appears to be inherited from

COMPARISON OF ANGIOTENSIN RESPONSIVENESS IN 192 PRIMIGRAVID WOMEN (1190 INFUSIONS)

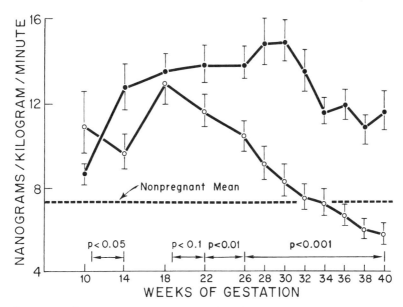

Figure 11.5. Comparison of the mean angiotensin II doses (in ng/kg/minute) required to evoke a pressor response in 120 primigravidas who remained normotensive *(filled circles)* and 72 primigravidas who ultimately developed pregnancy-induced hypertension *(unfilled circles)*. The nonpregnant mean is shown as a *dashed line*. The *vertical bars* represent the SEM. The difference between the two groups became significant after week 23, and the two groups continued to diverge widely after the 26th week. (From Gant NF, Daley GL, Chand S, Whalley PJ, MacDonald PC. A study of angiotensin II pressor response throughout primigravid pregnancy. *J Clin Invest* 1973;52:2682–2689.)

the mother, since preeclampsia is more frequent in the mothers but not the mothers-in-law of women with preeclampsia (Sutherland et al., 1981), and the frequency of eclampsia is increased in the daughters of women who had eclampsia (Cooper et al., 1988). Statistical modeling supports homozygosity for a single recessive gene shared by mother and fetus (Liston and Kilpatrick, 1992). A significantly higher incidence of preeclampsia in 25 pregnancies complicated by trisomy 13 suggests that a fetal factor also may be involved (Tuohy and James, 1992).

Intravascular Coagulation

As seen in Figure 11.6, activation of intravascular coagulation and subsequent fibrin deposition may be responsible for much of the eventual organ damage seen in severe preeclampsia. Increased plasma levels of indicators of platelet activation (bcta thromboglobulin), coagulation (thrombin-antithrombin III complexes), and endothelial cell damage (fibronectin and laminin) have been measured up to 4 weeks before the onset of clinical features of preeclampsia,

suggesting that these processes may be more involved than usually is credited (Ballegeer et al., 1992).

HELLP Syndrome.   A few women develop a more serious complication of preeclampsia: the HELLP syndrome, which involves hemolysis (H), elevated liver enzymes (EL), and low platelet (LP) counts (Weinstein, 1982). In one series of 454 pregnancies, with increasing degrees of thrombocytopenia below 150,000/ml, maternal and perinatal mortality increased and one in six patients developed eclampsia (Martin et al., 1992).

Immunologic Injury

An immunologic mechanism is supported by the decreased incidence of preeclampsia in women who have had prior term pregnancy (Campbell et. al., 1985) or blood transfusion (Feeney et al., 1977) and by the increased risk for users of contraceptives that prevent exposure to sperm (Klonoff-Cohen et al., 1989), suggesting that the disease is related to initial exposure of the patient to foreign antigens. Moreover, when multiparas develop preeclampsia, it is

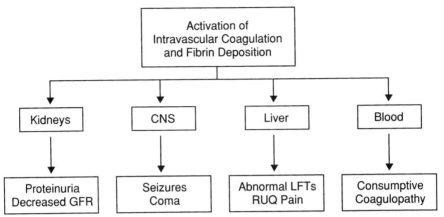

Figure 11.6. Proposed model to explain the consequences of activation of intravascular coagulation and fibrin deposition in the pathophysiology of preeclampsia. *CNS*, central nervous system; *GFR*, glomerular filtration rate; *LFT*, liver function test; *RUQ*, right upper quadrant. (From Friedman SA and reprinted with permission from The American College of Obstetricians and Gynecologists. *Obstetrics and Gynecology* 1988;71:122).

often in association with a new father (Ikedife, 1980), further suggesting an inadequate immune response to different fetal antigens.

Alterations in Sodium Transport

Some, but not all, of the alterations in sodium transport across cell membranes seen in normal pregnancy may be accentuated during pre-eclampsia. These include:

—Increased erythrocyte sodium-lithium countertransport (Seely et. al., 1992);
—Increased erythrocyte sodium-potassium cotransport (Miyamoto et. al., 1992);
—Increased plasma levels of a ouabain-like sodium pump inhibitor (Seely et al., 1992). However, no evidence of either sodium pump inhibition or increased intracellular sodium were found in 32 preeclamptic women (MacPhail et al., 1992);
—Increased plasma levels of atrial natriuretic factor (Malee et al., 1991).

Other Associations

Hyperinsulinemia. Among 16 women with nonproteinuric hypertension in the third trimester, eight had marked hyperinsulinemia in response to an oral glucose load (Bauman et al., 1988).

Plasma Endothelin. Plasma endothelin is found to be elevated by some (Schiff et al., 1992) but not by others (Benigni et al., 1992).

Sympathetic Nervous System Activity. Plasma catecholamines have been found to be elevated by some (Øian et al., 1986) but not by others (Rubin et al., 1986).

Serotonin. Increased urinary excretion of 5-hydroxyindole acetate, the major metabolite of serotonin, has been found (Filshie et al., 1992).

Calcium and Parathyroid Hormone. After noting that preeclampsia is usually associated with hypocalciuria, August et al. (1992) found decreased 1,25-dihydroxyvitamin D levels in preeclamptic women, which they assume lead to decreased intestinal absorption of calcium, stimulation of parathyroid hormone, and increased renal tubular reabsorption of calcium. The cause of the low 1,25-hydroxyvitamin D levels remains unknown. These findings complement the reports of reduced risks of developing preeclampsia with increased calcium intake (Villar et al., 1987; Marcoux et al., 1991).

Diagnosis

Hypertension developing after the 20th week of gestation with proteinuria and edema in a young nullipara is probably preeclampsia, particularly if she has a positive family history for the syndrome. Since patients usually have no symptoms due to the three main features of preeclampsia—hypertension, proteinuria, and edema—prenatal care is crucial in order to detect these features early and thereby prevent the dangerous sequelae of the fully developed syndrome.

Hypertension

The BP criterion is based either on readings of 140/90 mm Hg or higher or on rises of systolic blood pressure (SBP) of 30 mm Hg or more or diastolic blood pressure (DBP) of 15 mm Hg or more. These pressures should be recorded on at least two occasions, 6 hours or more apart. Obviously, it is not possible to reconfirm the pressure levels over many weeks, as is recommended in nonpregnant patients.

Overdiagnosis. Despite the greater overall perinatal mortality with even transient elevations in pressure, for the individual patient there is a significant chance of overdiagnosing preeclampsia on the basis of these values, which have been found to have only a 23% to 33% positive predictive value and an 81% to 85% negative predictive value (Dekker and Sibai, 1991). Therefore, multiple readings and careful follow-up over at least a few days or weeks are needed for women who display such findings in the absence of any other suggestive features before making the diagnosis or instituting therapy.

Consequences. On the other hand, the level of pressure may not be inordinately high for it to have serious consequences: women may convulse because of hypertensive encephalopathy with pressures of only 160/110. This may well reflect the relatively low pressure at which the breakthrough of cerebral blood flow occurs in previously normotensive patients, as described by Strandgaard et al. and detailed in Chapter 8. Since women with preeclampsia are usually young and, by definition, previously normotensive, their blood vessels would be particularly susceptible to the pressure-induced marked breakthrough vasodilation that leads to encephalopathy.

Proteinuria

The urine should contain more than 300 mg of protein in a 24-hour collection or 100 mg/dl in two random, cleanly voided specimens collected at least 4 hours apart.

Edema

Sudden and excessive weight gain of more than 2 lbs in 1 week due to extracellular fluid volume expansion is usually the earliest warning sign that preeclampsia is developing, and it is detectable before subcutaneous edema can be detected.

Progression of the Disease

Preeclampsia is considered to become progressively more severe with the appearance of the signs and symptoms listed in Table 11.2, which usually mandate hospitalization. Fetal distress is common, and preterm delivery often is needed.

Table 11.2. Ominous Signs and Symptoms in Women with Preeclampsia

Blood pressure ≥110 mm Hg diastolic

Proteinuria of new onset at a rate of ≥2 g per 24 hours or ≥100 mg per deciliter in a randomly collected specimen

Increasing serum creatinine levels (especially > 177 μmol per liter [2 mg per deciliter] unless the level was known to be elevated previously)

Platelet count <10 × 10⁹ per liter or evidence of microangiopathic hemolytic anemia

Upper abdominal pain, especially epigastric and right-upper-quadrant pain

Headache, visual disturbances, or other cerebral signs

Cardiac decompensation (e.g., pulmonary edema)

Retinal hemorrhage, exudates, or papilledema

Fetal growth retardation

From Cunningham FG, Lindheimer MD. Hypertension in pregnancy. *N Engl J Med* 1992;326:927–932.

Differential Diagnosis

The onset of preeclampsia before the 37th week of gestation increases the chance that not preeclampsia, but another form of hypertension—usually primary (essential) hypertension or chronic renal disease—is present (Ihle et al., 1987), as has been documented by renal biopsy findings (Packham et al., 1988).

The error can be minimized by recognition of the features that favor the diagnosis of primary hypertension over preeclampsia:

—Onset of hypertension before 20 weeks of gestation;
—Hypertension not caused by preeclampsia in a previous pregnancy;
—Failure to develop hypertension during the first pregnancy, but its appearance in subsequent ones;
—Absence of proteinuria and edema;
—Evidence of sustained and severe hypertension (systolic pressure of 200 mm Hg) with retinal hemorrhages and exudates or left ventricular hypertrophy (Thompson et al., 1986);
—Age of 30 years or more.

Early Detection

Women with the following features should be more closely watched, because they have a higher likelihood of developing preeclampsia: young primigravidas; a family history of preeclampsia; multiple fetuses; black race; preexisting hypertension, heart disease, or renal disease;

obesity, and preeclampsia in a previous pregnancy (Eskenazi et al., 1991).

A number of clinical and laboratory tests have been used in an attempt to recognize preeclampsia before it develops and to differentiate it from primary hypertension. As Dekker and Sibai (1991) note: "More than 100 clinical, biophysical, and biochemical tests have been recommended for predicting future development of preeclampsia. Results of the pooled data and the wide scatter therein suggest that none of these tests is sufficiently sensitive or specific for use as a screening test in clinical practice." Therefore, we are left with frequent determinations of BP and the appearance of proteinuria and edema as the best method of early detection.

Management

A succinct overview of the management of preeclampsia is provided by Redman and Roberts (1993):

... The cure is achieved by delivery, which removes the diseased tissue—the placenta. In short, the need is to deliver before it is too late. To achieve this apparently simple end the clinician must detect the symptomless prodromal condition by screening all pregnant women, admit to hospital those with advanced preeclampsia so as to keep track of an unpredictable situation, and time pre-emptive delivery to maximize the safety of mother and baby.

Nonpharmacologic Management

Monitoring. In the absence of any of the ominous manifestations listed in Table 11.2, frequent outpatient observations are continued; if these signs and symptoms appear, however, immediate hospitalization is indicated.

Modified Bed Rest. The value of bed rest has been widely accepted but little supported by clinical trials. As Brown (1990) observes: "The few data available suggest that in severe forms of [preeclampsia], bed rest confers some benefit upon fetal outcome, possibly by improving placental function, with little demonstrable benefit upon maternal outcome."

Diet. Current evidence favors maintenance of usual sodium intake in order to avoid further reducing placental perfusion (Steegers et al., 1991). Some favor plasma volume expansion, but this practice should be limited to those with documented volume reduction (Brown, 1990).

There is no need to restrict dietary protein or calories in patients who are not markedly overweight. Calcium supplements have been found to reduce the incidence of preeclampsia in populations with low calcium intake (Marcoux et al., 1991), but there is no evidence that they are useful in the treatment of established hypertension.

Pharmacologic Therapy

The 1990 National High Blood Pressure Education Program Working Group states:

The palliative management of preeclampsia remote from delivery is controversial. The sole rationale is to allow maturation of the fetus and, if attempted, it must not subject the mother to undue risk. An important part of safe management is control of elevated blood pressure. In the woman with diastolic blood pressure 100 mm Hg or greater, risk is sufficient to warrant pharmacologic therapy. The therapy is solely for maternal benefit; there is neither theoretic basis nor empiric evidence that such therapy is beneficial to the fetus.

This hesitation to use antihypertensive drugs in women with preeclampsia remote from term has received additional support from studies showing no advantage of drug therapies over bed rest alone (Plouin et al., 1990; Sibai et al., 1992).

The continued advocacy of methyldopa, a drug that has been largely abandoned in the treatment of hypertension in every setting save pregnancy, reflects the known ability of the drug to reduce midtrimester abortions and perinatal deaths while causing no physical or mental developmental difficulties in the offspring followed for up to 7.5 years (Redman, 1991a). Equal antihypertensive efficacy has been shown for other drugs (Lowe and Rubin, 1992), but there are reports of intrauterine growth retardation with the beta blocker atenolol (Butters et al., 1990) and concern that calcium entry blockers may interfere with myometrial contractions (Hennessy and Horvath, 1992). Only ACEIs are absolutely contraindicated because of their propensity to induce neonatal renal failure and hypotension (Rosa et al., 1989).

Therapy of Severe Preeclampsia

Often the BP increases abruptly as the woman goes into labor or during delivery. Guidelines for the treatment of severe hypertension in this setting are given in Table 11.3 (Cunningham and Lindheimer, 1992). More details about the individual agents are provided in Chapter 8 (Table 8.5) and by Remuzzi and Ruggenenti (1991). Few trials have compared the various drugs. In one trial, 24 patients received sublingual and oral nifedipine, and 25 received intravenous and oral hydralazine (Fenakel et al., 1991).

Table 11.3. Guidelines for Treating Severe Hypertension Near Term or During Labor

Regulation of blood pressure

The degree to which blood pressure should be decreased is disputed; we recommend maintaining diastolic levels between 90 and 110 mm Hg.

Drug therapy

Hydralazine administered intravenously is the drug of choice. Start with low doses (5 mg as an intravenous bolus), then administer 5 to 10 mg every 20 to 30 minutes to avoid precipitous decreases in pressure. Side effects include tachycardia and headache.

Dizoxide is recommended for women whose hypertension is refractory to hydralazine. Use 30-mg miniboluses since precipitous hypotension may result with higher doses. Side effects include arrest of labor and neonatal hypoglycemia.

The experience with labetalol is growing, and some physicians use this agent, instead of diazoxide, as a second-line drug.

Favorable results have been reported with calcium-channel blockers. If magnesium sulfate is being infused, magnesium may potentiate the effects of calcium channel blockers, resulting in precipitous and severe hypotension.

Refrain from using sodium nitroprusside, because fetal cyanide poisoning has been reported in animals. However, maternal well-being should dictate the choice of therapy.

Prevention of convulsions

Parenteral magnesium sulfate is the drug of choice for preventing eclamptic convulsions. Therapy should be continued for 12 to 24 hours post partum because one-third of women with eclampsia have convulsions during this period.

From Cunningham FG, Lindheimer MD. Hypertension in pregnancy. *N Engl J Med* 1992;326:927–932.

Nifedipine provided better control of the hypertension and induced less fetal distress than did hydralazine, but there were no differences in substantive neonatal outcomes. In another trial, intravenous labetalol and hydralazine were equally effective in lowering the BP, but labetalol appeared to cause beta blockade in the fetuses, an effect the authors consider potentially harmful (Harper and Murnaghan, 1991). Intravenous prostacyclin has also been shown to be as effective as hydralazine and to induce less tachycardia (Moodley and Gouws, 1992).

As seen in Table 11.3, Cunningham and Lindheimer advocate the prophylactic use of magnesium sulfate to prevent eclamptic convulsions in women with severe and advancing preeclampsia; magnesium sulfate has been shown to dilate small intracranial vessels and to relieve cerebral ischemia (Belfort and Moise, 1992). Diazepam or phenytoin often is used elsewhere (Hutton et al., 1992).

ECLAMPSIA

Eclampsia is defined by the occurrence of seizures due to hypertensive encephalopathy on the background of preeclampsia. This serious complication is becoming less common as better prenatal care is given: the present incidence in North America and Europe is estimated to be about 1 in every 2000 deliveries (Douglas and Redman, 1992). However, where prenatal care is neglected, eclampsia remains both common and deadly (Sibai, 1990).

Clinical Features

Eclampsia is a form of hypertensive encephalopathy, and is demonstrable by cerebral imaging (Dahmus et al., 1992). The convulsions that signify eclampsia are usually preceded by the clinical manifestations of preeclampsia. In as many as 20% of cases, seizures begin post partum, even as late as 6 days after delivery (Neiger and Rosene, 1992). Although patients may have preceding auras, epigastric pain, apprehension, and hyperreflexia, the convulsions often occur with little or no warning. After the intense tonic-clonic convulsion, patients become stuporous and usually comatose.

Other Features

Hypertension may be severe, although some patients may have only minimal pressure elevations. Proteinuria frequently is pronounced. Edema is variable and occasionally massive. Oliguria is invariable, and anuria may supervene if adequate fluid intake is not maintained (Sibai et al., 1990b). Pulmonary edema is common in fatal cases and probably represents direct damage to the capillary bed and heart failure. Blindness, usually from retinal edema but sometimes from retinal detachment, occurs rarely. Evidence of intravascular coagulation, often with the full

HELLP syndrome, is prominent and probably secondary to the widespread vascular damage (Miles et al., 1990).

Management

Delivery is delayed until convulsions are stopped, the BP is controlled, and reasonable fluid and electrolyte balance have been established. With the following standardized treatment of 245 consecutive cases of eclampsia, only one maternal death occurred, and all but one of the fetuses survived who were alive when treatment was started and who weighed 1800 g or more at birth (Pritchard et al., 1984):

1. Magnesium sulfate to control convulsions.
2. Control of severe hypertension (DBP 110 mm Hg) with intermittent intravenous injections of hydralazine.
3. Avoidance of diuretics and hyperosmotic agents.
4. Limitation of fluid intake unless fluid loss was excessive.
5. Delivery once convulsions were arrested and consciousness was regained.

Consequences

Considering the seriousness of eclampsia, many physicians have advised affected women that they should not become pregnant again. However, Chesley (1980) found that in 466 later pregnancies in 189 women who had had eclampsia, only 25% had recurrent hypertension, and only 4 had a second episode of eclampsia. In a 22- to 44-year follow-up of these women, the remote prognosis for those who had eclampsia during their first pregnancy was excellent (Chesley et al., 1976). The distribution of their BPs was identical to those of the general population.

CHRONIC HYPERTENSION AND PREGNANCY

Pregnant women may have any of the other types of hypertension listed in Table 1.6, in Chapter 1. Because the BP usually falls during the first half of pregnancy, preexisting hypertension may not be recognized if the woman is first seen during that time. If the pressure is high during the first 20 weeks, however, chronic hypertension and not preeclampsia is almost always present.

Essential Hypertension During Pregnancy

Pregnancy seems to bring out latent primary hypertension in certain women whose pressures

return to normal between pregnancies but eventually remain elevated. In most patients, such "transient hypertension" appears late in gestation, is not accompanied by significant proteinuria or edema, and recedes within 10 days after delivery. Transient hypertension usually recurs during subsequent pregnancies and is often the basis for the misdiagnosis of preeclampsia in multiparous women (National High Blood Pressure Education Program Working Group, 1990).

To elucidate the true nature of hypertension seen during a pregnancy, it is often necessary to follow the patient post partum. By 3 months, complete resolution of the various changes seen in pregnancy will have occurred so that, if indicated, further studies can be obtained.

Management

Women with severe hypertension should be advised not to become pregnant and should be warned of the possibility of superimposed preeclampsia (see below). Women with mild to moderate hypertension should be watched more closely, warned about signs of early preeclampsia, and delivered at 37 weeks of gestation. With current management, there is no increased risk for adverse fetal outcome (Ferrazzani et al., 1990). As to the issue of antihypertensive therapy: it may protect the mother and may improve the chances for successful outcome of the pregnancy (Phippard et al., 1991); however, in a randomized trial of 263 women with mild chronic hypertension at 6 to 13 weeks of gestation, the third who received a placebo did as well as the third who received methyldopa or the third who were given labetalol throughout pregnancy (Sibai et al., 1990a).

Furthermore, not only may it be unnecessary to start medication, but many patients may be able to discontinue therapy used before pregnancy: of 211 pregnant women with mild chronic hypertension who stopped their medications at the first prenatal visit, only 13% required reinstitution of therapy and only 10% had superimposed preeclampsia (Sibai et al., 1983). Among the 190 without superimposed preeclampsia, only 5.3% had small-for-age infants, and there was only one perinatal death.

Cunningham and Lindheimer (1992) recommend the use of drugs in the manner shown in Table 11.4 "at diastolic pressures above 100 mm Hg, but at lower pressures if there are risk factors (for example, renal disease or end-organ damage)." They concur with the continued use of diuretics if they were used before conception.

Table 11.4. Antihypertensive Drugs: Used to Treat Chronic Hypertension in Pregnancy

Alpha-adrenergic receptor agonists
Methyldopa is the most extensively used drug in this group. Its safety and efficacy are supported by evidence from randomized trials, and there is a 7.5-year follow-up study of children born to mothers treated with methyldopa.

Beta-adrenergic receptor antagonists
These drugs, especially atenolol and metoprolol, appear to be safe and efficacious in late pregnancy, but fetal growth retardation has been reported when treatment was started in early or mid-gestation. Fetal bradycardia can occur, and animal studies suggest that the fetus's ability to tolerate hypoxic stress may be compromised.

Alpha-adrenergic receptor of beta-adrenergic receptor antagonists
Labetalol appears to be as effective as methyldopa, but there are no follow-up studies of children born to mothers given labetalol, and there is concern about maternal hepatotoxicity.

Arteriolar vasodilator
Hydralazine is frequently used as adjunctive therapy with methyldopa and beta-adrenergic receptor antagonists. Rarely, neonatal thrombocytopenia has been reported. Trials with calcium channel blockers look promising. The experience with minoxidil is limited, and this drug is not recommended.

Angiotensin-converting enzyme inhibitors
Captopril causes fetal death in diverse animal species, and several converting-enzyme inhibitors have been associated with oligohydramnios and neonatal renal failure when administered to humans. *Do not use in pregnancy.*

Diuretics
Many authorities discourage the use of diuretics, but others continue these medications if they were prescribed before conception or if a woman with chronic hypertension appears quite sensitive to salt.

From Cunningham FG, Lindheimer MD. Hypertension in pregnancy. *N Engl J Med* 1992;326:927–932.

Preeclampsia Superimposed on Chronic Hypertension

Preeclampsia occurs more frequently in women with preexisting hypertension than in previously normotensive women; the incidence varies from as low as 10% to as high as 50% (Chesley, 1978). The diagnosis usually is based on the appearance of proteinuria and edema, and an increase in the level of BP. About 1% of these women develop eclampsia, and they are prone to redevelop preeclampsia with subsequent pregnancies: Chesley (1978) found a 71% recurrence rate of superimposed preeclampsia.

POSTPARTUM SYNDROMES

As noted earlier, preeclampsia and eclampsia may appear after delivery. In addition, other hypertension-related problems may develop post partum.

Postpartum Hypertension

In one study, 12% of 136 previously normotensive women had a DBP above 100 mm Hg over the first 4 days after delivery (Walters et al., 1986). In women who were preeclamptic, the hypertension may worsen during those first few days post partum (Crawford et al., 1987). These findings may relate to the fact that cardiac output remains elevated for at least 48 hours after normal delivery (Robson et al., 1987).

At 6 weeks post partum, 4% to 17% of women who were not hypertensive during the prior pregnancy or during the first few days after delivery are found to have hypertension (Piver et al., 1967). This likely represents the uncovering of early primary hypertension hidden by the hemodynamic and hormonal changes of pregnancy.

Other Syndromes

Cardiomyopathy may present in the last month of pregnancy or the during the first 6 months after delivery, without other identifiable causes (Marin-Neto et al., 1991), but often on the background of chronic hypertension or valvular disease (Cunningham et al., 1986). Fulminant nephrosclerosis may appear post partum and rapidly proceed into oliguric renal failure with severe hypertension (Strauss and Alexander, 1976).

Hypertension and Lactation

Breast feeding does not raise the mother's BP (Robson et al., 1989a), but bromocriptine mesylate used for suppression of lactation may induce hypertension (Watson et al., 1989). All antihypertensive drugs taken by mothers enter their breast milk. Most are present in very low concentrations, except beta blockers (other than propranolol) (White, 1984) and nifedipine (Penny and Lewis, 1989), which are present in concentrations similar to those in maternal plasma.

HYPERTENSION WITH ORAL CONTRACEPTIVES

Oral contraceptives (i.e., "the pill"), or OCs, have been used by millions of women since the early 1960s. The pill is safe for most women, but its use carries some risk: the BP increases a little in most users, and hypertension will appear in 5% who use it for 5 years.

Risks in Perspective

Various cardiovascular risks are increased with OC use, including myocardial infarction (Thorogood et al., 1991) and occlusive stroke (Thorogood et al., 1992). These risks, although real, have been overemphasized. The problem revolves around the very definite, statistically significant increase in risk associated with pill use on the one hand, but the failure to recognize that the absolute number of people afflicted is quite small on the other hand, and that the risk is not equal for all women who use the pill, being quite small for its primary audience.

Thus, in a large prospective study in England, a 40% higher death rate was found among women who used the pill (Royal College study, 1981). Virtually all of the excessive mortality was due to cardiovascular disease, with a four-fold greater risk of ischemic heart disease and subarachnoid hemorrhage. However, when the actual number of pill users who would suffer a vascular complication is calculated (the attributable risk), the fourfold excess turns out to be a relatively small number—about 2 deaths per 10,000 women per year (Stadel, 1981). Furthermore, the risk of myocardial infarction was concentrated in women 35 years or older and in smokers (Croft and Hannaford, 1989).

It should be further noted that the pill used today is safer than the pill used in the past. Smaller amounts of estrogen and progestogen are associated with fewer cardiovascular complications (Rosenberg et al., 1991).

To put the dangers of the pill in proper perspective, its use in women aged 15 to 34 who do not smoke is associated with less risk of death than most other contraceptive methods, particularly when its lower rate of failure to prevent pregnancy is considered (Ory, 1983). Only the condom, plus abortion if the condom fails, is safer and more effective than the pill.

The risk of pill use resolves with discontinuation: both the Royal College study and the massive Nurses' Health Study (Stampfer et al., 1990) found no excessive risk among former pill users.

Incidence

The BP rises a little in most women who take estrogen-containing oral contraceptives (Woods, 1988). The rise is enough to push the pressure beyond 140/90 in about 5% of users over a 5-year period of pill use (Royal College, 1974). In a very small number of users, the rise will be so abrupt and severe as to cause accelerated or malignant hypertension (Lim et al., 1987).

Though the first report of pill-induced hypertension appeared a few years after the pill's introduction (Brownrigg, 1962), the association was not clearly defined until 1967 (Laragh et al., 1967; Woods, 1967). Not until a prospective study was begun in Glasgow did it become apparent that the BP rose in most women who started OCs. Among 186 women who took estrogen-containing oral contraceptives for 2 years, SBP rose in 164 and DBP in 150 (Weir, 1982) (Fig. 11.7). Of these, 8 women had increases in SBP greater than 25 mm Hg, and two had increases in DBP of 24 to 34 mm Hg. The incidence of hypertension may be less with present-day, lower-dose formulations containing only 30 to 35 g of estrogen (Malatino et al., 1988).

Although, as we shall see, estrogen has been incriminated as the cause of pill-induced hypertension, the progestogen component may also be involved. When used alone, progestogens do not appear to raise the BP (Wilson et al., 1984), but when given with estrogens, they may potentiate the problem (Meade, 1988).

Predisposing Factors

Age and obesity are the only known predisposing factors to pill-induced hypertension. Women over age 35 are particularly susceptible. A positive family history of hypertension is noted in about half of women with pill-induced hypertension, but women with prior preeclampsia seem to carry little additional risk: only 9 of 180 women who had preeclampsia had a rise in DBP beyond 90 mm Hg after 6 months to 2 years of pill use (Pritchard and Pritchard, 1977). Similarly, women with preexisting primary

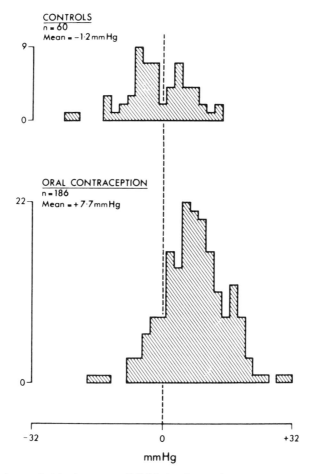

Figure 11.7. Changes in systolic blood pressure *(S.B.P.)* after 2 years in women taking estrogen-progestagen oral contraceptives and in controls. (From Weir RJ. Hypertension secondary to contraceptive agents. In: Amery A, Fagard R, Lijnen P, Staessen J, eds. *Hypertensive Cardiovascular Disease: Pathophysiology and Treatment.* The Hague/Boston/London: Martinus Nijhoff Publishers, 1982:612–628.)

hypertension do not appear to be particularly more susceptible (Tsai et al., 1985).

Clinical Course

In most women who develop hypertension, the disease is mild, and in more than half, the BP returns to normal when the pill is stopped (Weir, 1978). In a few women, the hypertension is severe, rapidly accelerating into a malignant phase and causing irreversible renal damage (Lim et al., 1987). Even in patients with reversible hypertension, considerable renal damage may be found by means of arteriography and renal biopsy (Boyd et al., 1975). A hemolytic

uremic syndrome may also follow pill use (Hauglustaine et al., 1981).

Mechanism

Whether the pill is causing hypertension de novo or simply uncovering the propensity toward primary hypertension that would eventually appear spontaneously is unknown. The mechanism for OC-induced hypertension also is unknown, particularly since endogenous estradiol appears to be vasodilatory (Sealey et al., 1992). Changes in hemodynamics, renin-angiotensin-aldosterone, insulin sensitivity, and erythrocyte cation transport have been identified. As noted, both the estrogen and the progestogen may be responsible.

Hemodynamic Changes

Walters and Lim (1970) and Lehtovirta (1974) found that body weight, plasma volume, and cardiac output were significantly increased in previously normal women after 2 to 3 months of pill intake. Crane and Harris (1978) found a 100- to 200-mEq increase in total body exchangeable sodium after 3 weeks' intake of stilbestrol, conjugated estrogens, estradiol, or mestranol. They also found that some of the progestogens used in the OCs, including norethindrone, caused comparable sodium retention when given to normal subjects.

Renin-Angiotensin-Aldosterone Changes

Estrogens increase the hepatic synthesis of renin substrate (Helmer and Judson, 1967) by inducing the expression of angiotensinogen mRNA (Gordon et al., 1992). The increase in substrate is accompanied by an increase in total renin activity but a fall in the concentration of renin (Derkx et al., 1986). Whether these changes in renin-angiotensin-aldosterone contribute to the hypertension is uncertain. With few exceptions (Saruta et al., 1970), most researchers have noted no significant differences in the direction or degree of these changes when comparing the majority of women who remain normotensive with the minority who become hypertensive.

In most women on the pill, the renal vasculature responds to the higher levels of angiotensin II with a reduction in renal blood flow (Hollenberg et al., 1976). Though the mean fall was 25% in this study, in some women it was as high as 50%. Perhaps women with the greatest renal vasoconstriction develop sodium retention and hypertension.

Insulin Resistance

In view of the potential role of insulin resistance in the pathogenesis of primary hypertension, as described in Chapter 3, it is noteworthy that OCs with 30 to 40 mg of ethinyl estradiol induce insulin resistance, and that progestin-only pills prolong the half-life of insulin (Godsland et al., 1992).

Guidelines for Use of OCs

When OCs are used, the following precautions should be taken:

—The lowest effective dose of estrogen and progestogen should be dispensed;

—No more than a 6-month supply should be provided at one time;

—The BP should be taken at least every 6 months or whenever the woman feels ill;

—If the BP rises significantly, the pill should be stopped and another form of contraceptive should be provided;

—If the BP does not become normal within 3 months, appropriate work-up and therapy should be provided;

—If no alternative form of contraception is feasible and the pill must be continued, antihypertensive therapy may be needed to control the BP.

POSTMENOPAUSAL ESTROGEN REPLACEMENT

In the future, an even larger number of women will likely begin postmenopausal estrogen replacement therapy (ERT) than will use estrogen-containing OCs. The increasingly strong evidence that ERT is associated with favorable changes in multiple cardiovascular risk factors (Nabulsi et al., 1993), which translates into significant protection against coronary disease (Rosenberg et al., 1993), stroke (Finucane et al., 1993), and overall mortality (Henderson et al., 1991), as well as osteoporosis (Prince et al., 1991), far outweighs the potential hazards of endometrial and breast cancer in the opinion of authorities worldwide (Barrett-Connor, 1992; Daly et al., 1992; Wren, 1992).

Hypertension and ERT

In view of the known prohypertensive effect of estrogens given in superphysiologic doses for contraception, there are concerns that the smaller doses for replacement might also raise the BP. Although hypertension rarely occurs with postmenopausal estrogen use (Crane et al., 1971), a prospective analysis of a large group of women aged 52 to 87 found that the use of oral estrogens for an average of 5 months did not alter the level or lability of the BP (Pfeffer et al., 1979). In fact, lower BPs among postmenopausal estrogen users than among nonusers have been reported (Hassager et al., 1987; Barrett-Connor et al., 1989), although the largest cross-sectional study found no difference after adjustment for multiple possible confounders (Nabulsi et al., 1993). The differences between OCs and ERT, as noted by McCaffrey (1985), are striking (Fig. 11.8). The lower pressures with ERT may reflect a number of antihypertensive effects of estrogen replacement, including:

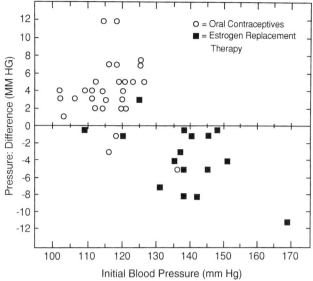

Figure 11.8. Effects of oral contraceptives and postmenopausal estrogens on systolic blood pressure as noted in longitudinal and cross-sectional studies reported up to 1985 (collated by Dr. T. A. McCaffrey, Cornell Medical Center, New York). (From McCaffrey TA. Estrogens and blood pressure: a theoretical review [Doctoral Thesis]. Purdue University, June 1985.)

—Vasodilation as measured by Doppler ultrasonography (Gangar et al., 1991) that may reflect increased endothelium-dependent relaxation (Williams et al., 1992);

—Effects on cation fluxes that reduce intracellular calcium that may involve the action of prostanoids (Stonier et al., 1992);

—Improvements in baroreceptor reflex sensitivity (Muneta et al., 1992);

—Reversal of the hyperinsulinemia seen after loss of ovarian function (Proudler et al., 1992).

Thus, the clinical and experimental evidence favoring ERT in the menopause continues to mount. Fortunately, hypertension is not a concern and may, in fact, be ameliorated.

We will turn next to less common causes of secondary hypertension involving the adrenal glands; although relatively rare, they often must be excluded.

References

Aalkjaer C, Johannesen P, Petersen EB, Rasmussen A, Mulvany MJ. Characteristics of resistance vessels in pre-eclampsia and normotensive pregnancy. *J Hypertens* 1984; 2(Suppl 3):183–185.

Abdul-Karim R, Assali NS. Pressor response to angiotonin in pregnant and nonpregnant women. *Am J Obstet Gynecol* 1961;82: 246–251.

Anonymous. Practice imperfect. *Lancet* 1991; 337:1195–1196.

Armanini D, Zennaro CM, Martella L, Scali M, Pratesi C, Grella PV, Mantero F. Mineralocorticoid effector mechanism in preeclampsia. *J Clin Endocrinol Metabol* 1992; 74:946–949.

August P, Marcaccio B, Gertner JM, Druzin ML, Resnick LM, Laragh JH. Abnormal 1,25-dihydroxyvitamin D metabolism in preeclampsia. *Am J Obstet Gynecol* 1992; 166:1295–99.

Baker PN, Broughton Pipkin F, Symonds EM. Comparative study of platelet angiotensin II binding and the angiotensin II sensitivity test as predictors of pregnancy-induced hypertension. *Clin Sci* 1992a;83: 89–95.

Baker PN, Broughton Pipkin F, Symonds EM. Longitudinal study of platelet angiotensin II binding in human pregnancy. *Clin Sci* 1992b;82:377–381.

Ballegeer VC, Spitz B, De Baene LA, Van Assche AF, Hidajat M, Criel AM. Platelet activation and vascular damage in gestational hypertension. *Am J Obstet Gynecol* 1992;166:629–633.

Barrett-Connor E. Risks and benefits of replacement estrogen. *Annu Rev Med* 1992; 43:239–251.

Barrett-Connor E, Wingard DL, Criqui MH. Postmenopausal estrogen use and heart disease risk factors in the 1980s. Rancho Bernardo, Calif. Revisited. *JAMA* 1989;261: 2095–2100.

Bauer TW, Moore GW, Hutchins GM. Morphologic evidence for coronary artery spasm in eclampsia. *Circulation* 1982; 65:255.

Bauman WA, Maimen M, Langer O. An association between hyperinsulinemia and hypertension during the third trimester of pregnancy. *Am J Obstet Gynecol* 1988; 159:446–450.

Belford MA, Moise KJ Jr. Effect of magnesium sulfate on maternal brain blood flow in preeclampsia: a randomized, placebo-controlled study. *Am J Obstet Gynecol* 1992; 167:661–666.

Benigni A, Orisio S, Gaspari F, Frusca T, Amuso G, Remuzzi G. Evidence against a pathogenetic role for endothelin in preeclampsia. *Br J Obstet Gynaecol* 1992;99: 798–802.

Bieniarz J, Yoshida T, Romero-Salinas G, Curuchet E, Caldeyro-Barcia R, Crottogini JJ. Aortocaval compression by the uterus in late human pregnancy. IV. Circulatory homeostasis by preferential perfusion of the placenta. *Am J Obstet Gynecol* 1969; 103:19–31.

Boyd WN, Burden RP, Aber GM. Intrarenal vascular changes in patients receiving oestrogen-containing compounds—a clinical, histological and angiographic study. *Q J Med* 1975;44:415–431.

Broughton-Pipkin F, Morrison R, O'Brien PMS. Effects of prostacyclin on the pressor response to angiotensin II in human pregnancy [Abstract]. *Eur J Clin Invest* 1984;14:3.

Brown JJ, Davies DL, Doak PD, Lever AF, Robertson JIS. Plasma-renin in normal pregnancy. *Lancet* 1963;2:900–902.

Brown MA. Non-pharmacological management of pregnancy-induced hypertension. *J Hypertens* 1990;8:295–301.

Brown MA, Gallery EDM, Ross MR, Esber RP. Sodium excretion in normal and hypertensive pregnancy: a prospective study. *Am J Obstet Gynecol* 1988;159:297–307.

Brown MA, Sinosich MJ, Saunders DM, Gallery EDM. Potassium regulation and progesterone-aldosterone interrelationships in human pregnancy: a prospective study. *Am J Obstet Gynecol* 1986;155:349–353.

Brown MA, Zammit VC, Mitar DA, Whitworth JA. Renin-aldosterone relationships in pregnancy-induced hypertension. *Am J Hypertens* 1992;5:366–371.

Brownrigg GM. Toxemia in hormone-induced pseudopregnancy. *Can Med Assoc J* 1962;87:408–409.

Butters L, Kennedy S, Rubin PC. Atenolol in essential hypertension during pregnancy. *Br Med J* 1990;301:587–589.

Campbell DM, MacGillivray I, Carr-Hill R. Pre-eclampsia in second pregnancy. *Br J Obstet Gynaecol* 1985;92:131–40.

Chamberlain G. Raised blood pressure in pregnancy. *Br Med J* 1991a;302:1454–1458.

Chamberlain G. The changing body in pregnancy. *Br Med J* 1991b;302:719–722.

Chesley LC. *Hypertensive Disorders in Pregnancy.* New York: Appleton-Century-Crofts, 1978.

Chesley LC. Hypertension in pregnancy: definitions, familial factor, and remote prognosis. *Kidney Int* 1980;18:234–240.

Chesley LC. Diagnosis of preeclampsia. *Obstet Gynecol* 1985;65:423–425.

Chesley LC, Annitto JE, Cosgrove RA. The remote prognosis of eclamptic women. *Am J Obstet Gynecol* 1976;124:446–459.

Christianson RE. Studies on blood pressure during pregnancy. *Am J Obstet Gynecol* 1976;125:509–513.

Contard S, Chanudet X, Coisne D, Battistella P, Marichal J-F, Pitiot M, de Gaudemaris R, Ribstein J. Ambulatory monitoring of blood pressure in normal pregnancy. *Am J Hypertens* 1993;6:880–884.

Cooper DW, Hill JA, Chesley LC, Bryans CI. Genetic control of susceptibility to eclampsia and miscarriage. *Br J Obstet Gynaecol* 1988;95:644–653.

Crane MG, Harris JJ. Estrogen and hypertension: effect of discontinuing estrogens on blood pressure, exchangeable sodium, and the renin-aldosterone system. *Am J Med Sci* 1978;276:33–55.

Crane MG, Harris JJ, Winsor W III. Hypertension, oral contraceptive agents, and conjugated estrogens. *Ann Intern Med* 1971;74:13–21.

Crawford JS, Lewis M, Weaver JB. Hypertension in the puerperium. *Lancet* 1987;2:693–694.

Croft P, Hannaford PC. Risk factors for acute myocardial infarction in women: evidence from the Royal College of General Practitioners' oral contraception study. *Br Med J* 1989;298:165–168.

Cugini P, Di Palma L, Battisti P, Leone G, Pachi A, Paesano R, Masella C, Stirati G, Pierucci A, Rocca AR, Morabito S. Describing and interpreting 24-hour blood pressure patterns in physiologic pregnancy. *Am J Obstet Gynecol* 1992;166:54–60.

Cunningham FG, Cox K, Gant NF. Further observations on the nature of pressor responsivity to angiotensin II in human pregnancy. *Obstet Gynecol* 1975;46:581–583.

Cunningham FG, Lindheimer MD. Hypertension in pregnancy. *N Engl J Med* 1992; 326:927–932.

Cunningham FG, Pritchard JA, Hankins DGV, Anderson PL, Lucas MJ, Armstrong KF. Peripartum heart failure: idiopathic cardiomyopathy or compounding cardiovascular events? *Obstet Gynecol* 1986;67:157–168.

Dahmus MA, Barton JR, Sibai BM. Cerebral imaging in eclampsia: magnetic resonance imaging versus computer tomography. *Am J Obstet Gynecol* 1992;167:935–941.

Daly E, Roche M, Barlow D, Gray A, McPherson K, Vessey M. HRT: an analysis of benefits, risks and costs. *Br Med Bull* 1992;48:368–400.

Davey DA, MacGillivray I. The classification and definition of the hypertensive disorders of pregnancy. *Am J Obstet Gynecol* 1988; 158:892–898.

Davison JM. The influence of pregnancy on renal function in humans. Proceedings of the 8th World Congress on Hypertension in Pregnancy, November 8–12, 1992, Buenos Aires, Argentina, p 75.

de Swiet M. Blood pressure measurement in pregnancy. *Br J Obstet Gynaecol* 1991;98:239–240.

Dekker GA, Sibai BM. Early detection of preeclampsia. *Am J Obstet Gynecol* 1991;165:160–172.

Dekker GA, Sibai BM. Low-dose aspirin in the prevention of preeclampsia and fetal growth retardation: rationale, mechanisms, and clinical trials. *Am J Obstet Gyecol* 1993; 168:214–227.

Delva P, Capra C, Degan M, Minuz P, Covi MG, Milan L, Steele A, Lechi A. High plasma levels of a ouabain-like factor in normal pregnancy and in pre-eclampsia. *Eur J Clin Invest* 1989;19:95–100.

Derkx FHM, Stuenkel C, Schalekamp MPA, Visser W, Huisveld IH, Schalekamp MADH. Immunoreactive renin, prorenin, and enzymatically active renin in plasma during pregnancy and in women taking oral contraceptives. *J Clin Endocrinol* 1986;63:1008–1015.

Douglas KA, Redman CWG. Eclampsia in the United Kingdom. The "best" way forward. *Br J Obstet Gynaecol* 1992;99:355–359.

Dudley L. Maternal mortality associated with hypertensive disorders of pregnancy in Africa, Asia, Latin America and the Caribbean. *Br J Obstet Gynaecol* 1992;99:547–553.

Easterling TR, Benedetti TJ. Preeclampsia: a hyperdynamic disease model. *Am J Obstet Gynecol* 1989;160:1447–1453.

Eneroth-Grimfors E, Bevegard S, Nilsson BA. Evaluation of three simple physiologic tests as predictors of pregnancy-induced hypertension. A pilot study: *Acta Obstet et Gynecol Scand* 1988;67:109–113.

Eskenazi B, Fenster L, Sidney S. A multivariate analysis of risk factors for preeclampsia. *JAMA* 1991;266:231–241.

Everett RB, Porter JC, MacDonald PC, Gant NF. Relationship of maternal placental blood flow to the placental clearance of maternal plasma dehydroisoandrosterone sulfate through placental estradiol formation. *Am J Obstet Gynecol* 1980;136:435–439.

Everett RB, Worley RJ, MacDonald PC, et al. Effect of prostaglandin synthetase inhibitors on pressor response to angiotensin II in human pregnancy. *J Clin Endocrinol Metab* 1978;46:1007–1010.

Feeney JG, Tovery LAD, Scott JS. Influence of previous blood-transfusion on incidence of pre-eclampsia. *Lancet* 1977;1:874–875.

Fenakel K, Fenakel G, Appleman Z, Lurie S, Katz Z, Schwartz ZS. Nifedipine in the treatment of severe preeclampsia. *Obstet Gynecol* 1991;77:331–337.

Ferrazzani S, Caruso A, De Carolis S, Martino IV, Mancuso S. Proteinuria and outcome of 44 pregnancies complicated by hypertension. *Am J Obstet Gynecol* 1990; 162:366–371.

Filshie GM, Maynard P, Hutter C, Cooper C, Robinson G, Rubin P. Urinary 5-hydroxyindole acetate concentration in pregnancy induced hypertension. *Br Med J* 1992; 304:1223.

Finucane FF, Madans JH, Bush TL, Wolf PH, Kleinman JC. Decreased risk of stroke among postmenopausal hormone users. *Arch Intern Med* 1993;153:73–79.

Friedman EA, Neff RK. Hypertension-hypotension in pregnancy. Correlation with fetal outcome. *JAMA* 1978;239:2249–2251.

Friedman SA. Preeclampsia: a review of the role of prostaglandins. *Obstet Gynecol* 1988;71:122–137.

Friedman SA, de Groot CJM, Taylor RN, Robert JM. Review of selected plasma and urinary predictors of preeclampsia [Abstract]. Presented at the 8th World Congress on Hypertension in Pregnancy, November 8–12, 1992, Buenos Aires, Argentina, p 101.

Gangar KF, Vyas S, Whitehead M, Crook D, Meire H, Campbell S. Pulsatility index in internal carotid artery in relation to transdermal oestradiol and time since menopause. *Lancet* 1991;338:839–842.

Gant NF, Daley GL, Chand S, Whalley PJ, MacDonald PC. A study of angiotensin II pressor response throughout primigravid pregnancy. *J Clin Invest* 1973;52:2682–2689.

Giles W, O'Callaghan S, Boura A, Walters W. Reduction in human fetal umbilical-placental vascular resistance by glyceryl trinitrate. *Lancet* 1992;340:856.

Godsland IF, Walton C, Felton C, Proudler A, Patel A, Wynn V. Insulin resistance, secretion, and metabolism in users of oral contraceptives. *J Clin Endocrinol Metab* 1992;74:64–70.

Goh JTW. First antenatal visit haematocrit and pregnancy induced hypertension. *Aust N Z J Obstet Gynecol* 1991;31:4:317–319.

Goldberg CA, Schrier RW. Hypertension in pregnancy. *Semin Nephrol* 1991;11:576–593.

Gordon MS, Chin WW, Shupnik MA. Regulation of angiotensinogen gene expression by estrogen. *J Hypertens* 1992;10:361–366.

Grady D, Rubin SM, Petitti DB, Fox CS, Black D, Ettinger B, Ernster VL, Cummings SR. Hormone therapy to prevent disease and prolong life in postmenopausal women. *Ann Intern Med* 1992;117: 1016–1037.

Halligan A, O'Brien E, O'Malley K, Mee F, Atkins N, Conroy R, Walshe JJ, Darling M. Twenty-four-hour ambulatory blood pressure measurement in a primigravid population. *J Hypertens* 1993;11:869–873.

Harper A, Murnaghan GA. Maternal and fetal haemodynamics in hypertensive pregnancies during maternal treatment with intravenous hydralazine or labetalol. *Br J Obstet Gynaecol* 1991;98:453–459.

Hassager C, Riis BJ, Strøm V, Guyene TT, Christiansen C. The long-term effect of oral and percutaneous estradiol on plasma renin substrate and blood pressure. *Circulation* 1987;76:753–758.

Hauglustaine D, Van Damme B, Vanrenterghem Y, Michielsen P. Recurrent hemolytic uremic syndrome during oral contraception. *Clin Nephrol* 1981;15:148–153.

Helmer OM, Judson WE. Influence of high renin substrate levels on renin-angiotensin system in pregnancy. *Am J Obstet Gynecol* 1967;99:9–17.

Henderson BE, Paganini-Hill A, Ross RK. Decreased mortality in users of estrogen replacement therapy. *Arch Intern Med* 1991;151:75–78.

Hennessy A, Horvath JS. Newer antihypertensive agents in pregnancy. *Med J Aust* 1992;156:304–305.

Hirvonen E, Idänpään-Heikkilä J. Cardiovascular death among women under 40 years of age using low-estrogen oral contraceptives and intrauterine devices in Finland from 1975 to 1984. *Am J Obstet Gynecol* 1990;163:281–284.

Hollenberg NK, Williams GH, Burger B, Chenitz W, Hoosmand I, Adams DF. Renal blood flow and its response to angiotensin II. An interaction between oral contraceptive agents, sodium intake, and the renin-angiotensin system in healthy young women. *Circ Res* 1976;38:35–40.

Hughes EC. *Obstetric Gynecologic Terminology.* Philadelphia: FA Davis, 1972: 422–423.

Hutton JD, James DK, Stirrat GM, Douglas KA, Redman CWG. Management of severe pre-eclampsia and eclampsia by UK consultants. *Br J Obstet Gynaecol* 1992;99: 554–556.

Ihle BU, Long P, Oats J. Early onset pre-eclampsia: recognition of underlying renal disease. *Br Med J* 1987;294:79–81.

Ikedife D. Eclampsia in multipara. *Br Med J* 1980;1:985–986.

Imperiale TF, Petrulis AS. A meta-analysis of low-dose aspirin for the prevention of pregnancy-induced hypertensive disease. *JAMA* 1991;266:260–265.

Italian Study of Aspirin in Pregnancy. Low-dose aspirin in prevention and treatment of intrauterine growth retardation and preg-nancy-induced hypertension. *Lancet* 1993;341:396–400.

Ito M, Nakamura T, Yoshimura T, Koyama H, Okamura H. The blood pressure response to infusions of angiotensin II during normal pregnancy: relation to plasma angiotensin II concentration, serum progesterone level, and mean platelet volume. *Am J Obstet Gynecol* 1992;166:1249–1253.

Itskovitz J, Rubattu S, Levron J, Sealey JE. Highest concentrations of prorenin and human chorionic gonadotropin in gestational sacs during early human pregnancy. *J Clin Endocrinol Metab* 1992;75:906–910.

Johenning AR, Barron WM. Indirect blood pressure measurement in pregnancy: Korotkoff phase 4 versus phase 5. *Am J Obstet Gynecol* 1992;167:577–580.

Kevin H, Stuart C. Transvaginal doppler studies of the uterine arteries in the early prediction of pre-eclampsia [Abstract]. Presented at the 8th World Congress on Hypertension in Pregnancy, November 8–12, 1992, Buenos Aires, Argentina, p 154.

Khong TY, Sawyer IH, Heryet AR. An immunohistologic study of endothelialization of uteroplacental vessels in human pregnancy—evidence that endothelium is focally disrupted by trophoblast in pre-eclampsia. *Am J Obstet Gynecol* 1992; 167:751–756.

Klonoff-Cohen HS, Savitz DA, Cefalo RC, McCann MF. An epidemiologic study of contraception and preeclampsia. *JAMA* 1989;262:3143–3147.

Laragh JG, Sealey JE, Ledingham JGG, Newton MA. Oral contraceptives. Renin, aldosterone, and high blood pressure. *JAMA* 1967;201:918–922.

Lehtovirta P. Haemodynamic effects of combined oestrogen/progestogen oral contraceptives. *J Obstet Gynaecol Br Commonwealth* 1974;81:517–525.

Lenox JW, Uguru V, Cibils LA. Effects of hypertension on pregnancy monitoring and results. *Am J Obstet Gynecol* 1990;163: 1173–1179.

Lenz T, Sealey JE, August P, James GD, Laragh JH. Tissue levels of active and total renin, angiotensinogen, human chorionic gonadotropin, estradiol, and progesterone in human placentas from different methods of delivery. *J Clin Endocrinol Metab* 1989;69:31–37.

Lim KG, Isles CG, Hodsman GP, Lever AF, Robertson JWK. Malignant hypertension in women of childbearing age and its relation to the contraceptive pill. *Br Med J* 1987;294:1057–1059.

Liston WA, Kilpatrick DC. Is genetic susceptibility to pre-eclampsia conferred by homozygosity for the same single recessive gene in mother and fetus? *Br J Obstet Gynaecol* 1991;98:1079–1086.

López M, Belizán JM, Elizalde E, Bergel E, Villar J, Lede R. Measurement of diastolic blood pressure during pregnancy: which phase should be used [Abstract]. Presented at the 8th World Congress on Hypertension in Pregnancy, November 8–12, 1992, Buenos Aires, Argentina, p 176.

Loquet P, Broughton Pipkin F, Symonds EM, Rubin PC. Influence of raising maternal blood pressure with angiotensin II on utero-placental and feto-placental blood velocity indices in the human. *Clin Sci* 1990;78:95–100.

Lowe SA, Macdonald GJ, Brown MA. Acute and chronic regulation of atrial natriuretic peptide in human pregnancy: a longitudinal study. *J Hypertens* 1992;10:821–829.

Lowe SA, Rubin PC. The pharmacological management of hypertension in pregnancy. *J Hypertens* 1992;10:201–207.

Lunell NO, Nylund LE, Lewander R, Sarby B. Uteroplacental blood flow in pre-eclampsia measured with indium-113m and a computer-linked gamma camera. *Clin Exp Hypertens* 1992;1:105–117.

MacPhail S, Thomas TH, Wilkinson R, Davison JM, Dunlop W. Pregnancy induced hypertension and sodium pump function in erythrocytes. *Br J Obstet Gynaecol* 1992; 99:803–807.

Magness RR, Hassan A, Rosenfeld CR, Shaul PW. Angiotensin II (AII) stimulates uterine artery (UA) cAMP and cGMP via endothelium-derived PGI$_2$ and nitric oxide (NO) in pregnancy [Abstract]. Presented at the 8th World Congress on Hypertension in Pregnancy, November 8–12, 1992, Buenos Aires, Argentina, p 163.

Malatino LS, Glen L, Wilson ESB. The effects of low-dose estrogen-progestogen oral contraceptives on blood pressure and the renin-angiotensin system. *Curr Ther Res* 1988;43:743–749.

Malee MP, Malee KM, Azuma SD, Taylor RN, Roberts JM. Increases in plasma atrial natriuretic peptide concentration antedate clinical evidence of preeclampsia. *J Clin Endocrinol Metab* 1992;74:1095–1100.

Marcoux S, Brisson J, Fabia J. Calcium intake from dairy products and supplements and the risks of preeclampsia and gestational hypertension. *Am J Epidemiol* 1991;133: 1266–1272.

Marin-Neto JA, Maciel BC, Urbanetz LLT, Gallo L Jr, Almeida-Filho OC, Amorim DS. High output failure in patients with peripartum cardiomyopathy: a comparative study with dilated cardiomyopathy. *Am Heart J* 1991;121:134–140.

Martin JN Jr, Magann EF, Blake PG, Martin RW, Perry KG Jr, Roberts WE. Severe preeclampsia/eclampsia with HELLP syndrome in 454 pregnancies: comparative analysis using the 3-class system of classification [Abstract]. Presented at the 8th World Congress on Hypertension in Pregnancy, November 8–12, 1992, Buenos Aires, Argentina, p 214.

McCaffrey TA. Estrogens and blood pressure: a theoretical review (Doctoral Thesis). Purdue University, June, 1985.

McCarthy AL, Raju KS, Poston L. Endothelium dependent relaxation in pre-eclampsia [Abstract]. *J Hypertens* 1992;10(Suppl 4):S45.

Meade TW. Risks and mechanisms of cardiovascular events in users of oral contraceptives. *Am J Obstet Gynecol* 1988;158: 1646–1652.

Meagher EA, FitzGerald GA. Disordered eicosanoid formation in pregnancy-induced hypertension. *Circulation* 1993;88: 1324–1333.

Miles JF Jr, Martin JN Jr, Blake PG, Perry KG Jr, Martin RW, Meeks GD. Postpartum eclampsia: a recurring perinatal dilemma. *Obstet Gynecol* 1990;76:328–331.

Miyamoto S, Makino N, Shimokawa H, Akazawa K, Wake N, Nakano H. The characteristics of erythrocyte Na^+ transport systems in normal pregnancy and pregnancy-induced hypertension. *J Hypertens* 1992;10: 367–372.

Moodley J, Gouws E. A comparative study of the use of epoprostenol and dihydralazine in severe hypertension in pregnancy. *Br J Obstet Gynaecol* 1992;99:727–730.

Mooney P, Dalton KJ, Swindells HE, Rushant S, Cartwright W, Juett D. Blood pressure measured telemetrically from home throughout pregnancy. *Am J Obstet Gynecol* 1990;163:30–36.

Morgan MA, Thurnau GR. Pregnancy-induced hypertension without proteinuria: is it true preeclampsia? *South Med J* 1988;81:210–213.

Moutquin JM, Rainville C, Giroux L, Raynauld P, Amyot G, Bilodeau R, Pelland N. A prospective study of blood pressure in pregnancy: prediction of preeclampsia. *Am J Obstet Gynecol* 1985;151:191–196.

Muneta S, Dazai Y, Iwata T, Hiwada K, Hamada K, Matsuura S, Murkami E, Sato Y, Imamura Y. Baroreceptor reflex impairment in climacteric and ovariectomized hypertensive women. *Hypertens Res* 1992; 15:27–32.

Nabulsi AA, Folsom AR, White A, Patsch W, Heiss G, Wu KK, Szklo M. Association of hormone-replacement therapy with various cardiovascular risk factors in postmenopausal women. *N Engl J Med* 1993; 328:1069–1075.

National High Blood Pressure Education Program Working Group. Report on high blood pressure in pregnancy. *Am J Obstet Gynecol* 1990;163:1689–1712.

Neiger R, Rosene K. Late postpartum eclampsia at 20 weeks' gestation: a case report and review of the literature. *Am J Perinatol* 1992;9:194–96.

Øian P, Lande K, Kjeldsen SE, Eide I, Maltau M. Increased arterial catecholamines in pre-eclampsia. *Acta Obstet Gynecol* Scand 1986;65:613–616.

Ory HW. Mortality associated with fertility and fertility control: 1983. *Fam Plan Perspect* 1983;15:57–63.

Packham DK, Mathews DC, Fairley KF, Whitworth JA, Kincaid-Smith PS. Morphometric analysis of pre-eclampsia in women biopsied in pregnancy and postpartum. *Kidney Int* 1988;34:704–711.

Penny WJ, Lewis MJ. Nifedipine is excreted in human milk. *Eur J Clin Pharmacol* 1989;36:427–428.

Perry IJ, Stewart BA, Brockwell J, Khan M, Davies P, Beevers DG, Luesley DM. Recording diastolic blood pressure in pregnancy. *Br Med J* 1990;301:1198.

Perry IJ, Wilkinson LS, Shinton RA, Beevers DG. Conflicting views on the measurement of blood pressure in pregnancy. *Br J Obstet Gynaecol* 1991;98:241–243.

Pfeffer RI, Kurosaki TT, Charlton SK. Estrogen use and blood pressure in later life. *Am J Epidcmiol* 1979;110:469–478.

Phippard AF, Fischer WE, Horvath JS, Child AG, Korda AR, Henderson-Smart D, Duggin GG, Tiller DJ. Early blood pressure control improves pregnancy outcome in primigravid women with mild hypertension. *Med J Aust* 1991;154:378–382.

Phippard AF, Horvath JS. Hypertension in pregnancy. In: Rubin PC, ed. *Handbook of Hypertension, Vol 10.* Amsterdam: Elsevier Science Publishers, 1988:168.

Pijnenborg R, Anthony J, Davey DA, Rees A, Tiltman A, Vercruysse L, Van Assche A. Placental bed spiral arteries in the hypertensive disorders of pregnancy. *Br J Obstet Gynaecol* 1991;98:648–655.

Pinto A, Sorrentino R, Sorrentino P, Guerritore T, Miranda L, Biondi A, Martinelli P. Endothelial-derived relaxing factor released by endothelial cells of human umbilical vessels and its impairment in pregnancy-induced hypertension. *Am J Obstet Gynecol* 1991;164:507–513.

Piver MS, Corson SL, Bolognese RJ. Hypertension 6 weeks post partum in apparently normal women. *Obstet Gynecol* 1967;30: 238–241.

Plouin P-F, Breart G, Llado J, Dalle M, Keller M-E, Goujon H, Berchel C. A randomized comparison of early with conservative use of antihypertensive drugs in the management of pregnancy-induced hypertension. *Br J Obstet Gynaecol* 1990;97:134–141.

Prince RL, Smith M, Dick IM, Price RI, Webb PG, Henderson NK, Harris MM. Prevention of postmenopausal osteoporosis. *N Engl J Med* 1991;325:1189–95.

Pritchard JA, Cunningham FG, Pritchard SA. The Parkland Memorial Hospital protocol for treatment of eclampsia: evaluation of 245 cases. *Am J Obstet Gynecol* 1984; 148:951–963.

Pritchard JA, Pritchard SA. Blood pressure response to estrogen-progestin oral contraceptive after pregnancy-induced hypertension. *Am J Obstet Gynecol* 1977;129: 733–739.

Pritchard JA, Weisman R, Ratnoff OD, Vosburgh GJ. Intravascular hemolysis, thrombocytopenia and other hematologic abnormalities associated with severe toxemia in pregnancy. *N Engl J Med* 1954:250–89.

Proudler AJ, Felton CV, Stevenson C. Ageing and the response of plasma insulin, glucose and C-peptide concentrations to intravenous glucose in postmenopausal women. *Clin Sci* 1992;83:489–494.

Redman CWG. Controlled trials of antihypertensive drugs in pregnancy. *Am J Kid Dis* 1991a;17:149–153.

Redman CWG. Current topic: pre-eclampsia and the placenta. *Placenta* 1991b;12:301–308.

Redman CWG, Roberts JM. Management of pre-eclampsia. *Lancet* 1993;341:1451–1454.

Remuzzi G, Ruggenenti P. Prevention and treatment of pregnancy-associated hypertension: what have we learned in the last 10 years? *Am J Kidney Dis* 1991;18:285–305.

Roberts JM, Redman CWG. Pre-eclampsia: more than pregnancy-induced hypertension. *Lancet* 1993;341:1447–1451.

Roberts JM, Taylor RN, Goldfien A. Clinical and biochemical evidence of endothelial cell dysfunction in the pregnancy syndrome preeclampsia. *Am J Hypertens* 1991;4:700–708.

Robson SC, Dunlop W, Hunter S. Haemodynamic changes during the early puerperium. *Br Med J* 1987;294:1065.

Robson SC, Dunlop W, Hunter S. Haemodynamic effects of breast-feeding. *Br J Obstet Gynaecol* 1989a;96:1106–1108.

Robson SC, Hunter S, Boys RJ, Dunlop W. Serial study of factors influencing changes in cardiac output during human pregnancy. *Am J Physiol* 1989b;256:H1060–H1065.

Rosa FW, Bosco LA, Graham CF, Milstien JB, Dreis M, Creamer J. Neonatal anuria with maternal angiotensin-converting enzyme inhibition. *Obstet Gynecol* 1989; 74:371–374.

Rosenberg L, Palmer JR, Shapiro S. Use of lower dose oral contraceptives and risk of myocardial infarction [Abstract]. *Circulation* 1991;83:8.

Rosenberg L, Palmer JR, Shapiro S. A case-control study of myocardial infarction in relation to use of estrogen supplements. *Am J Epidemiol* 1993;137:54–63.

Royal College of General Practitioners. Hypertension. In: *Oral Contraceptives and Health.* From the Oral Contraceptive Study of the Royal College of General Practice. New York: Pitman Publishing, 1974:37–42.

Royal College of General Practitioners. Further analyses of mortality in oral contraceptive users. Royal College of General Practitioners' Oral Contraception Study. *Lancet* 1981;1:541–546.

Rubin PC, Butters L, McCabe R, Reid JL. Plasma catecholamines in pregnancy induced hypertension. *Clin Sci* 1986;71: 111–115.

Saruta T, Saade GA, Kaplan NM. A possible mechanism for hypertension induced by oral contraceptives. *Arch Intern Med* 1970;127:621–626.

Schiff E, Ben-Baruch G, Peleg E, Rosenthal T, Alcalay M, Devir M, Mashiach S. Immunoreactive circulating endothelin-1 in normal and hypertensive pregnancies. *Am J Obstet Gynecol* 1992;166:624–628.

Sealey JE, Thaler I, Rubattu S, James GD, August P, Itskovitz I. Gross activation of the renin-aldosterone system in normal women by endogenous estradiol (E2) and progesterone (P4) without perturbation of electrolyte homeostasis [Abstract]. *J Hypertens* 1992;10(Suppl 4):48.

Sealey JE, Wilson M, Morganti AA, Zervoudakis I, Laragh JH. Changes in active and inactive renin throughout normal pregnancy. *Clin Exp Hypertens* 1982;A4: 237–2384.

Seely EW, Williams GH, Graves SW. Markers of sodium and volume homeostasis in pregnancy-induced hypertension. *J Clin Endocrinol* 1992;74:150–156.

Sibai BM. Eclampsia. VI. Maternal-perinatal outcome in 254 consecutive cases. *Am J Obstet Gynecol* 1990;163:1049–1055.

Sibai BM, Abdella TN, Anderson GD. Pregnancy outcome in 211 patients with mild chronic hypertension. *Obstet Gynecol* 1983;61:571–576.

Sibai BM, Barton JR, Aki S, Sarinoglu, Mercer B. A randomized prospective comparison of nifedipine and bed rest versus bed rest alone in the management of pre-eclampsia remote from term. *Am J Obstet Gynecol* 1992;167:879–884.

Sibai BM, Caritis SN, Thom E, Klebanoff M, McNellis D, Rocco L, Paul R, Romero R, Witter F, Rosen M, Depp R. Prevention of preeclampsia with low-dose aspirin in healthy, nulliparous pregnant women. *N Engl J Med* 1993;329:1213–1218.

Sibai BM, Mabie WC, Shamsa F, Villar MA, Anderson GD. A comparison of no medication versus methyldopa or labetalol in chronic hypertension during pregnancy. *Am J Obstet Gynecol* 1990a;162:960–977.

Sibai BM, Villar MA, Mabie BC. Acute renal failure in hypertensive disorders of pregnancy. *Am J Obstet Gynecol* 1990b;162: 777–783.

Speroff L. Toxemia of pregnancy. Mechanism and therapeutic management. *Am J Cardiol* 1973;32:582–586.

Stadel BV. Oral contraceptives and cardiovascular disease (second of two parts). *N Engl J Med* 1981;305:672–677.

Stampfer MJ, Willett WC, Colditz GA, Speizer FE, Hennekens CH. Past use of oral contraceptives and cardiovascular disease: a meta-analysis in the context of the Nurses' Health Study. *Am J Obstet Gynecol* 1990;163:285–291.

Steegers EA, Van Lakwijk HPJM, Jongsma HW, Fast JH, De Boo T, Eskes TKAB, Hein PR. (Patho)physiological implications of chronic dietary sodium restriction during pregnancy: a longitudinal prospective randomized study. *Br J Obstet Gynaecol* 1991;98:980–987.

Steel SA, Pearce JM, McParland P, Chamberlain GVP. Early doppler ultrasound screening in prediction of hypertensive disorders of pregnancy. *Lancet* 1990;335:1548–1551.

Stokes CG, Monaghan JC, Flemming CL, Johnston H, Jones M, Pinkerton G, Baber R. Effects of oral contraceptives containing oestrogen combined with norethisterone or levonorgestrel on erythrocyte cation transport in normal women. *Clin Sci* 1992;82: 505–512.

Stonier C, Bennett J, Messenger EA, Aber GM. Oestradiol-induced hypotension in spontaneously hypertensive rats: putative role for intracellular cations, sodium-potassium flux and prostanoids. *Clin Sci* 1992;82:389–395.

Strauss RG, Alexander RW. Postpartum hemolytic uremic syndrome. *Obstet Gynecol* 1976;47:169–173.

Sutherland A, Cooper DW, Howie PW, Liston WA, MacGillivray I. The incidence of severe pre-clampsia amongst mothers and mothers-in-law of pre-eclamptics and controls. *Br J Obstet Gynaecol* 1981;88: 785–791.

Svensson A. Hypertension in pregnancy. In: Hansson L, ed. *International Society of Hypertension 1988 Hypertension Annual.*

London: Gower Academic Journals Ltd, 1988:33–46.

Taufield PA, Mueller FB, Edersheim TG, Druzin ML, Laragh JH. Blood pressure regulation in normal pregnancy: unmasking the role of the renin angiotensin system with captopril [Abstract]. *Clin Res* 1988;36:433A.

Taylor RN, Musci TJ, Rodgers GM, Roberts JM. Preeclamptic sera stimulate increased platelet-derived growth factor mRNA and protein expression by cultured human endothelial cells. *Am J Reprod Immunol* 1991;25:105–108.

Thompson JA, Hays PM, Sagar KB, Cruickshank DP. Echocardiographic left ventricular mass to differentiate chronic hypertension from preeclampsia during pregnancy. *Am J Obstet Gynecol* 1986;155:994–999.

Thomson AM, Hytten FE, Billewicz WZ. The epidemiology of oedema during pregnancy. *J Obstet Gynaecol Br Commonwealth* 1967;74:1–10.

Thorogood M, Mann J, Murphy M, Vessey M. Fatal stroke and use of oral contraceptives: findings from a case-control study. *Am J Epidemiol* 1992;136:35–45.

Thorogood M, Mann J, Murphy M, Vessey M. Is oral contraceptive use still associated with an increased risk of fatal myocardial infarction? Report of a case-control study. *Br J Obstet Gynaecol* 1991;98:1245–1253.

Tsai CC, Williamson HO, Kirkland BH, Braun JO, Lam CF. Low-dose oral contraception and blood pressure in women with a past history of elevated blood pressure. *Am J Obstet Gynecol* 1985;151:28–32.

Tuohy JF, James DK. Pre-eclampsia and trisomy 13. *Br J Obstet Gynaecol* 1992;99: 891–894.

Villar J, Repke J, Belizan JM, Pareja G. Calcium supplementation reduces blood pressure during pregnancy: results of a randomized controlled clinical trial. *Obstet Gynecol* 1987;70:317–322.

Wallenburg HCS. Hemodynamics in hypertensive pregnancy. In: Rubin PC, ed. *Handbook of Hypertension, Vol 10: Hypertension in Pregnancy.* Amsterdam: Elsevier Science Publishers, 1988:66–101.

Walters BNJ, Thompson ME, Lee A, de Swiet M. Blood pressure in the puerperium. *Clin Sci* 1986;71:589–594.

Walters WAW, Lim YL. Haemodynamic changes in women taking oral contraceptives. *J Obstet Gynecol Br Commonwealth* 1970;77:1007–1012.

Wang Y, Walsh SW, Guo J, Zhang J. Maternal levels of prostacyclin, thromboxane, vitamin E, and lipid peroxides throughout

normal pregnancy. *Am J Obstet Gynecol* 1991;165:1690–1694.

Wang Y, Walsh SW, Kay HH. Placental lipid peroxides and thromboxane are increased and prostacyclin is decreased in women with preeclampsia. *Am J Obstet Gynecol* 1992;167:946–9.

Watson DL, Bhatia RK, Norman GS, Brindley BA, Sokol RJ. Bromocriptine mesylate for lactation suppression: a risk for postpartum hypertension? *Obstet Gynecol* 1989;74:573–576.

Weinstein L. Syndrome of hemolysis, elevated liver enzymes, and low platelet count: a severe consequence of hypertension in pregnancy. *Am J Obstet Gynecol* 1982;142:159–167.

Weir RJ. Hypertension secondary to contraceptive agents. In Amery A, Fagard R, Lijnen P, Staessen J, eds. *Hypertensive Cardiovascular Disease: Pathophysiology and Treatment.* The Hague/Boston/London: Martinus Nijhoff Publishers, 1982:612–628.

Weir RJ. When the pill causes a rise in blood pressure. *Drugs* 1978;16:522–527.

White WB. Management of hypertension during lactation. *Hypertension* 1984;6: 297–300.

Wilkes BM, Hollander AM, Sung SY, Mento PF. Cyclooxygenase inhibitors blunt thromboxane action in human placental arteries by blocking thromboxane receptors. *Am J Physiol* 1992;263:E718–E723.

Williams JK, Adams MR, Herrington DM, Clarkson TB. Short-term administration of estrogen and vascular responses of atherosclerotic coronary arteries. *J Am Coll Cardiol* 1992;20:452–457.

Wilson ESB, Cruickshank J, McMaster M, Weir RJ. A prospective controlled study of the effect on blood pressure of contraceptive preparations containing different types and dosages of progestogen. *Br J Obstet Gynaecol* 1984;91:1254–1260.

Woods JW. Oral contraceptives and hypertension. *Hypertension* 1988;11(Suppl 2):11–15.

Woods JW. Oral contraceptives and hypertension. *Lancet* 1967;2:653–654.

Wren BG. The effect of oestrogen on the female cardiovascular system. *Med J Aust* 1992;157:204–208.

Zhou Y, Damsky CH, Chiu K, Roberts JM, Fisher SJ. Preeclampsia is associated with abnormal expression of adhesion molecules by invasive cytotrophoblasts. *J Clin Invest* 1993;91:950–960.

Zuspan FP, Rayburn WF. Blood pressure self-monitoring during pregnancy: practical considerations. *Am J Obstet Gynecol* 1991;164:2–6.

12 Pheochromocytoma (with a Preface About Incidental Adrenal Masses)

THE INCIDENTAL ADRENAL MASS

Before considering adrenal causes of hypertension in this and the subsequent two chapters, the management of incidentally discovered adrenal masses will be covered. Such masses are being found increasingly during abdominal computed tomography (CT) and magnetic resonance imaging (MRI). They must be evaluated both because they may be functionally active and because they may be malignant (Rácz et al., 1993).

Incidence

Nonfunctioning adrenal masses have long been found in many people at autopsy: in one series, adrenal masses from 2 mm to 4 cm in size were found in 8.7% of 739 autopsies and in 12.4% of the patients known to have been hypertensive (Hedeland et al., 1968).

With the increasing use of CT and MRI scans, these previously unrecognized masses are now being recognized in many patients who have no clinical evidence of adrenal hyperfunction. At the Mayo Clinic, of 61,054 abdominal CT scans done from 1985 to 1990, 3.4% revealed adrenal masses: of these, over half were obviously metastatic cancer, 25% were other known lesions, and 7.5% were symptomatic tumors, leaving 16.5% as incidental tumors, defined as a well-circumscribed tumor greater than 1 cm in size (Herrera et al., 1991). Thus, 0.4% of all CT scans in this series revealed an incidental adrenal tumor. Ross and Aron (1990) estimate that an incidental adrenal mass will be discovered in at least 2% of patients undergoing abdominal CT scanning for an unrelated reason.

Evaluation

Since only a small percentage of these incidental tumors will be either malignant or functional, guidelines for the evaluation and treatment of patients with such lesions have been proposed (Francis et al., 1992), but controversy persists as to how much should be done.

Work-Up for Malignancy

Size. Most authors agree with Copeland (1983) that a lesion larger than 6 cm be surgically removed, since a large proportion will be cancerous. Since Herrera et al. (1991) found reports of at least 20 adrenal carcinomas that were between 4 and 6 cm in size, they recommend surgical removal of lesions larger than 4 cm, particularly in younger patients. This cutoff would have yielded a benign/malignant ratio of 8:1 among their patients, which they believe is a reasonable balance. They recommend simple observation of those with tumors less than 4 cm with a repeat CT scan in 3 months.

Adrenal Scintigraphy. Adrenal scintigraphy with an iodinated cholesterol derivative (NP-59) that localizes in functioning adrenal cortical tissue but not in most malignant adrenal masses has been used by Gross et al. (1988) in 119 euadrenal patients with unilateral masses found on CT scans. Those adrenal glands that took up the NP-59 were almost certainly benign; those that did not take up the NP-59 were mostly malignant, either metastatic or primary.

MRI and CT. MRI or CT may characterize the tissue adequately to predict the histologic type of the adrenal tumor: A hyperintense signal intensity as compared to the liver on a T_2-weighted MRI image is usually noted in adrenal carcinomas (Francis et al., 1992). However, 8 of 38 such tumors could not be differentiated (Reinig et al., 1986), so the use of NP-59 scintigraphy likely is the better approach for now. On the other hand, if the adrenal mass has a uniform configuration on CT indicating a high fat content, the diagnosis of myelolipoma can be reasonably assured, and no further work-up need be performed save a test to rule out a pheochromocytoma (Meaglia and Schmidt, 1992). Similarly, adrenal pseudocysts should be recognizable by MRI (Case Records, 1992).

Hypoaldosteronism. In a series of 15 patients with adrenal tumors, the seven malignant tumors had very low plasma aldosterone but elevated levels of aldosterone precursors, suggesting that this finding may be a useful diagnostic test (Aupetit-Faisant et al., 1993).

Work-Up for Functional Tumors

As for recognizing functional tumors, Ross and Aron (1990) argue that simple clinical criteria (such as shown in Table 12.1) be used to indicate the need for screening tests. These guidelines seem reasonable except for the need for a screening test to rule out subtle mineralocorticoid or glucocorticoid excess (Rácz et al.,

1993). Patients with normal basal plasma and urine glucocorticoid levels have been reported to have nonsuppressible steroid levels after dexamethasone (Rosen and Swartz, 1992). The danger is that removal of the subclinically functioning tumor may expose the patient to adrenal insufficiency from the prolonged suppression of the other gland. A dexamethasone suppression test, then, should be part of the evaluation.

Virilized patients with incidental adrenal tumors should also be screened for congenital adrenal hyperplasia (CAH), since adenomas may arise from such hyperplastic tissue (Jaresch et al., 1992).

Adrenal Hyperfunction in the Hypertensive Patient

Beyond the need to evaluate patients with incidentally discovered adrenal masses, an adrenal cause for hypertension will need to be considered much more frequently than the low prevalence—less than 0.5%—of these causes would suggest. The presence of adrenal hyperfunction is often considered in the evaluation of hypertensive patients because many of the symptoms and signs of adrenal hyperfunction are nonspecific and are encountered in patients with normal adrenal function. Recurrent ''spells'' suggestive of pheochromocytoma, hypokalemia pointing to primary aldosteronism, and cushingoid features are all encountered in many more patients than the relatively few who turn out to have these

Table 12.1. Evaluation of Incidental Adrenal Masses

Diagnosis	Suggestive Clinical Features	Laboratory Screening Tests
Pheochromocytoma	Paroxysmal hypertension Spells of sweating, headache, palpitations	Spot-urine metanephrine Normal: <1 μg or 5.5 μmol/mg of creatinine
Cushing's syndrome	Truncal obesity Thin skin Muscle weakness	8 A.M. plasma cortisol after 1 mg of dexamethasone at bedtime Normal: <5 μg/dl (140 nmol/L)
Primary aldosteronism	Weakness	Hypokalemia Urine potassium excretion Normal: <30 mmol/24 hour urine in presence of hypokalemia

Adrenocortical carcinoma	Virilization or feminization	Urine 17-ketosteroids
		Normal:
		  Men: 6–20 mg or 20–70 μmol/24 hours
		  Women: 6–17 mg or 20–60 μmol/24 hours
		Plasma androgens or estrogens

diseases. Of all of these, consideration of a pheochromocytoma is likely most important.

PHEOCHROMOCYTOMA

The presence of a pheochromocytoma (pheo) should be considered in all hypertensives since, if not recognized, a pheo may provoke fatal hypertensive crises during anesthesia and other stresses. Pheos are often unrecognized: at the Mayo Clinic from 1928 to 1977, of 54 pheos found at autopsy, only 13 had been diagnosed during life (Lie et al., 1980). Of the 41 previously unrecognized, death was related to the manifestations of the tumor in 30 patients. This experience with unrecognized pheos should be contrasted to the excellent results obtained at the Mayo Clinic on 138 patients with demonstrated pheos who underwent surgery during these years: the survival curve of those with a benign tumor was similar to that of the normal population (Sheps et al., 1990).

INCIDENCE

The incidence of pheos diagnosed during life or at autopsy among the residents of Rochester, Minnesota—the location of the Mayo Clinic— was found to be 0.95 cases per 100,000 person-years (Beard et al., 1983). This figure, the most accurate estimate of the incidence of the tumor now available, suggests that, if 15% of the adult population is hypertensive, only about six pheos would be expected to be found among 100,000 hypertensives each year. Even lower rates, approximately two cases per million people per year, have been estimated in Japan (Takeda et al., 1986), Sweden (Stenström and Svördsüdd, 1986), and Denmark (Andersen et al., 1988).

PATHOPHYSIOLOGY

Development

The cells of the sympathetic nervous system arise from the primitive neural crest as primordial stem cells, called sympathogonia (Fig. 12.1). The sympathogonia migrate out of the central nervous system to occupy a place behind the aorta. These stem cells may differentiate into either sympathoblasts, which give rise to sympathetic ganglion cells, or pheochromoblasts, which give rise to chromaffin cells. As seen in Figure 12.1, tumors may arise from each of these cell lines, often sharing histologic and biochemical characteristics. These include highly malignant neuroblastomas, arising from sympathoblasts, and ganglioneuromas, which are usually more benign. These tumors are rarely seen after adolescence and usually are recognized by the excretion of large amounts of homovanillic acid (HVA), the urinary metabolite of dopamine (Fig. 12.2).

The chromaffin cells, which have the capacity to synthesize and store catecholamines and therefore stain brown on treatment with chromium, are found mainly in the adrenal medulla. They also appear in the sympathetic ganglia and paraganglia that lie along the sympathetic chain and organ of Zuckerkandl, located anteriorly at the bifurcation of the aorta. In a developmental sense, the adrenal medulla may be considered a sympathetic ganglion that lacks postsynaptic fibers. In a functional sense, its chromaffin cells differ from the rest by having the capacity to convert norepinephrine (NE) to epinephrine (Epi) (Fig. 12.2).

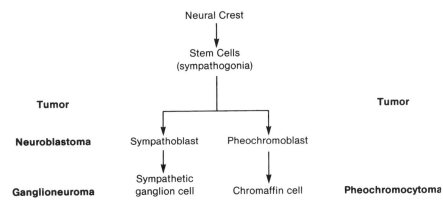

Figure 12.1. Developmental pathway for sympathetic ganglion and chromaffin cells and the tumors that may arise from them.

Location and Tumor Nomenclature

Chromaffin cell tumors (i.e., pheochromocytomas) can arise wherever these cells are found (Table 12.2). As many as 15% of pheos in adults and 30% in children are extraadrenal; they may be located anywhere along the sympathetic chain and, rarely, in aberrant sites (Whalen et al., 1992). Those functioning tumors arising outside the adrenal medulla are best termed *extraadrenal pheochromocytomas* (Whalen et al., 1992), whereas nonsecreting extraadrenal tumors are termed *paragangliomas* (Shapiro and Fig, 1989). Paragangliomas that arise from the specialized chemoreceptor tissue in the carotid body, glomus jugulare, and aortic body have been separately classified as *chemodectomas*. Glomus jugular tumors are fairly common in the middle ear and temporal bone, and they may secrete catecholamines (Blumenfeld et al., 1992).

Among the most frequent sites of extraadrenal pheos are the organ of Zuckerkandl and the urinary bladder (Nomura et al., 1991). However, they may arise wherever there are paraganglion cells, even within the heart (Aravot et al., 1992) or prostate (Dennis et al., 1989). Rarely, extraadrenal pheos are multiple (Reinholdt and Pedersen, 1988) or familial (Glowniak et al., 1985),

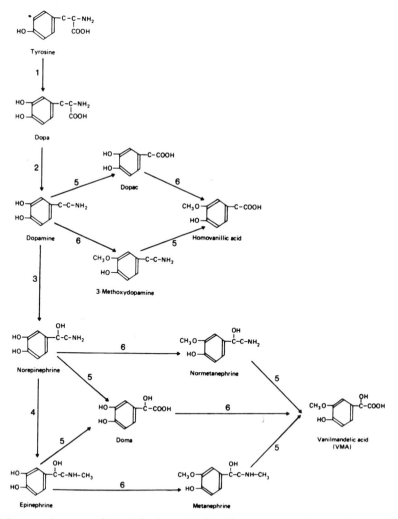

Figure 12.2. Pathways and enzymes of catecholamine metabolism. The excretory products are shown on the right of the vertically displayed biosynthetic pathway. *1*, tyrosine hydroxylase; *2*, aromatic amino acid decarboxylase; *3*, phenylamine beta-hydroxylase; *4*, phenylethanolamine N-methyltransferase; *5*, monamine oxidase plus aldehyde dehydrogenase; and *6*, catechol 0-methyltransferase. (From Sheps SG, Jiang N-S, Klee GG. Diagnostic evaluation of pheochromocytoma. *Endocrinol Metab Clin North Am* 1988;17:397–414.)

Table 12.2. Location of Pheochromocytoma

Location	%
Intraabdominal	97–99
Single adrenal tumor	50–70
Single extraadrenal tumor[a]	10–20
Multiple tumors[b]	15–40
Bilateral adrenal tumors	5–25
Multiple extraadrenal tumors	5–15
Outside abdomen	1–3
Intrathoracic[c]	2
In neck	< 1

[a]Sites along the sympathetic chain—lumbar, paravertebral, epigastrium, bladder.
[b]More common in children and in familial syndrome with medullary thyroid cancer.
[c]Usually in the posterior mediastinum.

and about 40% are malignant (Manger and Gifford, 1993).

Chromaffin Cell Secretion

The chromaffin cells synthesize catecholamines from the dietary amino acid tyrosine (Fig. 12.2); NE is the end-product, except in the adrenal medulla, where over 75% of the NE is methylated into Epi. Most adrenal medullary pheos secrete some Epi, but a few, usually small in size and having a rapid turnover of catecholamines, secrete only NE (Crout and Sjöerdsma, 1964). On the other hand, with rare exceptions (Mannix et al., 1972), extraadrenal pheos do not secrete Epi.

When catecholamines are released by exocytosis from adrenal storage vesicles, there is a coupled, proportional release of the enzyme dopamine beta-hydroxylase and the soluble protein chromogranin A. Plasma chromogranin A levels are elevated in patients with pheos and other endocrine tumors (Takiyyuddin et al., 1990).

Patterns of Catechol Secretion

Secretion from pheos varies considerably. Small pheos tend to secrete larger proportions of active catecholamines; larger pheos, with the capacity to store and metabolize large quantities of catecholamines, tend to secrete less of their content, and most of that may be secreted in inactive forms.

The frequency and severity of symptoms and signs likely relate to the secretory pattern of the pheo: those that continuously release large amounts of catecholamines may induce sustained hypertension with few paroxysms since the adrenergic receptors become desensitized after prolonged exposure to their agonists (Valet et al., 1988); those that are less active but cyclically release their catecholamine stores may induce striking paroxysms of hypertension with the classic symptoms of a pheo, since the receptors are more responsive.

The nature of the signs and symptoms also reflects the predominant catecholamine that is secreted: NE produces more alpha-mediated vasoconstriction with diastolic hypertension, Epi more beta-mediated cardiac stimulation with predominantly systolic hypertension, tachycardia, sweating, flushing, and tremulousness.

Dopa and Dopamine

Pheos that secreted large amounts of the vasodilating precursors dopa and dopamine may not manifest hypertension. This could explain the rarity of symptoms in patients with neuroblastomas and in some patients with malignant pheos who hypersecrete dopa and dopamine (Goldstein et al., 1986).

Other Secretions

Various peptide hormones may be released concomitantly with catecholamines from pheos, and their secretion may be associated with various clinical manifestations. These secretions include neuropeptide Y, which is not secreted by extraadrenal pheos (Senanayake et al., 1992); galanin (Bauer et al., 1986); opioid peptides (Bostwick et al., 1987); somatostatin (Reubi et al., 1992); insulin-like growth factor II (Gelato and Vassalotti, 1990); and parathyroid hormone-related protein (Mune et al., 1993). These secretions may give rise to a host of ancillary syndromes along with those related to catecholamines, including acromegaly (Roth et al., 1986), watery diarrhea (Salmi et al., 1988), and flushing (Sheps et al., 1988). The secretion of somatostatin may have suppressed release of catechols from a pheo in a patient whose blood and urine catechol levels were repeatedly normal despite frequent hypertensive paroxysms that were relieved by removal of the tumor (Morice et al., 1989).

Hemodynamics

The hemodynamics in 24 patients with a pheo were little diffcrent from those in age-, sex-, and weight-matched patients with essential hypertension, despite the 10-fold higher plasma NE levels in the pheo patients (Bravo et al., 1990).

The major finding in both was an increased peripheral resistance, whereas the pheo patients had lower blood volumes. Heart rate is usually around 90 beats per minute, even when the blood pressure (BP) is not high, but cardiac output is usually normal, except during surges of Epi release.

With ambulatory BP monitoring, pheo patients may not have a nocturnal fall in pressure and show a negative relation between pulse and pressure (Padfield et al., 1991).

CLINICAL FEATURES

Table 12.3 summarizes the varied and often dramatic symptoms and signs of catecholamine excess. Most patients have either headache, sweating, or palpitations, and many have all three occurring in paroxysms. On the other hand, rare patients may be virtually asymptomatic

Table 12.3. Symptoms and Signs of Pheochromocytoma[a]

Common (more than one-third of patients)
Hypertension—probably over 90%
   Intermittent only—2 to 50%
   Sustained—50 to 60%
   Paroxysms superimposed—about 50%
Hypotension, orthostatic—50 to 70%
Headache—40 to 80%
Sweating—40 to 70%
Palpitations and tachycardia—45 to 70%
Pallor—40 to 45%
Anxiety and nervousness—35 to 40%
Nausea and vomiting—10 to 50%
Funduscopic changes—50 to 70%
Weight loss—80%

Less Common (fewer than one-third)
Tremor
Anxiety
Abdominal pain
Chest pain
Polydipsia, polyuria
Acrocyanosis, cold extremities
Flushing
Dyspnea
Dizziness
Convulsions
Bradycardia
Fever (Kirby et al., 1983)
Thyroid swelling (Buckels et al., 1983)

[a]Data from Hume DM. *Am J Surg* 99:458, 1960; Stackpole RH, Melicow MM, Uson AC. *J Pediatr* 63:315, 1963; Hermann H, Mornex R. *Human Tumors Secreting Catecholamines.* New York: Pergamon Press, 1964; Moorhead EL, Caldwell JR, Kelly AR, et al. *JAMA* 196:1107, 1966; Manger WM. *Arch Intern Med* 145:229, 1985; Ross EJ, Griffith DNW. *Q J Med* 71:485, 1989.

despite having high levels of circulating catecholamines (Taubman et al., 1974). Although most patients have lost some weight, 8 of 22 patients in one series were 10% or more overweight, and 4 were definitely obese (Lee and Rousseau, 1967).

Symptoms

Paroxysms

The paroxysms represent the classic picture of the disease, but true paroxysmal hypertension with intervening normotension is relatively uncommon, and more than 50% of patients have sustained hypertension. In those with paroxysms, the spell can be brought on in multiple ways, including exercise, bending over, urination, defecation, taking an enema, induction of anesthesia, smoking, dipping snuff, palpation of the abdomen, or pressure from an enlarging uterus during pregnancy. Episodes may follow use of multiple drugs that either increase catecholamine synthesis (e.g., ACTH [Jan et al., 1990]) or release (e.g., histamine, opiates, or nicotine [McPhaul et al., 1984]); antagonize dopamine (e.g., droperidol [Montiel et al., 1986]); or inhibit catechol reuptake (e.g., tricyclic antidepressants [Achong and Keane, 1981]). Wide episodic fluctuations of BP may occur spontaneously (Ganguly et al., 1984) and may be related to an impaired baroreceptor reflex (Muneta et al., 1992).

In patients with predominant Epi secretion, beta blockers can raise the BP by blocking the beta$_2$-mediated vasodilator action of Epi, leaving the alpha-mediated vasoconstrictor action unopposed. Those with NE-producing pheos likely will not have a pressor response to beta blockers since NE has little action on vasodilatory beta$_2$ receptors (Plouin et al., 1979).

The episodes vary in frequency, duration, and severity. They may occur many times per day or only every few months, but most patients experience at least one episode per week. Patients are often considered psychoneurotic, particularly when they describe a sensation of tightness starting in the abdomen and rising into the chest and head, anxiety, tremors, sweating, and palpitations, followed by marked weakness. Overt psychiatric disturbances sometimes are found (Medvei and Cattell, 1988).

These episodes, sometimes with BP above 250/150, may lead to angina (Goldbaum et al., 1986), cardiomyopathy with acute congestive heart failure (Sardesai et al., 1990), noncardiogenic pulmonary edema (de Leeuw et al., 1986), or arrhythmias (Shimizu et al., 1992). Rarely, the presentation may be as an "acute abdomen" (Jones and Durning, 1985), sudden death after minor abdominal trauma (Primhak et al., 1986), lactic acidosis (Bornemann et al., 1986), or high fever and encephalopathy (Newell et al., 1988). Tumors arising in the wall of the bladder may cause symptoms only with micturition and, in about half of such cases, produce painless hematuria (Raper et al., 1977).

Hypotension

As noted, patients with a pheo secreting predominantly Epi may, though rarely, have profound hypotension with sweating, fever, and ventricular arrhythmias. Prolonged hypotension may also occur by spontaneous necrosis of the tumor (Atuk et al., 1977) or after administration of a phenothiazine (Lund-Johansen, 1962) or an alpha blocker (Watson et al., 1990). Much more commonly, patients have modest falls in BP with standing, associated with dizziness. The presence of postural hypotension in an untreated hypertensive may be a clue to the presence of a pheo.

Other Associated Diseases

Cholelithiasis was found in up to 30% of patients in the series of Manger and Gifford (1993).

Diabetes with fasting glucose levels above 125 mg/dl was present in 14 of 60 patients in the study of Stenström et al. (1984).

Hypercalcemia was found in the absence of hyperparathyroidism in the study of Kimura et al. (1990).

Polycythemia was ascribed to erythropoietin production in Waldmann and Bradley's study (1961), but the more likely cause of a patient's high hematocrit would be a shrunken plasma volume.

Renovascular hypertension occurred through compression of the renal artery by a pheo in the study of Ishibashi et al. (1975). Confusion may arise from high renin levels often seen in patients with a pheo (Plouin et al., 1988).

Adrenocortical hyperfunction was found in a patient with a pheo in one adrenal and a cortisol-secreting adenoma in the other, both of which were discovered incidentally (Ooi and Dardick, 1988).

Adrenocortical insufficiency has been recognized in rare patients preoperatively and has been implicated in postoperative hypotension (Mulrow et al., 1959).

Rhabdomyolysis has occurred with renal failure (Shemin et al., 1990).

Conditions Simulating a Pheochromocytoma (Table 12.4)

Most patients with hypertension and one or more of the manifestations of pheo turn out *not* to have that diagnosis. Some patients with highly suggestive symptoms have been found to have surges of dopamine or a decreased rate of inactivation of catecholamines, leading to increased free levels in the circulation that might account for their symptoms (Robertson et al., 1993). A few patients with severe hypertensive paroxysms have baroreceptor dysfunction (Kuchel et al., 1987) or prostaglandin-mediated catechol surges (Sato et al., 1988). The combined use

Table 12.4. Conditions That May Simulate Pheochromocytoma

Cardiovascular
Hyperdynamic, labile hypertension
Paroxysmal tachycardia
Angina, coronary insufficiency
Acute pulmonary edema
Eclampsia
Hypertensive crisis during or after surgery
Hypertensive crisis with MAO inhibitors
Rebound hypertension after abrupt cessation of clonidine and other antihypertensives

Psychoneurologic
Anxiety with hyperventilation
Panic attacks
Migraine and cluster headaches
Brain tumor
Basilar artery aneurysm
Stroke
Diencephallic seizures
Porphyria
Lead poisoning
Familial dysautonomia
Acrodynia
Autonomic hyperreflexia, as with quadriplegia

Endocrinologic
Menopausal symptoms
Thyrotoxicosis
Diabetes mellitus
Hypoglycemia
Carcinoid
Mastocytosis

Factitious: ingestion of sympathomimetics (Keiser, 1991)

of a monoamine oxidase (MAO) inhibitor (e.g., selegiline) with an antidepressant that inhibits serotonin receptors (e.g., fluoxetine) for treatment of Parkinson's disease may precipitate major hypertensive episodes that simulate a pheo (Montastruc et al., 1993).

Clinical confusion arises mostly from neurotic patients with hyperkinetic circulation. Patients having angina may have sudden rises in BP, possibly as a reflex from reduction of coronary blood flow. Various central nervous system lesions—tumors (Gabriel and Harrison, 1974), strokes (Mazey et al., 1974), and trauma (Wortsman et al., 1980)—may activate the sympathoadrenal pathway, produce neurogenic hypertension, and closely mimic pheo. On the other hand, increased thyroid function may be caused by a pheo, so the possibility should be considered before giving a beta blocker to control thyrotoxic symptoms (Ober, 1991).

Pheochromocytoma During Pregnancy

The association of pheochromocytoma and pregnancy may be greater than could be attributed to chance: more than 180 cases have been reported (Harper et al., 1989). When pheos are not recognized before delivery, the maternal mortality rate is about 40%, and the infant mortality rate is about 30%. Patients are usually thought to have preeclampsia, but their features and laboratory tests are fairly typical of pheo. When recognized and treated properly, the disease should pose no great problems to the pregnancy.

Pheochromocytoma in Children

The younger the patient, the more likely it is that the syndrome is familial, the pheos multiple and extraadrenal, and the hypertension persistent (Stackpole et al., 1963; Hodgkinson et al., 1980). The clinical manifestations are generally more severe in children; not infrequently, grade 3 or 4 funduscopic changes are present along with a history of convulsions. The youngest patient in Stackpole's series was only 1 month old. Catecholamine-induced hypertension is also seen in about 20% of children with neurogenic tumors (Weinblatt et al., 1983).

Familial Syndromes (Table 12.5)

The familial incidence of phco is almost certainly higher than the 6% reported by Hermann and Mornex in their 1964 survey of 507 cases. Often the search for the disease in other family members is either not made or not reported. Knowledge of the family history is obviously important since, if the disease is familial, inheritance is by a dominant gene that will cause a pheo in approximately 90% of the half of the offspring who inherit it (Knudson and Strong, 1972).

Of the familial cases, most become manifest by the fourth decade of life, and the average age of diagnosis is 20. The clinical features are similar to those of the sporadic, nonfamilial cases. There is a much greater tendency for bilateral adrenal tumors: fewer than 5% of sporadic cases are bilateral; 45% of familial cases are bilateral, with the locations often similar in the affected individuals.

Simple Familial Syndromes

About 60% of familial pheos occur without other glandular dysfunction. They occur in young people, usually before age 20; at least 40% of childhood cases represent the familial form. The simple familial gene is dominant with almost 100% penetrance. The child may be diagnosed before the parent.

Multiple Endocrine Neoplasia

The two most common combinations of multiple, familial endocrine tumors are:

1. Multiple endocrine neoplasia (MEN), type 1 (Wermer's syndrome), with tumors of the pituitary, pancreatic islet cells, and parathyroids; carcinoids of the gastrointestinal tract and lung; and frequently gastrinomas causing fulminant peptic ulcer disease (i.e., Zollinger-Ellison syndrome) (Marx et al., 1988).
2. Multiple endocrine neoplasia, type 2A (Sipple's syndrome), with medullary carcinoma of the thyroid, pheo, parathyroid hyperplasia or adenoma and, less frequently, bilateral adrenocortical hyperplasia with Cushing's syndrome.

A variant of MEN 2 has been identified with mucosal neuromas, bumpy lips, hypertrophied corneal nerves and, less commonly, skeletal defects and gastrointestinal abnormalities (Gorlin et al., 1968) and is characterized as an apparently distinct entity (MEN 2B) (Khairi et al., 1975).

Both MEN 2A and 2B are inherited as autosomal dominant traits with distinct phenotypes, but both appear to have mutations at the same locus on chromosome 10 (Nanes and Catherwood, 1992). The majority of patients with med-

Table 12.5. Types of Pheochromocytoma

	Usual Age of Diagnosis	Bilateral Tumors %
Nonfamilial	40	0[a]
Familial		
Simple	20	45
Multiple endocrine neoplasia, 2A and 2B	30–35	80
von Hippel–Lindau	25–30	45
Neurofibromatosis	40–45	12

[a]Hume (1960) reported 5% of nonfamilial tumors to be bilateral, but Knudson and Strong (1972) argue that such patients almost certainly represent unrecognized familial cases.

ullary thyroid cancer have the sporadic form that is not associated with pheos or other components of MEN 2A or 2B (Ponder et al., 1988). However, since penetrance of the MEN 2 gene is incomplete, only 40% of carriers present with symptoms before age 70 (Mathew et al., 1991). Therefore, all members of families with medullary thyroid cancer should have plasma calcitonin and urine catecholamine measurements frequently, and any family members who become hypertensive should be carefully evaluated for a pheo. Until the gene is identified, a genetic prediction can be made in families in which two or more affected members can be studied; the prediction is based on the linkage of DNA markers from the pericentromeric region of chromosome 10 to MEN 2, and can be at least 90% accurate (Lichter et al., 1992). Persons predicted to carry the gene can be selected earlier for more careful biochemical screening; those likely without the gene can be reassured (Calmettes et al., 1992).

Most of the pheos that are seen in the MEN 2A and 2B syndromes are bilateral (Lips et al., 1981), and there is increasing evidence that diffuse hyperplasia may precede the development of tumors (Carney et al., 1976). The hypertension in patients with MEN 2A or 2B is almost always paroxysmal, reflecting the predominant secretion of Epi demonstrable by urinary Epi levels above 20 μg per 24 hours (Hamilton et al., 1978).

Other Neurocutaneous Syndromes

About 1% of patients with multiple neurofibromatosis and café-au-lait spots (von Recklinghausen's disease) will have a pheo, accounting for about 5% of all pheos (Kalff et al., 1982). About 10% of these pheos are bilateral. The average age of onset of pheo symptoms is 40 to 45. Other family members may have neurofibromatosis, but no cases of familial pheos have been reported among them (Knudson and

Strong, 1972). About 15% of patients with von Hippel–Lindau disease (hemangioblastomas of the retinae and central nervous system) have a pheo (Lenz et al., 1992). With more extensive testing, 17 of 82 unselected pheo patients were found to be carriers of von Hippel–Lindau disease, and 38% of these carriers had a pheo as the only manifestation of their syndrome (Neumann et al., 1993).

Malignant Pheochromocytoma

As many as 10% of adrenal pheos and 40% of extraadrenal pheos are malignant (Manger and Gifford, 1993). To be classified as malignant, metastases must be found where aberrant chromaffin tissue does not occur, since benign pheos often show dysplasia and invasion of capsule and vessel. Routine histology is of little value, but analysis of nuclear DNA content is helpful since the normal diploid pattern almost always connotes a benign lesion, whereas a tetraploid or aneuploid pattern is seen in most patients with invasive, malignant tumors (Nativ et al., 1992). Most metastases are to skeleton, lymph nodes, liver, and lungs. Many secrete large amounts of dopamine, recognized from its metabolite homovanillic acid in the urine or serum dopamine levels. Tumor growth is often slow, and long survival is possible, likely enhanced by aggressive medical and surgical therapy, as will be described at the end of this chapter. The extent of metastatic disease may be determined by scintigraphy with [^{131}I]metaiodobenzylguanidine (Shapiro and Fig, 1989).

Death from Pheochromocytoma

Most deaths are related to failure to consider the disease in patients undergoing severe stress such as surgery or delivery. Many deaths are unexpected and sudden; this is likely related to catecholamine-induced effects on the cardiac muscle and conduction system. At least seven deaths have followed acute hemorrhagic necrosis of a pheo, most of them after phentolamine administration (van Way et al., 1976).

LABORATORY CONFIRMATION

Routine laboratory screening for pheochromocytoma in the work-up of every hypertensive is *not* recommended. Testing should be reserved for patients with features suggestive of pheo (Table 12.3) or those with incidentally found adrenal masses.

Making the Diagnosis

The simplest screening procedure is a metanephrine assay of a single voided (spot) urine specimen, preferably obtained while the patient is on no medication. The spot-urine metanephrine level was 0.35 ± 0.35 (2 SD) with a range of 0.06 to 1.18 μg per milligram of creatinine in 500 patients diagnosed with essential hypertension (Kaplan et al., 1977). Results with the single-voided specimen correlated closely to those found with 24-hour urine specimens.

In addition to urine metanephrine, assays of other catecholamines and their metabolites in urine and plasma are available (Table 12.6). In patients with a pheo, the levels of all of these are almost always elevated, although a rare patient with infrequent paroxysms may have high levels only for awhile after an episode. Such patients should be given a bottle with a few drops of HCl as a preservative and asked to collect a urine sample during and for a few hours after the next episode. The finding of normal blood and urine catecholamines during a paroxysm of hypertension almost certainly excludes pheo. Plasma catecholamines assays, though increasingly available, should not be used for screening purposes, since they are so frequently false-positive, either because of non-specific stimulation of catechol release by numerous activities or because of interference with the excretion of catechols, as seen when the glomerular filtration rate is below 20 ml/minute (Laederach and Weidmann, 1987).

A common and difficult current problem is the interference from metabolites of the antihypertensive drug labetalol, particularly with more severe forms of hypertension in which the drug is likely to be used and in which pheo may be more likely. Labetalol metabolites cause falsely high levels of urinary excretion of Epi by fluorometry, of NE by radioenzymatic or fluorometric assays, and of metanephrine by spectrophotometry or high-pressure liquid chromatography (HPLC) (Feldman, 1987), as well as of plasma catechol assays by HPLC (Bouloux and Perrett, 1985). Fortunately, these metabolites do not interfere with measurements of urine vanillylmandelic acid (VMA) or plasma catechols by radioenzymatic assay (Feldman, 1987) or of urine metanephrine by reversed-phase liquid chromatography coupled with electrochemical detection (Girerd et al., 1992). Samples should be collected before labetalol is used or 3 days after it is discontinued.

Urine Tests

Assays are available for each of the three urinary products of catecholamine metabolism: free catecholamines, metanephrines, and VMA (Fig 12.2). Patients with small, active tumors may excrete mainly free catecholamines; those with large, indolent tumors may excrete predominantly VMA. In most patients, excretion of all

Table 12.6. Normal Values (mean ± 2 S.D.) for Catecholamines and Their Metabolites

	Rosano et al. (1991) Normotensives	Duncan et al. (1988) Hypertensives
Plasma		
Dopamine	< 50 pg/ml	
Epinephrine	38–129 pg/ml	
Norepinephrine	250–620 pg/ml	140–1700 pg/ml
3,4-Dihydroxy-phenylglycol		420–2620 pg/ml
Urine		
Dopamine	308–681 μg/day	
Vanilmandelic acid (VMA)	5.3–9.4 mg/day	
Metanephrine	< 600 μg/day	
Epinephrine	3–37 μg/day	
Norepinephrine	41–135 μg/day	11–156 μg/day
3,4-Dihydroxy-phenylglycol		16–192 μg/day

Conversion factor for μg/ml to nmol/L: 5.5 for epinephrine, metanephrine, 3,4-Dihydroxy-phenylglycol; 5.9 for norepinephrine; 5.0 for VMA.

Table 12.7. Urinary Tests for Pheochromocytoma

Compound	Urinary Excretion (mg/day or μg/mg of creatinine)		No. of Patients with Pheo	% of Patients with Pheochromocytoma Correctly Identified
	Normal Adults	Pheochromocytoma		
Free catecholamines	<0.1	0.1–10.0	179	85
Metanephrine + normetanephrine	<1.2	1.0–100.0	282	96
Vanillylmandelic acid	<6.5	5–600	294	84

Data from Mann P, Runge LA. *Am J Epidemiol* 1984;120:788–790.

will be elevated, but normal values of one of the urinary products may be found in patients with proved tumors. Since pheos may secrete just Epi or just NE, both should be measured to confirm elevated metanephrine levels (Smythe et al., 1992).

A compilation of the findings in nine larger series documents the greater sensitivity of the urine metanephrine procedure (Table 12.7). False-negatives with the urine metanephrine assay may be attributable to the collection of the specimen soon after various radiographic procedures using the contrast medium methylglucamine (McPhaul et al., 1984). This chemical reacts with the reagent needed to convert metanephrine to vanillin, the end-product that is analyzed in the spectrophotometric assay. The interference can be removed by chromatography, but the better course is to obtain the urine before radiographic procedures are done. False-negative metanephrine assays by the Pisano procedure may also be caused by a 4-hydroxy metabolite of propranolol in the urine that, by producing a high blank level, spuriously decreases the level of the measured metanephrine (Chou et al., 1990).

The specificity of all three tests in the multiple series shown in Table 12.7 was 99%, so very few false-positives are to be expected with any of them. The few false-positives seen with the urine metanephrine assay may be related to drug intake (Table 12.8). An even longer list of factors that have been purported, sometimes with little validation, to interfere with these assays has been compiled by Young et al. (1975).

Improved assays, including HPLC, gas-liquid chromatography (GLC), and radioenzymatic methods are being increasingly used, thereby improving on the accuracy of the determinations (Rosano et al., 1991). Remember that patients under considerable stress (e.g., perioperatively, with acute myocardial infarction, or with severe congestive heart failure) may have high catechol levels, and they should be tested only after the stress has subsided for 5 to 7 days (Thomas and

Marks, 1978). The distinction between tumor-related and stress-induced rises in catechols may be helped by measurement of 3,4-dihydroxyphenylglycol (DHPG) along with NE (Duncan et al., 1988). NE released by neurons is subject to reuptake and converted to the deaminated metabolite DHPG. Sympathetic stimulation causes similar rises in NE and DHPG, with the ratio around 1.0. On the other hand, NE secreted from a pheo undergoes minimal conversion to DHPG, so that the ratio of NE to DHPG will be well above 2:1. However, Lenders et al. (1992) noted that with pheos that secrete only Epi, the ratio may be normal.

Children excrete more of these metabolites per milligram of creatinine, and their levels should be compared with those given in Table 12.9 (Gitlow et al., 1968).

Plasma Tests

Elevated basal plasma levels of both NE and Epi have been found in most patients with a pheo, sometimes with fewer false-negatives than either urinary VMA or metanephrine assays (Bravo and Gifford, 1984). However, most published series report that 10% to 30% of pheo patients have falsely normal values (Cryer et al., 1980; Plouin et al., 1981; Brown et al., 1981; Duncan et al., 1988). As previously noted, there are too many false-positive plasma NE and Epi levels to use plasma assays for screening purposes. Plasma levels may be elevated in patients with renal insufficiency, and falls are usually noted after hemodialysis (Musso et al., 1989). Measurement of platelet catecholamines also gives too many false-positives (Berent et al., 1990). Plasma levels of chromogranin A can be measured by immunoassay and may serve both as a diagnostic test and as a marker for the completeness of surgery (Deftos, 1991).

The use of plasma assays requires careful attention to the patient's circumstances: upright posture, sodium deprivation, exercise, fasting, and smoking all will elevate plasma catecholamines. The patient should be supine for 1 hour

Table 12.8. Factors That Interfere with Urine Tests for Catecholamines and Metabolites

Assay	Factors That Interfere	
	Increase	Decrease
Catecholamines	**Pharmacologic** Exogenous catecholamines L-dopa, methyldopa Theophylline **Analytic** Tetracycline, erythromycin Quinine, quinidine Chloral hydrate Chlorpromazine Labetalol	**Pharmacologic** Sympathetic nervous inhibitors (e.g., clonidine) Fenfluramine Mandelamine (destroys catecholamines in bladder urine)
Metanephrines	**Pharmacologic** Exogenous catecholamines MAO inhibitors Rapid withdrawal of sympathetic inhibitors **Analytic** Acetaminophen Benzodiazepines Triamterene Labetalol Sotalol	**Analytic** Methylglucamine (radiographic contrast) Propranolol
VMA	**Pharmacologic** Exogenous catecholamines L-dopa **Analytic** Nalidixic acid Anileridine Dietary phenolic acids (e.g., vanilla, bananas, coffee)	**Pharmacologic** MAO inhibitors Methyldopa Ethanol **Analytic** Clofibrate Disulfiram

Table 12.9. Urinary Excretion of VMA, HVA, and Total Metanephrines in Children

Age (yr)	VMA		HVA		Total Metanephrines	
	Mean	SD	Mean	SD	Mean	SD
<1	6.9[a]	3.2	12.9	9.6	1.6	1.3
1–2	4.6	2.2	12.6	6.3	1.7	1.1
2–5	3.9	1.7	7.6	3.6	1.2	0.8
5–10	3.3	1.4	4.7	2.7	1.1	0.8
10–15	1.9	0.8	2.5	2.4	0.6	0.5
15–18	1.3	0.6	1.0	0.6	0.2	0.2

[a]All values are given as micrograms per milligram of creatinine.
From Gitlow SE, Mendlowitz M, Wilk EK, et al. Excretion of catecholamine catabolites by normal children. *J Lab Clin Med* 1968;72:612–620.

after placement of an indwelling venous catheter. Blood should be immediately chilled, and the plasma should be separated quickly and frozen at -90°C until assayed.

Pharmacologic Tests

In view of the availability of accurate urinary assays, there is little need to subject patients to the discomfort and hazard of either provocative (histamine, tyramine, glucagon) or suppression (Regitine) tests. Moreover, these tests give both false-positive and false-negative results (Sheps and Maher, 1968; White et al., 1973).

Provocative Tests. The only rational use of the best of these provocative procedures, the glucagon stimulation test, is to identify bilateral medullary hyperplasia in patients with medullary carcinoma of the thyroid whose control urine metanephrine assays are normal, or to diagnose a pheo in the extremely rare patient with normal plasma and urine catecholamine levels. The safety of glucagon testing is improved by pretreatment with an alpha blocker that does not block the rise in plasma catecholamines (Elliott et al., 1989).

Suppression Tests. Suppression tests by nature seem more physiologic and are likely safer than provocative tests. One test uses a 2.5-mg intravenous dose of the preganglionic blocking agent pentolinium (Brown et al., 1981). Pheos do not have preganglionic nerve supply, and therefore pentolinium should not suppress their autonomous catechol secretion. The test was correct in separating all 18 patients with a pheo who did not suppress their plasma Epi or NE levels from 20 patients with intermittently elevated plasma catechols who did.

The second and more widely used test uses the effect of the centrally acting sympathetic inhibitor clonidine on plasma catechols (Bravo et al., 1981). Plasma NE and Epi are measured before and 2 and 3 hours after a single oral 0.3-mg dose of clonidine; NE + E levels fall to below the normal range in patients without a pheo but remain high in those with a pheo. The authors found a normal response (i.e., an absolute fall of plasma NE + E to below 500 pg/ml and a relative fall of at least 40% from the basal level) in all 70 nonpheo hypertensives but in only 1 of 32 patients with a pheo (Fig. 12.3) (Bravo and Gifford, 1984) The 2-hour sample almost always gives the best discrimination. To save money, the 3-hour sample can be frozen and analyzed only if the 2-hour sample is equivocal.

The test has performed well in most investigators' experience (Gross et al., 1987; Mannelli et al., 1987). A few false-positives have been reported because of diuretic therapy (Hui et al., 1986) or use of a radioimmunoassay that also measures slowly-turned-over conjugated catechols in plasma (Aron et al., 1983). More bothersome but even rarer false-negatives have been reported (Taylor et al., 1986).

Results as good as those with the plasma response have been reported with an overnight clonidine suppression test measuring urine catecholamines in urine collected from 2100 to 0700 hours after 0.3 mg of clonidine at 2100 (Macdougall et al., 1988).

Summary of Confirmatory Testing

The following guidelines should simplify the laboratory confirmation of pheo:

1. Obtain a metanephrine assay on a single-voided urine specimen on all patients with suggestive features, preferably while they are taking no medications. If the patient is on therapy with antihypertensive drugs, recall that falsely low values have been found in patients on propranolol and falsely high values with triamterene and labetalol.

   If the urine test is normal, the diagnosis has been excluded with a specificity of over 99%. However, if the patient has only paroxysmal symptoms, collect a urine sample during and after a hypertensive paroxysm and measure free catecholamines.

2. If the spot urine metanephrine assay is elevated, confirm the diagnosis by measuring metanephrine and total catecholamines in a 24-hour urine specimen.

3. If the urine assays are borderline, useful tests are clonidine suppression (if the patient is hypertensive) or glucagon provocation (if the patient is normotensive).

Localizing the Tumor

Computed tomography (CT) and magnetic resonance imaging (MRI) of the abdomen have simplified greatly the localization of pheochromocytomas (Fig. 12.4). Most pheos are big enough, larger than 2 cm, to be easily identified. Both CT and MRI provide high sensitivity and negative predictive value, but about one-third of the abnormal scans will be nonpheo lesions—thus, these modalities have only about a 70% positive predictive value (Case Records, 1991). Because of its greater sensitivity, MRI is preferred, since a pheo usually has a distinctive bright signal in T_2-weighted images (Edelman and Warach, 1993). CT and MRI can identify extraadrenal tumors (van Gils et al., 1991) and metastatic disease and have been of considerable help in evaluating patients with the MEN syndrome who may be normotensive and difficult to assess by biochemical tests (Shapiro and Fig, 1989).

The most accurate way to localize a pheo is by scintigraphy using an analogue of guanethidine (MIBG) labeled with ^{131}I, which concentrates in adrenergic vesicles and that has been found to be taken up preferentially by pheos (Sisson et al., 1981). At the University of Michigan, where 26% of 562 patients had a pheo, the ^{131}I-MIBG scan provided 88% sensitivity and 99% specificity, which translate into a 95% positive predictive value and a 98% negative predictive

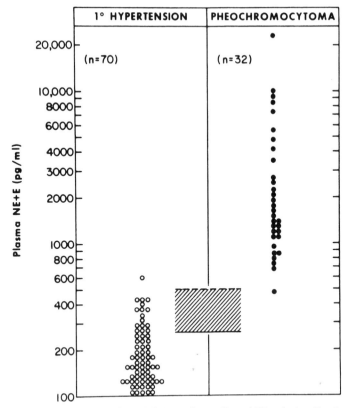

Figure 12.3. Plasma catecholamine (*NE* + *E*) levels in 32 patients with and 70 patients without a pheochromocytoma before and 2 or 3 hours after a single oral dose of clonidine, 0.3 mg. *Hatched area*, mean values obtained from 60 healthy adult subjects (+2 SD). (From Bravo EL, Gifford RW Jr. Pheochromocytoma: diagnosis, localization and management. *N Engl J Med* 1984;311:1298–1303, and by permission of *The New England Journal of Medicine*, 1984.)

value (Shapiro and Fig, 1989). The isotope is available through the Nuclear Medicine Pharmacy of the University of Michigan, and the scintigraphy equipment is widely available; thus, the procedure should be performed in any patient with abnormal biochemical tests and equivocal findings on a CT scan (Hanson et al., 1991). In addition to interfering with biochemical tests, labetalol reduces ^{131}I-MIBG uptake by pheos and normal tissues, presumably by blocking catechol reuptake and depleting storage vesicles (Khafagi et al., 1989).

With the widespread availability of CT and MRI, other procedures are rarely indicated. In a few cases, selective sampling of venous blood from multiple sites for plasma NE and Epi levels may be required (Newbould et al., 1991).

The few extraabdominal tumors can be localized by palpation of the neck, by routine radiographs of the chest and thoracic spine and, perhaps, by CT or MRI. Paragangliomas may be localized by scanning with a labeled analogue of somatostatin (Lamberts et al., 1990).

THERAPY FOR BENIGN PHEOCHROMOCYTOMAS

The symptoms of pheo can be controlled medically but, if possible, surgery should be done with the expectation that all symptoms will be relieved in the majority of patients who have benign tumors and in the hope that metastatic spread will be limited in the minority with malignant ones.

Before surgery, the patient should be treated medically for at least 1 week, preferably until hypertension and spells are controlled. In those who cannot be cured by surgery, medical therapy can be used chronically.

Medical Therapy

Acute

In a hypertensive crisis, the alpha-adrenergic blocker phentolamine (Regitine) is given intravenously, 2 to 5 mg every 5 minutes, until the BP is controlled. If serious tachycardia or arrhythmias are present, propranolol may then

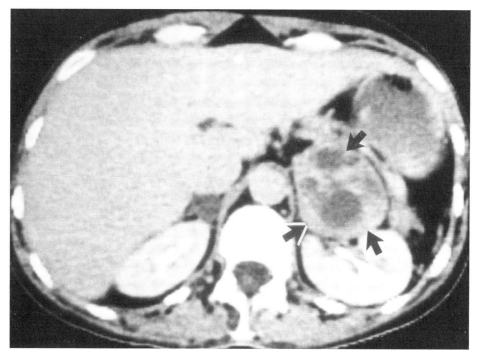

Figure 12.4. Computerized tomography scan of a 40-year-old woman with a large left adrenal pheochromocytoma. Note the multiple cystic areas within the tumor.

Table 12.10. Pharmacotherapy of Pheochromocytoma

Blockade of hormone receptor	Alpha adrenergic blockers: *Alpha₁ and alpha₂—phentolamine* *Alpha₁—prazosin, doxazosin* Beta-adrenergic blocker
Inhibition of hormone release	Calcium entry blockers
Inhibition of hormone synthesis	Alpha-methyl-para-tyrosine
Nonspecific cytotoxins	Chemotherapy: *cyclophosphamide,* *vincristine, dacarbazine*
Tissue specific cytotoxins	6-OH-dopamine (not clinically applicable)

Adapted from Shapiro B, Fig LM. Management of pheochromocytoma. *Endocrinol Metab Clin North Am* 1989;18:443.

be given intravenously, 1 to 2 mg over a 5- to 10-minute period. Control should be maintained by oral therapy until the patient is ready for surgery. Recall the potential for hemorrhagic necrosis of the tumor with alpha blockers (van Way et al., 1976).

Chronic

A number of drugs that act in different ways can be used to prepare a patient for surgery or, lacking that, to manage the disease in the long term (Shapiro and Fig, 1989) (Table 12.10).

Nonselective Alpha Blockers. Oral *phenoxybenzamine* (Dibenzyline) is preferred since it has a smoother and more prolonged action. The dose should be started at 10 mg once daily and increased slowly until the pressure is at the desired level. Side effects—postural hypotension, nasal stuffiness, and inhibition of ejaculation—are rarely bothersome. Since the presynaptic alpha₂ receptor also is blocked by this drug, the release of NE from adrenergic neurons may increase, leading to tachycardia, which may call for the use of a beta blocker.

Selective Alpha₁ *Blockers.* Oral prazosin, terazosin, or doxazosin will preferentially block the postsynaptic alpha$_1$ receptors on the vessel wall but will leave the presynaptic alpha$_2$ receptors on the neuronal surface open. Thereby, the feedback inhibition of neuronal release of NE is preserved, unlike the situation with phenoxybenzamine. Tachycardia should be less of a problem, so that a beta blocker may not be needed (Miura and Yoshinaga, 1988). Additional phentolamine may be needed during surgery (Havlik et al., 1988).

Beta Blockers. Beta blockers may be given to control tachycardia and arrhythmias but only after alpha blockers have been started. If inadvertently used alone, beta blockers may cause either a pressor response, since the beta blockade of the beta$_2$-mediated vasodilator actions of Epi leaves the alpha-mediated vasoconstrictor actions unopposed, or pulmonary edema, presumably by removal of beta-adrenergic drive to the heart (Sloand and Thompson, 1984).

The combined alpha- and beta-blocking drug labetalol has been used with good results (Reach et al., 1980). However, since it causes more beta blockage than alpha blockade, a rise in BP may be seen; thus, it should be used with great caution (Feek and Earnshaw, 1980) and only after the diagnostic tests are obtained: recall the false-positive catecholamine assays from labetalol.

Rare patients cannot be controlled on any alpha blocker (Hauptman et al., 1983), whereas a few cases have been reported to respond well to a calcium-entry blocker (Proye et al., 1989) or a converting enzyme inhibitor (Blum, 1987).

Alpha-Methyltyrosine. An inhibitor of catecholamine synthesis, *alpha*-methyl-*p*-tyrosine, or metyrosine, is now available (Demser; Merck, Sharp and Dohme). Though effective, it may cause sedation, diarrhea, and other side effects, so its primary use is for those whose tumors are inoperable. It should not be used without concomitant use of an alpha blocker (Ram et al., 1985).

Surgical Therapy

Patients with a pheo who are not under adequate BP control are at high risk during surgery, with mortality rates as high as 50%. With adequate preoperative control and intraoperative management, the risks should be little more than with other major surgical procedures. The details are well delineated by Shapiro and Fig (1989).

Preoperative Management

With the medical therapy previously described, the BP and symptoms can be controlled, the shrunken blood volume restored, and swings of pressure during surgery minimized.

Anesthesia

Certain anesthetic agents have been advocated because they tend not to cause a release of catecholamines or to sensitize the myocardium. However, in the extensive experience of Desmonts and Marty (1984), the type of anesthetic agent was of secondary importance to the control of operative hypotension by replacement of fluid volume. Neuromuscular relaxants (e.g., atracurium) should be avoided because they can cause severe hypertension (Pullertis et al., 1988).

Surgical Procedure

Most surgeons prefer an upper abdominal incision long enough to expose both adrenals, the entire periaortic sympathetic chain, and the urinary bladder. Although only one pheo may be found, exploration must be thorough, since as many as 20% of patients have multiple pheos. In familial cases, multiple pheos are almost always present. Rises in pressure during palpation may help locate small tumors. The need for such extensive exploration is less likely with the availability of CT and MRI scans.

After removal of the pheo, the BP may fall precipitously for one or more reasons (Fig. 12.5). The major factor seems to be the shrunken blood volume, which is no longer supported by intense vasoconstriction.

Postoperative Care

Patients may become hypoglycemic in the immediate postoperative period, presumably because the sudden decrease in catecholamines leads to an increase in insulin secretion while simultaneously decreasing the formation of glucose from glycogen and fat.

If the pressure remains high, some of the tumor may have been inadvertently left behind; less commonly, a renal artery may have been damaged, with induction of renovascular hypertension. The presence of residual tumor can be checked by the response to intravenous phentolamine, but reexploration should await repeated urine collection for catecholamine measures and appropriate CT or scintigraphy.

Long-Term Follow-Up

The prognosis is usually excellent for benign pheos. If the pheo is not totally resectable or the patient is a high surgical risk, long-term medical therapy can provide excellent control of all pheo

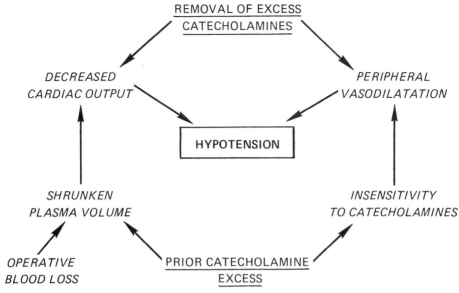

Figure 12.5. Possible causes of hypotension after removal of a pheochromocytoma.

manifestations (Pelegri et al., 1989). If the patient has a familial syndrome, repeated assays in conjunction with blood calcitonin levels and palpation of the neck for medullary thyroid cancer should be continued for life.

THERAPY FOR MALIGNANT PHEOCHROMOCYTOMAS

The prognosis is obviously not as good for those with inaccessible metastases. As much tumor mass as can be reached should be resected, and medical therapy should be provided to shrink the tumor and control the symptoms. Shrinkage of tumor mass has been reported with metyrosine (Serri et al., 1984), streptozocin (Feldman, 1983), and ^{131}I-MIBG (Krempf et al., 1991); skeletal metastases may respond to irradiation (Scott et al., 1982). The best response has been reported with chemotherapy combining cyclophosphamide, vincristine, and dacarbazine (Averbuch et al., 1988). Long-term control of symptoms is possible with alpha and beta blockers and metyrosine. With such aggressive therapy, long-term survival is possible.

We will next examine primary aldosteronism, another uncommon but fascinating adrenal cause of hypertension.

References

Achong MR, Keane PM. Pheochromocytoma unmasked by desipramine therapy. *Ann Intern Med* 1981;94:358–359.

Andersen GS, Toftdahl DB, Lund JO, Strandgaard S, Nielsen PE. The incidence rate of phaeochromocytoma and Conn's syndrome in Denmark, 1977–1981. *J Hum Hypertens* 1988;2:187–189.

Aravot DJ, Banner NR, Cantor AM, Theodoropoulos S, Yacoub MH. Location, localization and surgical treatment of cardiac pheochromocytoma. *Am Cardiol* 1992;69:283–285.

Aron DC, Bravo EL, Kapcala LP. Erroneous plasma norepinephrine levels with radioimmunoassay. *Ann Intern Med* 1983;98:1023.

Atuk NO, Teja K, Mondzelewski J, Turner SM, Selden RF. Avascular necrosis of pheochromocytoma followed by spontaneous remission. *Arch Intern Med* 1977;137:1073–1075.

Aupetit-Faisant B, Battaglia C, Zenatti M, Emeric-Blanchouin N, Legrand JC. Hypo-

aldosteronism accompanied by normal or elevated mineralocorticosteroid pathway steroid: a marker of adrenal carcinoma. *J Clin Endocrinol Metab* 1993;76:38–43.

Averbuch SD, Steakley CS, Young RC, Gelmann EP, Goldstein DS, Stull R, Keiser HR. Malignant pheochromocytoma: effective treatment with a combination of cyclophosphamide, vincristine, and dacarbazine. *Ann Intern Med* 1988;109:267–273.

Bauer FE, Hacker GW, Terenchi G, Adrian TE, Polak JM, Bloom SR. Localization and molecular forms of galanin in human adrenals: elevated levels in pheochromocytomas. *J Clin Endocrinol Metab* 1986;63:1372–1378.

Beard CM, Sheps SG, Kurland LT, Carney JA, Lie JT. Occurrence of pheochromocytoma in Rochester, Minnesota, 1950 through 1979. *Mayo Clin Proc* 1983;58:802–804.

Berent H, Uchman B, Wocial B, Januszewica W. Platelet norepinephrine and epineph-

rine concentration in patients with pheochromocytoma. *Am J Hypertens* 1990;3:618–621.

Blum R. Enalapril in pheochromocytoma. *Ann Intern Med* 1987;106:326–327.

Blumenfeld JD, Cohen N, Laragh JH, Ruggiero DA. Hypertension and catecholamine biosynthesis associated with a glomus jugulare tumor. *N Engl J Med* 1992;327:894.

Bornemann M, Hill SC, Kidd GS II. Lactic acidosis in pheochromocytoma. *Ann Intern Med* 1986;105:880–882.

Bostwick DG, Null WE, Holmes D, Weber E, Barchas JD, Bensch KG. Expression of opioid peptides in tumors. *N Engl J Med* 1987;317:1439–1443.

Bouloux P-MG, Perrett D. Interference of labetalol metabolites in the determination of plasma catecholamines by HPLC with electrochemical detection. *Clin Chimica Acta* 1985;150:111–117.

Bravo E, Fouad-Tarazi F, Rossi G, Imamura M, Lin W-W, Madkour MA, Wicker P,

Cressman MD, Saragoca M. A reevaluation of the hemodynamics of pheochromocytoma. *Hypertension* 1990;15(Suppl 1): 128–131.

Bravo EL, Gifford RW Jr. Pheochromocytoma: diagnosis, localization and management. *N Engl J Med* 1984;311:1298–1303.

Bravo EL, Tarazi RC, Fouad FM, Vidt DG, Gifford RW Jr. Clonidine-suppression test. A useful aid in the diagnosis of pheochromocytoma. *N Engl J Med* 1981;305: 623–626.

Bravo EL, Tarazi RC, Gifford RW, Stewart BH. Circulating and urinary catecholamines in pheochromocytoma. *N Engl J Med* 1979;301:682–686.

Brown MJ, Allison DR, Jenner DA, Lewis PJ, Dollery CT. Increased sensitivity and accuracy of phaeochromocytoma diagnosis achieved by use of plasma-adrenaline estimations and a pentolinium-suppression test. *Lancet* 1981;1:174–177.

Buckels JAC, Webb AMC, Rhodes A. Is paroxysmal thyroid swelling due to phaeochromocytoma a forgotten physical sign? *Br Med J* 1983;287:1206–1207.

Calmettes C, Ponder BAJ, Fischer JA, Raue F. Early diagnosis of the multiple endocrine neoplasia type 2 syndrome: consensus statement. *Eur J Clin Invest* 1992;22: 755–760.

Carney JA, Sizemore GW, Sheps SG. Adrenal medullary disease in multiple endocrine neoplasia, type 2. *Am J Clin Pathol* 1976;66:279–290.

Case Records of the Massachusetts General Hospital. Case 16-1991. Presentation of Case. *N Engl J Med* 1991;324:1119–1127.

Case Records of the Massachusetts General Hospital. Case 15-1992. Presentation of Case. *N Engl J Med* 1992;326:1008–1015.

Chou D, Tsuru M, Holtzman JL, Eckfeldt JH. Interference by the 4-hydroxylated metabolite of propranolol with determination of metanephrines by the Pisano method. *Clin Chem* 1990;26:776–777.

Copeland PM. The incidentally discovered adrenal mass. *Ann Intern Med* 1983; 98:940–945.

Crout JR, Sjöerdsma A. Turnover and metabolism and catecholamines in patients with pheochromocytoma. *J Clin Invest* 1964;43: 94–102.

Cryer PE, Rizza RA, Haymond WM, Gerich JE. Epinephrine and norepinephrine are cleared through beta-adrenergic, but not alpha-adrenergic, mechanisms in man. *Metabolism* 1980;29:1114–1118.

Deftos LJ. Chromogranin A: its role in endocrine function and as an endocrine and neuroendocrine tumor marker. *Endocrine Rev* 1991;12:181–187.

de Leeuw PW, Waltman FL, Birkenhäger WH. Noncardiogenic pulmonary edema as the sole manifestation of pheochromocytoma. *Hypertension* 1986;8:810–812.

Dennis PJ, Lewandowski AE, Rohner TJ Jr, Weidner WA, Mamourian AC, Stern DR. Pheochromocytoma of the prostate: an unusual location. *J Urol* 1989;141:130–132.

DeOreo GA Jr, Stewart GH, Tarazi RC, Gifford RW Jr. Preoperative blood transfusion in the safe surgical management of pheochromocytoma: a review of 46 cases. *J Urol* 1974;111:715–721.

Desmonts JM, Marty J. Anaesthetic management of patients with phaeochromocytoma. *Br J Anaesth* 1984;56:781–789.

Duncan MW, Compton P, Lazarus L, Smythe GA. Measurement of norepinephrine and 3,4-dihydroxyphenylglycol in urine and plasma for the diagnosis of pheochromocytoma. *N Engl J Med* 1988;319:136–142.

Edelman RR, Warach S. Magnetic resonance imaging. *N Engl J Med* 1993;328:785–791.

Elliott WJ, Murphy MB, Straus FH II, Jarabak J. Improved safety of glucagon testing for pheochromocytoma by prior α-receptor blockade. A controlled trial in a patient with a mixed ganglioneuroma/pheochromocytoma. *Arch Intern Med* 1989;149: 214–216.

Feek CM, Earnshaw PM. Hypertensive response to labetalol in phaeochromocytoma. *Br Med J* 1980;2:387.

Feldman JM. Treatment of metastatic pheochromocytoma with streptozocin. *Arch Intern Med* 1983;143:1799–1800.

Feldman JM. Falsely elevated urinary excretion of catecholamines and metanephrines in patients receiving labetalol therapy. *J Clin Pharmacol* 1987;27:288–292.

Francis IR, Gross MD, Shapiro B, Korobkin M, Quint LE. Intergrated imaging of adrenal disease. *Radiology* 1992;184:1–13.

Gabriel R, Harrison BDW. Meningioma mimicking features of a phaeochromocytoma. *Br Med J* 1974;2:312.

Ganguly A, Grim CE, Weinberger MH, Henry DP. Rapid cyclic fluctuations of blood pressure associated with an adrenal pheochromocytoma. *Hypertension* 1984;6: 281–284.

Gelato MC, Vassalotti J. Insulin-like growth factor-II: possible local growth factor in pheochromocytoma. *J Clin Endocrinol Metab* 1990;71:1168–1174.

Girerd X, Billaud EM, Sorrel-Dejerine A, Ropers J, Safavian A, Safar M, Laurent S. Labetalol does not interfere with urinary metanephrine determination in hypertensive patients [Abstract]. *J Hypertens* 1992;10:1295.

Gitlow SE, Mendlowitz M, Bertani LM. The biochemical techniques for detecting and establishing the presence of a pheochromocytoma. *Am J Cardiol* 1970;26:270–279.

Gitlow SE, Mendlowitz M, Wilk ED, Wilk S, Wolf RL, Bertani LM. Excretion of catecholamine catabolites by normal children. *J Lab Clin Med* 1968;72:612–620.

Glowniak JV, Shapiro B, Sisson JC, Thompson NW, Coran AG, Lloyd R, Kelsch RC, Beierwaltes WH. Familial extra-adrenal pheochromocytoma. A new syndrome. *Arch Intern Med* 1985;145:257–261.

Goldbaum TS, Henochowicz S, Mustafa M, Blunda M, Lindsay J Jr. Pheochromocytoma presenting with Prinzmetal's angina. *Am J Med* 1986;81:921–922.

Goldstein DS, Stull R, Eisenhofer G, Sisson JC, Weder A, Averbuch SD, Keiser HR. Plasma 3,4-dihydroxyphenylalanine (dopa) and catecholamines in neuroblastoma or pheochromocytoma. *Ann Intern Med* 1986;105:887–888.

Gorlin RJ, Sedano HO, Vickers RA, Cervenka J. Multiple mucosal neuromas, pheochromocytoma and medullary carcinoma of the thyroid—a syndrome. *Cancer* 1968;22:293–299.

Gross MD, Shapiro B, Bouffard JA, Glazer GM, Francis IR, Wilton GP, Khafagi F, Sonda LP. Distinguishing benign from malignant euadrenal masses. *Ann Intern Med* 1988;109:613–618.

Gross MD, Shapiro B, Sisson JC, Zweifler A. Clonidine-induced suppression of plasma catecholamines in states of adrenal medulla hyperfunction. *J Endocrinol Invest* 1987;10: 359–364.

Hamilton BP, Landsberg L, Levine RJ. Measurement of urinary epinephrine in screening for pheochromocytoma in multiple endocrine neoplasia type II. *Am J Med* 1978;65:1027–1032.

Hanson MW, Feldman JM, Beam CA, Leight GS, Coleman E. Iodine 131-labeled meta-iodobenzylguanidine scintigraphy and biochemical analyses in suspected pheochromocytoma. *Arch Intern Med* 1991;151: 1397–1402.

Harper MA, Murnaghan GA, Kennedy L, Hadden DR, Atkinson AB. Phaeochromocytoma in pregnancy. Five cases and a review of the literature. *Br J Obstet Gynaecol* 1989;96:594–606.

Hauptman JB, Modlinger RS, Ertel NH. Pheochromocytoma resistant to α-adrenergic blockade. *Arch Intern Med* 1983; 143:2321–2323.

Havlik RJ, Cahow E, Kinder BK. Advances in the diagnosis and treatment of pheochromocytoma. *Arch Surg* 1988;123:626–630.

Hedeland H, Östberg G, Hökfelt B. On the prevalence of adrenocortical adenomas in an autopsy material in relation to hypertension and diabetes. *Acta Med Scand* 1968;184:211.

Hermann H, Mornex R. *Human Tumors Secreting Catecholamines.* New York: Pergamon Press, 1964.

Herrera MF, Grant CS, van Heerden JA, Sheedy PF II, Ilstrup DM. Incidentally discovered adrenal tumors: an institutional perspective. *Surgery* 1991;110: 1014–1021.

Hodgkinson DJ, Telander RL, Sheps SG, Gilchrist GS, Crowe JK. Extra-adrenal intrathoracic functioning paraganglioma (pheochromocytoma) in childhood. *Mayo Clin Proc* 1980;55:271–276.

Hui TP, Krakoff LR, Felton K, Yeager K. Diuretic treatment alters clonidine suppression of plasma norepinephrine. *Hypertension* 1986;8:272–276.

Hume DM. Pheochromocytoma in the adult and in the child. *Am J Surg* 1960; 99:458–496.

Ishibashi M, Takeuchi A, Yokoyama S, Yamaji T, Tsuchimochi T, Tanaka T, Kurihara H, Ikeda M. Pheochromocytoma with renal artery stenosis and high plasma renin activity. *Jpn Heart J* 1975;16:741–748.

Jan T, Metzger BE, Baumann G. Epinephrine-producing pheochromocytoma with hypertensive crisis after corticotropin injection. *Am J Med* 1990;89:824–825.

Jaresch S, Kornely E, Kley H-K, Schlaghecke R. Adrenal incidentaloma and patients with homozygous or heterozygous congenital adrenal hyperplasia. *J Clin Endocrinol Metab* 1992;74:685–689.

Jones DH, Reid JL, Hamilton CA, Allison DJ, Welbourn RB, Dollery CT. The biochemical diagnosis, localization and follow up of phaeochromocytoma: the role of plasma and urinary catecholamine measurements. *Q J Med* 1980;49:341–361.

Jones DJ, Durning P. Phaechromocytoma presenting as an acute abdomen: report of two cases. *Br Med J* 1985;291:1267–1268.

Kalff V, Shapiro B, Lloyd R, Sisson JC, Holland K, Nakajo M, Beierwaltes WH. The spectrum of pheochromocytoma in hypertensive patients with neurofibromatosis. *Arch Intern Med* 1982;142:2092–2098.

Kaplan NM, Kramer NJ, Holland OB, Sheps SG, Gomez-Sanchez C. Single-voided urine metanephrine assays in screening for pheochromocytoma. *Arch Intern Med* 1977;137:190–193.

Keiser HR. Surreptitious self-administration of epinephrine resulting in "pheochromocytoma." *JAMA* 1991;266:1553–1555.

Khafagi FA, Shapiro B, Fig LM, Mallette S, Sisson JC. Labetalol reduces iodine-131 MIBG uptake by pheochromocytoma and normal tissues. *J Nucl Med* 1989;30: 481–489.

Khairi MRA, Dexter RN, Burzynski NJ, Johnston CC Jr. Mucosal neuroma, pheochromocytoma and medullary thyroid carcinoma: multiple endocrine neoplasia type 3. *Medicine* 1975;54:89–112.

Kimura S, Nishimura Y, Yamaguchi K, Nagasaki K, Shimada K, Uchida H. A case of pheochromocytoma producing parathyroid hormone-related protein and presenting with hypercalcemia. *J Clin Endocrinol Metab* 1990;70:1559–1563.

Kirby BD, Ham J, Fairley HB, Benowitz N, Schambelan M. Normotensive pheochromocytoma. Pharmacologic, paraneoplastic and anesthetic considerations. *West J Med* 1983;139:221–225.

Knudson AG Jr, Strong LC. Mutation and cancer: neuroblastoma and pheochromocytoma. *Am J Hum Genet* 1972;24:514–532.

Krempf M, Lumbroso J, Mornex R, Brendel AJ, Wemeau JL, Delisle MJ, Aubert B, Carpentier P, Fleury-Goyon MC, Gibold C, Guyot M, Lahneche B, Marchandise X, Schlumberger M, Charbonnel B, Chatal JF. Use of *m*-[¹³¹I]iodobenzylguanidine in the treatment of malignant pheochromocytoma. *J Clin Endocrinol Metab* 1991;72: 455–461.

Kuchel O, Buu NT, Larochelle P, Hamet P, Genest J Jr. Episodic dopamine discharge in paroxysmal hypertension. Page's syndrome revisited. *Arch Intern Med* 1986; 146:1315–1320.

Laederach K, Weidmann P. Plasma and urinary catecholamines as related to renal function in man. *Kidney Int* 1987; 31:107–111.

Lamberts SWJ, Bakker WH, Reubi J-C, Krenning EP. Somatostatin-receptor imaging in the localization of endocrine tumors. *N Engl J Med* 1990;323: 1246–1249.

Lee RE, Rousseau P. Pheochromocytoma and obesity. *J Clin Endocrinol Metab* 1967;27: 1050–1052.

Lenders JWM, Willemsen JJ, Beissel T, Kloppenborg PWC, Thien T, Benraad TJ. Value of the plasma norepinephrine/3,4-dihydroxyphenylglycol ratio for the diagnosis of pheochromocytoma. *Am J Med* 1992;92:147–152.

Lenz T, Thiede HM, Nussberger J, Atlas SA, Distler A, Schulte K-L. Hyperreninemia and secondary hyperaldosteronism in a patient with pheochromocytoma and von Hippel-Lindau disease. *Nephron* 1992;62: 345–350.

Lichter JB, Wu J, Genel M, Flynn SD, Pakstis AJ, Kidd JR, Kidd KK. Presymptomatic testing using DNA markers for individuals at risk for familial multiple endocrine neoplasia 2A. *J Clin Endocrinol Metab* 1992;74:368–373.

Lie JT, Olney BA, Spittel JA. Perioperative hypertensive crisis and hemorrhagic diathesis: fatal complication of clinically unsuspected pheochromocytoma. *Am Heart J* 1980;100:716–722.

Lips KJM, Veer JVDS, Struyvenberg A, Alleman A, Leo JR, Wittebol P, Minder WH, Kooiker CJ, Geerdink RA, Van Waes PFGM, Hackeng WHL. Bilateral occurrence of pheochromocytoma in patients with the multiple endocrine neoplasia syndrome type 2A (Sipple's syndrome). *Am J Med* 1981;70:1051–1060.

Lund-Johansen P. Shock after administration of phenothiazines in patients with pheochromocytoma. *Acta Med Scand* 1962;172:525–529.

Macdougall IC, Isles CG, Stewart H, Inglis GC, Finlayson J, Thomson I, Lees KR, McMillan NC, Morley P, Ball SG. Overnight clonidine suppression test in the diagnosis and exclusion of pheochromocytoma. *Am J Med* 1988;84:993–1000.

Manger WM. Psychiatric manifestations in patients with pheochromocytomas. *Arch Intern Med* 1985;145:229–230.

Manger WM, Gifford RW Jr. Pheochromocytoma: current diagnosis and management. *Clev Clin J Med* 1993;60:365–378.

Mannelli M, De Feo ML, Maggi M, Pupilli C, Opocher G, Valenza T, Baldi E, Serio M. Usefulness of basal catecholamine plasma levels and clonidine suppression test in the diagnosis of pheochromocytoma. *J Endocrinol Invest* 1987;10: 377–382.

Mannix H Jr, O'Grady WP, Gitlow SE. Extraadrenal pheochromocytoma-producing epinephrine. Its physiologic significance. *Arch Surg* 1972;104:216–218.

Manu P, Runge LA. Biochemical screening for pheochromocytoma. Superiority of urinary metanephrines measurements. *Am J Epidemiol* 1984;120:788–790.

Marx SJ, Sakaguchi K, Green J III, Aurbach GD, Brandi M-L. Mitogenic activity on parathyroid cells in plasma from members of a large kindred with multiple endocrine neoplasia type 1. *J Clin Endocrinol Metab* 1988;67:149–153.

Mathew CGP, Easton DF, Nakamura Y, Ponder BAJ. Presymptomatic screening for multiple endocrine neoplasia type 2A with linked DNA markers. *Lancet* 1991;337:7–11.

Mazey RM, Kotchen TA, Ernst CB. A syndrome resembling pheochromocytoma following a stroke. Report of a case. *JAMA* 1974;230:575–577.

McPhaul M, Punzi HA, Sandy A, Borganelli M, Rude R, Kaplan NM. Snuff-induced hypertension in pheochromocytoma. *JAMA* 1984;252:2860–2862.

Meaglia JP, Schmidt JD. Natural history of an adrenal myelolipoma. *J Urol* 1992;147: 1089–1090.

Medvei VC, Cattell WR. Mental symptoms presenting in phaeochromocytoma: a case report and review. *J R Soc Med* 1988;81: 550–551.

Miura Y, Yoshinaga K. Doxazosin: a newly developed, selective α_1-inhibitor in the management of patients with pheochromocytoma. *Am Heart J* 1988;116:1785–1789.

Montastruc JL, Chamontin B, Senard JM, Tran MA, Rascol O, Llau ME, Rascol A. Pseudophaeochromocytoma in parkinsonian patient treated with fluoxetine plus selegiline. *Lancet* 1993;341:555.

Montiel C, Artalejo AR, Bermejo PM, Sanchez-Garcia P. A dopaminergic receptor in adrenal medulla as a possible site of action for the droperidol-evoked hypertensive response. *Anesthesiology* 1986;65:474–479.

Moorhead EL, Caldwell JR, Kelly AR, Morales AR. The diagnosis of pheochromocytoma. *JAMA* 1966;196:1107–1113.

Morice AH, Price JS, Ashby MJ, Brown MJ. Phaeochromocytoma with associated somatostatin production. *Br Med J* 1989; 298:1358–1359.

Mulrow PJ, Cohn GL, Yesner R. Isolation of cortisol from a pheochromocytoma. *Yale J Biol Med* 1959;31:363–372.

Mune T, Katakami H, Kato Y, Yasuda K, Matsukura S, Miura K. Production and secretion of parathyroid hormone-related protein in pheochromocytoma. Participation of an α-adrenergic mechanism. *J Clin Endocinol Metab* 1993;76:757–762.

Muneta S, Kawada H, Iwata T, Murakami E, Hiwada K. Impairment of baroreceptor reflex in patients with phaeochromocytoma. *J Hum Hypertens* 1992;6:77–78.

Musso NR, Deferrari G, Pende A, Vergassola C, Saffioti S, Gurreri G, Litti G. Free and sulfoconjugated catecholamines in normotensive uremic patients: effects of hemodialysis. *Nephron* 1989;51:344–349.

Nanes MS, Catherwood BD. The genetics of multiple endocrine neoplasia syndromes. *Ann Rev Med* 1992;43:253–268.

Nativ O, Grant CS, Sheps SG, O'Fallon JR, Farrow GM, van Heerden JA, Lieber MM. The clinical significance of nuclear DNA ploidy pattern in 184 patients with pheochromocytoma. *Cancer* 1992;69:2683–2687.

Neumann HPH, Berger DP, Sigmund G, Blum U, Schmidt D, Parmer RJ, Volk B, Kirste G. Pheochromocytomas, multiple endocrine neoplasia type 2, and von Hippel–Lindau disease. *N Engl J Med* 1993; 329:1531–1538.

Newbould EC, Ross GA, Dacie JE, Bouloux PMG, Besser GM, Grossman A. The use of venous catheterization in the diagnosis and localization of bilateral phaeochromocytomas. *Clin Endocrinol* 1991;35:55–59.

Newell K, Prinz RA, Braithwaite S, Brooks M. Pheochromocytoma crisis. *Am J Hypertens* 1988;1:189S–191S.

Nomura A, Yasuda H, Katoh K, Kakinoki S, Takechi S, Kobayashi T, Shimono H. Continuous blood pressure recordings in patients with pheochromocytoma of the urinary bladder. *Am J Hypertens* 1991;4: 189–191.

Ober KP. Pheochromocytoma in a patient with hyperthyroxinemia. *Am J Med* 1991;90: 137–138.

Ooi TC, Dardick I. Coexisting pheochromocytomas and adrenocortical tumour discovered incidentally. *Can Med Assoc J* 1988; 139:869–871.

Padfield PL, Jyothinagaram SG, McGinley IM, Watson DM. Reversal of the relationship between heart rate and blood pressure in phaeochromocytoma: a non-invasive diagnostic approach? *J Hum Hypertens* 1991; 5:501–504.

Pelegri A, Romero R, Reguant M, Aisa L. Non-resectable phaeochromocytoma: long term follow-up. *J Hum Hypertens* 1989;3: 145–147.

Plouin P-F, Chatelleri G, Rougeot M-A, Comoy E, Menard J, Corvol P. Plasma renin activity in phaeochromocytoma: effects of beta-blockade and converting enzyme inhibition. *J Hypertens* 1988;6: 579–585.

Plouin P-F, Duclos JM, Menard J, Comoy E, Bohuon C, Alexandre JM. Biochemical tests for diagnosis of phaeochromocytoma: urinary versus plasma determinations. *Br Med J* 1981;281:853–854.

Plouin P-F, Menard J, Corvol P. Noradrenaline producing phaeochromocytomas with absent pressor response to beta-blockade. *Br Heart J* 1979;42:359–361.

Ponder BAJ, Ponder MA, Coffey R, Pembrey ME, Gagel RF, Telenius-Berg M, Semple P, Easton DF. Risk estimation and screening in families of patients with medullary thyroid carcinoma. *Lancet* 1:397, 1988.

Primhak RA, Spicer RD, Variend S. Sudden death after minor abdominal trauma: an unusual presentation of phaeochromocytoma. *Br Med J* 292;1986:95–96.

Proye C, Thevenin D, Cecat P, Petillot P, Carnaille B, Verin P, Sautier M, Racadot N. Exclusive use of calcium channel blockers in preoperative and intraoperative control of pheochromocytomas: hemodynamics and free catecholamine assays in ten consecutive patients. *Surgery* 1989;106: 1149–1154.

Pullertis J, Ein S, Balfe JW. Anaesthesia for phaeochromocytoma. *Can J Anaesth* 1988;35:526–534.

Rácz K, Pinet F, Marton T, Szende B, Gláz E, Corvol P. Expression of steroidogenic enzyme messenger ribonucleic acids and corticosteroid production in aldosterone-producing and "nonfunctioning" adrenal adenomas. *J Clin Endocrinol Metab* 1993; 77:677–682.

Ram CVS, Meese R, Hill SC. Failure of α-methyltyrosine to prevent hypertensive crisis in pheochromocytoma. *Arch Intern Med* 1985;145:2114–2115.

Raper AJ, Jessee EF, Texter JH Jr, Giffler RF, Hietala S-O. Pheochromocytoma of the urinary bladder: a broad clinical spectrum. *Am J Cardiol* 1977;40:820–824.

Reach G, Thibonnier M, Chevillard C, Corvol P, Milliez P. Effect of labetalol on blood pressure and plasma catecholamine concentrations in patients with phaeochromocytoma. *Br Med J* 1980;280:1300–1301.

Reinholdt S, Pedersen KE. A case of multiple extra-adrenal pheochromocytomas. *Acta Med Scand* 1988;223:285–287.

Reinig JW, Doppman JL, Dwyer AJ, Frank J. MRI of indeterminate adrenal masses. *Am J Radiol* 1986;147:493–496.

ReMine WH, Chong GC, Van Heerden JA, Sheps SG, Harrison EG Jr. Current management of pheochromocytoma. *Ann Surg* 1974;179:740–748.

Reubi JC, Waser B, Khosla S, Lvols L, Goellner JR, Krenning E, Lamberts S. *In vitro* and *in vivo* detection of somatostatin receptors in pheochromocytomas and paragangliomas. *J Clin Endocrinol Metab* 1992; 74:1082–1089.

Robertson D, Hollister AS, Biaggioni I, Netterville JL, Mosqueda-Garcia R, Roberston RM. The diagnosis and treatment of baroreflex failure. *N Engl J Med* 1993;329: 1449–1455.

Rosano TG, Swift TA, Hayes LW. Advances in catecholamine and metabolite measurements for diagnosis of pheochromocytoma. *Clin Chem* 1991;37:1854–1867.

Rosen HN, Swartz SL. Subtle glucocorticoid excess in patients with adrenal incidentaloma. *Am J Med* 1992;92:213–216.

Ross EJ, Griffith DNW. The clinical presentation of phaeochromocytoma. *Q J Med* 1989;71:485–496.

Ross NS, Aron DC. Hormonal evaluation of the patient with an incidentally discovered adrenal mass. *N Engl J Med* 1990;323: 1401–1405.

Roth KA, Wilson DM, Eberwine J, Dorin RI, Kovacs K, Bensch KG, Hoffman AR. Acromegaly and pheochromocytoma: a multiple endocrine syndrome caused by a plurihormonal adrenal medullary tumor. *J Clin Endocrinol* 1986;63:1421–1426.

Salmi J, Pelto-Huikko M, Auvinen O, Karvonen A-L, Saaristo J, Paronenm I, Pöyhönen L, Seppönen S. Adrenal pheochromocytoma-ganglioneuroma producing catecholamines and various neuropeptides. *Acta Med Scand* 1988;224:403–408.

Sardesai SH, Mourant AJ, Sivathandon Y, Farrow R, Gibbons DO. Phaeochromocytoma and catecholamine induced cardiomyopathy presenting as heart failure. *Br Heart J* 1990;63:234–237.

Sato T, Igarashi N, Minami S, Okabe T, Hashimoto H, Hasui M, Kato E. Recurrent attacks of vomiting, hypertension and psychotic depression: a syndrome of periodic catecholamine and prostaglandin discharge. *Acta Endocrinol (Copenh)* 1988; 117:189–197.

Scott HW, Reynolds V, Green N, Page D, Oates JA, Robertson D, Roberts S. Clinical experience with malignant pheochromocytomas. *Surg Gynecol Obstet* 1982;154: 801–818.

Senanayake PD, Denker JK, Graham RM, Bravo EL. Neuropeptide Y and chromogranin A in adrenal and extraadrenal pheochromocytoma [Abstract]. *Hypertension* 1992;20:27.

Serrı O, Comtois R, Bettez P, Gubuc G, Buu NT, Kuchel O. Reduction in the size of a pheochromocytoma pulmonary metastasis by metyrosine therapy. *N Engl J Med* 1984;310:1264–1265.

Shapiro B, Fig LM. Management of pheochromocytoma. *Endocrinol Metab Clin North Am* 1989;18:443–481.

Shemin D, Cohn PS, Zipin SB. Pheochromocytoma presenting as rhabdomyolysis and acute myoglobinuric renal failure. *Arch Intern Med* 1990;150:2384–2385.

Sheps SG, Jiang N-S, Klee GG. Diagnostic evaluation of pheochromocytoma. *Endocrinol Metab Clin North Am* 1988;17: 397–414.

Sheps SG, Jiang N-S, Klee GG, van Heerden JA. Recent developments in the diagnosis and treatment of pheochromocytoma. *Mayo Clin Proc* 1990;65:88–95.

Sheps SG, Maher FT. Histamine and glucagon tests in diagnosis of pheochromocytoma. *JAMA* 1968;205:895–902.

Shimizu K, Miura Y, Meguro Y, Noshiro T, Ohzeki T, Kusakari T, Akama H, Watanabe T, Honma H, Imai Y, Yoshinaga K, Totsuka H. QT prolongation with torsade de pointes in pheochromocytoma. *Am Heart J* 1992;124:235–239.

Sisson JC, Frager MS, Valk TW, Gross MD, Swanson DP, Wieland DM, Tobes MC, Beierwaltes WH, Thompson NW. Scintigraphic localization of pheochromocytoma. *N Engl J Med* 1981;305:12–7.

Sjöersdma A, Engelman K, Waldmann TA, Cooperman LH, Hammond WG. Pheochromocytoma: current concepts of diagnosis and treatment. Combined clinical staff conference at the National Institutes of Health. *Ann Intern Med* 1966;65: 1302–1326.

Sloand EM, Thompson BT. Propranolol-induced pulmonary edema and shock in a patient with pheochromocytoma. *Arch Intern Med* 1984;144:173–174.

Smythe GA, Edwards G, Graham P, Lazarus L. Biochemical diagnosis of pheochromocytoma by simultaneous measurement of urinary excretion of epinephrine and norepinephrine. *Clin Chem* 1992;38:486–492.

Stackpole RH, Melicow MM, Uson AC. Pheochromocytoma in children. *J Pediatr* 1963;63:315–336.

Stenström G, Sjöström L, Smith U. Diabetes mellitus in pheochromocytoma. Fasting blood glucose levels before and after surgery in 60 patients with pheochromocytoma. *Acta Endocrinol* 1984;106:511–515.

Stenström G, Svördsudd K. Pheochromocytoma in Sweden 1958–1981. *Acta Med Scand* 1986;220:225–232.

Stewart GH, Bravo EL, Meaney TF. A new simplified approach to the diagnosis of pheochromocytoma. *J Urol* 1979;122: 579–581.

Takeda K, Yashuhara S, Miyamori I, Sato T, Miura Y. Phaeochromocytoma in Japan: analysis of 493 cases during 1973–1982. *J Hypertens* 1986;4(Suppl 5):397–399.

Takiyuddin MA, Cervenka JH, Hsiao RJ, Barbosa JA, Parmer RJ, O'Connor DT. Chromogranin A. Storage and release in hypertension. *Hypertension* 1990;15:237–246.

Taubman I, Pearson OH, Anton AH. An asymptomatic catecholamine-secreting pheochromocytoma. *Am J Med* 1974;57: 953–956.

Taylor HC, Mayes D, Anton AH. Clonidine suppression test for pheochromocytoma:

examples of misleading results. *J Clin Endocrinol Metab* 1986;63:238–242.

Thomas JA, Marks BH. Plasma norepinephrine in congestive heart failure. *Am J Cardiol* 1978;41:233–243.

Valet P, Damase-Michel C, Chamontin B, Durand D, Chollet F, Montastruc JL. Platelet α_2 and leucocyte β_2-adrenoceptors in phaechromocytoma: effect of tumour removal. *Eur J Clin Invest* 1988;18:481–485.

van Gils APG, Falke THM, van Erkel AR, Arndt J-W, Sandler MP, van der Mey AGL, Hoogma RPLM. MR imaging and MIBG scintigraphy of pheochromocytomas and extraadrenal functioning paragangliomas. *RadioGraphics* 1991;11:37–57.

van Way CE III, Faraci RP, Cleveland HC, Foster JF, Scott HW Jr. Hemorrhagic necrosis of pheochromocytoma associated with phentolamine administration. *Ann Surg* 1976;184:26–30.

Waldmann T, Bradley JE. Polycythemia secondary to a pheochromocytoma with production of an erythropoiesis stimulating factor by the tumor. *Proc Soc Exp Biol Med* 1961;108:425–427.

Watson JP, Hughes EA, Bryan RL, Lawson N, Barnett AH. A predominantly adrenaline-secreting phaeochromocytoma. *Q J Med* 1990;76:747–752.

Weinblatt ME, Heisel MA, Siegel SE. Hypertension in children with neurogenic tumors. *Pediatrics* 1983;71:947–951

Whalen RK, Althausen AF, Daniels GH. Extra-adrenal pheochromocytoma. *J Urol* 1992;147:1–10.

White LW, Levy RP, Anton AH. Comparison of biochemical and pharmacological testing for pheochromocytoma. *Res Commun Chem Pathol Pharmacol* 1973;5:252–262.

Wortsman J, Brns G, Van Beek AL, Couch J. Hyperadrenergic state after trauma to the neuroaxis. *JAMA* 1980;243:1459–1460.

Young DS, Pestaner LC, Gibberman V. Effects of drugs on clinical laboratory tests. *Clin Chem* 1975;21:1D–432D.

13 Primary Aldosteronism

Interest in the latest of all the major hypertensive syndromes to be recognized, primary aldosteronism, has heightened over the past few years with increasingly easier recognition of milder presentations of the classic syndrome and elucidation of the pathophysiology of two relatively rare but fascinating forms of mineralocorticoid excess: glucocorticoid-remediable aldosteronism (Lifton et al., 1992) and apparent mineralocorticoid excess (Ulick, 1991). The unraveling of the latter condition has led to an understanding of how licorice and other sources of glycyrrhetinic acid induce hypertension (Walker and Edwards, 1991; Walker, 1993).

This chapter will cover the syndromes listed in Table 13.1, in which secretion of the physiologic mineralocorticoid aldosterone is primarily increased. The next chapter will cover syndromes caused by increased secretion of other mineralocorticoids (e.g., congenital adrenal hyperplasias) or by cortisol acting on mineralo-

corticoid receptors (e.g., licorice-induced mineralocorticoid excess).

Before proceeding, a caveat is in order. Most clinicians, even those who see a large number of hypertensive patients, will see only a very few with primary aldosteronism. As will be described later in this chapter, when large groups of these patients are carefully assessed at centers with special interest in mineralocorticoid hypertension, 10% or more will have aberrant findings, either in pathophysiologic or radiologic findings that, if not recognized, could lead to mistaken management. Fortunately, most clinicians, simply on the basis of chance, will never encounter such aberrant patients, but all should be aware that aberrancies do occur. Therefore, when the relatively easy diagnosis of primary aldosteronism is made and an imaging procedure demonstrates either a single tumor or two enlarged glands, some additional matching between function and anatomy should be made before deciding on surgery or medical therapy, respectively.

DEFINITIONS

Primary aldosteronism is the syndrome resulting from the secretion of excessive amounts of aldosterone from the adrenal cortex, usually by a solitary adenoma, sometimes by bilateral hyperplasia, rarely by variants of these two (Irony et al., 1990; Tunny et al., 1991) (Table 13.1).

Most aldosteronism seen in clinical practice is *secondary* to an increase in renin-angiotensin activity. A classification of the various forms of secondary aldosteronism, by mechanism, is virtually the same as the right side of Table 3.7, Clinical Conditions Affecting Renin Levels. The ability to measure plasma renin activity (PRA)

Table 13.1. Syndromes of Primary Aldosterone Excess

I. Aldosterone-producing adenoma (APA)
  A. Usual: Angiotensin-unresponsive
  B. Atypical
    1. Angiotensin-responsive (AP-RA)
    2. Familial
II. Bilateral Adrenal hyperplasia
  A. Usual: Angiotensin-responsive
    (Idiopathic hyperaldosteronism: IHA)
  B. Atypical: Angiotensin-unresponsive
    (Primary adrenal hyperplasia: PAH)
III. Glucocorticoid-remediable aldosteronism
  (GRA)
IV. Adrenal carcinoma
V. Extra-adrenal tumors

has made the differentiation much easier since it is elevated in secondary aldosteronism and suppressed in primary aldosteronism.

INCIDENCE

Soon after the first cases were described, apparently by a Polish physician writing in an obscure journal (Litynski, 1953), Jerome Conn (1955) fully characterized this fascinating syndrome. Over the next decade, Conn and coworkers broadened the scope of primary aldosteronism so that it covered almost 20% of the hypertensive patients at the University of Michigan (Conn et al., 1965). This high prevalence was subsequently shown to reflect the nature of the patients referred to that center, highly selected and suspected of having the disease. In most series of unselected patients, classic primary aldosteronism was found in fewer than 0.5% of hypertensives (Kaplan, 1967; Gifford, 1969; Sinclair et al., 1987). Throughout Denmark from 1977 to 1981, only 19 cases were identified, corresponding to 0.8 cases per million people per year (Anderson et al., 1988). During the same period, 47 cases of pheochromocytoma were identified.

On the other hand, using a relatively simple screening test—the plasma aldosterone/plasma renin ratio—one group of investigators in Brisbane, Australia found 48 patients with primary aldosteronism in 1 year (Gordon et al., 1992). Therefore, the condition may be more common than the formerly published series would suggest.

CLINICAL FEATURES

The disease is usually seen in patients between the ages of 30 and 50, though cases have been found in patients from age 3 to 75, and in women more frequently than in men. The syndrome has been recognized during pregnancy in hypokalemic patients with even higher aldosterone levels than expected and, most importantly, suppressed PRA (Gordon and Tunny, 1982).

The classic clinical features of primary aldosteronism, outlined in Figure 13.1, are hypertension, hypokalemia, excessive urinary potassium excretion, hypernatremia, and metabolic alkalosis. The usual presence of these features reflects the pathophysiology of aldosterone excess.

Hypertension

Patients with primary aldosteronism have been hypertensive, with very few exceptions (Matsunaga et al., 1983). The BP may be quite

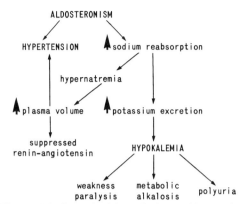

Figure 13.1. Pathophysiology of primary aldosteronism. (From Kaplan NM. Primary aldosteronism. In: Astwood EB, Cassidy CE, eds. *Clinical Endocrinology, vol. 2.* New York: Grune & Stratton, 1968:468–472.)

high—the mean in one series of 136 patients was 205/123 (Ferriss et al., 1978b). In another series of 140 patients, 28 had severe, resistant hypertension (Bravo et al., 1988). More than a dozen cases have had malignant hypertension (Kaplan, 1963; Sunman et al., 1992). Unlike the high renin levels seen with other causes of malignant hypertension, renin levels are low in those who have primary aldosteronism (Baxter and Wang, 1974; Sunman et al., 1992).

Complications

In the Medical Research Council (MRC) series, 31 of 136 patients with primary aldosteronism had experienced either a stroke or myocardial infarction (Beevers et al., 1976). Significant renal damage may be present (Young et al., 1991) along with considerable left ventricular enlargement and an increased end-diastolic internal dimension index (Pringle et al., 1988).

Hemodynamics

The hypertension is hemodynamically characterized by an increased peripheral resistance, a slightly expanded plasma volume, and an increased total body and exchangeable sodium content (Williams et al., 1984). When 10 patients with primary aldosteronism, previously well controlled on spironolactone, were studied 2 weeks after the drug was stopped and the hypertension reappeared, cardiac output and sodium content (both plasma volume and total exchangeable sodium) rose initially (Wenting et al., 1982) (Fig. 13.2). Between weeks 2 and 6, the hemodynamic patterns separated into two types: in five patients, the hypertension was maintained through increased cardiac output; in

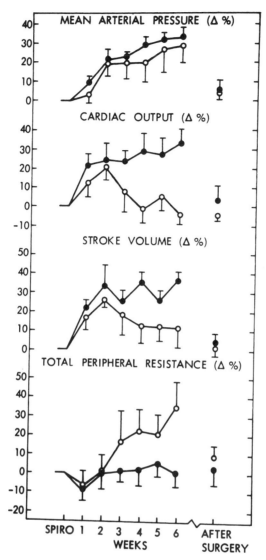

Figure 13.2. Changes (mean ± SEM) in systemic hemodynamics after discontinuation of spironolactone treatment *(SPIRO)* and after surgery in 10 patients with primary aldosteronism. Note the fall of stroke volume and cardiac output after 2 weeks in the five patients with "high-resistance" hypertension *(open circles)*, as compared with the five with "high-flow" hypertension *(closed circles)*. (From Wenting GJ, Man in't Veld AJ, Derkx FHM, Schalekamp MADH. Recurrence of hypertension in primary aldosteronism after discontinuation of spironolactone. Time course of changes in cardiac output and body fluid volumes. *Clin Exp Hypertens [A]* 1982;4:1727–1748.)

the other five, cardiac output and blood volume returned to their initial values, but total peripheral resistance rose markedly. Total body sodium space remained expanded in both groups, though more so in those with increased cardiac output (Man in't Veld et al., 1984). After surgery, the cardiac output fell in the "high flow" patients, and the peripheral resistance fell in the "high resistance" patients.

Mechanism of Sodium Retention. The pressor actions of aldosterone are generally related to its effects on sodium retention via its action on renal mineralocorticoid receptors (Fig. 13.3). The human kidney mineralocorticoid receptor has been cloned, sequenced, and expressed and shown to be equally receptive to glucocorticoids and to mineralocorticoids (Arriza et al., 1987). Relatively small concentrations of aldosterone are able to bind to the mineralocorticoid receptor in the face of much higher concentrations of glucocorticoids (mainly cortisol) because of the action of the 11-beta-

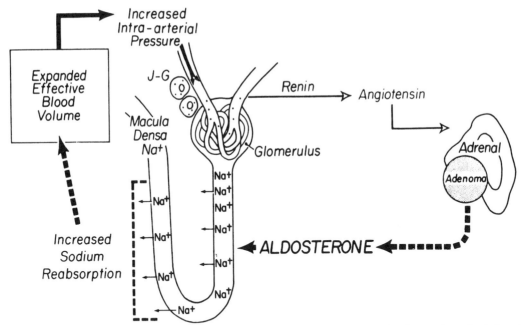

Figure 13.3. Mechanism for the manifestations of primary aldosteronism. The increased sodium reabsorption induced by the excess aldosterone expands blood volume and increases pressure at the juxtaglomerular (J-G) cells, thereby suppressing the release of renin (From Kaplan NM. In: Stollerman GH, ed. *Curable Hypertension: Advances in Internal Medicine*. Chicago: Year Book, 1969;15:95–115.)

hydroxysteroid dehydrogenase enzyme, which converts the cortisol (which has potent mineralocorticoid effects) into cortisone (which is impotent) (Walker, 1993).

In the presence of excess mineralocorticoid, sodium reabsorption in the distal tubule is increased by a number of effects on ion transport (Horisberger and Rossier, 1992). After a certain amount of volume expansion, the increases in renal perfusion pressure and atrial natriuretic factor inhibit sodium reabsorption so that ''escape'' from progressive sodium retention occurs despite continued aldosterone excess (Gonzalez-Campoy et al., 1989).

Aldosterone's actions, moreover, are not limited to renal sodium retention. Others include:

—Myocardial fibrosis: in hypertensive rats, the usual collagen accumulation and myocardial fibrosis were prevented by the aldosterone antagonist, spironolactone (Brilla and Weber, 1992);

—Direct hypertensive effects when administered into the brain, increasing total peripheral resistance (Kageyama and Bravo, 1988);

—An increase in sodium influx into vascular smooth muscle (Friedman and Tanaka, 1987);

—An increase in the number of cardiac calcium channels (Fukuda et al., 1988);

—An enhancement of vasopressin effects in the kidney (Jeffries et al., 1988).

Hypokalemia

Incidence

Although some patients have been recognized as persistently normokalemic (Conn et al., 1965; Bravo et al., 1983), the majority are hypokalemic. In the MRC series, hypokalemia occurred in all 62 patients with a proved adenoma and was persistent in 53; among the 17 with hyperplasia, plasma potassium was persistently normal in only 3 patients (Ferriss et al., 1983b). On the other hand, some patients with an adenoma are normokalemic on presentation: 5 of 40 (12%) in a series from Indiana (Weinberger et al., 1979), and 17 of 70 (24%) in a series from Cleveland Clinic (Bravo et al., 1983). Of 48 patients in a referred population who were diagnosed as having primary aldosteronism by the sensitive plasma aldosterone/renin ratio, 34 (71%) were normokalemic on presentation (Gordon et al., 1992).

Significance

Although persistent hypokalemia may be less common in patients diagnosed early in the course of the disease, the argument can be made that the search for primary aldosteronism need only be undertaken in those with hypokalemia. The few who might initially be missed because of a normal potassium level will almost certainly show up subsequently with diuretic-induced or spontaneous hypokalemia. In the interim, a few patients may have had a delay in their diagnosis, but many more will be saved the expense and discomfort of unnecessary work-ups. In hypertensives with *unprovoked* hypokalemia, perhaps half will turn out to have primary aldosteronism; thus, they must have a complete evaluation.

Mechanism

Considering the effects of persistent aldosterone excess, hypokalemia is certainly to be expected. Whereas with continued exposure to excessive mineralocorticoids the renal retention of sodium ''escapes,'' the renal wastage of potassium is unrelenting (Young and Guyton, 1977). The aldosterone-driven increase in potassium secretion also involves an exchange of hydrogen for sodium so that metabolic alkalosis is generated; increased proximal and distal reabsorption of bicarbonate maintains the alkalosis, the severity of which is related to the degree of hypokalemia.

Clinical Features

The effects of hypokalemia include muscle weakness and easy fatigability, polyuria from a loss of renal concentrating ability, a high incidence of renal cysts (Torres et al., 1990), increased ventricular ectopy, blunting of circulatory reflexes with postural falls in pressure without compensatory tachycardia, impaired insulin secretion with decreased carbohydrate tolerance (Ferrannini et al., 1992), and suppression of aldosterone synthesis, even from presumably autonomous adenomas.

Suppression of Renin Release

As a consequence of the initial expansion of vascular volume and the elevated blood pressure (BP), the baroreceptor mechanism in the walls of the renal afferent arterioles suppresses the secretion of renin (Conn et al., 1964) to the point that renin mRNA may be undetectable in the kidney (Shionoiri et al., 1992). Patients with primary aldosteronism usually have low levels of PRA that respond poorly to upright posture and diuretics, two maneuvers that usually raise PRA.

Other Effects

Hypernatremia is usual, unlike most forms of edematous secondary aldosteronism wherein the sodium concentration is low.

Hypomagnesemia from excessive renal excretion of magnesium may produce tetany.

Sodium retention and *potassium wastage* may be demonstrable wherever such exchange is affected by aldosterone: sweat, saliva, and stool.

Atrial natriuretic factor (ANF) levels are appropriately elevated for a state of volume expansion (Opocher et al., 1992).

DIAGNOSIS

The diagnosis of primary aldosteronism should be easy to make in patients with unprovoked hypokalemia and other manifestations of the fully expressed syndrome. It can be much more difficult in patients with minimal findings. The decision to perform a diagnostic work-up is based on the attitude that the less wrong with the patient, the lesser the need for a prolonged and expensive evaluation.

As noted earlier, unprovoked hypokalemia must be thoroughly evaluated, following the scheme shown in Figure 13.4. However, patients with persistent normokalemia rarely need be evaluated for the very unlikely presence of primary aldosteronism. No instances of primary aldosteronism were found among 400 patients with uncomplicated hypertension carefully evaluated in three centers (Kaplan, 1967; Ledingham et al., 1967; Beevers et al., 1974). In the Syracuse series of 1028 patients referred for study, only eight cases of adenomatous hyperaldosteronism were found (Streeten et al., 1979). With plasma renin/aldosterone ratios, more normokalemic patients may be recognized (Gordon et al., 1992), but the cost-effectiveness of such testing remains to be shown.

Screening Tests

Plasma Potassium

Caution should be used to ensure that hypokalemia is not inadvertently missed:

—A very low sodium diet will stop renal potassium wastage, and blood potassium levels will rise;

—If obtaining the blood is difficult, requiring the patient to close and open the fist repeatedly, potassium may enter the blood from the exercised muscles;

—Even the slightest degree of hemolysis will raise the plasma level;

—Blood potassium levels increase on changing from the supine to the upright position (Sonkodi et al., 1981);

—The lower level of normal for plasma, which is usually used for automated chemistry anal-

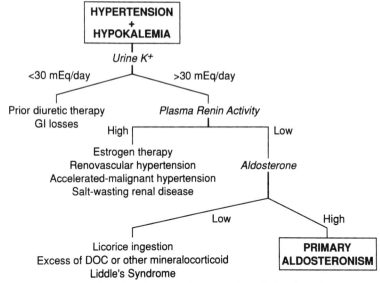

Figure 13.4. Flow diagram for the differential diagnosis of hypertension with hypokalemia.

yses, is 3.2 mmol/L, as compared to 3.4 mmol/L in serum (Hyman and Kaplan, 1985)

Urine Potassium

If hypokalemia is present, a 24-hour urine sample should be collected for sodium and potassium levels before starting potassium replacement therapy but 3 to 4 days after diuretics have been stopped. If the urine sodium is above 100 mmol/24 hours (to ensure that enough sodium is present to allow potassium wastage to express itself), the presence of a potassium level above 30 mmol indicates a driven wastage of potassium through the kidneys. In addition to the action of excess mineralocorticoid in the syndromes of primary aldosteronism, a number of other conditions may require consideration, conditions in which hypokalemia is coupled with renal potassium wastage (Table 13.2). If the urine potassium is less than 30 mmol/24 hours, mineralocorticoid excess is much less likely, and other causes of hypokalemia may be responsible (Table 13.3).

In the presence of hypokalemia with urinary potassium wastage, it may be preferable to correct the hypokalemia with potassium supplements, 40 to 80 mmol/day, after discontinuation of diuretics before performing additional workup. To restore body potassium deficits after prolonged diuretic use, a minimum of 3 weeks is needed, and it may take months. After a suitable interval, the supplemental potassium should be stopped for at least 3 days and the plasma potassium level should be rechecked. If plasma potassium is normal, plasma renin and aldosterone levels should be measured.

In practice, a more rapid screening protocol may be used: once hypokalemia is recognized, proceed to the plasma aldosterone/renin ratio. If the ratio is definitely abnormal, despite the

Table 13.2. Causes of Renal Loss of Potassium

1. Ongoing diuretic therapy
2. Osmotic diuresis: glucose, nonreabsorbable anions
3. Drugs: barium, amphotericin, licorice
4. Primary renal disease
   a. Renal tubular disease
   b. Fanconi syndrome
   c. K^+-wasting renal disease
      1. With hypomagnesemia
      2. With Na^+ conservation
      3. Bartter's syndrome
5. Metabolic alkalosis
6. Hypercalcemia
7. Adrenocortical hormone excess
   a. Primary aldosteronism
   b. Exogenous glucocorticoid
   c. Endogenous cortisol: Cushing's syndrome, 11-beta-hydroxylase deficiency
   d. Excess DOC or other mineralocorticoid
   e. Secondary aldosteronism
      1. Accelerated hypertension
      2. Renovascular hypertension
      3. Renin-secreting tumor

Table 13.3. Causes of Hypokalemia without Urinary Potassium Wastage

A. Prior diuretic use
B. Cellular shifts
  1. Rapid tumor growth
  2. Alkalosis (e.g., hyperventilation)
  3. Hormones: insulin, beta agonists
  4. Periodic paralysis
C. Decreased intake: starvation
D. Increased nonrenal loss
  1. Gastrointestinal
    a. Vomiting and drainage
    b. Diarrhea and laxatives
  2. Skin
    a. Sweating
    b. Burns

aberrant and uncontrolled circumstances, the diagnosis of primary aldosteronism is strongly supported. However, hypokalemia will suppress aldosterone secretion, so the aldosterone/renin ratio may not be abnormal. As a reasonable compromise, the blood for renin and aldosterone could be drawn, the plasma separated and frozen, and the analyses done only if the 24-hour urine sample displays excessive potassium wastage. Regardless, if the aldosterone/renin ratio is not definitely abnormal in the presence of hypokalemia, it may need to be repeated after potassium replenishment.

Plasma Aldosterone/Renin ratio

Plasma aldosterone and PRA are measured in a peripheral venous blood sample preferably obtained while the patient is on no antihypertensive drugs but without prior manipulation of diet (Hiramatsu et al., 1981). The values are put into a ratio, dividing the plasma aldosterone (normal, 5 to 20 ng/dl) by the plasma renin activity (normal, 1 to 3 ng/ml/hour). The normal ratio would be around 10, whereas patients with primary aldosterone are usually well above 20 (Weinberger and Fineberg, 1993). If plasma aldosterone is measured in pmol/L, as in Figure 13.5, an abnormal ratio would be above 900.*

This simple procedure that requires one blood sample and no special conditions has proved to

be quite useful as a screening test (McKenna et al., 1991) and should be performed *before any therapy is given* to any patient suspected of having primary aldosteronism (Fig. 13.5). The only patients with a high ratio who did not have primary aldosteronism were 5 of 17 patients with chronic renal failure, in whom PRA was suppressed by loss of juxta-glomerular (J-G) cells and hypervolemia and plasma aldosterone were elevated by hyperkalemia. Since plasma aldosterone levels in patients with aldosterone-producing adenomas usually fall during the day in concert with adrenocorticotropic hormone (ACTH) and cortisol, the blood sample should be obtained early in the morning, if possible.

Definitive Tests

If the plasma aldosterone/renin ratio is abnormal, many would proceed to computed tomography (CT) or magnetic resonance imaging (MRI) of the adrenal glands. However, more definitive proof of the presence of primary aldosteronism may be justified before proceeding to the more expensive scans, particularly since they may be either falsely negative, missing perhaps 10% of adrenal abnormalities, or falsely positive, finding incidental adrenal masses, as described at the beginning of Chapter 12. Nonetheless, if the scan shows a definite lesion in the presence of unprovoked hypokalemia and a high plasma aldosterone/renin ratio, the rest of the definitive tests may be superfluous.

Suppressed PRA

Suppressed PRA is confirmed most simply by obtaining a blood sample after 2 hours of upright posture immediately before beginning the saline suppression test of plasma aldosterone. A low-sodium diet or a diuretic may be used to demonstrate renin suppression (Fig. 13.6), but the extra trouble hardly seems necessary.

Elevated and Nonsuppressible Aldosterone

The easiest way to document that aldosterone levels are elevated and do not suppress normally is by the saline suppression test of plasma aldosterone (Kem et al., 1971). Plasma aldosterone is measured before and after the infusion of 2 L of normal saline over 4 hours. Patients with primary aldosteronism have higher basal levels but, more importantly, fail to suppress these levels after saline to below 10 ng/dl (Fig. 13.6). Some patients with adrenal hyperplasia may suppress to a level between 5 and 10 ng/dl after saline, so that the normal level may need to

---

*Conversion of laboratory values from traditional units to SI units can be performed as follows: *Plasma aldosterone* from nanograms per deciliter to picomoles per liter: multiply by 27.7; *Urine aldosterone* from micrograms per day to nanomoles per day: multiply by 2.77; *Plasma renin activity* from nanograms per milligram per hour to nanograms per liter: multiply by 0.278.

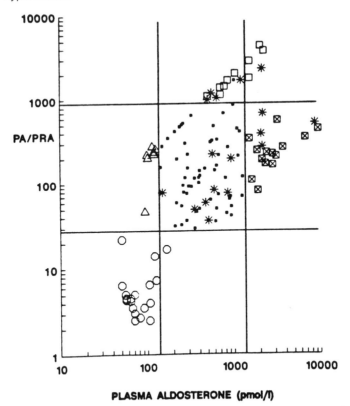

Figure 13.5. Distribution of patients with primary and secondary adrenal disorders and nonadrenal disorders according to the plasma aldosterone (PA):plasma renin activity (PRA) ratio plotted against the plasma aldosterone level. *Unfilled squares,* Primary hyperaldosteronism; *Squares with X,* secondary hyperaldosteronism; *Open circles,* primary aldosterone deficiency; *Triangles,* secondary aldosterone deficiency, *Asterisks,* renal failure; *Dots,* nonadrenal disorders. (From McKenna TJ, Sequeira SJ, Heffernan A, Chambers J, Cunningham S. Diagnosis under random conditions of all disorders of the renin-angiotensin-aldosterone axis, including primary hyperaldosteronism. *J Clin Endocrinol Metab* 1991;73:952–957.)

be set at 5 ng/dl when screening is done for hyperplasia (Holland et al., 1984).

Captopril Suppression. Whereas plasma aldosterone levels were markedly suppressed 3 hours after oral intake of 1 mg of captopril per kilogram of body weight in patients with essential hypertension or renovascular hypertension, they remained elevated in patients with primary hyperaldosteronism (Thibonnier et al., 1982). The response to captopril provides good sensitivity but lacks specificity (Hambling et al., 1992).

Other Tests. Less commonly used are suppression tests of urinary aldosterone. In the Cleveland series, a urine aldosterone level above 14 μg/24 hours after 3 days of salt loading provided the best separation between primary aldosteronism and essential hypertension (Bravo et al., 1983).

Response to Spironolactone

Spark and Melby (1968) showed that patients with primary aldosteronism had a fall of at least 20 mm Hg in their diastolic BP after 5 weeks of spironolactone, 100 mg 4 times a day for 5 weeks. The procedure is no longer needed as a diagnostic test, although Biglieri and Kater (1991) note that patients with autonomous forms of primary aldosteronism do not show an increase in steroid levels, whereas those with nonautonomous forms have a marked rise after spironolactone. The response to spironolactone may have prognostic value, since the response to spironolactone in patients with an adenoma closely resembled their subsequent response to surgery (Ferriss et al., 1978a).

Rule Out Glucocorticoid-Remediable Aldosteronism

As will be described in the next section, glucocorticoid-remediable aldosteronism (GRA) should be considered in the absence of an adenoma, particularly if other family members have aldosteronism.

A 10-day course of dexamethasone, 0.5 mg 4 times daily, will identify the rare patient with glucocorticoid-remediable aldosteronism, whose hypertension and hyperaldosteronism should be completely relieved (Fallo et al., 1987). However, as will be seen, now that the mechanism for GRA has been elucidated, the measurement of increased amounts of 18-hydroxylated cortisol derivatives in a 24-hour urine sample is far easier and more certain (Rich et al., 1992) and can be obtained in some steroid reference laboratories such as the Mayo Clinic.

Measure Other Steroids

The precursor of aldosterone, 18-hydroxycorticosterone (18-OHB), may be elevated even more than the aldosterone level (Biglieri and Schambelan, 1979). Serum levels are useful both in establishing the diagnosis and in separating the two major types of adrenal pathology, as will be discussed later in this chapter.

Excluding Other Diseases

Various causes of secondary aldosteronism are easily excluded by the presence of edema and high levels of peripheral blood PRA. In addition, there are a number of "pseudoaldosteronism" conditions that should be identified by history and by the presence of low levels of aldosterone. Two rare syndromes have hypokalemia and marked hyperaldosteronism but normal BP: Bartter's syndrome (Bartter et al., 1962), caused by a defect in the renal transport of chloride (Kurtzman and Gutierrez, 1975), and Gitelman's syndrome (Gitelman et al., 1966), a familiar disorder with renal wastage of potassium and magnesium.

Conditions with Low PRA

Unlike conditions with high PRA, others more closely simulate primary aldosteronism because PRA is low, either because of abnormal renal sodium retention or because another mineralo-

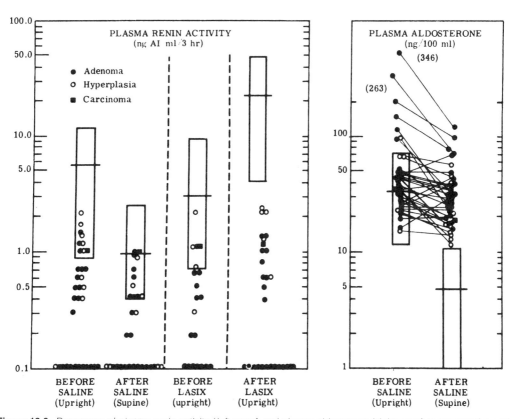

Figure 13.6. Responses of plasma renin activity (*left panel*) and plasma aldosterone (*right panel*) to suppressive and stimulating maneuvers. Scales are logarithmic to accommodate the range of values. Normal values (114 subjects) are represented as mean (*bars*) ±95% confidence limits (*boxes*). Values for patients with primary aldosteronism are indicated by symbols (see *key*); connecting lines for plasma aldosterone represent values of a given patient. AI, angiotensin I. (From Weinberger MH, Grim CE, Hollifield JW, Kem DC, Ganguly A, Kramer NJ, Yune HY, Wellman H, Donohue JP. Primary aldosteronism. Diagnosis, localization, and treatment. *Ann Intern Med* 1979;90:386–395.)

corticoid is present, including deoxycorticosterone (Irony et al., 1987) and cortisol (see Chapter 14). In all of these, aldosterone levels should also be low, whereas they are high in primary aldosteronism.

Iatrogenic Mineralocorticoid Excess. As with Cushing's syndrome induced by exogenous glucocorticoids, aldosteronism may be induced by exogenous mineralocorticoids, even when absorbed through the skin in an ointment for the treatment of dermatitis (Lauzurica et al., 1988).

Excessive Renal Sodium Conservation. Liddle et al. (1963) described members of a family with hypertension, hypokalemic alkalosis, and negligible aldosterone secretion, apparently resulting from an unusual tendency of the kidneys to conserve sodium and excrete potassium even in the virtual absence of mineralocorticoids. Such patients appear to have a generalized defect in sodium transport (Gardner et al., 1971).

Another syndrome has been described with increased renal sodium and chloride retention that causes hypertension and suppression of the renin-aldosterone mechanism, but with *hyperkalemia* (Gordon, 1986). The syndrome is familial and may be associated with short stature and poor dentition.

This long listing of various diseases, most involving hypokalemia and many with hypertension, should not imply the need for a long and complicated work-up to diagnose primary aldosteronism. By following the flow diagram shown in Figure 13.4, one can usually make the correct diagnosis with relative ease.

ESTABLISHING THE TYPE OF ADRENAL PATHOLOGY

Once the diagnosis of primary aldosteronism is made, the type of adrenal pathology must be ascertained, since the choice of therapy is different: surgical for an adenoma, medical for hyperplasia.

Types of Adrenal Pathology

Aldosterone-Producing Adenomas (APAs)

Unilateral solitary benign adenomas (Fig. 13.7) are present in most patients with classic primary aldosteronism. The tumor is almost always unilateral and most are small, weighing less than 6 g and measuring less than 3 cm in diameter. Histologically, most adenomas are composed of lipid-laden cells arranged in small acini or cords, similar in appearance and arrangement to the normal zona fasciculata, the middle

zone of the adrenal cortex. Moreover, focal or diffuse hyperplasia as seen in Figure 13.7 is usually present in both the remainder of the adrenal with the adenoma and the contralateral gland (Lack et al., 1990).

Gordon et al. (1992) postulate that such histologic hyperplasia outside the adenoma "suggests a genetic abnormality not limited to the adenoma cells." These same investigators have also identified seven families, each with two members who had adenomas that were not suppressed by glucocorticoids (Stowasser et al., 1991). Thus, genetics may be involved in more of primary aldosteronism than now is appreciated. Nonetheless, most patients with an adenoma do not have a family history or features that indicate a genetic basis for their condition.

Bilateral Adrenal Hyperplasia (Idiopathic Hyperaldosteronism)

In the early 1970s, reports of hyperaldosteronism with no adenoma but rather with bilateral adrenal hyperplasia began to appear (George et al., 1970; Baer et al., 1970). This has been referred to as "idiopathic hyperaldosteronism," abbreviated as IHA. Overall, such cases represent about one-quarter of all cases of primary aldosteronism. These patients tend to have milder biochemical and hormonal abnormalities that are less obvious that those seen with adenomas. The wide availability of hormonal assays and even wider availability of adrenal imaging techniques have made it much easier to recognize hyperplasia. At the Mayo Clinic, hyperplasia was found in 30% of cases before 1978 but in 46% from 1978 to 1987 (Young et al., 1990).

However, the better detail provided by newer imaging procedures may lead to confusion: because the hyperplasia that often accompanies an adenoma can be recognized, bilateral hyperplasia may be mistakenly diagnosed; because nodularity is often seen with hyperplasia, an adenoma may be mistakenly diagnosed. Moreover, the clear separation between adenoma and hyperplasia may also be blurred by the recognition that, in response to suppression or stimulation tests, a solitary adenoma occasionally behaves like bilateral hyperplasia (Tunny et al., 1991), and bilateral hyperplasia occasionally mimics the responses of a solitary adenoma (Biglieri, 1991). Therefore, anatomic evidence must be correlated with functional data to ensure the correct diagnosis (Blevins and Wand, 1992).

The presence of bilateral hyperplasia suggests a secondary response to some stimulatory mech-

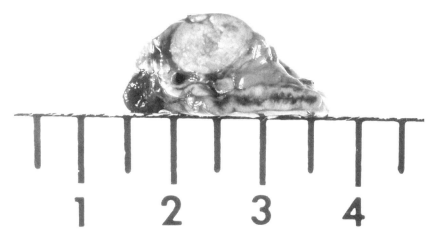

Figure 13.7. Solitary adrenal adenoma with diffuse hyperplasia removed from a patient with primary aldosteronism.

anism rather than a primary neoplastic growth. Although claims have been made for novel aldosterone-stimulating substances in patients with hyperplasia (Komiya et al., 1991), none has been identified.

Unilateral Hyperplasia. Even more difficult to explain than the presence of bilateral hyperplasia are the few cases of hyperaldosteronism that apparently are caused by hyperplasia of only one adrenal gland (Irony et al., 1990).

Glucocorticoid-Remediable Aldosteronism (GRA)

Early Observations. In 1966, Sutherland et al. described a father and son with classic features of primary aldosteronism whose entire syndrome was completely relieved by dexamethasone, 0.5 mg 4 times a day (i.e., "glucocorticoid remediable"). Subsequently, the syndrome was shown to follow an autosomal dominant mode of inheritance. In the early 1980s, Ulick et al. (1983) and Gomez-Sanchez et al. (1984) found increased levels of 18-hydroxylated cortisol in such patients. The presence of high levels of 18-hydroxylated steroids (normally secreted only from the outer zona glomerulosa because it alone normally possesses the aldosterone synthase enzyme needed for C-18 oxygenation) in association with the suppression of the features by exogenous glucocorticoid (normally characterizing the control of the middle zona fasciculata by ACTH) led Ulick et al. (1990a) to postulate that the syndrome was due to the acquisition of aldosterone synthase enzymatic activity by cells of the zona fasciculata.

Genetic Confirmation. The correctness of Ulick et al.'s postulate was proven in a striking manner by Lifton et al. (1992). Using restriction fragment length polymorphism analysis of cells from eight affected members of a large kindred, these investigators found "complete linkage of glucocorticoid-remediable aldosteronism to a gene duplication arising from unequal crossing over, fusing the 5' regulatory region of 11-beta-hydroxylase to the 3' coding sequences of aldosterone synthase" (Lifton et al., 1992).

This chimeric 11-beta-hydroxylase/aldosterone synthase gene produces an enzyme that catalyzes the formation of 18-hydroxylated steroids beyond the zona glomerulosa with excessive secretion of aldosterone and, even more so, of hormones such as 18-hydroxycortisol. The enzyme is very sensitive to ACTH; thus, normal levels of ACTH lead to excessive production of 18-hydroxylated steroids, while at the same time the syndrome is completely remediable by glucocorticoid suppression of ACTH.

Clinical and Laboratory Features. Additional clinical studies were done on 11 of 18 at-risk patients in this kindred who displayed the phenotype (Rich et al., 1992). All with GRA were hypertensive before age 21 and had low PRA levels, but they were all normokalemic unless given thiazide diuretic therapy, which induced severe hypokalemia. As a measure of the increased secretion of 18-hydroxylated cortisol from the zona fasciculata, their 24-hour urinary tetrahydro-18-oxocortisol (TH-18-oxoF) levels were markedly elevated as were the TH-18-oxoF/TH-Aldo ratios. The authors suggest that measurement of these steroids in a 24-hour urine sample should replace the dexamethasone suppression of mineralocorticoid effects, the traditional diagnostic procedure. Obviously, hypertensive children are the prime suspects, particularly if other family members had developed hypertension at an early age.

Significance. Elucidation of this mutation represents the first description of a genetic basis of a form of hypertension in otherwise phenotypically normal humans (or animals). Lifton et al. (1992) predict that other mutations may be involved in mendelian forms of human hypertension. Though few such forms of hypertension are known, excessive amounts of 18-hydroxylated steroids have been reported in 30 of 436 Japanese patients (Komiya et al., 1991) and in a group of young normotensive adults whose personal and parental BPs were the highest within a large population (Watt et al., 1992).

Spectrum of Adenomas and Hyperplasias

Gordon et al. (1992) and Biglieri (1991) have stressed the variable features of both adenomas and hyperplasias, as will be described later in this chapter. Gordon et al. have gone so far as to hypothesize that all of these features are induced by genetic mutations, calling particular attention to the similarities between most adenomas and autosomal dominant GRA. These variants are certainly of interest academically. Their clinical importance is less certain, since the documentation of aldosterone excess and visualization of the adrenal glands remain the keys to diagnosis. However, as will be noted, knowledge of the functional characteristics of the lesion is needed to ensure that therapy is appropriate (surgery for adenomas and medical therapy for hyperplasias).

Carcinoma

Aldosterone-producing carcinomas are rare. Most are associated with concomitant hypersecretion of other adrenal hormones, but a few may hypersecrete only aldosterone (Luton et al., 1990).

Other Pathologies

Associated Conditions. Patients have been reported with primary aldosteronism caused by an adrenal adenoma in association with acromegaly (Dluhy and Williams, 1969), primary hyperparathyroidism (Ferriss et al., 1983a) and the multiple endocrine neoplasia I syndrome (Beckers et al., 1992). An aldosterone-producing adenoma may coexist with a nonfunctioning contralateral adrenal tumor (Hollak et al., 1991).

Extra-Adrenal Tumors. Single ectopic aldosterone-producing tumors have been found in the lower pole of the right kidney (Flanagan and McDonald, 1967) and in an ovary (Jackson et al., 1986).

Diagnosing the Type of Adrenal Pathology

Various procedures are available for diagnosing the type of adrenal pathology (Table 13.4). The percentages given for six of the procedures are taken from Young et al.'s (1990) review of 47 published reports. The figure for dexamethasone scintigraphy is taken from Gross and Shapiro's (1989) review of 317 scans in 13 reports. The large number of techniques recommended gives witness to the problems in making the differentiation in the past. Fortunately, the resolution offered by CT and MRI has made these noninvasive techniques the first and best way to diagnose the type of adrenal pathology. Current CT and MRI technology usually permits visualization of even small adenomas and bilateral hyperplasia. However, variants such as nodular hyperplasia and bilateral adenomas may be noted by adrenal imaging, which make it mandatory to correlate the imaging findings with hormonal studies (Blevins and Wand, 1992).

In general, autonomous lesions that are cured by surgery (adenomas and the very rare primary adrenal hyperplasia) display their autonomy from the normal control by the renin-angiotensin mechanism by having (*a*) very high levels of aldosterone and its precursor 18-OH-corticosterone along with more severe clinical features of aldosteronism, (*b*) little or no response to stimulation of renin-angiotensin such as during an upright posture test, and (*c*) the production of hybrid steroids such as 18-OH-cortisol (Blumenfeld, 1993).

Aldosterone and Renin Levels

Although adenomas tend to be associated with higher BP and aldosterone levels but lower PRA and potassium levels than hyperplasia, these alone cannot make the differentiation.

Other Steroids

Most adenomas, but not hyperplastic glands, secrete excess amounts of both normal precursors (e.g., 18-OH-corticosterone [B]), and hybrid steroids (e.g., 18-oxo-cortisol [F]) (Ulick et al., 1993). In this series, 18-oxo-F levels were above 16 μg/day in 19 of 21 patients with an adenoma and below 16 μg/day in all 20 patients

Table 13.4. Techniques to Differentiate Adrenal Adenoma (APA) from Bilateral Hyperplasia (IHA) in Patients with Primary Aldosteronism

Technique	Adenoma	Hyperplasia	Discriminatory Value
Basal aldosterone levels	High	Less high	Poor
Basal renin levels	Low	Less low	Poor
Basal plasma 18-OH-B	>65 ng/dl	<65 ng/dl	Excellent (82%)[a]
Basal 18-oxo-F, 18-OH-F	Increased	Normal	Excellent
Upright posture (rise in PA)	<30%	>30%	Excellent (85%)
Suppression test (Change in PA)			
DOC administration	None	Fall	Poor
Florinef administration	None	Fall	Poor
Response to spironolactone	None	Rise	Good
Stimulation tests (change in PA)			
ACTH	Rise	Less rise	Poor
Saralasin	No change	Increase	Good (only one report)
Adrenal venography	Tumor	Bilateral enlargement	Good (66%)
Adrenal venous aldosterone	Increased on side of adenoma	Equal	Excellent (95%)
Adrenal scintiscan with			
[131I]cholesterol	Unilateral update	Bilateral update	Good (72%)
Plus dexamethasone	Persistent	Suppressed	Excellent (90%)
Adrenal computed tomography and MRI	Unilateral mass	Bilaterally enlarged	Good (73%) (>90% in 1993)

PA, plasma aldosterone; *18-OH-B,* 18-hydroxycorticosterone; *18-oxo-F,* 18-oxycortisol; *18-OH-F,* 18-hydroxy-cortisol.
[a]Values in parentheses are from multiple references as reported by Young et al. (1990).

with bilateral hyperplasia. The level of 18-OH-B that provides the best separation appears to be 65 ng/dl, somewhat lower than the originally recommended 100 ng/dl (Kater et al., 1989).

Suppression and Stimulation Tests

Upright Posture.   This test depends on changes in plasma aldosterone in response to variations in endogenous stimuli during 2 to 4 hours of upright posture (Ganguly et al., 1973). The premise is that adenomas are not responsive to postural increases in angiotensin (which stay suppressed anyway) but are exquisitely sensitive to the diurnal fall in plasma ACTH, whereas hyperplasia is very responsive to even small postural changes in angiotensin. Thus, patients with hyperplasia should have an even greater than normal *rise* in plasma aldosterone after 4 hours of standing, whereas patients with an adenoma show an anomalous *fall* in plasma aldosterone, in parallel with the falling plasma ACTH levels during the early morning hours.

The major advocates of this procedure, Biglieri and coworkers, have found the discriminatory power of the 2-hour posture test to be improved by subtracting the percentage of cortisol change from the percentage of aldosterone change (Fontes et al., 1991). This is appropriate: if, for whatever reason, ACTH levels rise during the test rather than fall as expected, aldosterone levels will rise even from an adenoma. A corrected aldosterone increase of less than 30% identified 76 of 89 adenomas but was present in 11 of 57 hyperplasias (Fig. 13.8). These investigators define the relatively few adenomas that respond to posture as "renin responsive" (Irony et al., 1990); such adenomas do not overproduce hybrid steroids and contain fewer zona fasciculata–type cells (Tunny et al., 1991).

In addition, Irony et al. (1990) define hyperplasias that behave like adenomas as "primary adrenal hyperplasia" and report that relief of the aldosteronism may follow removal of one hyperplastic gland. Despite these findings, the prudent approach remains to remove adenomas (renin-responsive or not) and to medically treat hyperplasias. Moreover, there are reports that the discrimination of the postural test is not good (Nomura et al., 1992).

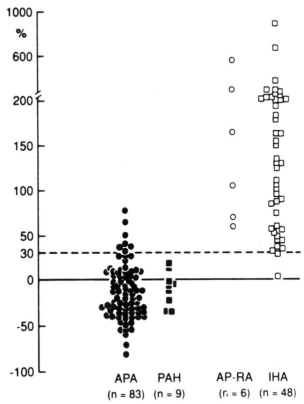

Figure 13.8. Individual plasma aldosterone responses to postural stimulation (as percentage of change from baseline lying values) in patients with primary aldosteronism. *APA*, aldosterone-producing adenoma; *PAH*, primary adrenal hyperplasia; *AP-RA*, aldosterone-producing renin-responsive adenoma; *IHA*, idiopathic hyperaldosteronism). The *dashed line* is the cutoff point (30%) used to define responses. (From Fontes RG, Kater CE, Biglieri EG, Irony I. Reassessment of the predictive value of the postural stimulation test in primary aldosteronism. *Am J Hypertens* 1991;4:786–791.)

Other Procedures.   Other tests utilize ACTH or various mineralocorticoids to suppress or stimulate the adrenal (Table 13.4). These have not worked well since some adenomas remain responsive to angiotensin II, and hyperplasias are responsive to ACTH.

Localizing Techniques

The accuracy provided by CT, MRI, and scintigraphy relegate the other procedures to infrequent use in the few cases not so identified by the imaging procedures.

Adrenal CT or MRI.   Most aldosterone-producing adenomas are identified, at least those down to 1.0 cm in diameter (Gross and Shapiro, 1989) (Fig. 13.9). However, since some aldosterone-producing adenomas are smaller, some as small as 3 mm, the CT and MRI scans may miss them. MRI may provide greater specificity, and continued improved technology may make it superior to CT scans (Edelmann and Warach, 1993).

Bilateral nodularity may suggest bilateral hyperplasia when a unilateral adenoma is the cause (Doppman et al., 1992). Similarly, what appears to be a solitary nodule may be the only visible feature of diffuse hyperplasia (Radin et al., 1992). Therefore, equivocal or minimal abnormalities by CT/MRI should be correlated with hormonal studies, as noted below.

Adrenal Scintigraphy.   If the CT or MRI scan is not revealing, adrenal scintiscans with the isotope, 6-beta-[^{131}I]-iodomethyl-19-norcholesterol (NP-59), offer discrimination as good as found by adrenal vein catheterization, with less discomfort. Even better results have been achieved with suppression scintiscans using 0.5 or 1 mg of dexamethasone every 6 hours to discriminate between adenomas, which remain visible, and bilateral hyperplasia, which fades after a few days of dexamethasone (Hattner, 1993).

Although small adenomas with relatively low uptake of the tracer may give false-negative results (Nomura et al., 1990), the published experiences with adrenal scintiscans have shown discrimination between adenoma and hyperplasia in 90% of cases (Gross and Shapiro, 1989).

Adrenal Venography. This procedure identifies most adenomas. However, the smaller size and variation in the position of the right adrenal vein, which usually empties directly into the vena cava, may preclude its catheterization. Moreover, intraadrenal hemorrhage occurs in 10% or more of patients despite careful injection of dye (Miller, 1993).

Adrenal Venous Plasma Aldosterone Assays. In most series, patients with adenomas not only have a high aldosterone/cortisol ratio from the affected gland but also a lower ratio from the nonaffected gland than in the lower caval blood, which indicates contralateral suppression of aldosterone secretion. In cases with hyperplasia, the ratio from both adrenals is higher than that found in the lower caval blood (Takasaki et al., 1987; Miller, 1993).

Overall Plan

Once the presence of aldosterone excess has been established, the algorithm shown in Figure 13.10 should determine the type of pathology. The algorithm starts with a CT or MRI scan of the adrenals. Even if a unilateral mass or two symmetrically enlarged glands are clearly seen, a posture study, measurements of serum 18-OH-B and, if available, a urine 18-oxo-F assay should be performed. If they do not correlate with the CT/MRI findings, adrenal venous sampling or adrenal scintigraphy should be obtained, preferably in a center with considerable experience with these procedures. If the CT or MRI scan is normal, the patient should be treated medically and the scan repeated in 6 to 12 months. Fortunately, most adenomas and hyperplasia will be correctly identified by the CT or MRI scan.

Remember that patients found to have neither an adenoma nor hyperplasia should have a measurement of urinary 18-oxo-cortisol, looking for

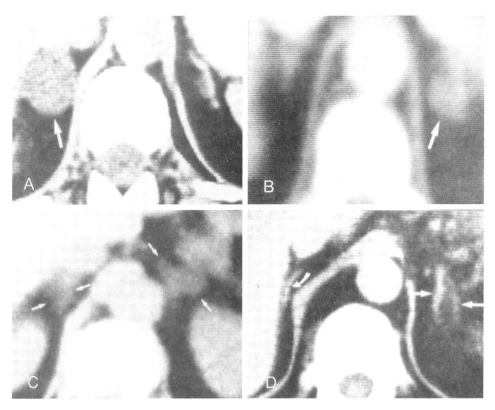

Figure 13.9. Computed tomograms showing the typical appearance of a unilateral adrenal adenoma (*A* and *B*), of bilateral adrenal hyperplasia (*C*), and of normal adrenal glands (*D*). (From White EA, Schambelan M, Rost CR, Biglieri EG, Moss AA, Korobkin M. Use of computed tomography in diagnosing the cause of primary aldosteronism. *N Engl J Med* 1980;303:1503–1507.)

the rare glucocorticoid-remediable syndrome, wherein much higher levels are found than in patients with an adenoma (Blumenfeld, 1993). The problem of excluding adrenal hyperfunction in adrenal glands found incidentally to have a mass or to be enlarged by abdominal CT done for other reasons is addressed in the first portion of Chapter 12.

THERAPY

The CT or MRI scan coupled with the appropriate hormonal studies (Fig. 13.10) should establish the type of adrenal pathology with virtual certainty. If the diagnosis is *adenoma*, surgery should be done; if it is *bilateral hyperplasia*, medical therapy is indicated. Although there are reports of relief of aldosteronism by removal of a unilaterally hyperplastic gland or one of two hyperplastic glands (Irony et al., 1990), surgery should rarely be performed if an adrenal adenoma is not visualized by scan or scintigraphy.

Surgical Treatment

Preoperative Management

Once the diagnosis is made, a 3- to 5-week course of spironolactone therapy may be given, both as an additional diagnostic study and as a guide to the probable response of the hypertension to removal of an adenoma if that is the lesion, or to chronic medical therapy if hyperplasia is the lesion (Ferriss et al., 1978a). For patients with an adenoma, the various disturbances of electrolyte composition and fluid volume should also be normalized, easing anesthetic, surgical, and postoperative management (Morimoto et al., 1970).

Surgical Technique

With improved preoperative diagnosis of an adenoma, a unilateral extraperitoneal approach seems preferable (Auda et al., 1980).

If bilateral hyperplasia is found at surgery despite the preoperative diagnosis of an adenoma, only a unilateral adrenalectomy should be done. In view of the poor overall results with bilateral adrenalectomy and its complications, one gland should be left intact.

Postoperative Complications

Hypoaldosteronism. The patient, even if given spironolactone preoperatively, may develop hypoaldosteronism with an inability to conserve sodium and excrete potassium. This may persist for some time after renin levels return to normal, analogous to the slowness of the return of cortisol production after prolonged ACTH suppression by exogenous glucocorticoids (Conn et al., 1964).

The aldosterone deficiency is usually not severe or prolonged and can be handled simply by providing adequate salt without the need for

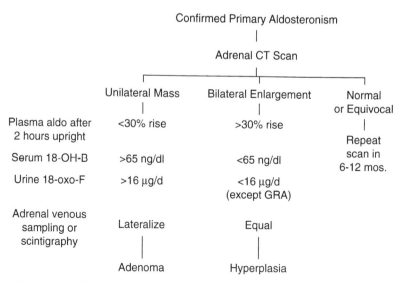

Figure 13.10. A flow diagram for the progressive work-up of confirmed primary aldosteronism, with additional steps for when initial studies are aberrant. Rare, angiotensin II–responsive adenomas may demonstrate features of hyperplasia but lateralize by venous sampling or scintigraphy. On the other hand, primary adrenal hyperplasia may demonstrate features of an adenoma except for equally high steroid levels by venous sampling. *18-OH-B*, 18-hydroxycorticosterone; *18-oxo-F*, 18-hydrocortisol; *GRA*, glucocorticoid-remediable aldosteronism.

exogenous glucocorticoid or mineralocorticoid therapy. However, 5 of 37 patients who underwent unilateral adrenalectomy for an adenoma were symptomatically hypotensive 1 year later, some with low plasma cortisol, others with low plasma aldosterone and adrenaline levels (Gordon et al., 1989).

Sustained Hypertension. The hypertension may persist for some time; a few patients require years for return of normal BP. In 13 series published since 1978, 64% of 466 patients were cured of hypertension, and 33% were improved (Shenker, 1989). Persistence of hypertension was seen more commonly in patients over age 50, in males, and in patients with multiple adenomas or macronodules (Obara et al., 1992).

If the BP fails to respond, hyperfunctioning adrenal tissue may have been left. More likely is the presence of coincidental primary hypertension, as would be expected in at least 20% of cases, or the occurrence of significant renal damage from the prolonged secondary hypertension (Danforth et al., 1977). Few patients with bilateral hyperplasia respond to unilateral (Groth et al., 1985) or even to bilateral adrenalectomy (Ferriss et al., 1978a).

Medical Treatment

Chronic medical therapy with spironolactone or, if that is not tolerated, amiloride with or without a thiazide diuretic (Griffing et al., 1982) is the treatment of choice for patients with hyperplasia, patients with an adenoma who are unable or unwilling to have surgery, patients who remain hypertensive after surgery, and patients with equivocal findings.

For patients with hyperplasia, spironolactone usually lowers the BP and keeps it down (Ferriss et al., 1978a). Doses of 100 to 200 mg a day may be needed initially, but a satisfactory

response may then be maintained with as little as 50 mg a day. The combination of spironolactone with a thiazide diuretic may provide even better control and allow for smaller doses of spironolactone. With these lower doses, the various side effects are generally minor, and in only three of 95 cases were they severe enough to lead to withdrawal of the drug (Ferriss et al., 1978a). Aspirin should be avoided since it will antagonize the effects of spironolactone (Tweeddale and Ogilvie, 1973). If additional antihypertensive therapy is needed, calcium blockers or angiotensin-converting enzyme (ACE) inhibitors may be used (Young, 1993).

For patients with an adenoma who are not candidates for surgery, long-term control can be provided with spironolactone (Takeda et al., 1992). In the future, even more potent mineralocorticoid inhibitors with fewer antiandrogenic side effects may be available (Opoku et al., 1991).

Adrenal Cancer

Various inhibitors of steroidogenesis may be useful in patients with adrenal cancer. The only proven effective agent is o,p'-DDD (mitotane) (Luton et al., 1990). Others that may be useful include *trilostane*, a competitive inhibitor of adrenal 3-beta-hydroxysteroid dehydrogenase (Nomura et al., 1986), and *ketoconazole*, an inhibitor of the P-450–dependent enzymes 11-beta- and 18-hydroxylase (Leal-Cerro et al., 1988).

CONCLUSIONS

Primary aldosteronism remains a fascinating disease that has probably generated a number of publications equal to the number of patients in whom it is the cause of hypertension. We turn from it to other adrenal causes of hypertension, some induced by other mineralocorticoids.

References

Andersen GS, Toftdahl DB, Lund JO, Strandgaard S, Nielsen PE. The incidence rate of phaeochromocytoma and Conn's syndrome in Denmark, 1977–1981. *J Hum Hypertens* 1988;2:187–189.

Arriza JL, Weinberger C, Cerelli G, Glaser TM, Handelin BL, Housman DE, Evans RM. Cloning of human mineralocorticoid receptor complementary DNA: structural and functional kinship with the glucocorticoid receptor. *Science* 1987;237:268–275.

Auda SP, Brennan MF, Gill JR Jr. Evolution of the surgical management of primary aldosteronism. *Ann Surg* 1980;191:1–7.

Baer L, Sommers SC, Krakoff KR, Newton MA, Laragh JH. Pseudo-primary aldosteronism. An entity distinct from true primary aldosteronism. *Circ Res* 1970; 26–27(Suppl 1):203–220.

Bartter FC, Pronove P, Gill JR Jr, MacCardle RC. Hyperplasia of the juxtaglomerular complex with hyperaldosteronism and hypokalemic alkalosis. *Am J Med* 1962;33:811–828.

Baxter RH, Wang I. Malignant hypertension in a patient with Conn's syndrome. *Scott Med J* 1974;19:161–163.

Beckers A, Abs R, Willems PJ, van der Auwera B, Kovacs K, Reznik M, Stevenaert A. Aldosterone-secreting adrenal adenoma as part of multiple endocrine neoplasia type 1 (MEN1): loss of heterozygosity for polymorphic chromosome 11 deoxyribonucleic acid markers, including the MEN1 locus. *J Clin Endocrinol Metab* 1992;75:564–570.

Beevers DG, Brown JJ, Ferriss JB, Fraser R, Lever AF, Robertson JIS, Tree M. Renal abnormalities and vascular complications in primary hyperaldosteronism. Evidence on tertiary hyperaldosteronism. *Q J Med* 1976;45:401–410.

Beevers DG, Nelson CS, Padfield PL, Barlow DH, Duncan S, Greaves DA, Hawthorne VM, Morton JJ, Young GAR, Young J. The prevalence of hypertension in an unselected population, and the frequency of abnormalities of potassium, angiotensin II and aldosterone in hypertensive subjects. *Acta Clin Belg* 1974;29:276–280.

Biglieri EG. Spectrum of mineralocorticoid hypertension. *Hypertension* 1991; 17:251–261.

Biglieri EG, Kater CE. Steroid characteristics of mineralocorticoid adrenocortical hypertension. *Clin Chem* 1991;37:1843–1848.

Biglieri EG, Schambelan M. The significance of elevated levels of plasma 18-hydroxycorticosterone in patients with primary aldosteronism. *J Clin Endocrinol Metab* 1979;49:87–91.

Blevins LS Jr, Wand GS. Primary aldosteronism: an endocrine perspective. *Radiology* 1992;184:599–600.

Blumenfeld JD. Hypertension and adrenal disorders. *Curr Opin Nephrol Hypertens* 1993;2:274–282.

Bravo EL, Fouad-Tarazi FM, Tarazi RC, Pohl M, Gifford RW, Vidt DG. Clinical implications of primary aldosteronism with resistant hypertension. *Hypertension* 1988;11(Suppl 1):207–211.

Bravo EL, Tarazi RC, Dustan HP, Fouad FM, Textor SC, Gifford RW, Vidt DG. The changing clinical spectrum of primary aldosteronism. *Am J Med* 1983;74: 641–651.

Brilla CG, Weber KT. Reactive and reparative myocardial fibrosis in arterial hypertension in the rat. *Cardiovasc Res* 1992;26:671–677.

Conn JW. Part I. Painting background. Part II. Primary aldosteronism, a new clinical syndrome. *J Lab Clin Med* 1955;43:3–17.

Conn JW, Cohen E, Rovner DR. Suppression of plasma renin activity in primary aldosteronism. Distinguishing primary from secondary aldosteronism in hypertensive disease. *JAMA* 1964;190:213–225.

Conn JW, Cohen ED, Rovner DR, Nesbit RM. Normokalemic primary aldosteronism. A detectable cause of curable "essential" hypertension. *JAMA* 1965;193: 200–206.

Danforth DW, Orlando MM, Bartter FC, Javadpour N. Renal changes in primary aldosteronism. *J Urol* 1977;117:140–144.

Dluhy RG, Williams GH. Primary aldosteronism in a hypertensive acromegalic patient. *J Clin Endocrinol* 1969;29: 1319–1324.

Doppman JL, Gill JR Jr, Miller DL, Chang R, Gupta R, Friedman TC, Choyke PK, Feuerstein IM, Dwyer AJ, Jicha DL, Walther MM, Norton JA, Linehan WM. Distinction between hyperaldosteronism due to bilateral hyperplasia and unilateral aldosteronoma: Reliability of CT. *Radiology* 1992;184:677–682.

Edelman RR, Warach S. Magnetic resonance imaging. *N Engl J Med* 1993;328: 785–791.

Fallo F, Sonino N, Boscaro M, Aramanini D, Mantero F, Dörr HG, Knorr D, Kuhnle U. Dexamethasone-suppressible hyperaldosteronism: Pathophysiology, clinical aspects, and new insights into the pathogenesis. *Klin Wochenschr* 1987;65:437–444.

Ferrannini E, Galvan AQ, Santoro D, Natali A. Potassium as a link between insulin and the renin-angiotensin-aldosterone system. *J Hypertens* 1992;10(Suppl 1):5–10.

Ferriss JB, Beevers DG, Boddy K, Brown JJ, Davies DL, Fraser R, Kremer D, Lever AF, Robertson JIS. The treatment of low-renin ("primary") hyperaldosteronism. *Am Heart J* 1978a;96:97–109.

Ferriss JB, Beevers DG, Brown JJ, Davies DL, Fraser R, Lever AF, Mason P, Neville AM, Robertson JIS. Clinical, biochemical and pathological features of low-renin ("primary") hyperaldosteronism. *Am Heart J* 1978b;95:375–388.

Ferriss JB, Brown JJ, Cumming AMM, Fraser R, Lever AF, Peacock M, Robertson JIS. Primary hyperparathyroidism associated with primary hyperaldosteronism. *Acta Endocrinol* 1983a;103:365–370.

Ferriss JB, Brown JJ, Fraser R, Lever AF, Robertson JIS. Primary aldosterone excess: Conn's syndrome and similar disorders. In: Robertson JIS, ed. *Handbook of Hypertension, vol. 2: Clinical Aspects of Secondary Hypertension*. New York: Elsevier, 1983b:132–161.

Flanagan MJ, McDonald JH. Heterotopic adrenocortical adenoma producing primary aldosteronism. *J Urol* 1967; 98:133–139.

Fontes RG, Kater CE, Biglieri EG, Irony I. Reassessment of the predictive value of the postural stimulation test in primary aldosteronism. *Am J Hypertens* 1991;4: 786–791.

Friedman SM, Tanaka M. Increased sodium permeability and transport as primary events in the hypertensive response to deoxycorticosterone acetate (DOCA) in the rat. *J Hypertens* 1987;5:341–345.

Fukuda K, Baba A, Kuchii M, Nakamura Y, Nishio I, Masuyama Y. Increased concentration of calcium channel and intracellular free calcium in the acute phase of deoxycorticosterone acetate salt hypertension. *J Hypertens* 1988;6(Suppl 4):261–263.

Ganguly A, Dowdy AJ, Luetscher JA, Melada GA. Anomalous postural response of plasma aldosterone concentration in patients with aldosterone-producing adrenal adenoma. *J Clin Endocrinol Metab* 1973;36:401–404.

Gardner JD, Lapey A, Simopoulos AP, Bravo EL. Abnormal membrane sodium transport in Liddle's syndrome. *J Clin Invest* 1971;50:2253–2258.

George JM, Wright L, Bell NH, Bartter FC. The syndrome of primary aldosteronism. *Am J Med* 1970;48:343–356.

Gifford RW Jr. Evaluation of the hypertensive patient with emphasis on detecting curable causes. *Milbank Mem Fund Q* 1969;47:170–186.

Gitelman HJ, Graham JB, Welt LG. A new familial disorder characterized by hypokalemia and hypomagnesemia. *Trans Assoc Am Phys* 1966;79:221–235.

Gomez-Sanchez CE, Montgomery M, Ganguly A, Holland OB, Gomez-Sanchez EP, Grim CE, Weinberger MH. Elevated urinary excretion of 18-oxocortisol in glucocorticoid-suppressible aldosteronism. *J Clin Endocrinol Metab* 1984;59: 1022–1024.

Gonzalez-Campoy JM, Romero JC, Knox FG. Escape from the sodium-retaining effects of mineralocorticoids: role of ANF and intrarenal hormone systems. *Kidney Int* 1989;35:767–777.

Gordon RD. Syndrome of hypertension and hyperkalemia with normal glomerular filtration rate. *Hypertension* 1986;8:93–102.

Gordon RD, Hawkins PG, Hamlet SM, Tunny TJ, Klemm SA, Bachmann AW, Finn WL. Reduced adrenal secretory mass after unilateral adrenalectomy for aldosterone-producing adenoma may explain unexpected incidence of hypotension. *J Hypertens* 1989;7(Suppl 6):210–211.

Gordon RD, Klemm SA, Tunny TJ, Stowasser M. Primary aldosteronism: hypertension with a genetic basis. *Lancet* 1992; 340:159–161.

Gordon RD, Tunny TJ. Aldosterone-producing-adenoma (A-P-A): effect of pregnancy. *Clin Exp Hypertens [A]* 1982;4: 1685–1693.

Griffing GT, Cole AG, Aurecchia SA, Sindler BH, Komanicky P, Melby JC. Amiloride in primary hyperaldosteronism. *Clin Pharmacol Ther* 1982;31:56–61.

Gross MD, Shapiro B. Scintigraphic studies in adrenal hypertension. *Semin Nucl Med* 1989;19:122–143.

Groth H, Vetter W, Stimpel M, Greminger P, Tenschert W, Klaiber E, Vetter H. Adrenalectomy in primary aldosteronism: a long-term follow-up study. *Cardiology* 1985;72(Suppl 1):107–116.

Hambling C, Jung RT, Gunn A, Browning MCK, Bartlett WA. Re-evaluation of the captopril test for the diagnosis of primary hyperaldosteronism. *Clin Endocrinol* 1992;36:499–503.

Hattner RS. Practical considerations in the scintigraphic evaluation of endocrine hypertension. *Radiol Clin North Am* 1993;31:1029–1038.

Hiramatsu K, Yamada T, Yukimura Y, Komiya I, Ichikawa K, Ishihara M, Nagata H, Izumiyama T. A screening test to identify aldosterone-producing adenoma by measuring plasma renin activity. Results in hypertensive patients. *Arch Intern Med* 1981;141:1589–1593.

Hollak CEM, Prummel MF, Tiel-Van Buul MMC. Bilateral adrenal tumours in primary aldosteronism: localization of a unilateral aldosteronoma by dexamethasone suppression scan. *J Intern Med* 1991; 229:545–548.

Holland OB, Brown H, Kuhnert L, Fairchild C, Risk M, Gomez-Sanchez CE. Further evaluation of saline infusion for the diagnosis of primary aldosteronism. *Hypertension* 1984;6:717‑723.

Horisberger J-D, Rossier BC. Aldosterone regulation of gene transcription leading to control of ion transport. *Hypertension* 1992;19:221–227.

Hyman D, Kaplan NM. The difference between serum and plasma potassium. *N Engl J Med* 1985;313:642.

Irony I, Biglieri EG, Perloff D, Rubinoff H. Pathophysiology of deoxycorticosterone-secreting adrenal tumors. *J Clin Endocrinol Metab* 1987;65:836–840.

Irony I, Kater CE, Biglieri EG, Shackleton CHL. Correctable subsets of primary aldosteronism. Primary adrenal hyperplasia and renin responsive adenoma. *Am J Hypertens* 1990;3:576–582.

Jackson B, Valentine R, Wagner G. Primary aldosteronism due to a malignant ovarian tumour. *Aust N Z J Med* 1986;16:69–71.

Jeffries WB, Wang Y, Pettinger WA. Enhanced vasopressin (V$_2$-receptor)-induced sodium retention in mineralocorticoid hypertension. *Am J Physiol* 1988;254:F739–F746.

Kageyama Y, Bravo EL. Hypertensive mechanisms associated with centrally administered aldosterone in dogs. *Hypertension* 1988;11:750–753.

Kaplan NM. Primary aldosteronism with malignant hypertension. *N Engl J Med* 1963;269:1282–1286.

Kaplan NM. Hypokalemia in the hypertensive patient. With observation on the incidence of primary aldosteronism. *Ann Intern Med* 1967;66:1079–1090.

Kaplan NM. Primary aldosteronism. In: Astwood EB, Cassidy CE, eds. *Clinical Endocrinology, vol. 2.* New York: Grune & Stratton, 1968:468–472.

Kater CE, Biglieri EG, Brust N, Chang B, Hirai J, Irony I. Stimulation and suppression of the mineralocorticoid hormones in normal subjects and adrenocortical disorders. *Endocrin Rev* 1989;10:149–164.

Kem DC, Weinberger MH, Mayes DM, Nugent CA. Saline suppression of plasma aldosterone in hypertension. *Arch Intern Med* 1971;128:380–386.

Komiya I, Yamada T, Aizawa T, Takasu N, Niwa A, Maruyama Y, Ogawa A. Inappropriate elevation of the aldosterone/plasma renin activity ratio in hypertensive patients with increases of 11-deoxycorticosterone and 18-hydroxy-11-deoxycorticosterone: A subtype of essential hypertension? *Cardiology* 1991;78:99–110.

Kurtzman NA, Gutierrez LF. The pathophysiology of Bartter syndrome. *JAMA* 1975;234:758–759.

Lack EE, Travis WD, Oertel JE. Adrenal cortical nodules, hyperplasia, and hyperfunction. In: Lack EE, ed. *Contemporary Issues in Surgical Pathology, vol 14: Pathology of the Adrenal Glands.* New York: Churchill Livingstone, 1990:75–113.

Lauzurica R, Bonal J, Bonet J, Romero R, Teixido J, Serra A, Caralps A. Rhabdomyolysis, oedema and arterial hypertension: different syndromes related to topical use of 9-alpha-fluoroprednisolone. *J Hum Hypertens* 1988;2:183–186.

Leal-Cerro A, Garcia-Luna P, Villar J, Sampalo A, Calero M, Zamora E, Astorga R. Ketoconazole as an inhibitor of steroid production [Letter]. *N Engl J Med* 1988;318:710–711.

Ledingham JGG, Bull MB, Laragh JH. The meaning of aldosteronism in hypertensive disease. *Circ Res* 1967;20–21(Suppl 2):177–186.

Liddle GW, Bledsoe T, Coppage WS Jr. A familial renal disorder simulating primary aldosteronism but with negligible aldosterone secretion. *Trans Assoc Am Phys* 1963;76:199–213.

Lifton RP, Dluhy RG, Powers M, Rich GM, Cook S, Ulick S, Lalouel J-M. A chimaeric 11β-hydroxylase/aldosterone synthase gene causes glucocorticoid-remediable aldosteronism and human hypertension. *Nature* 1992;355:262–265.

Litynski M. Nadcisnienie tetnicze wywolane guzami korowo-nad-nerczowymi. *Pol Tyg Lek* 1953;8:204–208.

Luton J-P, Cerdas S, Billaud L, Thomas G, Guilhaume B, Bertagna X, Laudat M-H, Louvel A, Chapuis Y, Blondeau P, Bonnin A, Bricaire H. Clinical features of adrenocortical carcinoma, prognostic factors, and the effects of mitotane therapy. *N Engl J Med* 1990;322:1195–1201.

Man in't Veld AJ, Wenting GJ, Schalekamp MADH. Distribution of extracellular fluid over the intra- and extravascular space in hypertensive patients. *J Cardiovasc Pharmacol* 1984;6:S143–S150.

Matsunaga M, Hara A, Song TS, Hashimoto M, Tamori S, Ogawa K, Morimoto K, Pak CH, Kawai C, Yoshida O. Asymptomatic normotensive primary aldosteronism. *Hypertension* 1983;5:240–243.

McKenna TJ, Sequeira SJ, Heffernan A, Chambers J, Cunningham S. Diagnosis under random conditions of all disorders of the renin-angiotensin-aldosterone axis, including primary hyperaldosteronism. *J Clin Endocrinol Metab* 1991;73:952–957.

Miller DL. Endocrine angiography and venous sampling. *Radiol Clin North Am* 1993;31:1051–1067.

Morimoto S, Takeda R, Murakami M. Does prolonged pretreatment with large doses of spironolactone hasten a recovery from juxtaglomerular-adrenal suppression in a primary aldosteronism? *J Clin Endocrinol Metab* 1970;31:659–664.

Nomura K, Demura H, Horiba N, Shizume K. Long-term treatment of idiopathic hyperaldosteronism using trilostane. *Acta Endocrinol (Copenh)* 1986;113:104–110.

Nomura K, Kusakabe K, Maki M, Ito Y, Aiba M, Demura H. Iodomethylnorcholesterol uptake in an aldosteronoma shown by dexamethasone-suppression scintigraphy: relationship to adenoma size and functional activity. *J Clin Endocrinol Metab* 1990;71:825–830.

Nomura K, Toraya S, Horiba N, Ujihara M, Aiba M, Demura H. Plasma aldosterone response to upright posture and angiotensin II infusion in aldosterone-producing adenoma. *J Clin Endocrinol Metab* 1992;75:323–327.

Obara T, Ito Y, Okamoto T, Kanaji Y, Yamashita T, Aiba M, Fujimoto Y. Risk factors associated with postoperative persistent hypertension in patients with primary aldosteronism. *Surgery* 1992;112:987–993.

Opocher G, Rocco S, Carpené G, Vettoretti A, Cimolato M, Mantero F. Usefulness of atrial natriuretic peptide assay in primary aldosteronism. *Am J Hypertens* 1992;5:811–816.

Opoku J, Kalimi M, Agarwal M, Qureshi D. Effect of a new mineralocorticoid antagonist mespirenone on aldosterone-induced hypertension. *Am J Physiol* 1991;260:E269–E271.

Pringle SD, Macfarlane PW, Isles CG, Cameron HL, Brown IA, Lorimer AR, Dunn FG. Regression of electrocardiographic left ventricular hypertrophy following treatment of primary hyperaldosteronism. *J Hum Hypertens* 1988;2:157–159.

Radin DR, Manoogian C, Nadler JL. Diagnosis of primary hyperaldosteronism: importance of correlating CT findings with endocrinologic studies. *Am J Radiol* 1992;158:553–557.

Rich GM, Ulick S, Cook S, Wang JZ, Lifton RP, Dluhy RG. Glucocorticoid-remediable aldosteronism in a large kindred: clinical spectrum and diagnosis using a characteristic biochemical phenotype. *Ann Intern Med* 1992;116:813–820.

Shenker Y. Medical treatment of low-renin aldosteronism. *Endocrin Metab Clin North Am* 1989;18:415–442.

Shionoiri H, Hirawa N, Ueda S-I, Himeno H, Gotoh E, Noguchi K, Fukamizu A, Seo MS, Murakami K. Renin gene expression in the adrenal and kidney of patients with primary aldosteronism. *J Clin Endocrinol Metab* 1992;74:103–107.

Sinclair AM, Isles CG, Brown I, Cameron H, Murray GD, Robertson JMK. Secondary hypertension in a blood pressure clinic. *Arch Intern Med* 1987;147:1289–1293.

Sonkodi S, Nicholls MG, Cumming AMM, Robertson JIS. Effects of change in body posture on plasma and serum electrolytes in normal subjects and in primary aldosteronism. *Clin Endocrinol* 1981;14:613–620.

Spark RF, Melby JC. Aldosteronism in hypertension. The spironolactone response test. *Ann Intern Med* 1968;69:685–691.

Stowasser M, Gordon RD, Tunny TJ, Klemm SA, Finn WL, Krek AL. Primary aldosteronism: implications of a new familial variety. *J Hypertens* 1991;9(Suppl 6):264–265.

Streeten DHP, Tomycz N, Anderson GH Jr. Reliability of screening methods for the diagnosis of primary aldosteronism. *Am J Med* 1979;67:403–413.

Sunman W, Rothwell M, Sever PS. Conn's syndrome can cause malignant hypertension. *J Hum Hypertens* 1992;6:75–76.

Sutherland DJA, Ruse JL, Laidlaw JC. Hypertension, increased aldosterone secretion and low plasma renin activity relieved by dexamethasone. *Can Med Assoc J* 1966;95:1109–1119.

Takasaki I, Shionoiri H, Yasuda G, Miyajima E, Umemura S, Gotoh E, Kaneko Y. Preoperative lateralisation of aldosteronomas by aldosterone/cortisol ratios in adrenal venous plasma. *J Hum Hypertens* 1987;1:95–99.

Takeda R, Yamazaki T, Ito Y, Koshida H, Morise T, Miyamori I, Hashimoto T, Morimoto S. Twenty-four year spironolactone therapy in an aged patient with aldosterone-producing adenoma. *Acta Endocrinol* 1992;126:186–190.

Thibonnier M, Sassano P, Joseph A, Plouin PF, Corvol P, Menard J. Diagnostic value of a single dose of captopril in renin- and aldosterone-dependent, surgically curable hypertension. *Cardiovasc Rev Rep* 1982;3:1659–1667.

Torres VE, Young WF Jr, Offord KP, Hattery RR. Association of hypokalemia, aldosteronism, and renal cysts. *N Engl J Med* 1990;322:345–351.

Tunny TJ, Gordon RD, Klemm SA, Cohn D. Histological and biochemical distinctiveness of atypical aldosterone-producing adenomas responsive to upright posture and angiotensin. *Clin Endocrinol* 1991;34:363–369.

Tweeddale MG, Ogilvie RI. Antagonism of spironolactone-induced natriuresis by aspirin in man. *N Engl J Med* 1973;289: 198–200.

Ulick S. Two uncommon causes of mineralocorticoid excess. Syndrome of apparent mineralocorticoid excess and glucocorticoid-remediable aldosteronism. *Endocrinol Metab Clin North Am* 1991;20: 269–276.

Ulick S, Blumenfeld JD, Atlas SA, Wang JZ, Vaughan ED. The unique steroidogenesis of the aldosteronoma in the differential diagnosis of primary aldosteronism. *J Clin Endocrinol Metab* 1993;76:873–878.

Ulick S, Chan CK, Gill JR, Gutkin M, Letcher L, Mantero F, New MI. Defective fasciculata zone function as the mechanism of glucocorticoid-remediable aldosteronism. *J Clin Endocrinol Metab* 1990;71: 1151–1157.

Ulick S, Chu MD, Land M. Biosynthesis of 18-oxocortisol by aldosterone-producing adrenal tissue. *J Biol Chem* 1983;258: 5498–5502.

Walker BR. Defective enzyme-mediated receptor protection: novel mechanisms in the pathophysiology of hypertension. *Clin Sci* 1993;85:257–263.

Walker BR, Edwards CRW. 11β-hydroxysteroid dehydrogenase and enzyme-mediated receptor protection: life after liquorice? *Clin Endocrinol* 1991;35:281–289.

Watt GCM, Harrap SB, Foy CJW, Holton DW, Edwards HV, Davidson HR, Connor JM, Lever AF, Fraser R. Abnormalities of glucocorticoid metabolism and the renin-angiotensin system: a four-corners approach to the identification of genetic determinants of blood pressure. *J Hypertens* 1992;10:473–482.

Weinberger MH, Fineberg NS. The diagnosis of primary aldosteronism and separation of two major subtypes. *Arch Intern Med* 1993;153:2125–2129.

Weinberger MH, Grim CE, Hollifield JW, Kem DC, Ganguly A, Kramer NJ, Yune HY, Wellman H, Donohue JP. Primary aldosteronism. Diagnosis, localization, and treatment. *Ann Intern Med* 1979; 90:386–395.

Wenting GJ, Man in't Veld AJ, Derkx FHM, Schalekamp MADH. Recurrence of hypertension in primary aldosteronism after discontinuation of spironolactone. Time course of changes in cardiac output and body fluid volumes. *Clin Exp Hypertens* 1982;A4:1727–1748.

White EA, Schambelan M, Rost CR, Biglieri EG, Moss AA, Korobkin M. Use of computed tomography in diagnosing the cause of primary aldosteronism. *N Engl J Med* 1980;303:1503–1507.

Williams ED, Boddy K, Brown JJ, Cumming AMM, Davies DL, Harvey IR, Haywood JK, Lever AF, Robertson JIS. Body elemental composition, with particular reference to total and exchangeable sodium and potassium and total chlorine, in untreated and treated primary hyperaldosteronism. *J Hypertens* 1984; 2:171–176.

Young DB, Guyton AC. Steady state aldosterone dose-response relationships. *Circ Res* 1977;40:138–145.

Young WF Jr. Primary aldosteronism. In: Rakel RE, ed. *Conn's Current Therapy.* Philadelphia: WB Saunders, 1993: 610–614.

Young WF Jr, Hogan MJ, Klee GG, Grant CS, van Heerden JA. Primary aldosteronism: diagnosis and treatment. *Mayo Clin Proc* 1990;65:96–110.

Young S-C, Shionoiri H, Takasaki I, Kihara M, Gotoh E. Hypertensive complications in patients with primary aldosteronism. *Curr Ther Res* 1991;50:317–325.

14 Hypertension Induced by Cortisol or Deoxycorticosterone

The preceding chapter described the syndromes of hypertension induced by primary aldosterone excess. This chapter will cover syndromes in which hypertension is induced by other adrenal steroids: *cortisol,* either in excess (Cushing's syndrome) or with increased binding to mineralocorticoid receptors (apparent mineralocorticoid excess, licorice ingestion); or *deoxycorticosterone* (congenital adrenal hyperplasias).

CUSHING'S SYNDROME

Cushing's syndrome is a serious disease with a mortality rate, even after successful therapy, 4 times above that of an age- and sex-matched population (Ross and Linch, 1982). Much of the excessive mortality is caused by cardiovascular disease; marked left ventricular hypertrophy is common (Sugihara et al., 1992). Hypertension is present in over 80% of patients with Cushing's syndrome and is a major risk factor contributing to that excessive mortality.

Etiology

The syndrome is caused by excess glucocorticoid: endogenous cortisol with the idiopathic form, various exogenous steroids with the iatrogenic form. As shown in Figure 14.1, the idiopathic disease may be caused either by ACTH-dependent mechanisms with bilateral adrenal hyperplasia, which may be macronodular in 12% to 15% (Doppman, 1993):

—Pituitary hypersecretion of adrenocorticotrophic hormone (ACTH)—that is, Cushing's *disease* (about 70% of all cases), *or*
—Ectopic tumors secreting ACTH (about 12%) (Limper et al., 1992) or, rarely, corticotrophin-releasing factor (O'Brien et al., 1992);

or by ACTH-independent mechanisms:

—Adrenal tumors, either benign or malignant (about 12%) *or*
—Primary adrenal hyperplasia (about 5%), which may be familial (Findlay et al., 1993) or caused by unusual non-ACTH stimuli such as gastric inhibitory polypeptide (Lacroix et al., 1992).

As noted in Chapter 12, the number of adrenal tumors found incidentally by abdominal computed tomography (CT) or magnetic resonance imaging (MRI) is increasing. A surprising 12% of 68 such "incidentalomas" were found to be autonomous cortisol-secreting tumors with subclinical features of Cushing's syndrome (Reincke et al., 1992).

Other interesting variants have been reported, including these:

—Spontaneously remitting disease (Dickstein et al., 1991);
—Cyclic or episodic disease (Shapiro and Shenkman, 1991);
—An association with overt hypothalamic disorders (Stewart et al., 1992);
—Transition from pituitary-dependent to pituitary-independent disease (Hermus et al., 1988);
—ACTH-independent bilateral macronodular hyperplasia, which may be familial (Findlay et al., 1993);
—Familial micronodular adrenocortical dysplasia (Hodge and Froesch, 1988);
—Unilateral nodular hyperplasia (Josse et al., 1980);
—Bilateral adrenal adenomas (Mimou et al., 1985).

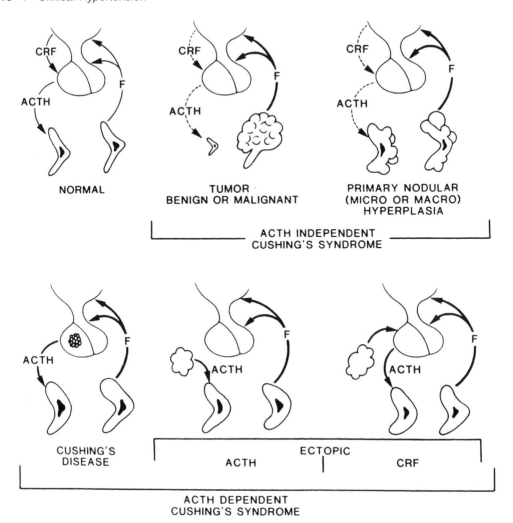

Figure 14.1. Etiologies of endogenous Cushing's syndrome. The lesions on the top arise within the adrenal. Those on the bottom arise within the pituitary (Cushing's disease) or from ectopic production of ACTH or corticotropin-releasing factor (CRF). *F,* cortisol. (From Carpenter PC. Diagnostic evaluation of Cushing's syndrome. *Endocrinol Metab Clin North Am* 1988;17:445–472.)

Hypertension in Cushing's Syndrome

Hypertension is present in about 80% of patients with Cushing's syndrome. It may be severe; in the series of Ross and Linch (1982), 10 of 70 patients had blood pressure (BP) exceeding 200/120 mm Hg, and all but one of these patients died despite treatment of the Cushing's syndrome. Among all 70 patients, 55% had an abnormal electrocardiogram and 28% had cardiomegaly. The severity of the hypertension may be related to the abolition of the normal nocturnal fall in BP seen after exogenous glucocorticoid administration and in patients with Cushing's syndrome (Imai et al., 1988).

Incidence of Hypertension with Exogenous Steroids

Hypertension is relatively rare in patients who take exogenous glucocorticoids (Sanders et al., 1992) because of the use of steroid derivatives with less mineralocorticoid activity than cortisol. Even less trouble will be seen with alternate-day therapy or with low doses: continuous therapy in the range of 10 mg/day of prednisone did not induce hypertension (Jackson et al., 1981).

However, significant rises of BP can occur within 5 days of the administration of glucocorticoids or ACTH in fairly high doses (Whitworth, 1992). These rises in BP developed in the absence of sodium retention or volume expansion, suggesting some direct "hypertensinogenic" effect of adrenal steroids beyond the mechanisms held responsible for the development of hypertension in endogenous Cushing's syndrome.

Mechanisms for the Hypertension

Multiple mechanisms may be responsible for the hypertension so common in Cushing's disease. They are:

1. The salt-retaining action of the high levels of cortisol, either through binding to mineralocorticoid receptors (Ulick et al., 1992a) or nonreceptor mechanisms (Montrella-Waybill et al., 1991). Although cortisol is 300 times less potent a mineralocorticoid as aldosterone, 200 times more cortisol is normally secreted, and this level is increased by 2 times or more in Cushing's disease.
2. Increased production of mineralocorticoids. Though usually noted only in patients with adrenal tumors, increased levels of 19-nordeoxycorticosterone (Ehlers et al., 1987), deoxycorticosterone (DOC) and, less commonly, aldosterone (Cassar et al., 1980) have been found in patients with all forms of the syndrome.
3. Increased levels of renin substrate (Saruta et al., 1986).
4. Increased cardiac sensitivity to catecholamines (Ritchie et al., 1990). However, hydrocortisone raised BP even when a rise in cardiac output was prevented by concomitant administration of a beta blocker (Pirpiris et al., 1993).
5. Increased responsiveness to various pressors (Pirpiris et al., 1992) likely by effects on vascular receptors (Sato et al., 1992) that may, in turn, be mediated by an overwhelming of the 11-beta-hydroxysteroid dehydrogenase capacity to convert cortisol to cortisone in vascular tissue (Walker et al., 1992).
6. Other mechanisms may also be involved:
   —Suppression of response to atrial natriuretic factor (Yasunari et al., 1990);
   —Inhibition of the production of vasodilatory prostaglandins and kinins (Nakamoto et al., 1992);
   —Hyperinsulinemia secondary to insulin resistance (Rebuffé-Scrive et al., 1988).

Clinical Features

Many more patients with cushingoid features are seen than the relatively few who have the syndrome. The syndrome is more likely in patients with the clinical features shown in the top portion of Table 14.1 (Ross and Linch, 1982).

Various neuropsychiatric disturbances, ranging from a mild decrease in energy to severe depression, were found in 62% of patients in Ross and Linch's series. Non-Cushing's patients with endogenous depression may have poorly suppressible hypercortisolism related to increased ACTH pulse frequency (Mortola et al., 1987), but their basal cortisol levels are usually normal and they do not hyperrespond to corticotrophin-releasing hormone (Gold et al., 1986).

Alcoholics often display numerous features suggestive of Cushing's syndrome, including hypertension and a failure to suppress plasma cortisol after overnight dexamethasone (Stewart et al., 1993). Alcohol should not be consumed for at least 2 weeks before studies are done.

Pregnant women often have features suggestive of Cushing's syndrome; the rare appearances of Cushing's syndrome during pregnancy may pose diagnostic dilemmas (Aron et al., 1990).

Laboratory Diagnosis*

The extent of the work-up of patients suspected of having Cushing's syndrome varies with the clinical situation: an overnight 1-mg dexamethasone suppression test will be adequate for most patients with only minimally suggestive features; patients with highly suggestive features should have both the low-dose urinary suppression test and a 24-hour urine-free cortisol measurement (Kaye and Crapo, 1990) (Fig. 14.2). The urine-free cortisol measurement is an excellent discriminator: None of 48 patients with Cushing's syndrome but 96% of 95 obese patients excreted less than 120 μg per day (Mengden et al., 1992).

Overnight Plasma Suppression

For screening of patients with cushingoid features, the single bedtime 1-mg-dose dexamethasone suppression test, measuring the plasma cortisol at 8 A.M. the next morning, has worked very well, with fewer than 2% false-negative results

---

*The data to be presented all use the traditional units of μg/dl or mg/day. To convert to SI units:
—*Plasma cortisol* from μg/dl to nmol/L: multiply by 27.6;
—*Urine cortisol* from μg/24 hour to nmol/day: multiply by 2.76;
—*Urine 17-hydroxycorticoids* from mg/day to μmol/day; multiply by 2.76;
—*Plasma ACTH* from pg/ml to pmol/L: multiply by 0.22.

Table 14.1. Discriminant Indices of Clinical Features in Cushing's Syndrome[a]

	Discriminant Index in Series	
Clinical Features	Present (70 Cases)	Collected (711 Cases)
Strong discriminatory value		
Bruising	10.3	10.5
Myopathy	8.0	7.1
Hypertension	4.4	5.1
Plethora	3.0	3.6
Edema	2.9	3.3
Hirsutism in women	2.8	2.7
Red striae	2.5	3.1
Less discriminatory value		
Menstrual irregularity	1.6	1.6
Truncal obesity	1.6	
Headaches	1.3	1.1
No discriminatory value		
Acne	0.9	
Generalized obesity	0.8	
Impaired glucose tolerance	0.7	0.7

[a]The index is obtained by dividing the prevalence of each feature in the separate series of patients with Cushing's syndrome, the authors' 70 cases, and the 711 cases collected from the literature by its prevalence in the series of Nugent et al. (1964) of 159 mostly obese patients in whom the diagnosis of Cushing's syndrome was suspected but not biochemically substantiated. From Ross EJ, Linch DC. Cushing's syndrome—killing disease: discriminatory value of signs and symptoms aiding early diagnosis.

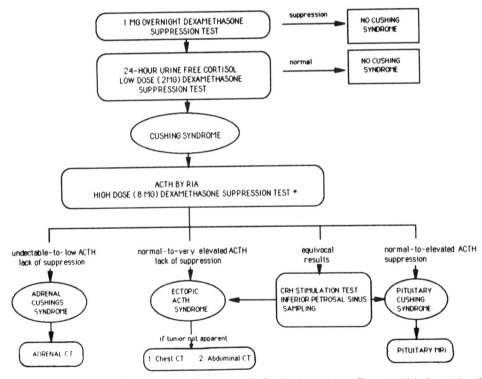

Figure 14.2. An algorithm for the evaluation of a patient with Cushing's syndrome. The *asterisk* indicates that if the overnight high-dose dexamethasone suppression test is validated in the outpatient setting, it should be used at this point. Currently, the classic high-dose dexamethasone suppression test or the corticotropin-releasing hormone *(CRH)* stimulation test may be used. (From Kaye TB, Crapo L. The Cushing syndrome: an update on diagnostic tests. *Ann Intern Med* 1990;112:434–444.)

(Cronin et al., 1990). Most consider a level of less than 5 μg/dl as an indication of normal suppression, but some use a value of 2 μg/dl (Trainer and Grossman, 1991).

False-positive results are seen in 12.5% of non-Cushing's patients (Cronin et al., 1990). One reason is too-rapid inactivation of the exogenous dexamethasone to produce suppression of ACTH by drugs that stimulate the hepatic drug-metabolizing enzymes such as diphenylhydantoin, barbiturates, tolbutamide, rifampin, and perhaps alcohol (Trainer and Grossman, 1991).

Another reason may be the overriding effect of stress or endogenous depression. Patients in a hospital frequently fail to suppress the pituitary-adrenal system nearly as well as they do when restudied as outpatients (Connolly et al., 1968). Patients with endogenous depression may also fail to respond to dexamethasone (Mortola et al., 1987).

Low-Dose Dexamethasone Suppression

If the overnight screening test is abnormal or the clinical evidence is very strong, the presence of hypercortisolism can be virtually assured by the finding that plasma or urine levels of cortisol cannot be normally suppressed by a "low dose" of 0.5 mg of dexamethasone every 6 hours for 2 days (Liddle, 1960). This amount of dexamethasone is equivalent to about 40 mg of cortisol, approximately twice the normal daily secretion rate. In Crapo's 1979 review, 240 of 241 controls without Cushing's syndrome suppressed below 4.0 mg/day of urinary 17-hydroxycorticosteroid (17-OHCS) or 25 μg/day of urine-free cortisol, whereas only 9 of 154 patients with Cushing's syndrome suppressed below those levels.

To circumvent the need for multiple 24-hour urine collections, plasma cortisol may be measured. When blood was obtained at 8 A.M. on the morning after the 2 days of low-dose dexamethasone, serum cortisol was below 2.2 μg/dl in 31 of 32 patients without Cushing's syndrome and above 9.1 μg/dl in 12 of 13 patients with Cushing's syndrome (Kennedy et al., 1984).

Dexamethasone suppression tests may give anomalous results because excessive hormone secretion may be cyclic or variable (Shapiro and Shenkman, 1991). One patient has been described whose hypothalamic-pituitary feedback mechanism failed to recognize dexamethasone but did suppress with cortisol (Carey, 1980).

Establishing the Cause of the Syndrome

Once Cushing's syndrome has been diagnosed, the mechanism needs to be accurately determined to guide therapy. Easier and more accurate visualization of both the pituitary and the adrenals using CT and MRI has greatly enhanced our diagnostic accuracy.

Laboratory Studies

The longest and largest experience has been with high-dose dexamethasone suppression. Kaye and Crapo (1990) recommend the measurement of plasma ACTH along with dexamethasone suppression as the first maneuvers in determining the cause (Fig. 14.2).

High-Dose Dexamethasone Suppression (Fig. 14.2). The high-dose test is an extension of the low-dose test, predicated on the resetting of the pituitary-cortisol feedback mechanism at a higher level in those with ACTH-dependent Cushing's disease arising in the pituitary: whereas a low dose of dexamethasone (i.e., the equivalent of 40 mg of cortisol per day) will not suppress the hyperfunctioning pituitary, a high dose (i.e., the equivalent of 160 mg of cortisol per day) usually will. On the other hand, not even the high dose will usually suppress an adrenal tumor or an ectopic ACTH-producing tumor. With <u>suppression</u> indicated by a <u>40% decrease</u> from baseline <u>urinary cortisol</u> on the <u>second day</u> of 2.0 mg every 6 hours, 84 of 91 patients with pituitary Cushing's syndrome suppressed, whereas only one of 44 with an adrenal tumor and four of 20 with ectopic ACTH tumor suppressed (Crapo, 1979).

The diagnostic accuracy of the high-dose dexamethasone test is improved by measuring both urine free cortisol and 17-hydroxycorticoid (17-HOCS) excretion: when urine free cortisol was suppressed by more than 90% and 17-HOCS by more than 64%, specificity was 100% and correct predictions were found in 86% of 112 patients with Cushing's syndrome (Flack et al., 1992).

Plasma ACTH. Plasma ACTH levels should clearly separate the three major forms of Cushing's syndrome (Figs. 14.1 and 14.2), with adrenal tumors having very low levels, pituitary hyperfunction having "normal" levels (which are abnormally high in the presence of elevated plasma cortisol), and ectopic Cushing's syndrome having very high levels (Orth, 1991). ACTH and lipotropins (LPH) are synthesized through a common precursor, proopiomelanocortin, in the pituitary. Kuhn et al. (1989) have found that assays of plasma ACTH and LPH give excellent separation between the three forms of Cushing's syndrome, with even better results from the LPH assay, perhaps because LPH is more stable in blood.

Petrosal Sinus Sampling. Increasingly, sampling of inferior petrosal venous sinus blood is being used to localize ACTH-secreting pituitary microadenomas and to distinguish them from ectopic ACTH tumors when standard approaches have failed (Oldfield et al., 1991).

Corticotorpin-Releasing Factor Test. The availability of ovine or human corticotropin-releasing factor (CRF) will provide another way to differentiate various forms of cortisol excess. A marked rise in plasma ACTH and cortisol occurs after an intravenous bolus of CRF in patients with pituitary Cushing's syndrome, but no change is seen in either ACTH or cortisol in patients with ectopic ACTH secretion (Trainer and Grossman, 1991).

Radiologic Studies

If the hormonal tests indicate ACTH-independent disease, the adrenal glands should be scanned by CT or MRI. ^{131}I-6-beta-iodomethylnorcholesterol (NP-59) scintigraphy will identify some lesions that are too small to be seen on CT (Fig et al., 1988). Bilateral macronodular hyperplasia is seen in 12% to 15% of patients with ACTH-dependent disease (Doppman, 1993).

If the hormonal tests indicate ACTH-dependent disease, CT or preferably MRI scans should look for a pituitary tumor. CT scans of the pituitary have only a 47% sensitivity and a 74% specificity in identifying a pituitary adenoma (Kaye and Crapo, 1990). MRI scans, especially with gadolinium contrast, have given better results (Orth, 1991).

If the hormonal tests indicate ectopic tumor, CT scans of the chest and abdomen should be performed.

Treatment of Cushing's Syndrome

Treatment of the Hypertension

Until definitive therapy is provided, the hypertension that accompanies Cushing's syndrome can temporarily be treated with the usual antihypertensive agents described in Chapter 7. Since excess fluid volume is likely involved, a diuretic, perhaps in combination with the aldosterone antagonist spironolactone, is an appropriate initial choice.

Treatment of the Syndrome in General

The choice of definitive therapy depends on the cause of the syndrome; many choices are available (Table 14.2):

—For benign adrenal tumors, surgical removal is indicated (Välimäki et al., 1984);
—For adrenal cancers and ectopic ACTH tumors that cannot be resected, removal of the adrenal may be helpful, but chemotherapy is usually needed (Miller and Crapo, 1993);
—For pituitary tumors, trans-sphenoidal microsurgical removal of pituitary tumors has become the treatment of choice (Klibanski and Zervas, 1991). The syndrome may recur in as many as 20% of patients, so yearly follow-up cortisol measurements are recommended (Tahir and Sheeler, 1992). The pituitary can be irradiated from an external source (Ahmed et al., 1984) or from yttrium-90 interstitial implants (Sandler et al., 1987). The long-term use of reserpine may cure a larger percentage of patients after pituitary irradiation (Murayama et al., 1992). A few patients with bilateral adrenal hyperplasia have been successfully treated by total adrenalectomies with autotransplantation of part of one gland (Xu et al., 1992).

Table 14.2. Therapies for Cushing's Syndrome

Surgery
Pituitary: Trans-sphenoidal microresection
Transfrontal hypophysectomy
Adrenal: Unilateral adrenalectomy
Bilateral adrenalectomy

Radiation
External: High-voltage x-ray (cobalt) ±
mitotane, etc., alpha-particle, proton beam (cyclotron)
Internal: Implants of yttrium-90, gold-198

Drugs
Acting on CNS neurotransmission
Bromocriptine (Parlodel)
Cyproheptadine (Periacten)
Sodium valproate
Acting on adrenocortical steroid synthesis
o,p'-DDD (mitotane, Lysodren)
Metyrapone (Metopirone)
Aminoglutethimide (Elipten)
Trilostane (WIN 24,540)
Ketoconazole (Nizoral)
Acting as a competitive glucocorticoid antagonist (RU 486)

In the future, drugs that selectively inhibit corticotropin-releasing factor may have a primary place. At present, such drugs are a secondary line of therapy (Miller and Crapo, 1993); such drugs include bromocriptine (Lamberts et al., 1980) and cyproheptadine (Wiesen et al., 1983). Patients in whom pituitary surgery is inappropriate or who have recurrent disease can be successfully treated with inhibitors of adrenal steroid synthesis, often combined with external irradiation. The largest experience has been with mitotane (*o,p'*-DDD) (Schteingart, 1989), but results with the inhibitor of cytochrome P-450–dependent adrenal enzymes, ketoconazole, for long-term therapy of ACTH-dependent disease have been generally excellent (Sonino et al., 1991). In the future, glucocorticoid antagonists such as RU-486 may be more widely used since they are so well tolerated (van der Lely et al., 1991). Miller and Crapo (1993) estimate that one-third of all patients with Cushing's syndrome will need medical therapy.

Course of Hypertension

As with most secondary causes of hypertension, the BP may remain elevated despite removal of the cause. In the series of Ross and Linch (1985), 29% of patients relieved of their hypercortisolism remained hypertensive; the mortality rate of the 57 patients was 4 times greater than expected.

SYNDROMES WITH INCREASED CORTISOL BINDING TO MINERALOCORTICOID RECEPTORS

Less common than Cushing's syndrome caused by cortisol excess are a variety of fascinating syndromes wherein normal (or increased) levels of cortisol exert a mineralocorticoid effect by binding to the renal mineralocorticoid receptors. As noted in Chapter 13, the normal renal mineralocorticoid receptor is as receptive to glucocorticoids as to mineralocorticoids. The 11-beta-hydroxysteroid dehydrogenase (11-beta-OHSD) enzyme in the renal tubules upstream to these receptors normally converts the large amounts of fully active cortisol to the inactive cortisone, thereby leaving the mineralocorticoid receptors open to the effects of aldosterone.

However, there are both congenital and acquired deficiencies of the 11-beta-OHSD enzyme, so that the normal levels of cortisol remain fully active, flooding the mineralocorticoid receptor and inducing the full syndrome of mineralocorticoid excess: sodium retention, potassium wastage, and hypertension with virtually complete suppression of renin and aldosterone secretion.

Apparent Mineralocorticoid Excess (AME)

The handful of children and one adult known to have this syndrome have provided the substrate for studies that have elucidated the 11-beta-OHSD directed cortisol/cortisone shuttle. Soon after the first case was described (Werder et al., 1974), New, Ulick, and coworkers (Ulick et al., 1979) recognized that these children did not metabolize cortisol normally. Some years later, Stewart et al. (1988), in studies on a 20-year-old with the syndrome, recognized a defect in the renal cortisol/cortisone shuttle and demonstrated the deficiency of the 11-beta-OHSD enzyme that was presumably responsible for what became known as the type 1 form of AME. Later, Ulick et al. (1990) described three patients with AME who had normal cortisol/cortisone ratios, labeling them as type 2. More recently, Ulick et al. (1992a) showed that both forms of the syndrome involve defective ring A reduction of cortisol from a deficiency in the 5-beta-reductase enzyme that normally converts cortisol to the inactive tetrahydrocortisol metabolite, thereby keeping the mineralocorticoid receptors flooded with cortisol in the same manner as when 11-beta-OHSD is deficient.

Glycyrrhetenic Acid

Since the early 1950s, glycyrrhetenic acid, the active ingredient in licorice extract, has been known to cause sodium retention, potassium wastage, and hypertension. Stewart, Edwards, and coworkers (Stewart et al., 1987; Edwards et al., 1988) recognized the similarities between the syndrome induced by licorice and the syndrome of apparent mineralocorticoid excess and documented that licorice inhibited the same renal 11-beta-OHSD enzyme that was deficient in type 1 AME. In addition, central mechanisms may be involved in the rise of BP (Gomez-Sanchez and Gomez-Sanchez, 1992)

Relatively small amounts of confectionery licorice, 200 g daily for 10 days, produce sodium retention, kaliuresis, and suppression of renin and aldosterone in normal people (Stewart et al., 1987). The syndrome has been induced by the licorice extracts in chewing tobacco and gum (Rosseel and Schoors, 1993). These effects are accompanied by a fall in cortisone and a rise in cortisol excretion, reflecting the inhibition of renal 11-beta-OHSD activity.

The potential for an expanded role of inhibitors of 11-beta-OHSD and 5-beta-reductase activity far beyond that related to ingestion of licorice has been raised. Morris et al. (1992a) provided preliminary evidence for the presence of glycyrrhetenic acid-like factors (GALFs) in the urine of normal people, with increased levels during pregnancy. They also reported higher levels in patients with essential hypertension (Morris et al., 1992b). In addition, some patients with "essential hypertension" (Walker et al., 1993) or chronic renal insufficiency (Vierhapper et al., 1991) have been found to have impaired conversion of cortisol to cortisone.

Massive Cortisol Excess

The capacity of the 11-beta-OHSD directed cortisol/cortisone shuttle and of 5-beta-reductase inactivation may be overcome by massive amounts of cortisol. Ulick et al. (1992b) have shown this to be the mechanism responsible for the significant features of mineralocorticoid excess—profound hypokalemia and hypertension—that are seen in patients with ectopic ACTH tumors wherein cortisol levels are higher than in other causes of Cushing's syndrome.

PRIMARY CORTISOL RESISTANCE

A small number of patients have been found to have a primary resistance to cortisol and other glucocorticoids, usually resulting from a defect in the glucocorticoid receptor (Werner et al., 1992). The resultant increased secretion of ACTH may lead to an increased secretion of mineralocorticoids with hypertension (Chrousos et al., 1983) or sexual precocity (Malchoff et al., 1990).

DEOXYCORTICOSTERONE EXCESS

DOC-Secreting Tumors

In addition to hypertension induced by either excessive amounts of cortisol or increased binding of cortisol to mineralocorticoid receptors, excessive amounts of the mineralocorticoid deoxycorticosterone (DOC) may cause hypertension (Biglieri and Kater, 1991). Excess DOC can arise either from hyperplastic adrenals with enzymatic deficiencies or from DOC-secreting tumors (Gröndal et al., 1990).

Congenital Adrenal Hyperplasia (CAH)

Defects in all of the enzymes involved in adrenal steroid synthesis shown in Figure 14.3 have been recognized. These defects are inherited in an autosomal recessive manner; the specific molecular defects are being recognized (Helmberg et al., 1992). Their manifestations result from inadequate levels of the end-products of steroid synthesis—in particular, cortisol. The low levels of cortisol call forth increased secretion of ACTH, further increasing the accumulation of the precursor steroids proximal to the enzymatic block and stimulating steroidogenesis in pathways that are not blocked (Table 14.3).

The clinical manifestations, often obvious at birth, vary with the degree of enzymatic deficiency and the mix of steroids secreted by the hyperplastic adrenal glands. Therapy is with glucocorticoid, usually cortisol, though dexamethasone may provide more prolonged ACTH suppression with fewer systemic side effects in adults (Miller, 1991).

The most common type, the 21-hydroxylase deficiency, responsible for perhaps 90% of all CAH, is not associated with hypertension but is accompanied by a high prevalence of benign adrenal tumors (Jaresch et al., 1992).

The two forms of CAH in which hypertension occurs are the 11-hydroxylase defect, wherein 11-DOC is present in excess along with adrenal androgens, and the 17-hydroxylase defect, which also has an excess of DOC but a deficiency of androgen production. Though these are rare causes of hypertension, partial enzymatic deficiencies have been observed in hirsute women (Lucky et al., 1986), so some hypertensive adults may have unrecognized, subtle forms of CAH. A pattern suggesting a partial deficiency of adrenal 11-hydroxylase with high levels of DOC and deoxycortisol, both basal and after ACTH stimulation, was reported in 15 patients with what appears to be ordinary primary hypertension (de Simone et al., 1985), but there has been no further documentation of this pattern.

11-Hydroxylase Deficiency

The 11-hydroxylase deficiency syndrome is usually recognized in infancy because, as shown in Figure 14.4, the defect sets off production of excessive androgens. The enzyme deficiency prevents the hydroxylation of 11-deoxycortisol, resulting in cortisol deficiency. The defect also prevents the conversion of DOC to corticosterone and aldosterone. The high levels of DOC induce hypertension and hypokalemia, the expected features of mineralocorticoid excess.

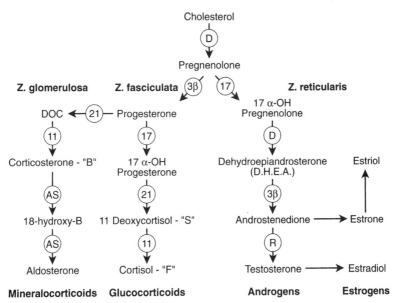

Figure 14.3. Major biosynthetic pathways in the three zones of the adrenal cortex. The enzymes involved are shown within the circles: *D*, desmolase; *3β*, 3-beta-ol-dehydrogenase; *17*, 17-hydroxylase; *11*, 11-beta-hydroxylase; *21*, 21-hydroxylase; *AS*, aldosterone synthase (also referred to as CMO I and II, corticosterone methyl oxidase I and II); *R*, 17-beta-hydroxysteroid dehydrogenase.

Table 14.3 Syndromes of Congenital Adrenal Hyperplasia

	Site of Defect		Steroid Levels[a]				Clinical Features	
	Increased Precursor	Decreased Product	17-KS	17-OH-P or P'triol	DOC	Aldo	Virilization	Hypertension
21-hydroxylase:								
Nonsalt-wasting	17-hydroxypro-gesterone	11-deoxycortisol, cortisol	↑	↑	N	↑	+ + + +	No
Salt-wasting	Progesterone	11-deoxycorti-costerone, cortisol	↑	↑	↓	↓	+ + + +	No
11-hydroxylase	11-deoxycortisol 11-deoxycorti-costerone	Cortisol Cortisterone	↑	↑	↑	↓	+ + + +	Yes
17-hydroxylase	Progesterone Pregnenolone	Cortisol 17-hydroxypreg-nenolone	↓	↓	↑	↓	0	Yes
3-beta-ol-dehydrogenase	Pregnenolone	Progesterone, cortisol	↑	↓	↓	↓	+	No

[a]*17-KS*, 17-ketosteroids; *17-OH-P*, 17-hydroxyprogesterone; *P'triol*, pregnanetriol; *DOC*, deoxycorticosterone; *Aldo*, aldosterone; *N*, normal; ↑, increased; ↓, decreased; +, slight; + + + +, marked; 0, absent.

Thus, the syndrome features virilization of the infant, hypertension, and hypokalemia.

The syndrome is diagnosed by finding high levels of 11-deoxycortisol and DOC in urine and plasma (Zachmann et al. 1983). Treatment, as for all of the syndromes of CAH, is with glucocorticoid, which should relieve the hypertension and hypokalemia and allow the child to develop normally. Since aldosterone synthesis is blocked, when glucocorticoid therapy is insti-

tuted, the resultant decrease in DOC production may be manifested by sodium wastage (Zadik et al., 1984).

17-Hydroxylase Deficiency

Unlike the 21-hydroxylase and 11-hydroxylase deficiencies, CAH caused by a 17-hydroxylase deficiency is associated with an absence of sex hormones, leading to incomplete masculinization in males and primary amenorrhea in

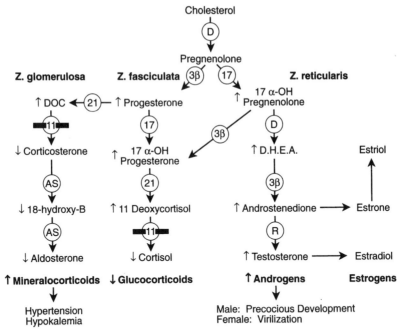

Figure 14.4. Defect in adrenal steroid synthesis in the syndrome of congenital adrenal hyperplasia caused by a deficiency of the 11-hydroxylase enzyme. The enzymes involved are shown within the circles: *D*, desmolase; *3β*, 3-beta-ol-dehydrogenase; *17*, 17-hydroxylase; *11*, 11-beta-hydroxylase; *21*, 21-hydroxylase; *AS*, aldosterone synthase (also referred to as CMO I and II, corticosterone methyl oxidase I and II); *R*, 17-beta-hydroxysteroid dehydrogenase.

females. Since 17-hydroxylase activity is also lacking in the gonads, the defect prevents conversion of the precursor pregnenolone into androgens and estrogens (Fig. 14.5). Though most affected 46,XY males are phenotypically females, some may appear as partially virilized males at birth, presumably because they have less severe enzyme deficiency (Dean et al., 1984). The syndrome usually is not recognized until after the age of puberty when sexual development does not progress in a normal manner in patients who are phenotypically female. Only about 40 cases have been recognized, but adolescents with hypertension and abnormal sexual development should be considered suspect (Cottrell et al., 1990).

Since the 17-hydroxylase deficiency interferes with cortisol synthesis, the resultant increase in ACTH stimulates the adrenal to do what it can—synthesize large amounts of the potent mineralocorticoid DOC, as well as other precursors (Cottrell et al., 1990). Hypertension and hypokalemia supervene. The hypertension can be very severe (Fraser et al., 1987).

Increased aldosterone synthesis would be expected in the presence of large amounts of its precursor corticosterone. However, low levels of aldosterone have been found in most cases. This could result from one or both of the mechanisms shown on the left in Figure 14.5. An additional deficiency of the aldosterone synthase enzyme, which is needed to convert corticosterone to aldosterone, has been suggested (Waldhäusl et al., 1978). On the other hand, the salt retention induced by the high levels of DOC produced by continuous ACTH stimulation would be expected to suppress the renin-angiotensin mechanism, the primary stimulus for aldosterone synthesis in the zona glomerulosa, so no additional biosynthetic defects other than the 17-hydroxylase deficiency need be evoked.

Regardless of the details, the entire syndrome can be corrected with glucocorticoid therapy—usually cortisol in doses of 10 to 30 mg/day.

Now that the various renal and adrenal causes of hypertension have been covered, we shall turn to an even larger variety of less common forms.

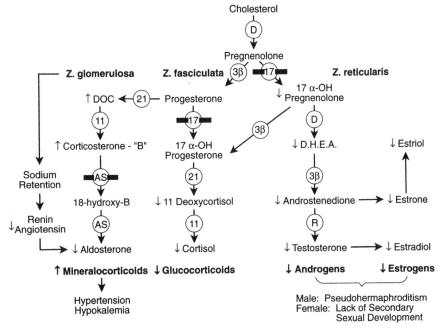

Figure 14.5. Defect in adrenal steroid synthesis in the syndrome of congenital adrenal hyperplasia caused by a deficiency of the 17-hydroxylase and, perhaps, the 18-ol-dehydrogenase enzymes. The enzymes involved are shown within the circles: *D,* desmolase; 3β, 3-beta-ol-dehydrogenase; *17,* 17-hydroxylase; *11,* 11-beta-hydroxylase; *21,* 21-hydroxylase; *AS,* aldosterone synthase (also referred to as CMO I and II, corticosterone methyl oxidase I and II); *R,* 17-beta-hydroxysteroid dehydrogenase.

References

Ahmed SR, Shalet SM, Beardwell CG, Sutton ML. Treatment of Cushing's disease with low dose radiation therapy. *Br Med J* 1984;289:643–646.

Aron DC, Schnall AM, Sheeler LR. Cushing's syndrome and pregnancy. *Am J Obstet Gynecol* 1990;162:244–252.

Biglieri EG, Kater CE. Steroid characteristics of mineralocorticoid adrenocortical hypertension. *Clin Chem* 1991;37:1843–1848.

Carey RM. Suppression of ACTH by cortisol in dexamethasone-nonsuppressible Cushing's disease. *N Engl J Med* 1980; 302:275–279.

Cassar J, Loizou S, Kelly WF, Joplin GF. Deoxycorticosterone and aldosterone excretion in Cushing's syndrome. *Metabolism* 1980;29:115–119.

Chrousos GP, Vingerhoeds ADM, Loriaux DL, Lipsett MB. Primary cortisol resistance: a family study. *J Clin Endocrinol Metab* 1983;56:1243–1245.

Connolly CK, Gore MBR, Stanley N, Wills MR. Single-dose dexamethasone suppression in normal subjects and hospital patients. *Br Med J* 1968;2:665–667.

Cottrell DA, Bello FA, Falko JM. Case report: 17 alpha-hydroxylase deficiency masquerading as primary hyperaldosteronism. *Am J Med Sci* 1990;300:380–382.

Crapo L. Cushing's syndrome: a review of diagnostic tests. *Metabolism* 1979; 28:955–977.

Cronin C, Igoe D, Duffy MJ, Cunningham SK, McKenna TJ. The overnight dexa-

methasone test is a worthwhile screening procedure. *Clin Endocrinol* 1990; 33:27–33.

Dean HJ, Shackleton CHL, Winter JSD. Diagnosis and natural history of 17-hydroxylase deficiency in a newborn male. *J Clin Endocrinol Metab* 1984; 59:513–520.

de Simone G, Tommaselli AP, Rossi R, Valentino R, Lauria R, Scopacasa F, Lombardi G. Partial deficiency of adrenal 11-hydroxylase. A possible cause of primary hypertension. *Hypertension* 1985; 7:204–210.

Dickstein G, Spindel A, Shechner C, Adawi F, Gutman H. Spontaneous remission in Cushing's disease. *Arch Intern Med* 1991;151:185–189.

Doppman JL. The dilemma of bilateral adrenocortical nodularity in Conn's and Cushing's syndromes. *Radiol Clin North Am* 1993;31:1039–1050.

Edwards CRW, Burt D, McIntyre MA, de Kloet ER, Stewart PM, Brett L, Sutanto WS, Monder C. Localisation of 11β-hydroxysteroid dehydrogenase– tissue specific protector of the mineralocorticoid receptor. *Lancet* 1988;2:986–989.

Ehlers ME, Griffing GT, Wilson TE, Melby JC. Elevated urinary 19-nor-deoxycorticosterone glucuronide in Cushing's syndrome. *J Clin Endocrinol Metab* 1987;64:926–930.

Fig LM, Gross MD, Shapiro B, Ehrmann DA, Freitas JE, Schteingart DE, Glazer GM,

Francis IR. Adrenal localization in the adrenocorticotropic hormone-independent Cushing syndrome. *Ann Intern Med* 1988;109:547–553.

Findlay JC, Sheeler LR, Engeland WC, Aron DC. Familial adrenocorticotropin-independent cushing's syndrome with bilateral macronodular adrenal hyperplasia. *J Clin Endocrinol Metab* 1993;76:189–191.

Flack MR, Oldfield EH, Cutler GB Jr, Zweig MH, Malley JD, Chrousos GP, Loriaux DL, Nieman LK. Urine free cortisol in the high-dose dexamethasone suppression test for the differential diagnosis of the Cushing syndrome. *Ann Intern Med* 1992; 116:211–217.

Fraser R, Brown JJ, Mason PA, Morton JJ, Lever AF, Robertson JIS, Lee HA, Miller H. Severe hypertension with absent secondary sex characteristics due to partial deficiency of steroid 17-hydroxylase activity. *J Hum Hypertens* 1987;1:53–58.

Gold PW, Loriaux DL, Roy A, Kling MA, Calabrese JR, Kellner CH, Nieman LK, Post RM, Pickar D, Gallucci W, Avgerinos P, Paul S, Oldfield EH, Cutler GB Jr, Chrousos GP. Responses to corticotropin-releasing hormone in the hypercortisolism of depression and Cushing's disease. *N Engl J Med* 1986;314:1329–1335.

Gomez-Sanchez EP, Gomez-Sanchez CE. Central hypertensinogenic effects of glycyrrhizic acid and carbenoxolone. *Am J Physiol* 1992;263:E1125–E1130.

Gröndal S, Eriksson B, Hagenäs L, Werner S, Curstedt T. Steroid profile in urine: a useful tool in the diagnosis and follow up of adrenocortical carcinoma. *Acta Endocrinologica (Copenh)* 1990;122:656–663.

Helmberg A, Ausserer B, Kofler R. Frame shift by insertion of 2 basepairs in codon 394 of CYP11B1 causes congenital adrenal hyperplasia due to steroid 11β-hydroxylase deficiency. *J Clin Endocrinol Metab* 1992;75:1278–1281.

Hermus AR, Pieters GF, Smals AG, Pesman GJ, Lamberts SW, Benraad TJ, van Haelst UJ, Kloppenborg PW. Transition from pituitary-dependent to adrenal-dependent Cushing's syndrome. *N Engl J Med* 1988;318:966–970.

Hodge BO, Froesch TA. Familial Cushing's syndrome. Micronodular adrenocortical dysplasia. *Arch Intern Med* 1988; 148:1133–1136.

Imai Y, Abe K, Sasaki S, Minami N, Nihei M, Munakata M, Murakami O, Matsue K, Sekino H, Miura Y, Yoshinaga K. Altered circadian blood pressure rhythm in patients with Cushing's syndrome. *Hypertension* 1988;12:11–19.

Jackson SHD, Beevers DG, Myers K. Does long-term low-dose corticosteroid therapy cause hypertension? *Clin Sci* 1981; 61:381s–383s.

Jaresch S, Kornely E, Kley H-K, Schlaghecke R. Adrenal incidentaloma and patients with homozygous or heterozygous congenital adrenal hyperplasia. *J Clin Endocrinol Metab* 1992;74:685–689.

Josse RG, Bear R, Kovacs K, Higgins HP. Cushing's syndrome due to unilateral nodular adrenal hyperplasia: a new pathophysiological entity? *Acta Endocrinol* 1980;92:495–504.

Kaye TB, Crapo L. The Cushing syndrome: an update on diagnostic tests. *Ann Intern Med* 1990;112:434–444.

Kennedy L, Atkinson AB, Johnston H, Sheridan B, Hadden DR. Serum cortisol concentrations during low dose dexamethasone suppression test to screen for Cushing's syndrome. *Br Med J* 1984;289:1188–1191.

Klibanski A, Zervas NT. Diagnosis and management of hormone-secreting pituitary adenomas. *N Engl J Med* 1991; 324:822–831.

Kuhn JM, Proeschel MF, Seurin DJ, Bertagna XY, Luton JP, Girard FL. Comparative assessment of ACTH and lipotropin plasma levels in the diagnosis and follow-up of patients with Cushing's syndrome: a study of 210 cases. *Am J Med* 1989; 86:678 684.

Lacroix A, Bolté E, Tremblay J, Dupré J, Poitras P, Fournier H, Garon J, Garrel D, Bayard F, Taillefer R, Flanagan RJ, Hamet P. Gastric inhibitory polypeptide-dependent cortisol hypersecretion—a new cause of cushing's syndrome. *N Engl J Med* 1992;327:974–980.

Lamberts SWJ, Klijn JGM, de Quijada M, Timmermans HAT, Uitterlinden P, de Jong FH, Birkenhäger JC. The mechanism of the suppressive action of bromocriptine on adrenocorticotropin secretion in patients with Cushing's disease and Nelson's syndrome. *J Clin Endocrinol Metab* 1980;51:307–311.

Liddle GW. Tests of pituitary-adrenal suppressibility in the diagnosis of Cushing's syndrome. *J Clin Endocrinol Metab* 1960;20:1539–1560.

Limper AH, Carpenter PC, Scheithauer B, Staats BA. The Cushing syndrome induced by bronchial carcinoid tumors. *Ann Intern Med* 1992;117:209–214.

Lucky AW, Rosenfield FL, McGuire J, Rudy S, Helke J. Adrenal androgen hyperresponsiveness to adrenocorticotropin in women with acne and/or hirsutism: adrenal enzyme defects and exaggerated adrenarche. *J Clin Endocrinol Metab* 1986; 62:840–848.

Malchoff CD, Javier EC, Malchoff DM, Martin T, Rogol A, Brandon D, Loriaux DL, Reardon GE. Primary cortisol resistance presenting as isosexual precocity. *J Clin Endocrinol* 1990;70:503–507.

Mengden T, Hubmann P, Müller J, Greminger P, Vetter W. Urinary free cortisol versus 17-hydroxycorticosteroids: a comparative study of their diagnostic value in Cushing's syndrome. *Clin Invest* 1992;70:545–548.

Miller JW, Crapo L. The medical treatment of Cushing's syndrome. *Endocrinol Rev* 1993;14:443–458.

Miller WL. Congenital adrenal hyperplasias. *Endocrinol Metab Clin North Am* 1991;20:721–749.

Mimou N, Sakato S, Nakabayashi H, Saito Z, Takeda R, Matsubara F. Cushing's syndrome associated with bilateral adrenal adenomas. *Acta Endocrinol* 1985; 108:245-254.

Montrella-Waybill M, Clore JN, Schoolwerth AC, Watlington CO. Evidence that high dose cortisol-induced Na⁺ retention in man is not mediated by the mineralocorticoid receptor. *J Clin Endocrinol Metab* 1991;72:1060–1066.

Morris DJ, Semafuko WEB, Latif SA, Vogel B, Grimes CA, Sheff MF. Detection of glycyrrhetinic acid-like factors (GALFs) in human urine. *Hypertension* 1992a; 20:356–360.

Morris DJ, Semafuko WEB, Grimes CA, Latif SA, Sheff MF, Levinson P, Walker BR, Edwards CRW. Measurement of glycyrrhetinic acid (GA)/liquorice-like factors (GALFs), in urine from essential hypertensives [Abstract]. *Hypertension* 1992b; 20:407–408.

Mortola JF, Liu JH, Gillin JC, Rasmussen DD, Yen SSC. Pulsatile rhythms of adrenocorticotropin (ACTH) and cortisol in women with endogenous depression: evidence for increased ACTH pulse frequency. *J Clin Endocrinol Metab* 1987;65:962–968.

Murayama M, Yasuda K, Minamori Y, Mercado-Asis LB, Yamakita N, Miura K. Long term follow-up of Cushing's disease treated with reserpine and pituitary irradiation. *J Clin Endocrinol Metab* 1992; 75:935–942.

Nakamoto H, Suzuki H, Kageyama Y, Murakami M, Ohishi A, Naitoh Ichihara A, Saruta T. Depressor systems contribute to hypertension induced by glucocorticoid excess in dogs. *J Hypertens* 1992; 10:561–569.

O'Brien T, Young WF, Davila DG, Scheithauer BW, Kovacs K, Horvath E, Vale W, van Heerden JA. Cushing's syndrome associated with ectopic production of corticotrophin-releasing hormone, corticotrophin and vasopressin by a phaeochromocytoma. *Clin Endocrinol* 1992; 37:460–467.

Oldfield EH, Doppman JL, Nieman LK, Chrousos GP, Miller DL, Katz DA, Cutler GB Jr, Loriaux DL. Petrosal sinus sampling with and without corticotropin-releasing hormone for the differential diagnosis of Cushing's syndrome. *N Engl J Med* 1991;325:897–905.

Orth DN. Differential diagnosis of Cushing's syndrome. *N Engl J Med* 1991;325: 957–959.

Pirpiris M, Sudhir K, Yeung S, Jennings G, Whitworth JA. Pressor responsiveness in corticosteroid-induced hypertension in humans. *Hypertension* 1992;19:567–574.

Pirpiris M, Yeung S, Dewar E, Jennings GL, Whitworth JA. Hydrocortisone-induced hypertension in men. *Am J Hypertens* 1993;6:287–294.

Rebuffé-Scrive M, Krotkiewski M, Elfverson J, Björntorp P. Muscle and adipose tissue morphology and metabolism in Cushing's syndrome. *J Clin Endocrinol Metab* 1988;67:1122–1128.

Reincke M, Nieke J, Krestin GP, Saeger W, Allolio B, Winkelmann W. Preclinical Cushing's syndrome in adrenal "incidentalomas": Comparison with adrenal Cushing's syndrome. *J Clin Endocrinol Metab* 1992;75:826–832.

Ritchie CM, Sheridan B, Fraser R, Hadden DR, Kennedy AL, Riddell J, Atkinson AB. Studies on the pathogenesis of hypertension in Cushing's disease and acromegaly. *Q J Med* 1990;76:855–867.

Ross EJ, Linch DC. Cushing's syndrome—killing disease: discriminatory value of signs and symptoms aiding early diagnosis. *Lancet* 1982;2:646–649.

Ross EJ, Linch DC. The clinical response to treatment in adult Cushing's syndrome following remission of hypercortisolaemia. *Postgrad Med J* 1985;61:205–211.

Rosseel M, Schoors D. Chewing gum and hypokalaemia. *Lancet* 1993;341:175.

Sanders BP, Portman RJ, Ramey RA, Hill M, Strunk RC. Hypertension during reduction of long-term steroid therapy in young subjects with asthma. *J Allergy Clin Immunol* 1992;89:816–821.

Sandler LM, Richards NT, Carr DH, Mashiter K, Joplin GF. Long term follow-up of patients with Cushing's disease treated by interstitial irradiation. *J Clin Endocrinol Metab* 1987;65:441–447.

Saruta T, Suzuki H, Handa M, Igarashi Y, Kondo K, Senba S. Multiple factors contribute to the pathogenesis of hypertension in Cushing's syndrome. *J Clin Endocrinol Metab* 1986;62:275–279.

Sato A, Suzuki H, Iwaita Y, Nakazato Y, Kato H, Saruta T. Potentiation of inositol trisphosphate production by dexamethasone. *Hypertension* 1992;19:109–115.

Shapiro MS, Shenkman L. Variable hormonogenesis in Cushing's syndrome. *Q J Med* 1991;79:351–363.

Sonino N, Boscaro M, Paoletta A, Mantero F, Ziliotto D. Ketoconazole treatment in Cushing's syndrome: experience in 34 patients. *Clin Endocrinol* 1991;35: 347–352.

Stewart PM, Burra P, Shackleton CHL, Sheppard MC, Elias E. 11β-hydroxysteroid dehydrogenase deficiency and glucocorticoid status in patients with alcoholic and non-alcoholic chronic liver disease. *J Clin Endocrinol Metab* 1993;76:748–751.

Stewart PM, Corrie JET, Shackleton CHL, Edwards CRW. Syndrome of apparent mineralocorticoid excess. A defect in the cortisol-cortisone shuttle. *J Clin Invest* 1988;82:340–349.

Stewart PM, Penn R, Gibson R, Holder R, Parton A, Ratcliffe JG, London DR. Hypothalamic abnormalities in patients with pituitary-dependent Cushing's syndrome. *Clin Endocrinol* 1992;36:453–458.

Stewart PM, Wallace AM, Valentino R, Burt D, Shackleton CHL, Edwards CRW. Mineralocorticoid activity of liquorice: 11-beta-hydroxysteroid dehydrogenase deficiency comes of age. *Lancet* 1987;2: 821–824.

Sugihara N, Shimizu M, Kita Y, Shimizu K, Ino H, Miyamori I, Nakabayashi H, Takeda R. Cardiac characteristics and postoperative courses in Cushing's syndrome. *Am J Cardiol* 1992;69:1475–1480.

Tahir AH, Sheeler LR. Recurrent Cushing's disease after transsphenoidal surgery. *Arch Intern Med* 1992;152:977–981.

Trainer PJ, Grossman A. The diagnosis and differential diagnosis of Cushing's syndrome. *Clin Endocrinol* 1991;34:317–330.

Ulick S, Levine LS, Gunczler P, Zanconato G, Ramirez LC, Rauh W, Rosler A, Bradlow HL, New MI. A syndrome of apparent mineralocorticoid excess associated with defects in the peripheral metabolism of cortisol. *J Clin Endocrinol Metab* 1979;49:757–764.

Ulick S, Tedde R, Mantero F. Pathogenesis of the type 2 variant of the syndrome of apparent mineralocorticoid excess. *J Clin Endocrinol Metab* 1990;70:200–206.

Ulick S, Tedde R, Wang JZ. Defective ring A reduction of cortisol as the major metabolic error in the syndrome of apparent mineralocorticoid excess. *J Clin Endocrinol Metab* 1992a;74:593–599.

Ulick S, Wang JZ, Blumenfeld JD, Pickering TG. Cortisol inactivation overload: a mechanism of mineralocorticoid hypertension in the ectopic adrenocorticotropin syndrome. *J Clin Endocrinol Metab* 1992b;74:963–967.

Välimäki M, Pelkonen R, Porkka L, Sivula A, Kahri A. Long-term results of adrenal surgery in patients with Cushing's syndrome due to adrenocortical adenoma. *Clin Endocrinol* 1984;20:229–236.

van der Lely A-J, Foeken K, van der Mast RC, Lamberts SWJ. Rapid reversal of acute psychosis in the Cushing syndrome with the cortisol-receptor antagonist mifepristone (RU 486). *Ann Intern Med* 1991;114:143–144.

Vierhapper H, Derfler K, Nowotny P, Hollenstein U, Waldhäusl W. Impaired conversion of cortisol to cortisone in chronic renal insufficiency—a cause of hypertension or an epiphenomenon? *Acta Endocrinologica* 1991;125:160–164.

Waldhäusl W, Herkner K, Nowotny P, Bratusch-Marrain P. Combined 17- and 18-hydroxylase deficiency associated with complete male pseudohermaphroditism and hypoaldosteronism. *J Clin Endocrinol Metab* 1978;46:236–246.

Walker BR, Connacher AA, Webb DJ, Edwards CRW. Glucocorticoids and blood pressure: a role for the cortisol/cortisone shuttle in the control of vascular tone in man. *Clin Sci* 1992;83:171–178.

Walker BR, Stewart PM, Shackleton CHL, Padfield PL, Edwards CRW. Deficient inactivation of cortisol by 11β-hydroxysteroid dehydrogenase in essential hypertension. *Clin Endocrinol* 1993;39:221–227.

Werder E, Zachmann M, Völlmin JA, Veyrat P, Prader A. Unusual steroid excretion in a child with low-renin hypertension. *Res Steroids* 1974;6:385–395.

Werner S, Thorén M, Gustafsson J-Å, Brönnegård M. Glucocorticoid receptor abnormalities in fibroblasts from patients with idiopathic resistance to dexamethasone diagnosed when evaluated for adrenocortical disorders. *J Clin Endocrinol Metab* 1992;75:1005–1009.

Whitworth JA. Adrenocorticotrophin and steroid-induced hypertension in humans. *Kidney Int* 1992;41(Suppl 37):34–37.

Wiesen M, Ross F, Krieger DT: Prolonged remission of a case of Cushing's disease following cessation of cyproheptadine therapy. *Acta Endocrinol* 1983;102: 436–438.

Xu Y-M, Chen Z-D, Qiao Y, Jin N-T. The value of adrenal autotransplantation with attached blood vessels for the treatment of Cushing's disease: a preliminary report. *J Urol* 1992;147:1209–1211.

Yasunari K, Kohno M, Murakawa K-i, Yokokawa K, Takeda T. Glucocorticoids and atrial natriuretic factor receptors on vascular smooth muscle. *Hypertension* 1990;16:581–586.

Zachmann M, Tassinari D, Prader A. Clinical and biochemical variability of congenital adrenal hyperplasia due to 11β-hydroxylase deficiency. A study of 25 patients. *J Clin Endocrinol Metab* 1983;56:222–229.

Zadik Z, Kahana L, Kaufman H, Benderli A, Hochberg Z. Salt loss in hypertensive form of congenital adrenal hyperplasia (11-β-hydroxylase deficiency). *J Clin Endocrinol Metab* 1984;58:384–387.

15 Other Forms of Secondary Hypertension

The preceding chapters covered the major types of hypertensive diseases listed in Table 1.6 (Chapter 1), accounting for perhaps 98% of the total. Others that deserve consideration will be covered in this chapter. Coarctation, described in this chapter, and congenital adrenal hyperplasia, covered in Chapter 14, are seen mainly in children; additional coverage of hypertension in childhood follows in Chapter 16.

COARCTATION OF THE AORTA

Constriction of the lumen of the aorta may occur anywhere along its length but most commonly just beyond the origin of the left subclavian artery, at or below the insertion of the ligamentum arteriosum. This lesion makes up about 7% of all congenital heart disease and presents either an infantile or an adult form, differing in pathologic and clinical features. Hypertension in the upper extremities with diminished or absent femoral pulses is the usual presentation (Table 15.1).

Infantile Coarctation

The narrowing involves a larger segment of the aorta and is usually accompanied by serious cardiac anomalies. If the coarctation is proximal to the ductus arteriosus, pulmonary hypertension, congestive failure, and cyanosis of the lower half of the body occur early in life. From 45% to 84% of infants found to have coarctation died during their first year of life (Campbell, 1970), but better results are possible with surgery (Bobby et al., 1991).

Adult Coarctation

Patients born with less severe postductal lesions may have no difficulties during childhood. However, they almost always develop premature cardiovascular disease; in the two largest series of autopsied cases seen prior to effective surgery, the mean age of death was 34 years (Campbell, 1970). The causes of death reflect the load on the heart and the associated cardiac and cerebral lesions:

—Congestive heart failure   25%
—Rupture of the aorta   21%
—Bacterial endocarditis   18%
—Intracranial hemorrhage   11%

Coarctation may affect the abdominal aorta,

Table 15.1. Symptoms and Signs of Coarctation

Symptoms	Signs
Headache	Hypertension Hyperdynamic apical impulse
Cold feet	Murmurs in front or back of chest
Pain in legs with exercise	Pulsations in neck Weak femoral pulse

either as a congenital lesion (Bergqvist et al., 1988) or as an acquired form of arterial fibroplasia (Keech et al., 1988).

Mechanism of Hypertension

Beyond the obvious obstruction to blood flow, the coarctation may lead to a generalized increase in vascular resistance in tissues below the stenosis, suggesting a systemic vasoconstrictor mechanism (Liard and Spadone, 1985). In experimental models, the normotensive vessels below the aorta also thicken (Stacy and Prewitt, 1989), which could explain the persistence of arterial stiffness and hypertension after repair of the lesion (Ong et al., 1992).

In experimental models, the renin-angiotensin system is inappropriately turned on in the presence of an expanded body fluid volume (Bagby and Mass, 1980). In patients, plasma renin levels may not be elevated under basal conditions (Sehested et al., 1983), but both catechol and renin levels may rise excessively during exercise (Ross et al., 1992).

Recognition of Coarctation

Hypertension in the arms with weak femoral pulses in a young person strongly suggests coarctation. With minimal constriction, symptoms may not appear until late in life. Often the heart is large and shows left ventricular strain on the electrocardiogram. The chest radiograph can be diagnostic, with the "3 sign" from dilation of the aorta above and below the constriction and notching of the ribs by enlarged collateral vessels. The diagnosis is now usually made by echocardiography and color Doppler flow mapping (Simpson et al., 1988). Neither magnetic resonance imaging (MRI) nor angiography is usually needed.

Atypical aortic coarctations in adults most likely represent aortitis (Lande, 1976). Takayasu's arteritis, or pulseless disease, usually affects the aortic arch and may also involve the descending aorta (Ishikawa, 1988). This large-vessel vasculitis may be successfully treated with glucocorticoids, cytotoxins, and surgery (Shelhamer et al., 1985).

Management of Coarctation

Surgery

If the disease is associated with other cardiac defects and induces heart failure in the first few weeks of life, early repair is necessary. If the infant is less afflicted, the operation should be performed electively between 6 months and 1 year of age; if postponed, hypertension is more likely to persist despite relief of aortic obstruction. If the disease is milder and no troubles occur during infancy, surgery should be performed before age 9 (Cohen et al., 1989).

Immediately after surgical repair, the blood pressure (BP) may paradoxically rise. In most patients, this is transient and likely represents both renin-angiotensin and sympathetic nervous hyperactivity (Choy et al., 1987). For many, an upper-body hypertensive response to exercise may persist (Cyran et al., 1993).

The long-term outcome of patients following surgery for coarctation is certainly better than it is for those who do not undergo repair, but survival following surgery is less than in the general population (Bobby et al., 1991) (Fig. 15.1). The continuing risks involve arterial aneurysms in various sites, recurrence of coarctation, and persistence or recurrence of hypertension in as many as 70% of patients 30 years or longer after surgery (Clarkson et al., 1983; Stewart et al., 1993). The prevalence of hypertension is related to the age of repair: 7% in patients undergoing surgery as infants but 33% in those undergoing surgery after age 14 (Cohen et al., 1989).

Angioplasty

Balloon dilation angioplasty is being increasingly used and may become the treatment of choice, but concerns about subsequent aneurysm formation persist (Shaddy et al., 1993). Rarely, an acute, severe rise in pressure follows angioplasty (Tani et al., 1993).

HORMONAL DISTURBANCES

Hypothyroidism

Incidence

Among 40 patients prospectively followed over the time they became hypothyroid after radioiodine therapy for thyrotoxicosis, 16 (40%) developed a diastolic BP (DBP) above 90 mm Hg (Streeten et al., 1988). These investigators found hypothyroidism in 3.6% of 688 consecutively seen, referred hypertensive patients; the hypertension was reversed in one-third of these patients given thyroid hormone replacement therapy.

Mechanism of Hypertension

Hypothyroid patients tend to have a low cardiac output due to a fall both in heart rate and in stroke volume. To maintain tissue perfusion,

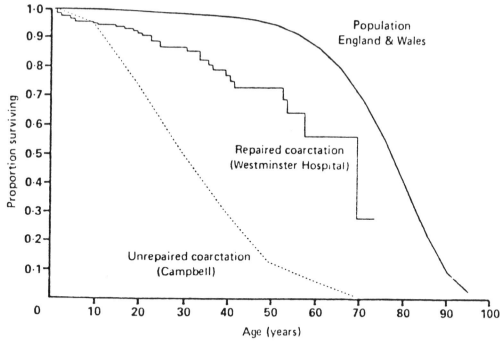

Figure 15.1. Comparative survival, excluding deaths in the first year of life, of the general population of England and Wales, 161 patients with unrepaired coarctation from M. Campbell's 1970 report on the natural history of the disease (*Br Heart J* 1970;32:633–630), and 223 patients surgically repaired at Westminister Hospital between 1946 and 1981. (From Bobby JJ, Emami JM, Farmer RDT, Newman CGH. Operative survival and 40 year follow up of surgical repair of aortic coarctation. *Br Heart J* 1991;65:271–276.)

they have a high peripheral resistance, from a combination of increased responsiveness of alpha-adrenergic receptors and an increased level of sympathetic nervous activity (Fraser et al., 1989). These would tend to raise diastolic pressures more than systolic pressures, the usual pattern seen in hypothyroidism.

Hyperthyroidism

An elevated systolic but lowered diastolic pressure is usual in patients with hyperthyroidism, and is associated with a high cardiac output and reduced peripheral resistance (Fraser et al., 1989).

Hyperparathyroidism

Beyond a possible role for increased levels of parathyroid hormone in the pathogenesis of primary hypertension described in Chapter 3, the presence of autonomous hyperfunction of the parathyroid glands—primary hyperparathyroidism—is associated with at least a doubling of the rate of hypertension, particularly in patients with a parathyroid adenoma (Lind et al., 1991a). From the other perspective, there is an increased prevalence of hyperparathyroidism,

as high as 1%, among patients with hypertension (Rosenthal and Roy, 1972). Patients with previously unrecognized primary hyperparathyroidism may have a sharp rise in plasma calcium levels after thiazide therapy is started; if the calcium level is above 10.5 mg/dl on thiazides and if hypercalcemia persists after the thiazide is stopped, the diagnosis of hyperparathyroidism should be considered.

Mechanism

The interactions between a number of vasoactive calcium-regulating hormones may be involved: vitamin D_3 may constrict vessels, calcitonin gene-related peptide is a potent vasodilator, and a recently described parathyroid hypertensive factor (Benishin et al., 1993) may be increased. Hypercalcemia raises the BP, probably by a direct effect on peripheral resistance that may be caused by an increased vascular reactivity to sympathetic nervous stimulation. Little difference was seen in the renin-aldosterone mechanism and whole-body exchangeable sodium between hypertensive and normotensive hyperparathyroid patients (Salahudeen et al., 1989).

Postoperative Course

After successful correction of the hypercalcemia by removal of a parathyroid adenoma, most find that hypertension does *not* remit (Salahudeen et al., 1989; Dominiczak et al., 1990; Lind et al., 1991b). Others find that it does remit in about half of patients (Diamond et al., 1986). Obviously, the relations between parathyroid disease and BP are complicated (Jespersen et al., 1993).

Pseudohypoparathyroidism

Half of a group of adults with pseudohypoparathyroidism type I, caused by target organ resistance to parathyroid hormone, were hypertensive (Brickman et al., 1988).

Acromegaly

Hypertension is found in about 35% of patients with acromegaly and may disappear when the disease is successfully treated (Fraser et al., 1989). The BP is elevated because of sodium retention caused by the high levels of growth hormone (Ritchie et al., 1990). The volume expansion, in turn, stimulates the secretion of the digitalis-like factor (Deray et al., 1987) postulated to be the natriuretic hormone (see Chapter 3). The heart is enlarged, and cardiac output is increased by 50% (Thuesen et al., 1988).

The diagnosis of acromegaly is made by finding high and usually nonsuppressible levels of growth hormone and insulin-like growth factor I (Melmed, 1990).

Acromegaly remains difficult to cure: the best results are with trans-sphenoidal surgery (Melmed, 1990). The somatostatin analogue octreotide may provide long-term suppression of growth hormone secretion and clinical improvement (James et al., 1992).

Carcinoid Syndrome

Among 34 patients with carcinoid, 9 had hypertension, and most of these had significant renal damage (Schwartz, 1970). In most patients, however, the BP is not high; occasionally hypotension may be noted (Klein and Ojamaa, 1992).

SLEEP APNEA

Sleep apnea may be one of the more frequent causes of reversible hypertension, likely more common than the various adrenal hyperfunction states that have received so much more attention. Among habitual loud snorers, who frequently have sleep apnea, hypertension is perhaps 3 times more common than among nonsnorers (Gislason et al., 1993).

Repetitive loud snoring followed by silent periods of apnea usually represents the syndrome of obstructive sleep apnea (OSA). OSA in turn is associated with a higher prevalence of persistent hypertension (Levinson and Millman, 1991) and a significantly greater risk of coronary disease (Hung et al., 1990) and stroke (Palomäki, 1991). Moreover, patients with OSA have more left ventricular hypertrophy (Hedner et al., 1990), dilated cardiomyopathy (Malone et al., 1991), and resistance to antihypertensive therapy (Isaksson and Svanborg, 1991). Many of these relationships may mainly reflect the presence of obesity.

Definition and Prevalence

Sleep apnea is usually defined as the occurrence of at least five periods of respiratory cessation lasting 10 or more seconds per hour. Three types have been defined: *central* sleep apnea, wherein no breathing efforts occur; the most common form, *obstructive*, wherein breathing efforts continue but, because of upper airway obstruction, air movement ceases; and *mixed*, wherein both central and obstructive elements are present. About 4% of adult men and 2% of adult women have sleep apnea (Young et al., 1993).

Clinical Features

The syndrome can only be diagnosed with certainty by an overnight sleep study involving continuous recordings of respiration, electroencephalogram (EEG), electromyograph (EMG), and eye movements along with electrocardiogram (ECG) and oxygen saturation measurements (Fig. 15.2) (Levinson and Millman, 1991).

The syndrome should be suspected in any patient who snores loudly, particularly overweight, middle-aged men who have repetitive episodes of gasping, choking, or loud snorting during sleep (often only recognized by the patient's bed partner) that are often accompanied by excessive daytime sleepiness and morning headaches. The presence of repetitive bradycardia (during apnea) and tachycardia (when breathing restarts) on a nighttime continuous ECG monitor may be a tip-off to the diagnosis. Although the history and physical examination will only identify about half of patients with OSA, the routine examinations can be used to indicate the need for nighttime oximetry studies

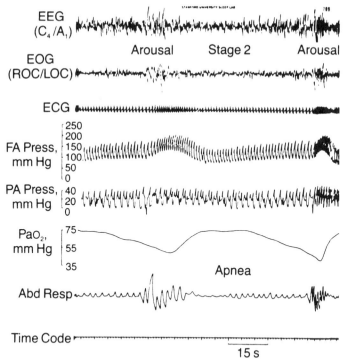

Figure 15.2. Direct polygraphic recording during sleep of repetitive obstructive apnea showing the cyclic variations in pressures, Pao₂, and heart rate. Airflow is represented in the abdominal respiration *(Abd Resp)* recording by exaggerated amplitude of abdominal excursions. *EEG*, electroencephalogram; *EOG*, electro-oculogram; *ECG*, electrocardiogram; *FA Press*, femoral artery pressure; *PA Press*, pulmonary artery pressure. (From Levinson PD, Millman RP. Causes and consequences of blood pressure alterations in obstructive sleep apnea. *Arch Intern Med* 1991;151:455–462.)

or, for a small number, a complete (and expensive) sleep study (Viner et al., 1991).

The prevalence of daytime hypertension in patients with OSA varies widely in different series but is almost certainly increased over the general population (Levinson and Millman, 1991). However, the obesity that almost always accompanies OSA is more closely correlated to the higher prevalence of hypertension than is sleep apnea (Rauscher et al., 1992).

Mechanism of Hypertension

As seen in Figure 15.2, systemic and pulmonary BPs rise with each episode of apnea. The hypoxemia that develops during apnea has been shown to be related to the rise in BP by some researchers (van den Aardweg and Karemaker, 1992) but not by others (Ringler et al., 1990). The frequency of snoring but not the degree of oxygen saturation was correlated with BP during sleep, each period of snoring ablating the normal fall in pressure associated with slow-wave sleep (Mateika et al., 1992). The scheme shown in

Figure 15.3 is supported by data (Somers et al., 1992) but many connections have not been established.

Treatment

Persons who are massively overweight or who have obvious obstructive defects in the upper airways may get relief from weight loss and nasal continuous positive airway pressure (nCPAP) with an accompanying decrease in BP (Mayer et al., 1991). The 5-HT reuptake inhibitor fluoxetine, by abolishing REM sleep, improved nocturnal oxygenation in 11 asymptomatic, extremely obese subjects with sleep hypoventilation (Kopelman et al., 1992). Corrective surgery may be needed for patients with severe sleep apnea, and it may be followed by prompt and dramatic relief of hypertension (Kaplan and Staats, 1990).

NEUROLOGIC DISORDERS

A number of seemingly different disorders of the central and peripheral nervous system may

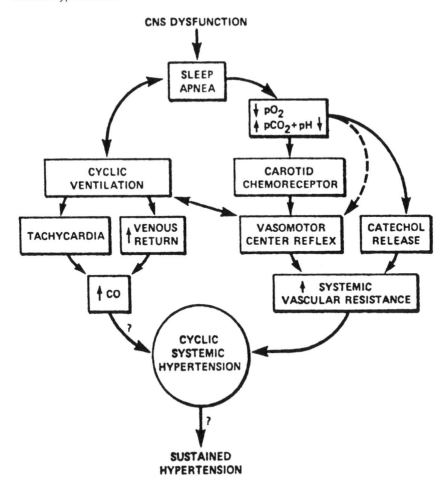

Figure 15.3. Proposed mechanism for cyclic systemic hypertension with sleep apnea that may lead to sustained hypertension. (From Schroeder JS, Motta J, Guilleminault C. *Sleep Apnea Syndromes.* New York: Alan R. Liss, 1978:191.)

cause hypertension. Many may do so by a common mechanism involving sympathetic nervous system discharge from the vasomotor centers in response to an increased intracranial pressure. The rise in systemic pressure is useful in restoring cerebral perfusion (Plets, 1989).

Unlike the situation in many neurologic diseases, hypertension is *less* common in patients with Alzheimer's disease, apparently receding as the process worsens even without an associated weight loss (Garbarino et al., 1989).

As noted in Chapters 4 and 7, patients with acute stroke may have transient marked elevations in BP. Rarely, episodic hypertension suggestive of a pheochromocytoma may occur after cerebral infarction (Funck-Brentano et al., 1987).

Brain Tumors

Intracranial tumors, especially those arising in the posterior fossa, may cause hypertension.

In some patients, paroxysmal hypertension and other features that suggest catecholamine excess may point mistakenly to the diagnosis of pheochromocytoma (Bell and Doig, 1983). The problem may be confounded by the increased incidence of neuroectodermal tumors, some within the central nervous system in patients with pheochromocytoma. Unlike patients with a pheochromocytoma who always have high catechol levels, patients with a brain tumor may have increased catecholamines during a paroxysm of hypertension but normal levels at other times.

Quadriplegia

Patients with transverse lesions of the cervical spinal cord above the origins of the thoracolumbar sympathetic neurons lose central control of their sympathetic outflow. Stimulation of nerves below the injury, as with bladder or bowel distension, may cause reflex sympathetic activity via the isolated spinal cord, inducing hypertension, sweating, flushing, piloerection, and headache, a syndrome described as autonomic hyperreflexia. Such patients have markedly exaggerated pressor responses to various stimuli (Krum et al., 1992).

The hypertension may be so severe and persistent as to cause cerebral vascular accidents and death. During hypertensive episodes in five patients whose mean arterial BP rose from 95 to 154, the heart rate fell from 72 to 45, cardiac output was unchanged, and peripheral resistance rose markedly (Naftchi et al., 1978). Plasma volume was reduced by 10% to 15%, which may explain the propensity of these patients to develop hypotension when the hypertensive stimulus is removed.

Severe Head Injury

Immediately after severe head injury, the BP may rise because of a hyperdynamic state mediated by excessive sympathetic nervous activity (Simard and Bellefleur, 1989). If the hypertension is persistent and severe, a short-acting beta blocker (e.g., esmolol) should be given. Caution is needed in the use of vasodilators such as hydralazine and nitroprusside, which may increase cerebral blood flow and intracranial pressure (Van Aken et al., 1989).

Other Neurologic Disorders

Hypertension related to high catechol levels may occur during Guillain-Barré syndrome (Ventura et al., 1986). Meningitis and other acute neurologic diseases may cause transient hypertension (Fan-Havard et al., 1992). Paroxysmal hypertension may develop after sinoaortic baroreceptor denervation (Aksamit et al., 1987) or dysfunction (Kuchel et al., 1987). Severe volatile hypertension has been described in patients with baroreceptor failure, with excellent control by clonidine (Robertson et al., 1993).

PSYCHOGENIC HYPERVENTILATION

During acute hyperventilation (Todd et al., 1993) or panic attacks (White and Baker, 1987), the BP may rise acutely and significantly. The recurrent spells, often associated with tremor, tachycardia, and headache, may suggest a pheochromocytoma. Even more commonly, hyperventilation is responsible for many of the symptoms noted by recently discovered hypertensives who are anxious over their diagnosis. Along with the symptoms, hyperventilation may cause myocardial and vascular contractions, leading to coronary spasm (DeGuire et al., 1992), as well as to a rise in systemic BP (Fig. 15.4).

ACUTE STRESS

Hypertension may appear during various acute stresses, usually reflecting an intense sympathetic discharge and sometimes the contribution of increased renin-angiotensin from volume contraction. Problems related to anesthesia and surgery are covered in Chapter 7.

Medical Conditions

Significant hypertension has been observed in patients with various medical conditions, including:

—Hypoglycemia, particularly if it develops in diabetics receiving noncardioselective beta blockers, wherein alpha-mediated vasoconstriction may be unopposed (Lloyd-Mostyn and Oram, 1975);

—Acute pancreatitis (Greenstein et al., 1987);

—Acute intermittent porphyria (Church et al., 1992);

—After exposure to cold (Wilmhurst et al., 1989).

Surgical Conditions

Burns

Hypertension appears in about 25% of patients with significant second- and third-degree burns (Brizio-Molteni et al., 1979). The BP usually rises within 3 to 5 days, may last 2 weeks, and occasionally induces encephalopathy (Lowrey, 1967).

Perioperative Hypertension

In addition to those mentioned in the coverage of anesthesia and hypertension in Chapter 7, there are numerous reasons why hypertension may be a problem during and soon after surgery. For example, the application of a tourniquet during lower limb surgery was accompanied by hypertension in 11% of patients (Kaufman and Walts, 1982). In 60 patients with transient postoperative readings in excess of 190/100 in the recovery room, the probable causes were pain (36%), hypoxia and hypercarbia (19%), and physical and emotional excitement (32%) (Gal and Cooperman, 1975).

Cardiovascular Surgery

Hypertension may accompany various cardiovascular surgical procedures for various reasons (Estafanous and Tarazi, 1980) (Table 15.2).

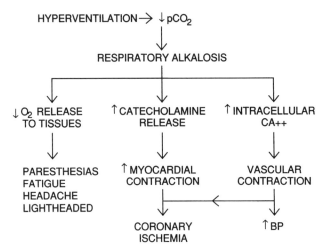

Figure 15.4. The mechanisms by which acute hyperventilation may induce various symptoms, coronary ischemia, and a rise in blood pressure.

Table 15.2. Hypertension Associated with Cardiac Surgery[a]

Preoperative
Anxiety, angina, etc.
Discontinuation of antihypertensive therapy
"Rebound" from beta blockers in patients with coronary artery disease

Intraoperative
Induction of anesthesia: tracheal intubation; nasopharyngeal, urethral, or rectal manipulation
Precardiopulmonary bypass (during sternotomy and chest retraction)
Cardiopulmonary bypass
Postcardiopulmonary bypass (during surgery)

Postoperative
Early—within 2 hours
    Obvious cause: hypoxia, hypercarbia, ventilatory difficulties, hypothermia, shivering, arousal
        from anesthesia
    With no obvious cause: after myocardial revascularization; less frequently after valve
        replacement; after resection of aortic coarctation
Late—weeks to months: after aortic valve replacement by homografts

[a]Data from Estafanous FG, Tarazi RC. *Am J Cardiol* 1980;46:685.

Coronary Bypass. About one-third of patients will have hypertension after coronary artery bypass grafting (CABG), usually starting within the first 2 postoperative hours and lasting 4 to 6 hours (Colvin and Kenny, 1989). The hypertension reflects an increase in peripheral resistance resulting from sympathetic overactivity (Cooper et al., 1985). Immediate therapy may be important to prevent postoperative heart failure or myocardial infarction. Besides stellate ganglion blockade, various parenteral antihypertensives have been found to work, including nitroprusside, nitroglycerin (Colvin and Kenny, 1989), trimethapan (Corr et al., 1986), nifedipine (van Wezel et al., 1987), labetalol (Orlowski et al., 1989), and esmolol (Gray et al., 1987).

Other Cardiac Surgery. Hypertension may also occur, though less frequently, after other operations on the heart, including closure of atrial septal defects (Cockburn et al., 1975) and valve replacement (Estafanous et al., 1978). Closure of a peripheral arteriovenous shunt may precipitate acute hypertension by various mechanisms, including activation of the renin-angiotensin mechanism (Rocchini et al., 1978).

Virtually all patients who undergo heart transplant develop hypertension and lose the usual nocturnal fall in pressure, likely from cyclosporine-induced generalized sympathetic activation that may be accentuated by the cardiac denervation (Scherrer et al., 1990). Despite higher BP and increased body weight, left ventricular mass may decrease and remain normal, perhaps because of the absence of cardiac sympathetic innervation, which may be needed for hypertrophy to develop (Leenen et al., 1991). The hypertension of fewer than half of patients was effectively controlled by either a calcium antagonist or an ACE inhibitor in the study of Brozena et al. (1993).

Carotid Endarterectomy. Postoperative hypertension may be particularly serious in patients with known cerebrovascular disease who have carotid endarterectomy, perhaps because of sudden exposure of the damaged intracerebral vessels to both high pressure and blood flow (Caplan et al., 1978). Treatment most logically should be with a short-acting beta blocker (esmolol) or labetalol (Orlowski et al., 1988) rather than with a vasodilator that might further increase cerebral blood flow.

INCREASED INTRAVASCULAR VOLUME

If vascular volume is raised a significant degree over a short period, the renal natriuretic response may not be able to excrete the load, particularly if renal function is also impaired.

Erythropoietin Therapy

Recombinant human erythropoietin is now being widely used to correct the anemia of chronic renal failure. As the hematocrit rises, so do blood viscosity and BP; 21% of patients developed clinically important hypertension in one study (Abraham and Macres, 1991). There is a need to correct the anemia slowly so as not to induce such severe, even malignant, hypertension, which may mandate phlebotomy (Fahal et al., 1992).

Polycythemia

Patients with primary polycythemia are often hypertensive, and some hypertensives have a relative polycythemia that may go away when the BP is lowered (Chrysant et al., 1976). A high hematocrit may significantly reduce cerebral blood flow, which puts the patient at additional risk (Hudak et al., 1986). With venesection and a fall in hematocrit, cerebral blood flow increases (Humphrey et al., 1979).

Hyperviscosity

The hypertension seen in polycythemic states could also reflect increased blood viscosity. One striking example of malignant hypertension has been reported in a patient with marked hyperviscosity caused by myeloma (Rubio-Garcia et al., 1989).

After Transfusions and Marrow Transplants

A syndrome of hypertension, convulsions, and cerebral hemorrhage was seen in eight patients with thalassemia after multiple blood transfusions (Wasi et al., 1978). Since the episodes often developed days after the transfusions, they were considered not to reflect volume overload, but rather the presence of unknown vasopressor substances. Similar episodes have been reported in others receiving multiple transfusions, particularly in the presence of renal insufficiency (Eggert and Stick, 1988).

Hypertension has developed after autologous bone marrow transplantation (Sugarman et al., 1990) and is seen in 75% of those who are given cyclosporine and other immunosuppressants with allogenic bone marrow transplants (Kone et al., 1988).

Inappropriate Antidiuretic Hormone

Hypertension has been reported in patients with inappropriate secretion of antidiuretic hormone, and is presumably related to an overexpanded vascular volume (Whitaker et al., 1979).

DRUGS AND OTHER SUBSTANCES THAT CAUSE HYPERTENSION

A variety of drugs, a few foods, and poisons may cause hypertension in various ways (Oren et al., 1988) (Table 15.3). Some of these substances, such as sodium-containing antacids, alcohol, insulin, licorice, oral contraceptives, and monoamine oxidase inhibitors, are covered elsewhere because of their frequency or special features.

Drugs

Cyclosporine

The introduction of this fungal metabolite in 1983 greatly improved the long-term survival of patients undergoing organ transplants. However, two major complications soon became obvious: nephrotoxicity and hypertension, and the two were assumed to be connected (Porter et al., 1990).

Hypertension develops in half or more of the patients who receive cyclosporin for immunosuppression after renal transplantation or treatment of various autoimmune diseases (Deray et al., 1992). On the other hand, virtually all

Table 15.3. Hypertension Induced by Chemical Agents

Mechanism	Examples
Expansion of fluid volume	
Increased sodium intake	Antacids, processed foods (Chapter 6)
Mineralocorticoid effects	Licorice (Chapter 13), cortisone (Chapter 14), anabolic steroids (Kuipers et al., 1991)
Stimulation of renin-angiotensin	Estrogens (oral contraceptives) (Chapter 11)
Inhibition of prostaglandins	Nonsteroidal anti-inflammatory agents (Oates et al., 1988)
Stimulation of sympathetic nervous activity	
Sympathomimetic agents	Cocaine (Om, 1992)
	Nose drops: phenylephrine (Saken et al., 1979)
	Nasal decongestants: pseudoephedrine (Chua et al., 1991)
	Appetite suppressants: phenylpropanolamine (Lake et al., 1990)
	Methylphenidate (Ritalin) (Ballard et al., 1976)
	Phencyclidine (Sernulan) (Eastman and Cohen, 1975)
Interactions with monamine oxidase inhibitors	Foods with high tyramine content (red wines, aged cheese, etc.) (Liu and Rustgi, 1987)
	Sympathomimetics (Thomas et al., 1991)
Anesthetics	Ketamine (Pipkin and Waldron, 1983)
Narcotic antagonist	Naloxone (Levin et al., 1985)
Ergot alkaloids	Ergometrine (Browning, 1974)
Dopamine receptor agonist	Bromocriptine (Parlodel) (ADR, 1983)
Antidopaminergic	Metoclopamide (Roche et al., 1985)
Interference with antihypertensive drugs	
Inhibition of prostaglandin synthesis	Nonsteroidal anti-inflammatory drugs (Oates et al., 1988)
Inhibition of neuronal uptake (block guanethidine, clonidine, methyldopa)	Tricyclic antidepressants (van Zwieten, 1975)
Paradoxical response to antihypertensive drugs	
Withdrawal, followed by increased catechols	Clonidine (Metz et al., 1987)
Unopposed alpha-adrenergic vasoconstriction	Beta blockers (Drayer et al., 1976)
Intrinsic sympathomimetic activity	Pindolol (Collins and King, 1972)
Combination of beta blocker and alpha agonist	Propranolol plus clonidine (Warren et al., 1979) or methyldopa (Nies and Shand; 1973)
Unknown mechanisms	
Heavy metal poisoning	Lead (Bertel et al., 1978)
	Thallium (Bank et al., 1972
Chemicals	Ethylene glycol dinitrate (Carmichael and Lieben, 1963)
	Methyl chloride (Scharnweber et al., 1974)
	Polychlorinated biphenyl (Kreiss et al., 1981)
Insecticides	Parathion (Tsachalinas et al., 1971)
Insect bites	Spiders (Weitzman et al., 1977)
	Scorpion (Gueron and Yaron, 1970)
Diagnostic agents	Indigo carmine (Wu and Johnson, 1969)
	Pentagastrin (Merguet et al., 1968)
	Thyrotropin-releasing hormone (Rosenthal et al., 1987)
Therapeutic agents	Lithium (Michaeli et al., 1984)
	Digitalis (Cohn et al., 1969)
	Cyclosporine (Porter et al., 1990)
	Disulfiram (Volicer and Nelson, 1984)
	Eryropoietin (Abraham and Macres, 1991)

patients given the drug after a heart transplant develop hypertension, possibly reflecting the inability of the denervated heart to respond to the increased sympathetic activity induced by cyclosporine (Scherrer et al., 1990).

The mechanisms for cyclosporine-induced hypertension have been found to include marked renal vasoconstriction (Garr and Paller, 1990), activation of the sympathetic nervous system (Scherrer et al., 1990), inhibition of endothelium-derived relaxation (Richards et al., 1990), increased calcium influx (Meyer-Lehnert and Schrier, 1989), volume retention with suppression of renin-angiotensin (Curtis et al., 1988), and perhaps other mechanisms (Luke, 1991).

Control of the elevated BP may be essential for preservation of transplant function and long-term cardiovascular health. Diuretics may be useful but, particularly in renal transplant patients, may accentuate the underlying increased propensity to urate retention and gout (Lin et al., 1989). The hemodynamic profile of volume expansion with suppressed renin and increased peripheral vascular resistance with sympathetic overactivity recommends the use of vasodilators and sympatholytics rather than beta blockers or angiotensin-converting enzyme (ACE) inhibitors. Preliminary evidence from controlled trials suggests that calcium entry blockers (CEBs) are effective but no more so than ACE inhibitors (Castelao et al., 1992). A combination of CEB and beta blocker was effective in a group of renal transplant recipients (Brouwer et al., 1992).

Other Drugs

Perhaps the most commonly encountered form of chemically induced hypertension is that related to the use of foods and drugs containing large amounts of sodium. More dramatic effects will be seen with the use of sympathomimetic agents. Large amounts of these drugs, available over-the-counter for use as nasal decongestants (e.g., pseudoephrine) and appetite suppressants (e.g., phenylpropanolamine), may raise the BP enough to induce, on rare occasions, hypertensive encephalopathy, strokes, and heart attacks (Lake et al., 1990).

The multiple interferences with the effectiveness of various antihypertensive agents are covered in Chapter 7. With increasing use of prostaglandin inhibitors, the possibility of interference with the effects of virtually all antihypertensive drugs (Oates et al., 1988) should be kept in mind. Tricyclic antidepressants may induce postural hypotension or supine hypertension and interfere with the antihypertensive effect of certain drugs (Walsh et al., 1992).

Perhaps the safest way to prevent these various interactions and interferences is to advise hypertensives to avoid all over-the-counter drugs and to inform their physicians who prescribe other medications about their antihypertensive drug regimens.

Street Drugs

Marijuana, or delta-9-tetrahydrocannabinol (THC), in moderate amounts will increase the heart rate but usually lowers the BP (Hollister, 1986).

Heroin and other drugs taken intravenously may lead to severe renal damage, likely from an immunologic response (Rao et al., 1974).

Cocaine and amphetamines may cause transient but significant hypertension that may cause strokes (Kaku and Lowenstein, 1990) and serious cardiac damage (Om, 1992). Most cocaine-related deaths are associated with myocardial injury similar to that seen from catecholamine excess and aggravated by acute hypertension.

The next and last chapter, written by Dr. Ellin Lieberman, looks further at hypertension in children and adolescents.

References

Abraham PA, Macres MG. Blood pressure in hemodialysis patients during amelioration of anemia with erythropoietin. *J Am Soc Nephrol* 1991;2:927–936.

ADR Highlight No. 83-12, FDA (HFN-730), 5600 Fishers La., Rockville, MD 20857, 1983.

Aksamit TR, Floras JS, Victor RG, Aylward PE. Paroxysmal hypertension due to sinoaortic baroreceptor denervation in humans. *Hypertension* 1987;9:309–314.

Bagby SP, Mass RD. Abnormality of the renin/body-fluid-volume relationship in serially-studied inbred dogs with neonatally-induced coarctation hypertension. *Hypertension* 1980;2:631–642.

Ballard JE, Boileau RA, Sleator EK, Massey BH, Sprague RL. Cardiovascular responses of hyperactive children to methylphenidate. *JAMA* 1976;236:2870–2874.

Bank WJ, Pleasure DE, Suzuki K, Nigro M, Katz R. Thallium poisoning. *Arch Neurol* 1972;26:456–464.

Bell GM, Doig A. Hypertension and intracranial tumor. In: Robertson JIS, ed. *Handbook of Hypertension, Clinical Aspects of Secondary Hypertension.* New York: Elsevier, 1983:291–303.

Benishin CG, Labedz T, Guo DD, Lewanczuk RZ, Pang PKT. Identification and purification of parathyroid hypertensive factor from organ culture of parathyroid glands from spontaneously hypertensive rats. *Am J Hypertens* 1993;6:134–140.

Bergqvist D, Bergentz S-E, Ekberg M, Jonsson K, Takolander R. Coarctation of the abdominal aorta in elderly patients. *Acta Med Scand* 1988;223:275–280.

Bertel O, Buhler FR, Ott J. Lead-induced hypertension: blunted beta-adrenoreceptor-mediated functions. *Br Med J* 1978;1:551.

Bobby JJ, Emami JM, Farmer RDT, Newman CGH. Operative survival and 40 year follow up of surgical repair of aortic coarctation. *Br Heart J* 1991;65:271–276.

Brickman AS, Stern N, Sowers JR. Hypertension in pseudohypoparathyroidism type I. *Am J Med* 1988;85:785–792.

Brizio-Molteni L, Molteni A, Cloutier LC, Rainey S. Incidence of post burn hypertensive crisis in patients admitted to two burn centers and a community hospital in the United States. *Scand J Plast Reconstr Surg* 1979;13:21–28.

Brozena SC, Johnson MR, Ventura JO, Naftel DC. Effectiveness of diltiazem or lisinopril for treatment of hypertension in cardiac transplant patients: a prospective, randomized multi-center trial [Abstract]. *Circulation* 1993;88(Part 2):480.

Brouwer RML, Wenting GJ, Schalekamp MADH, Man in 't Veld AJ. Diurnal blood pressure load and control in cyclosporine treated hypertensive renal transplant recipients [Abstract]. *J Hypertens* 1992; 10(Suppl 4):132.

Browning DJ. Serious side effects of ergometrine and its use in routine obstetric practice. *Med J Aust* 1974;1:957–959.

Campbell M. Natural history of coarctation of the aorta. *Br Heart J* 1970;32:633–640.

Caplan LR, Skillman J, Ojemann R, Fields WS. Intracerebral hemorrhage following carotid endarterectomy: a hypertensive complication. *Stroke* 1978;9:457–460.

Carmichael P, Lieben J. Sudden death in explosives workers. *Arch Environ Health* 1963;7:424–439.

Castelao AM, Grino JM, Galceran JM, Andres E, GilVernet S, Amenos M, Seron D, Alsina J. Verapamil vs enalapril in the treatment of hypertension (Hy) of kidney transplanted patients (KTP) under cyclosporin A (CsA) immunosuppression. A randomized study [Abstract]. *J Hypertens* 1992;10(Suppl 4):136.

Choy M, Rocchini AP, Beekman RH, Rosenthal A, Dick M, Crowley D, Behrendt D, Snider AR. Paradoxical hypertension after repair of coarctation of the aorta in children: balloon angioplasty versus surgical repair. *Circulation* 1987;75:1186–1191.

Chrysant SG, Frohlich ED, Adamopoulos PN, Stein PD, Whitcomb WH, Allen EW, Neller G. Pathophysiologic significance of "stress" or relative polycythemia in essential hypertension. *Am J Cardiol* 1976;37:1069–1072.

Chua SS, Benrimoj SI, Gordon RD, Williams G. Cardiovascular effects of a chlorpheniramine/paracetamol combination in hypertensive patients who were sensitive to the pressor effect of pseudoephedrine. *Br J Clin Pharmacol* 1991;31:360–362.

Church SE, McColl KEL, Moore MR, Youngs GR. Hypertension and renal impairment as complications of acute porphyria. *Nephrol Dial Transplant* 1992;7:986–990.

Clarkson PM, Nicholson MR, Barratt-Boyes BG, Neutze JM, Whitlock RM. Results after repair of coarctation of the aorta beyond infancy: a 10 to 28 year follow-up with particular reference to late systemic hypertension. *Am J Cardiol* 1983;51:1481–1488.

Cockburn JS, Benjamin IS, Thomson RM, Bain WH. Early systemic hypertension after surgical closure of atrial septal defect. *J Cardiovasc Surg* 1975;16:1–7.

Cohen M, Fuster V, Steele PM. Coarctation of the aorta. Long-term follow-up and prediction of outcome after surgical correction. *Circulation* 1989;80:840–845.

Cohn JN, Tristani FE, Khatri IM. Cardiac and peripheral vascular effects of digitalis in clinical cardiogenic shock. *Am Heart J* 1969;78:318–330.

Collins IS, King IW. Pindolol (Visken LB46): A new treatment for hypertension: report of a multicentric open study. *Curr Ther Res* 1972;14:185–194.

Colvin JR, Kenny GNC. Automatic control of arterial pressure after cardiac surgery. *Anaesthesia* 1989;44:37–41.

Cooper TJ, Clutton-Brock TH, Jones SN, Tinker J, Treasure T. Factors relating to the development of hypertension after cardiopulmonary bypass. *Br Heart J* 1985;54:91–95.

Corr L, Grounds RM, Brown MJ, Whitwam JG. Plasma catecholamine changes during cardiopulmonary bypass: a randomised double blind comparison of trimetaphan camsylate and sodium nitroprusside. *Br Heart J* 1986;56:89–93.

Curtis JJ, Luke RG, Jones P, Diethelm AG. Hypertension in cyclosporine-treated renal transplant recipients is sodium dependent. *Am J Med* 1988;85:134–138.

Cyran SE, Grzeszczak M, Kaufman K, Weber HS, Myers JL, Gleason MM, Baylen BG. Aortic "recoarctation" at rest versus at exercise in children as evaluated by stress doppler echocardiography after a "good" operative result. *Am J Cardiol* 1993;71:963–970.

DeGuire S, Gevirtz R, Kawahara Y, Maguire W. Hyperventilation syndrome and the assessment of treatment for functional cardiac symptoms. *Am J Cardiol* 1992;70:673–677.

Deray G, Benhmida M, Hoang PL, Maksud P, Aupetit B, Baumelou A, Jacobs C. Renal function and blood pressure in patients receiving long-term, low-dose cyclosporine therapy for idiopathic autoimmune uveitis. *Ann Intern Med* 1992;117:578–583.

Deray G, Rieu M, Devynck MA, Pernollet MG, Chanson P, Luton JP, Meyer P. Evidence of an endogenous digitalis-like factor in the plasma of patients with acromegaly. *N Engl J Med* 1987;316:575–580.

Diamond TW, Botha JR, Wing J, Meyers AM, Kalk WJ. Parathyroid hypertension. A reversible disorder. *Arch Intern Med* 1986;146:1709–1712.

Dominiczak AF, Lyall F, Morton JJ, Dargie HJ, Boyle IT, Tune TT, Murray G, Semple PF. Blood pressure, left ventricular mass and intracellular calcium in primary hyperparathyroidism. *Clin Sci* 1990;78:127–132.

Drayer JIM, Keim JH, Weber MA, Case DB, Laragh JH. Unexpected pressor response to propranolol in essential hypertension: an interaction between renin-aldosterone and sympathetic activity. *Am J Med* 1976;60:897–893.

Eastman JW, Cohen SN. Hypertensive crisis and death associated with phencyclidine poisoning. *JAMA* 1975;231:1270–1271.

Eggert P, Stick C. Blood pressure increase after erythrocyte transfusion in end-stage renal disease. *Lancet* 1988;1:1343–1344.

Estafanous FG, Tarazi RC. Systemic arterial hypertension associated with cardiac surgery. *Am J Cardiol* 1980;46:685–694.

Estafanous FG, Tarazi RC, Buckley S, Taylor PC. Arterial hypertension in immediate postoperative period after valve replacement. *Br Heart J* 1978;40:718–724.

Fahal IH, Yaqoob M, Ahmad R. Phlebotomy for erythropoietin-induced malignant hypertension. *Nephron* 1992;61:214–216.

Fan-Havard P, Yamaguchi E, Smith SM, Eng RHK. Diastolic hypertension in AIDS patients with cryptococcal meningitis. *Am J Med* 1992;93:347–348.

Findlay JC, Sheeler LR, Engeland WC, Aron DC. Familial adrenocorticotropin-independent Cushing's Syndrome with bilateral macronodular adrenal hyperplasia. *J Clin Endocrinol Metab* 1993;76:189–191.

Fraser R, Davies DL, Connel JMC. Hormones and hypertension. *Clin Endocrinol* 1989;31:701–746.

Funck-Brentano C, Pagny J-Y, Menard J. Neurogenic hypertension associated with an excessively high excretion rate of catecholamine metabolites. *Br Heart J* 1987;57:487–489.

Gal TJ, Cooperman LH. Hypertension in the immediate postoperative period. *Br J Anaesth* 1975;47:70–74.

Garbarino KA, Levitt JR, Feinsod FM. Resolution of systemic hypertension in Alzheimer's disease. *Am J Med* 1989;86:734–735.

Garr MD, Paller MS. Cyclosporine augments renal but not systemic vascular reactivity. *Am J Physiol* 1990;258:F211–F217.

Gislason T, Benediktsdóttir B, Björnsson JK, Kjartansson G, Kjeld M, Kristbjarnarson H. Snoring, hypertension, and the sleep apnea syndrome. *Chest* 1993;103:1147–1151.

Gray RJ, Bateman TM, Czer LSC, Conklin C, Matloff JM. Comparison of esmolol and nitroprusside for acute post-cardiac surgical hypertension. *Am J Cardiol* 1987;59:887–891.

Greenstein RJ, Krakoff LR, Felton K. Activation of the renin system in acute pancreatitis. *Am J Med* 1987;82:401–404.

Gueron M, Yaron R. Cardiovascular manifestations of severe scorpion sting. *Chest* 1970;57:156–162.

Hedner J, Ejnell H, Caidahl K. Left ventricular hypertrophy independent of hypertension in patients with obstructive sleep apnoea. *J Hypertens* 1990;8:941–946.

Hollister LE. Health aspects of cannabis. *Pharmacol Rev* 1986;38:1–20.

Hudak ML, Koehler RC, Rosenberg AA, Traystman RJ, Jones MD Jr. Effect of hematocrit on cerebral blood flow. *Am J Physiol* 1986;251:H63–H70.

Humphrey PRD, Marshall J, Russell RWR, Wetherley-Mein G, Du Boulay GH, Pearson TC, Symon L, Zilkha E. Cerebral blood-flow and viscosity in relative polycythaemia. *Lancet* 1979;3:873–877.

Hung J, Whitford EG, Parsons RW, Hillman DR. Association of sleep apnoea with myocardial infarction in men. *Lancet* 1990;336:261–264.

Isaksson H, Svanborg E. Obstructive sleep apnea syndrome in male hypertensives, refractory to drug therapy. Nocturnal automatic blood pressure measurements—an aid to diagnosis? *Clin Exp Hypertens [A]* 1991;13:1195–1212.

Ishikawa K. Diagnostic approach and proposed criteria for the clinical diagnosis of Takayasu's arteriopathy. *J Am Coll Cardiol* 1988;12:964–972.

James RA, White MC, Chatterjee S, Marciaj H, Kendall-Taylor P. A comparison of octreotide delivered by continuous subcutaneous infusion with intermittent injection in the treatment of acromegaly. *Eur J Clin Invest* 1992;22:554–561.

Jespersen B, Brock A, Charles P, Danielsen H, Sørensen SS, Pedersen EB. Unchanged noradrenaline reactivity and blood pressure after corrective surgery in primary hyperparathyroidism. *Scand J Clin Lab Invest* 1993;53:470–486.

Kaku DA, Lowenstein DH. Emergence of recreational drug abuse as a major risk factor for stroke in young adults. *Ann Intern Med* 1990;113:821–827.

Kaplan J, Staats BA. Obstructive sleep apnea syndrome. *Mayo Clin Proc* 1990;65: 1087–1094.

Kaufman RD, Walts LF. Tourniquet-induced hypertension. *Br J Anaesth* 1982;54:333–336.

Keech AC, Westlake GW, Wallis PL, Hamer AWF. An acquired case of aortic coarctation. *Am Heart J* 1988;115:1328–1332.

Klein I, Ojamaa K. Cardiovascular manifestations of endocrine disease. *J Clin Endocrinol Metab* 1992;75:339–342.

Kone BC, Whelton A, Santos G, Saral R, Watson AJ. Hypertension and renal dysfunction in bone marrow transplant recipients. *Q J Med* 1988;69:985–995.

Kopelman PG, Elliott MW, Simonds A, Cramer D, Ward S, Wedzicha JA. Short term use of fluoxetine in asymptomatic obese subjects with sleep-related hypoventilation. *Int J Obesity* 1992;16:825–830.

Kreiss K, Zack MM, Kimbrough RD, Needham LL, Smrek AL, Jones BT. Association of blood pressure and polychlorinated biphenyl levels. *JAMA* 1981;245:2505–2509.

Krum H, Louis WJ, Brow DJ, Howes LG. Pressor dose responses and baroreflex sensitivity in quadriplegic spinal cord injury patients. *J Hypertens* 1992;10:245–250.

Kuchel O, Cusson JR, Larochelle P, Buu NT, Genest J. Posture- and emotion- induced severe hypertensive paroxysms with baroreceptor dysfunction. *J Hypertens* 1987;5: 277–283.

Kuipers H, Wijnen JAG, Hartgens F, Willems SMM. Influence of anabolic steroids on body composition, blood pressure, lipid profile and liver functions in body builders. *Int J Sports Med* 1991;12:413–418.

Lacroix A, Bolté E, Tremblay J, Dupré J, Poitras P, Fournier H, Garon J, Garrei D, Bayard F, Taillefer R, Flanagan RJ, Hamet P. Gastric inhibitory polypeptide-dependent cortisol hypersecretion—a new cause of Cushing's syndrome. *N Engl J Med* 1992;327:974–980.

Lake CR, Gallant S, Masson E, Miller P. Adverse drug effects attributed to phenylpropanolamine: a review of 142 case reports. *Am J Med* 1990;89:195–208.

Lande A. Takayasu's arteritis and congenital coarctation of the descending thoracic and abdominal aorta: a critical review. *Am J Radiol* 1976;127:227–233.

Leenen FHH, Holliwell DL, Cardella CJ. Blood pressure and left ventricular anatomy and function after heart transplantation. *Am Heart J* 1991;122:1087–1094.

Levin ER, Sharp B, Drayer JIM, Weber MA. Case report: Severe hypertension induced by naloxone. *Am J Med Sci* 1985;290: 70–72.

Levinson PD, Millman RP. Causes and consequences of blood pressure alterations in obstructive sleep apnea. *Arch Intern Med* 1991;151:455–462.

Liard J-F, Spadone J-C. Regional circulations in experimental coarctation of the aorta in conscious dogs. *J Hypertens* 1985;3: 281–291.

Lin H-Y, Rocher LL, McQuillan MA, Schmaltz S, Palella TD, Fox IH. Cyclosporine-induced hyperuricemia and gout. *N Engl J Med* 1989;321:287–292.

Lind L, Hvarfner A, Palmer M, Grimelius L, Åkerström G, Ljunghall S. Hypertension in primary hyperparathyroidism in relation to histopathology. *Eur J Surg* 1991a;157: 457–459.

Lind L, Jacobsson S, Palmer M, Lithell H, Wengle B, Ljunghall S. Cardiovascular risk factors in primary hyperparathyroidism: a 15-year follow-up of operated and unoperated cases. *J Intern Med* 1991b;230: 29–35.

Liu L, Rustgi AK. Cardiac myonecrosis in hypertensive crisis associated with monoamine oxidase inhibitor therapy. *Am J Med* 1987;82:1060–1064.

Lloyd-Mostyn RH, Oram S. Modification by propranolol of cardiovascular effects of induced hypoglycemia. *Lancet* 1975;1: 1213–1215.

Lowrey GH. Hypertension in children with burns. *J Trauma* 1967;7:140–144.

Luke RG. Mechanism of cyclosporine-induced hypertension. *Am J Hypertens* 1991; 4:468–471.

Maheswaran R, Gill JS, Davies P, Beevers DG. High blood pressure due to alcohol. A rapidly reversible effect. *Hypertension* 1991;17:787–792.

Malone S, Liu PP, Holloway R, Rutherford R, Xie A, Bradley TD. Obstructive sleep apnoea in patients with dilated cardiomyopathy: effects of continuous positive airway pressure. *Lancet* 1991;338:1480–1484.

Mateika JH, Mateika S, Slutsky AS, Hoffstein V. The effect of snoring on mean arterial blood pressure during non-REM sleep. *Am Rev Respir Dis* 1992;145:141–146.

Mayer J, Becker H, Brandenburg U, Penzel T, Peter JH, Wichert Pv. Blood pressure and sleep apnea: results of long-term nasal continuous positive airway pressure therapy. *Cardiology* 1991;79:84–92.

Melmed S. Acromegaly. *N Engl J Med* 1990;322:966–977.

Merguet P, Ewers HR, Brouwers HP. Blutdruck und Herzfrequenz von Normotonikern nach maximaler Stimulation der Magensekretion mit Pentagastrin. *Kongr Innere Med* 1968;80:561–564.

Metz S, Klein C, Morton N. Rebound hypertension after discontinuation of transdermal clonidine therapy. *Am J Med* 1987; 82:17–19.

Meyer-Lehnert H, Schrier RW. Potential mechanism of cyclosporine A-induced

vascular smooth muscle contraction. *Hypertension* 1989;13:352–360.

Michaeli J, Ben-Ishay D, Kidron R, Dasberg H. Severe hypertension and lithium intoxication [Letter]. *JAMA* 1984;251:1680.

Naftchi NE, Demeny M, Lowman EW, Tuckman J. Hypertensive crises in quadriplegic patients. Changes in cardiac output, blood volume, serum dopamine-β-hydroxylase activity, and arterial prostaglandin PGE$_2$. *Circulation* 1978;57:336–341.

Nies AS, Shand DG. Hypertensive response to propranolol in a patient treated with methyldopa—a proposed mechanism. *Clin Pharmacol Ther* 1973;14:823–826.

Oates JA, FitzGerald GA, Branch RA, Jackson ED, Knapp HR, Roberts LJ II. Clinical implications of prostaglandin and thromboxane A$_2$ formation. *N Engl J Med* 1988;319:761–767.

O'Brien T, Young WF Jr, Davilla DG, Scheithauer BW, Kovacs K, Horvath E, Vale W, van Heerden JA. Cushing's syndrome associated with ectopic production of corticotrophin-releasing hormone, corticotrophin and vasopressin by a phaeochromocytoma. *Clin Endocrinol* 1992;37: 460–467.

Om A. Cardiovascular complications of cocaine. *Am J Med Sci* 1992;303:333–339.

Ong CM, Canter CE, Gutierrez FR, Sekarski DR, Goldring DR. Increased stiffness and persistent narrowing of the aorta after successful repair of coarctation of the aorta: relationship to left ventricular mass and blood pressure at rest and with exercise. *Am Heart J* 1992;123:1594–1600.

Oren S, Grossman E, Messerli FH, Frohlich ED. High blood pressure: side effects of drugs, poisons, and food. *Cardiol Clin* 1988;6:467–474.

Orlowski JP, Shiesley D, Vidt DG, Barnett GH, Little JR. Labetalol to control blood pressure after cerebrovascular surgery. *Crit Care Med* 1988;16:765–768.

Orlowski JP, Vidt DG, Walker S, Haluska JF. The hemodynamic effects of intravenous labetalol for postoperative hypertension. *Clev Clin J Med* 1989;56:29–34.

Palomäki H. Snoring and the risk of ischemic brain infarction. *Stroke* 1991;22:1021–1025.

Pipkin FB, Waldron BA. Ketamine hypertension and the renin-angiotensin system. *Clin Exp Hypertens* 1983;5:875–883.

Plets C. Arterial hypertension in neurosurgical emergencies. *Am J Cardiol* 1989;63: 40C–42C.

Porter GA, Bennett WM, Sheps SG. Cyclosporine-associated hypertension. *Arch Intern Med* 1990;150:280–283.

Rao TKS, Nicastri AD, Friedman EA. Natural history of heroin-associated nephropathy. *N Engl J Med* 1974;190:19–23.

Rauscher H, Popp W, Zwick H. Systemic hypertension in snorers with and without sleep apnea. *Chest* 1992;102:367–371.

Richards NT, Poston L, Hilton PJ. Cyclosporin A inhibits endothelium-dependent, prostanoid-induced relaxation in human subcutaneous resistance vessels. *J Hypertens* 1990;8:159–163.

Ringler J, Basner RC, Shannon R, Schwartzstein R, Manning H, Weinberger SE, Weiss JW. Hypoxemia alone does not explain blood pressure elevations after obstructive apneas. *J Appl Physiol* 1990;69:2143–2148.

Ritchie CM, Sheridan B, Fraser R, Hadden DR, Kennedy AL, Riddell J, Atkinson AB. Studies on the pathogenesis of hypertension in Cushing's disease and acromegaly. *Q J Med* 1990;76:855–867.

Robertson D, Hollister AS, Biaggioni I, Netterville JL, Mosqueda-Garcia R, Robertson RM. The diagnosis and treatment of baroreceptor failure. *N Engl J Med* 1993;329: 1449–1455.

Rocchini AP, Rosenthal A, Schuster S, Fellows KE Jr, Nadas AS. Systemic hypertension after surgical treatment of a congenital arteriovenous malformation. *Am Heart J* 1978;95:497–501.

Roche H, Hyman G, Nahas G. Hypertension and intravenous antidopaminergic drugs. *N Engl J Med* 1985;312:1125–1126.

Rosenthal E, Najm YC, Maisey MN, Curry PVL. Pressor effects of thyrotrophin releasing hormone during thyroid function testing. *Br Med J* 1987;294:806–807.

Rosenthal FB, Roy S. Hypertension and hyperparathyroidism. *Br Med J* 1972;4: 396–397.

Ross RD, Clapp SK, Gunther S, Paridon SM, Humes RA, Farooki ZQ, Pinsky WW. Augmented norepinephrine and renin output in response to maximal exercise in hypertensive coarctectomy patients. *Am Heart J* 1992;123:1293–1298.

Rubio-Garcia R, de Garcia-Diaz J, Ortiz MC, Praga M. IgG myeloma with hyperviscosity presenting as malignant arterial hypertension. *Am J Med* 1989;87:119.

Saken R, Kates GL, Miller K. Drug-induced hypertension in infancy. *J Pediatr* 1979;95:1077–1079.

Salahudeen AK, Thomas TH, Sellars L, Tapster S, Keavey P, Farndon JR, Johnston IDA, Wilkinson R. Hypertension and renal dysfunction in primary hyperparathyroidism: effect of parathyroidectomy. *Clin Sci* 1989;76:289–296.

Scharnweber HC, Spears GN, Cowles SR. Chronic methyl chloride intoxication in six industrial workers. *J Occup Med* 1974;16: 112–113.

Scherrer U, Vissing SF, Morgan BJ, Rollins JA, Tindall RSA, Ring S, Hanson P, Mohanty PK, Victor RG. Cyclosporine-induced sympathetic activation and hypertension after heart transplantation. *N Engl J Med* 1990;323:693–699.

Schroeder JS, Motta J, Guilleminault C. Hemodynamic studies in sleep apnea. In: Guilleminault C, Dement WC, eds. *Sleep Apnea Syndromes*. New York: Alan R. Liss, 1978:177–196.

Schwartz DT. Relation of intestinal carcinoid to renal hypertension. *Angiology* 1970;21: 568–574.

Sehested J, Kornerup HG, Pedersen EB, Christensen NJ. Effects of exercise on plasma renin, aldosterone and catechola-

mines before and after surgery for aortic coarctation. *Eur Heart J* 1983;4:52–58.

Shaddy RE, Boucek MM, Sturtevant JE, Ruttenberg HD, Jaffe RB, Tani LY, Judd VE, Veasy LG, McGough EC, Orsmond GS. Comparison of angioplasty and surgery for unoperated coarctation of the aorta. *Circulation* 1993;87:793–799.

Shelhamer JH, Volkman DJ, Parrillo JE, Lawley TJ, Johnston MR, Fauci AS. Takayasu's arteritis and its therapy. *Ann Intern Med* 1985;103:121–126.

Simard JM, Bellefleur M. Systemic arterial hypertension in head trauma. *Am J Cardiol* 1989;63:32C–35C.

Simpson IA, Sahn DJ, Valdes-Cruz LM, Chung KJ, Sherman FS, Swensson RE. Color doppler flow mapping in patients with coarctation of the aorta: new observations and improved evaluation with color flow diameter and proximal acceleration as predictors of severity. *Circulation* 1988; 77:736–744.

Somers VK, Dyken ME, Mark AL, Abboud FM. Autonomic and hemodynamic responses during sleep in normal and sleep apneic humans [Abstract]. *J Hypertens* 1992;10(Suppl 4):4.

Stacy DL, Prewitt RL. Attenuated microvascular alterations in coarctation hypertension. *Am J Physiol* 1989;256:H213–H221.

Stewart AB, Ahmed R, Travill CM, Newman CGH. Coarctation of the aorta life and health 20–44 years after surgical repair. *Br Heart J* 1993;69:65–70.

Streeten DHP, Anderson GH Jr, Howland T, Chiang R, Smulyan H. Effects of thyroid function on blood pressure. Recognition of hypothyroid hypertension. *Hypertension* 1988;11:78–83.

Sugarman J, Bashore TM, Ohman EM, Jones R, Peters WP. Hypertension and reversible myocardial depression associated with autologous bone marrow transplantation. *Am J Med* 1990;88(Suppl 1):52N–55N.

Tani LY, Orsmond GS, Boucek MM, Shaddy RE. Acute life-threatening hypertension following balloon angioplasty of native coarctation of the aorta. *Am Heart J* 1993;125:907–908.

Thomas SHL, Clark KL, Allen R, Smith SE. A comparison of the cardiovascular effects of phenylpropanolamine and phenylephrine containing proprietary cold remedies. *Br J Clin Pharmacol* 1991;32:705–711.

Thuesen L, Christensen SE, Weeke J, rskov H, Henningsen P. A Hyperkinetic heart in uncomplicated active acromegaly. *Acta Med Scand* 1988;223:337–343.

Todd GPA, Chadwick IG, Yeo WM, Jackson PR, Ramsay LE. Pressor effect of hyperventilation in healthy subjects [Abstract]. *J Hypertens* 1993;11:1152.

Tsachalinas D, Logaras G, Paradelis A. Observations on 246 cases of acute poisoning with parathion in Greece. *Eur J Toxicol Environ Hyg* 1971;4:46–49.

Van Aken H, Cottrell JE, Anger C, Puchstein, C. Treatment of intraoperative hypertensive emergencies in patients with intracranial disease. *Am J Cardiol* 1989;63:43C–47C.

van den Aardweg JG, Karemaker JM. Repetitive apneas induce periodic hypertension in normal subjects through hypoxia. *J Appl Physiol* 1992;72:821–827.

van Wezel HB, Bovill JG, Koolen JJ, Barendse GAM, Fiolet JWT, Dijkhuis JP. Myocardial metabolism and coronary sinus blood flow during coronary artery surgery: effects of nitroprusside and nifedipine. *Am Heart J* 1987;113:266–273.

Van Zwieten PA. Interaction between centrally acting hypotensive agents and tricyclic antidepressants. *Arch Inter Pharmacodyn* 1975;214:12–30.

Ventura HO, Messerli FH, Barron RE. Norepinephrine-induced hypertension in Guillain Barré syndrome. *J Hypertens* 1986;4: 265–267.

Viner S, Szalai JP, Hoffstein V. Are history and physical examination a good screening test for sleep apnea? *Ann Intern Med* 1991;115:356–359.

Volicer L, Nelson KL. Development of reversible hypertension during disulfiram therapy. *Arch Intern Med* 1984;144: 1294–1296.

Walsh BT, Hadigan CM, Wong LM. Increased pulse and blood pressure associated with desipramine treatment of bulimia nervosa. *J Clin Psychopharmacol* 1992;12: 163–168.

Warren SE, Ebert E, Swerdlin A-H, Steinberg SM, Stone R. Clonidine and propranolol paradoxical hypertension. *Arch Intern Med* 1979;139:253.

Wasi P, Pootrakul P, Piankijagum A, Na-Nakorn S, Sonakul D, Pacharee P. A syndrome of hypertension, convulsion, and cerebral haemorrhage in thalassaemic patients after multiple blood-transfusions. *Lancet* 1978;2:602–604.

Weitzman S, Margulis G, Lehmann E. Uncommon cardiovascular manifestations and high catecholamine levels due to "black widow" bite. *Am Heart J* 1977; 93:89–90.

Whitaker MD, McArthur RG, Corenblum B, Davidman M, Haslam RH. Idiopathic, sustained, inappropriate secretion of ADH with associated hypertension and thirst. *Am J Med* 1979;67:511–515.

White WB, Baker LH. Ambulatory blood pressure monitoring in patients with panic disorder. *Arch Intern Med* 1987;147: 1973–1975.

Wilmshurst PT, Nuri M, Crowther A, Webb-Peploe MM. Cold-induced pulmonary oedema in scuba divers and swimmers and subsequent development of hypertension. *Lancet* 1989;1:62–65.

Wu CC, Johnson AJ. The vasopressor effect of indigo carmine. *Henry Ford Hosp Med J* 1969;17:131–134.

Young T, Palta M, Dempsey J, Skatrud J, Weber S, Badr S. The occurrence of sleep-disorder breathing among middle-aged adults. *N Engl J Med* 1993;328:1230–1235.

16 Hypertension in Childhood and Adolescence

Ellin Lieberman, M.D.

A separate discussion of pediatric hypertension is needed in a book focused primarily on the disease as seen in adults because (*a*) many physicians care for children and adults, (*b*) criteria for the diagnosis of hypertension in an individual less than 16 years of age are based on techniques and data that differ from those used in adults, (*c*) techniques for the evaluation and treatment of children and adolescents also differ, (*d*) the existence of primary (essential) hypertension in parents has important implications for their offspring, (*e*) primary hypertension may have its origins in childhood and adolescence, and (*f*) attention to cardiovascular risk factors during the first two decades of life may prevent or retard the development of vascular complications associated with hypertension.

This chapter focuses on the problems of measurements and of interpretation of blood pressure (BP) levels in children, on the significance of elevated BP levels, and on special issues including neonatal hypertension, reflux nephropathy, and hypertensive emergencies. A discussion of major nonrenal causes has been excluded because they are covered elsewhere in this text: coarctation of the aorta in Chapter 15, adrenocortical disorders in Chapters 13 and 14, and pheochromocytoma in Chapter 12.

With the expanded knowledge concerning the epidemiology, evaluation, and treatment of childhood hypertension that has become available during the past two decades, clinicians now have an opportunity to apply this information to their medical practice. Long-term data concerning outcome variables are still lacking and require extrapolation from experience with adults. Areas that remain controversial and uncertain are identified so that the reader can distinguish assumptions from facts.

BLOOD PRESSURE MEASUREMENTS

Accurate recording and interpretation of BP levels in infants, children, and adolescents require appropriate equipment, agreement concerning which Korotkoff sounds are used for diastolic pressure and, most importantly, the availability of adequate data from large numbers of normal children examined with similar techniques. The following is an adaptation for children of the portion of Chapter 2 that deals with BP measurements in adults.

Technique

The fewest errors result if the observer employs the technique outlined below, recording the levels, the position of the child, and the size of the cuff used. The mercury manometer should be in place at eye level to avoid errors introduced by parallax, and the child's arm should be placed at heart level.

Cuff Size

The choice of BP cuff depends on the size and not on the age of the child. The appropriate BP cuff is one with a bladder that completely and comfortably encircles the girth of the arm, with or without overlap. At least three-fourths of the length of the child's upper arm should be covered by the bladder with adequate space in the antecubital fossa to allow proper placement of the head of the stethoscope. An alternative standard is that the cuff bladder width should be 40% of the mid-upper arm circumference (Gomez-Marin et al., 1992). Available commercial cuffs have bladders with varying dimensions, as shown in Table 16.1 (Report of the Second Task Force on Blood Pressure Control in Children, 1987).

If the ideal cuff and bladder are not available, a larger cuff is recommended to avoid spuriously high levels (Moss, 1981). The large adult cuff with large bladder dimensions is frequently required to obtain accurate measurements in a youngster with fat or muscular upper arms.

Ultrasonography

Measurement of BP in newborns and small infants is easy with Doppler ultrasonography. The appropriate-sized cuff is wrapped around the upper arm with a transducer directly over the brachial artery. The systolic pressure is recorded when the intensity of reflected sound waves increases and the observer hears a sound. Continued deflation of the cuff results in a distinct muffling of the ultrasound signal that is interpreted as the diastolic pressure. This method provides data comparable to those of other noninvasive indirect procedures (Kirkland and Kirkland, 1972; Dweck et al., 1974) and direct intraarterial measurements (Moss, 1981), but accuracy of this method for diastolic levels remains undocumented (Weismann, 1988).

Procedure

Children, especially in the toddler age group, are often anxious and restless. They require time to relax and to familiarize themselves with their surroundings and with the examiner. Younger children often respond favorably to a simple demonstration of the equipment and to the realization that pain is not involved. Children often are more at ease in the sitting position than in

a supine position. Even when these steps are taken and the child is quiet and cooperative, the Korotkoff sounds are often difficult to hear because they are softer in children than in adults.

When the child is relaxed and comfortable, the antecubital fossa is placed at heart level. By convention (Report of the Second Task Force, 1987), the right arm and seated position have been selected so that measurements can be compared over time. Inflation and deflation of the cuff are done in the same manner as with adults. The major difference is that the fourth Korotkoff phase (K4) (i.e., point of muffling) has been selected as the best indirect measure of diastolic pressure in infants and children, up to 13 years of age (Report of the Second Task Force, 1987). Use of the K4 phase is known to produce overestimation, and use of the fifth phase (K5) (i.e., disappearance of the sounds) to produce underestimation of the diastolic pressure in children as compared with direct intraarterial recordings (Moss, 1981).

Recording

To avoid confusion, the BP measurement should be recorded as follows: right arm, sitting position, 9-cm cuff: 100/70/40 (i.e., K1, K4, and K5). Recording the measurement in this manner reduces the likelihood of extraneous variability in repeated measurements and allows comparisons of subsequent readings. Nonetheless, the onset of the muffling sound (K4) may not be heard easily, and observer bias may cause repetitive recordings of the same numbers. Periodic quality control checks will assure that such errors are not introducing and perpetuating mistakes.

Interpretation

Consensus has been reached concerning the interpretation of BP levels in children and adolescents. The recommendations of the Second Task Force on BP Control in Children (1987) now form the basis for categorizing measurements as normal or abnormal. Figures 16.1 through 16.3 represent distribution curves for boys; similar curves for girls are available in the Report. Unfortunately, only the first BP reading was used to derive the BP distribution curves, but they were obtained on over 70,000 white, black, and Latino children from nine separate sources. The three sets of curves include systolic and diastolic pressure levels for boys and girls at birth to 12 months of age and from 1 to 13 years of age using K4 as the best indirect

Table 16.1. Dimensions of Bladders of Commercially Available Cuffs

	Range of Dimensions of Bladder (cm)	
	Width	Length
Newborn	2.5–4.0	5.0–9.0
Infant	4.0–6.0	11.5–18.0
Child	7.5–9.0	17.0–19.0
Adult	11.5–13.0	22.0–26.0
Large adult arm	14.0–15.0	30.5–33.0
Adult thigh	18.0–19.0	36.0–38.0

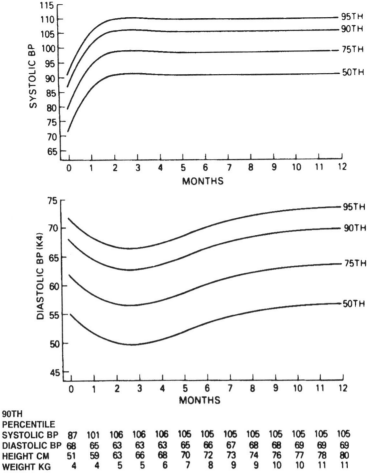

90TH PERCENTILE													
SYSTOLIC BP	87	101	106	106	106	105	105	105	105	105	105	105	105
DIASTOLIC BP	68	65	63	63	63	65	66	67	68	68	69	69	69
HEIGHT CM	51	59	63	66	68	70	72	73	74	76	77	78	80
WEIGHT KG	4	4	5	5	6	7	8	9	9	10	10	11	11

Figure 16.1. Age-specific percentiles of blood pressure measurements in boys—birth to 12 months of age; Korotkoff phase IV (K4) was used for diastolic blood pressure. (From Report of the Second Task Force on Blood Pressure Control in Children—1987. *Pediatrics* 1987;79:1–25.)

reflection of diastolic pressure, and curves for both boys and girls from 13 to 18 years of age utilizing K5. Data are supplied for integration of height and weight into the interpretation of the curves. If a child is taller and heavier than the 90th percentile and his or her BP level falls into that decile, the child is *not* considered hypertensive. On the other hand, if the child is short and lean, the same BP level is considered abnormal (Report of the Second Task Force, 1987).

Significance of Elevated Readings

The report of the 1987 Second Task Force on Blood Pressure Control in Children reflects a conservative approach to labeling children as hypertensive and of investigating abnormal levels. The definitions provided by the Task Force are shown in Table 16.2.

With these curves, children can be categorized as normotensive (i.e., less than the 90th percentile), high normal (between the 90th and 95th percentile), or hypertensive (three recorded BPs exceeding the 95th percentile), providing clear reference standards for the clinician to use in assessing the BP pattern of a specific child. The choice of 90th and 95th percentiles for identification of a systolic or diastolic pressure as high-normal or abnormal is arbitrary, as are the numbers presented for significant and severe hypertension (Table 16.3). Nonetheless, this approach provides a basis for clinical decision making that heretofore was lacking.

EPIDEMIOLOGIC DATA AND SURVEYS

Surveys of BP patterns in children have sought to identify infants and children destined

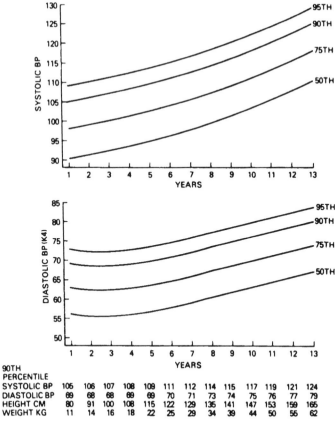

Figure 16.2. Age-specific percentiles of blood pressure measurements in boys—1 to 13 years of age; Korotkoff phase IV (K4) was used for diastolic blood pressure. (From Report of the Second Task Force on Blood Pressure Control in Children—1987. *Pediatrics* 1987;79:1–25.)

for hypertension in later life. Studies on neonates (deSwiet et al., 1980), and on children and adolescents from diverse backgrounds (Gutgesell et al., 1981; Levinson et al., 1985; Sinaiko et al., 1989) have not resulted in the identification of significant abnormalities detectable early in childhood to explain why some racial groups are at increased risk from cardiovascular disease (Anderson 1989). Studies that have focused on cardiovascular reactivity induced by physical and psychosocial stressors have demonstrated increased reactivity in black children and adolescents (Anderson, 1989; Murphy et al., 1992). McDonald et al. (1987) reported that sodium-lithium countertransport was positively associated with systolic BP in black children. In their review of racial aspects and BP, Alpert and Fox (1993) hypothesize that blacks may have an inherited congenital defect in sodium metabolism.

Of all factors, the most predictive one for sustained BP elevation is an antecedent elevated BP (Shear et al., 1986; Berenson et al., 1989). However, Lauer et al. (1984) have shown that children whose initial BP levels fall within the highest quartile may, on follow-up, fall into a lower quartile. Although an initial elevated recording during childhood may not evolve into later sustained elevations (Lauer et al., 1984), Lauer has shown that 24% of young adults whose pressures ever exceeded the 90th percentile as children had adult levels greater than the 90th percentile (2.4 times the expected, p < .001) (Lauer et al., 1993). The predictability of adult BP elevations is strengthened considerably if elevated childhood BP levels are combined with childhood obesity (Voors et al., 1977; Grobbee, 1992; Lauer et al., 1993). If there is a positive family history for hypertension and/or obesity these childhood abnormalities become more significant (Grobbee, 1992). These observations present both an opportunity and a challenge for preventing the evolution of hypertension.

Tracking

The pattern of BP over time is known as *tracking*. Multiple studies of different age groups followed for varied periods in different settings have led to the following conclusions (Rossner et al., 1977; Zinner et al., 1978; Shear et al., 1986; Michaels et al., 1987; Gillman et al., 1991): BP levels in children do track; however, the consistency of observations is greater for systolic than for diastolic pressures. Most significantly, BP patterns have much greater stability the longer the follow-up, especially if the subjects are followed through adolescence. As noted in Chapter 3, Lever and Harrap (1992) hypothesized that the pressure set during adolescence actually carries forward and determines the potential for adult hypertension and cardiovascular hypertrophy. These authors propose that growth and factors that play a role in the complex set of circumstances resulting in maturation may be interrelated. Accordingly, growth

hormone, IGF1, and insulin are growth-promoting compounds that may significantly influence not only general growth, but more specifically growth, hypertension, and cardiovascular abnormalities (Lever and Harrap, 1992). Longitudinal studies of children with BP patterns in the 95th percentile have revealed more consistent tracking when the study group is of adolescent age, obese, or the offspring of hypertensive parents, or if echocardiographic changes exhibiting increased left ventricular wall mass are present (deLeonardis et al., 1988; Falkner, 1989; Hansen et al., 1992).

Factors Determining BP

Increasing attention is being paid to an examination of factors that correlate with BP levels during childhood in the hope of identifying which of these are determinants of the rise in BP. In particular, the frequently observed, but until recently poorly studied, change in BP with

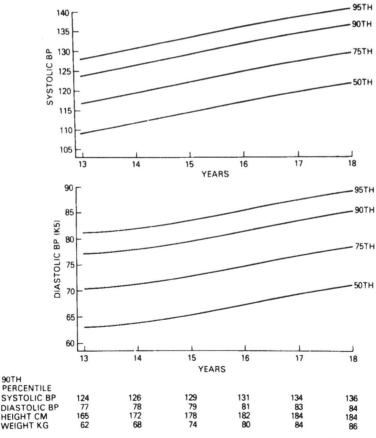

90TH PERCENTILE						
SYSTOLIC BP	124	126	129	131	134	136
DIASTOLIC BP	77	78	79	81	83	84
HEIGHT CM	165	172	178	182	184	184
WEIGHT KG	62	68	74	80	84	86

Figure 16.3. Age-specific percentiles of blood pressure measurements in boys—13 to 18 years of age; Korotkoff phase V (K5) was used for diastolic blood pressure. (From Report of the Second Task Force on Blood Pressure Control in Children—1987. *Pediatrics* 1987;79:1–25.)

Table 16.2. Definitions from Second Task Force on Blood Pressure Control in Children

Term	Definition
Normal BP	Systolic and diastolic BPs < 90th percentile for age and sex
High normal BP[a]	Average systolic and/or average diastolic BP between 90th and 95th percentiles for age and sex
High BP (hypertension)	Average systolic and/or average diastolic BPs ≥ 95th percentile for age and sex with measurements obtained on at least three occasions

[a] If the BP reading is high normal for age, but can be accounted for by excess height for age or excess lean body mass for age, such children are considered to have normal BP. Modified from the Report of the Second Task Force on Blood Pressure Control in Children—1987. *Pediatrics* 1987;79:1.

study of racial differences relating to BP in children. It is now clear that white and black youngsters react differently to specific stimuli, and that with maturation their BP patterns and cardiac reactivity differ (Table 16.5).

The various factors listed in Table 16.4 are the major ones that correlate with BP levels in young people; the single best correlate is body mass. Most factors can be categorized as either genetic or environmental, but some have features of both. Height, body mass, and muscular development depend not only on genetic influences but also on nutrition and exercise. Salt intake may exert its effect on BP in salt-sensitive persons genetically predisposed to higher BP levels. Obese adolescents have also demonstrated heightened responsiveness to salt intake (Rocchini et al., 1989). BP reactivity to some forms of stress varies with family history for hypertension (Falkner et al., 1979; Parker et al., 1987). Mongeau (1987) (Fig. 16.4) reviewed data from the Montreal adoption study, which led to a statistical assessment of the variability of BP in children attributable to genetic (30 ± 9%), nonfamilial (39% ± 9), environmental

Table 16.3. Classification of Hypertension by Age Group

	Significant Hypertension		Severe Hypertension	
	Systolic	Diastolic	Systolic	Diastolic
Age (yr)	(BP greater than, in mm Hg)		(BP greater than, in mm Hg)	
Infants (<2)	112	74	118	82
Children (3–5)	116	76	124	84
Children (6–9)	122	78	130	86
Children (10–12)	126	82	134	90
Adolescents (13–15)	136	86	144	92
Adolescents (16–18)	142	92	150	98

Modified from the Report of the Second Task Force on Blood Pressure Control in Children—1987. *Pediatrics* 1987;79:1.

the onset of puberty is now being investigated intensively (Lever and Harrap, 1992). The importance of the recognition of such factors lies in the generally accepted view that, if they were identified in childhood and adolescence, primary prevention of adult-onset hypertension might become a realistic public health and clinical goal.

Multiple factors have been reported to correlate with BP levels in children (Table 16.4). In addition to those listed, age (Lauer et al., 1984), gender (Goldring et al., 1977), and race (Anderson, 1989; Berenson et al., 1989; Alpert and Fox, 1993) have been shown to relate to BP in children. Berenson and coworkers (1989) summarized their observations from the Bogalusa

(20% ± 3), and shared environmental factors across generations (11% ± 3).

Genetic Factors

The influence of genetic factors on BP has been shown by the finding of a correlation of BP levels between parents and their natural offspring (Zinner et al., 1971; Munger et al., 1988), the lack of correlation of BP levels between parents and their adopted children (Mongeau, 1987), and comparisons of siblings (Zinner et al., 1971) and twins (monozygotic and dizygotic) and their families (Havlik et al., 1979; Rose et al., 1979). Overall, the studies indicate that genetic factors play a strong but still ill-defined role (Mongeau, 1987).

Table 16.4. Epidemiologic Factors Related to Blood Pressure Levels in Children and Adolescents

Genetic
Parental and sibling blood pressure levels (Mongeau, 1987)
Erythrocyte sodium flux (McDonald et al., 1987)
Haptoglobin phenotype 1-1 (Weinberger et al., 1987)
Increased salt sensitivity in blacks (Luft et al., 1988)

Environmental
Socioeconomic status (Macintyre et al., 1991)
Rural versus urban residence (Kotchen and Kotchen, 1978)
Pulse rate (Macintyre et al., 1991)
Small for Gestational Age (SGA) (Williams et al., 1992)
Exercise (Macintyre et al., 1991)

Mixed genetic and environmental
Height (Macintyre et al., 1991)
Weight (Macintyre et al., 1991)
Body mass (Grobbee, 1992; Lauer et al., 1993)
Obesity and response to sodium (Rocchini et al., 1989)
Sodium/potassium excretion (Geleijnse et al., 1990)
Stress (Falkner et al., 1979)
Skinfold thickness (Aristimuno et al., 1984)

A number of differences between normotensive children with normotensive parents (FH-) and normotensive offspring of hypertensive parents (FH+) have been examined in an attempt to identify which child may be destined for future development of hypertension. FH+ children have been found to have these features:

—Higher ambulatory diastolic BP levels during school hours (Wilson et al., 1988);
—Exaggerated BP responses with submaximal exercise on a bicycle ergometer (Molineux and Steptoe, 1988);
—Greater rise in diastolic BP and 24-hour urinary catecholamine excretion in response to isometric hand grip (Ferrara et al., 1988);
—A greater response to a 10-minute arithmetic test (Falkner et al., 1979). When these studies were extended to include 2 weeks of salt loading, mental stress induced an even greater pressor response in the FH+ group (Falkner et al., 1981);
—Increased forearm vascular resistance and decrease in forearm blood flow in response to a short math test (Anderson et al., 1987);
—Higher platelet alpha$_2$—adrenoceptor density (Michel et al., 1989);
—Higher PRA (Shibutani et al., 1988);
—Higher rate of sodium-lithium countertransport (McDonald et al., 1987);
—Lower erythrocyte membrane calcium-magnesium ATPase (Huai-yong et al., 1990);
—Higher interventricular septum/posterior wall mass ratio on M-mode echocardiograms

Table 16.5. Racial Differences Related to BP of Children

Whites[a]	Blacks[a]
All blood pressure strata	
Percentage of body fat	
Plasma renin activity	
Serum dopamine beta hydroxylase (DBH)	
24-hr urine K^+	
Fasting serum glucose	
High blood pressure strata	
Resting heart rate	Positive association of 24-hr urine Na^+ versus sitting blood pressure
Cardiac output	Systolic blood pressure in boys
Renin activity and DBH combined	Peripheral resistance
1-hr serum glucose	Negative association of plasma renin versus systolic blood pressures (black boys only)

[a]For each racial group, the characteristics listed are higher in that group than the other.
From Berenson GS, Lawrence M, Soto L: The heart and hypertension in childhood. *Semin Nephrol* 1989;9:234–246.

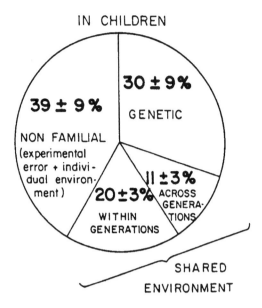

IN CHILDREN

Figure 16.4. Explanation of phenotypic variability of diastolic blood pressure in children (ISE). (From Mongeau J-G. Heredity and blood pressure in humans: an overview. *Pediatr Nephrol* 1987;1:69.)

(deLeonardis et al., 1988) and increased thickness of the interventricular septum during systole (Hansen et al., 1992).

As noted in Chapter 3, some studies of red blood cells from hypertensive individuals and their normotensive offspring reveal altered sodium fluxes as compared with normotensives and their offspring (Canessa et al., 1980; Garay et al., 1980). Trevisan et al. (1988) did not find that a positive family history determined intra-erythrocytic sodium or sodium-lithium countertransport in children. Abnormal whole-body and erythrocyte handling of $^{22}Na^+$ has been demonstrated in first-degree relatives of hypertensives (Henningsen et al., 1979), but Prineas et al. (1984) did not find the rate of $^{22}Na^+$ flux to be related to the BP levels in children or to parental BP levels. Mongeau (1985) reported studies of erythrocyte sodium handling in FH+ offspring as follows: 9/15 had decreased cotransport, 5/11 had increased countertransport, and 5/12 had a sodium leak. Trevisan et al. (1988) observed that sodium-lithium countertransport was related to systolic and diastolic BP in boys, but the associations lost significance when height and weight were considered. It therefore remains unclear whether the transmission of primary hypertension is related to the transmission of markers for sodium transport in red blood cell

membranes in children. Similar uncertainty was noted in Chapter 3 concerning adults.

Environmental Factors

Of the environmental factors, increased body mass has increasingly been recognized as a major determinant of higher BP levels throughout childhood and adolescence (Table 16.4). One study (Johnson et al., 1987) correlated suppressed anger in black adolescents with an increase in BP, whereas Gillum et al. (1985) did not find any correlation between BP and personality. The trend toward increasing levels of BP in childhood and adolescence is not understood and cannot be attributed to the hormonal changes of puberty (Lever and Harrap, 1992).

Sodium Intake. The subject of salt and its relation to BP was comprehensively reviewed in Chapter 3. Few studies have involved infants, children, and adolescents. During the first 6 months of life, infants randomized to a low-salt diet had a mean systolic pressure 2 mm below that of infants on a normal diet (Hofman et al., 1983). After a 4-year follow-up, however, no significant differences were found (Grobbee and Bak, 1989). A study of children in Massachusetts revealed that youngsters in a community with higher sodium content in their drinking water had higher BP levels than their peers from a low-salt water community (Calabrese and Tuthill,

1982). When the high-salt water children were placed on bottled water for 12 weeks, significant reductions in BP were observed only in girls (Calabrese and Tuthill, 1982). A study involving adolescents did not reveal a BP-lowering effect with sodium restrictions (Cooper et al., 1984). Therefore, the role of sodium as a sensitizing agent during early childhood has not been proven.

The most that can be gleaned from current pediatric experience is that the effect of sodium on BP may only reveal itself in a subset of salt-sensitive, hypertensive adolescents who achieve improved control with salt limitation. Accordingly, excessive sodium intake may exert its effect in a selected group of hypertensive individuals with a genetic predisposition to hypertension. The response of BP to a mathematical stress was measured before and after a 2-week period on 10 g of extra salt in 40 individuals who had participated in longitudinal studies (Falkner et al., 1986). When blacks were grouped according to family history there was a significant difference in weight gain after sodium load. Before sodium loading there was no difference in the BP response to mental stress. After sodium load, individuals displaying a rise in diastolic BP $\geq$ 5 mm Hg were regarded as sodium-sensitive (SS) and had a greater BP response to stress testing after the load. The greatest response occurred in SS individuals with a positive family history.

Sodium Plus Potassium

When the effects of sodium and potassium intakes are combined, preliminary evidence suggests that potassium-enriched diets may exert a protective effect (Gelenijnse et al., 1990). In a 7-year longitudinal study of Dutch children, the mean yearly change in systolic pressure was 1.4 mm Hg in those on higher potassium as compared with a mean of 2.4 mm Hg in children with low potassium intakes. Furthermore, the ratio of urinary sodium to potassium also showed an inverse relation to BP, whereas there was no effect attributable to sodium alone. Additional studies are needed to assess the potential beneficial effects of supplemental potassium.

Other Nutrients. Analyses of the response of children to magnesium, calcium, fats, or carbohydrates are inadequate. Therefore, it is premature to recommend wide-scale changes in nutrient intakes for children for the goal of prevention of hypertension. On the other hand, it is prudent to implement the recommendations

of the Subcommittee on Atherosclerosis and Hypertension in Childhood on a broad scale with the overall goal of reduction of cardiovascular risk factors in adulthood (Subcommittee, 1992).

Cardiovascular Risk Factors

As in adults, hypertension in childhood acts in combination with other risk factors to exert a deleterious effect on the cardiovascular system (Newman et al., 1986; Becque et al., 1988; Subcommittee, 1992). The relationship of hypertension and serum lipoprotein levels to early atherosclerosis in children and adolescents was assessed in an autopsy study of 35 persons who had, as children, been part of the Bogalusa Heart Study (Newman et al., 1986). Mean systolic BP tended to be higher in the four subjects with coronary-artery fibrous plaques than in those without them. Aortic fatty streaks were strongly related to antemortem levels of total and low-density lipoprotein (LDL) cholesterol and were universally correlated with the ratio of LDL cholesterol to LDL plus very-low-density lipoprotein (VLDL) cholesterol.

The additive effects of cardiovascular risk factors, including hypertension, to which children and adolescents are exposed forms the basis for the advocacy of noninvasive health-promoting behaviors starting in early childhood (Subcommittee, 1992). The Subcommittee on Atherosclerosis and Hypertension in Childhood emphasized the health hazards of smoking, lack of physical activity, obesity, and hyperlipidemia. These phenomena lend themselves to prevention or amelioration during critical childhood years when the stage is being set for later, irreversible cardiovascular disease. The Subcommittee provides step-by-step healthful interventions to inculcate healthy lifestyles from early childhood (Subcommittee, 1992).

Preventive Measures

Because the natural course for children with persistently elevated BP remains uncertain, definitive recommendations for prevention of fixed hypertension cannot be made. As noted earlier, sustained obesity is a definite risk factor for fixed hypertension in young people. Reduction of excess weight, moderation of salt intake, avoidance of smoking and pressor agents, plus an active dynamic sports program may prove beneficial. Sodium intake should be assessed; excessive intakes of sodium should be reduced in children if salt-sensitive hypertension is suspected. Supplemental potassium intake, in the form of natural fruits and vegetables, may prove beneficial, and certainly their ingestion has no adverse effects. Fat calories should make up 30% or less of caloric intake. All suggestions must be presented in a positive, nonthreatening manner to avoid an unnatural concern about hypertension and its sequelae and to promote healthy changes in lifestyle that will enhance the quality of life for the child and his or her family.

OBESITY AND HYPERTENSION

Obesity-associated hypertension is separated from primary and secondary hypertension because observations in pediatrics suggest that this group represents a subtype among pediatric populations (Report of the Second Task Force 1987; Rocchini et al., 1988). The clinical definition of obesity is a weight that exceeds normal for a given height by 20% or more; for practical purposes, such an approach is usually all that is needed. The association of excessive body weight for height and elevated BP levels has been observed by investigators and clinicians for many years (Court et al., 1974; Voors, 1977; Aristimuno et al., 1984). In addition, normalization of abnormal BP levels has occurred with acute weight reduction (Court et al., 1974; Rames et al., 1978; Rocchini et al., 1988, 1989), although prolonged follow-up studies have not been reported. Becque et al. (1988) also recorded that childhood obesity was associated with abnormal lipid patterns. In 1991, Steinberger correlated obesity with an increase in plasma insulin levels and elevated lipid levels. Rocchini (1993) proposed that obesity is associated with elevated insulin levels that selectively enhance renal sodium retention; moreover, sodium responsiveness is altered with weight reduction, as was shown earlier (Rocchini et al., 1989). The importance for care providers of obese children is that obesity-associated hypertension is preventable and, even if not prevented, amenable to treatment.

EVALUATION OF CHILDREN AND ADOLESCENTS WITH ELEVATED BLOOD PRESSURE

General Guidelines

Asymptomatic children and adolescents who have a single casual BP recording that exceeds the 90th percentile for systolic or diastolic pressure according to age-specific distributions of BP for boys and girls should have their BP remeasured within 3 months. A BP value exceeding the 90th percentile but below the 95th

percentile may be regarded as normal if height is increased above the 90th percentile, but may be abnormal if associated with adiposity. According to data derived from screening programs (Fixler et al., 1979; Hediger et al., 1984) and epidemiologic surveys (Rames et al., 1978), the likelihood of repeated measurements being elevated is small, unless the child is obese or has a hypertensive parent. However, if an adolescent has had repeated high-decile recordings and is consistently overweight for height, the chances of his or her BP remaining elevated and of developing fixed hypertension are greatly increased.

Evaluation

Ambulatory Recordings

One approach to the evaluation of abnormal BP measurements in children and adolescents is to obtain ambulatory BP levels. A study of 84 hypertensive children ages 6 to 23 years with ambulatory recordings revealed that application to pediatrics was limited because (*a*) the pressurometer only detected K5, (*b*) the Second Task Force (1987) recommended that BP be measured in a sitting position, (*c*) the full range of cuff sizes needed for children is not available for ambulatory BP monitors, and (*d*) ambulatory standards for normal BP measurements currently do not exist (Daniels et al., 1987). Until more data are available with improved technology, ambulatory recordings have little role in pediatric hypertension.

History

Evaluation of children with persistently elevated BP (i.e., over the 95th percentile on three occasions) includes ascertainment of these historical features: (*a*) primary or essential hypertension, or complications of uncontrolled hypertension (i.e., stroke, heart attack, and kidney failure of unknown origin) in first-degree relatives, (*b*) familial obesity, (*c*) familial hyperlipidemia, (*d*) BP levels of siblings, and (*e*) past events or present occurrences that might influence BP, such as prior renal disease, urologic surgery, or use of pressor agents (i.e., sympathomimetics and, in some cases, oral contraceptives). Attention should be focused on drug abuse with an emphasis on street drugs known to elevate BP, such as amphetamines, phencyclidine (PCP), and cocaine.

Physical Examination

The physical examination should include the patient's height and weight because of the association of obesity with elevated BP levels in childhood and adolescence (Report of the Second Task Force, 1987). The pulse should be recorded because of the reported association of an increased pulse rate with higher levels of pressure (Hediger et al., 1984, Macintyre et al., 1991). The physical examination is oriented toward clues for secondary causes of hypertension such as decreased femoral pulses, abdominal bruits, and cushingoid stigmata. In children, in contrast to adults, retinal arteriolar tortuosity, arteriovenous crossing, and increased arterial light reflex more likely reflect long-standing hypertension than atherosclerosis.

Laboratory Studies

Children with persistently elevated BP are usually not sick. Limited laboratory studies are needed (Report of the Second Task Force, 1987); these include urinalysis, serum urea nitrogen, and serum creatinine. The likelihood of an asymptomatic, nonobese child with persistently elevated BP having a recognizable cause for the BP elevation is remote. Secondary causes of hypertension are usually revealed by the history and the physical examination. Therefore, detailed diagnostic studies of children without suggestive evidence of secondary hypertension are not warranted. Emphasis in the literature on rare secondary causes that require detailed and sophisticated investigative studies has led some to advocate all-inclusive evaluations.

Echocardiography

The 1987 Second Task Force Report also recommends obtaining an echocardiogram, especially if pharmacologic intervention is contemplated, so that reversal of abnormalities can be monitored and correlated with adequacy of BP control.

Echocardiographic abnormalities found in adolescents with persistently elevated BP levels include increased left ventricular wall thickness (Laird and Fixler, 1981), increased left ventricular wall mass (Schieken et al., 1982; Daniels et al., 1990), and indices reflecting abnormal ventricular performance (Johnson et al., 1983). Observations by Daniels and coworkers (1990) using gender-specific 95th percentile criteria led to identification of left ventricular hypertrophy in 40 of 104 children and adolescents with elevated BP.

PRIMARY HYPERTENSION

Increasing numbers of children and adolescents with persistently elevated pressure are being identified as having primary (essential) hypertension. Ogborn et al. (1987) reported that 43 of 103 hypertensive children and adolescents had primary hypertension. Conclusive information as to the incidence and prevalence of primary hypertension in the United States is still lacking. This problem is compounded by the immigration of different ethnic groups, whose BP patterns may change after entry into this country.

Family History

Approximately 50% of children with primary hypertension come from families with a positive family history for primary hypertension or its complications in a first-degree relative (Londe et al., 1971). Although all children whose parents have primary hypertension are at greater risk than their peers, not all offspring are at the same risk. The development of primary hypertension and its complications is more likely when the BP tracks in the highest percentiles. The monitoring of such high-risk children includes serial BP recordings, serial height/weight measurements, and assessments of dietary intake. Echocardiograms at intervals of 1 to 2 years may also prove valuable.

Symptoms

Primary hypertension in childhood and adolescence is usually asymptomatic. The most frequent symptom is headache, which has no particular features that distinguish it from other pediatric causes. In adolescent athletes, headaches often occur after strenuous exercise. Occasionally a child complains of severe, throbbing frontal headaches that may or may not be relieved by analgesics. Symptoms such as seizures, nosebleeds, dizziness, or syncope are rare. Their presence suggests that hypertension has been exacerbated by pressor agents (i.e., sympathomimetics) or by an emotional crisis, particularly in adolescents. Otherwise, these symptoms are most often a reflection of severe secondary hypertension.

Physical Findings

Obesity is the most frequently detected abnormality and has been noted in as many as 50% of pediatric hypertensives (Londe et al., 1971), with the highest prevalence among black female adolescents. Careful physical examination is unlikely to reveal any other positive physical findings. A child occasionally has early changes of hypertensive retinopathy, including arteriolar narrowing and mild tortuosity, when hypertension is chronic and moderate. Clues to secondary causes of hypertension should be systematically sought.

Laboratory Studies

If no secondary cause of hypertension has been identified by history and physical examination, routine recommended studies include urinalysis, serum urea nitrogen, creatinine, and echocardiogram. The latter study may have two uses: to help identify anatomic changes and to evaluate hemodynamic alterations. Routine radiographs of the chest and electrocardiograms are no longer recommended because they are not as sensitive as echocardiograms (Laird and Fixler, 1981). In asymptomatic *adolescents* whose BP levels are distinctly elevated (e.g., diastolic levels consistently greater than 100 mm Hg) but who have unremarkable histories and physical examinations, additional tests are often obtained, even though the yield is low (Aschinberg et al., 1977; Loggie, 1974; Silverberg et al., 1975). In a small group of adolescent patients with primary hypertension at CHLA, there has been a tendency toward a high hemoglobin and hematocrit, as reported by Tochikubo et al. (1986). Secondary hypertension has been said to be more frequent among white female teenagers (Loggie, 1975), but our experience does not confirm this view.

The rationale for obtaining an all-inclusive diagnostic evaluation is the same as that for adults, based on the concept that an occult secondary cause may be detected. However, the data base on which to base an opinion is much smaller among children. Review of experience at Childrens Hospital Los Angeles (CHLA) and elsewhere with hypertensive adolescent patients suggests that the number of occult cases of secondary hypertension is small (Loggie, 1974; Silverberg et al., 1975; Levine et al., 1976). In other words, the majority of secondary causes of hypertension reveal themselves with a careful history, methodical physical examination, and minimal laboratory studies. Recommendations in pediatric patients also take into account the severity of hypertension and the age of the patient. The younger the patient and the higher the BP, the more likely an underlying etiology will be found. At CHLA, initial laboratory evaluation includes urinalysis, blood count, blood urea nitrogen (BUN) and creatinine, renal scan, renal ultrasonography, and echocardiogram (Table 16.6). As seen in Table 16.6, other experts have recommended more extensive evaluations.

In adolescents with moderate hypertension, the performance of a rapid sequence of hypertensive intravenous pyelograms has been abandoned because it is insensitive for the detection of renal arterial disease (RAD) (Korobkin et al., 1976). Ultrasonography coupled with radionuclide scans is helpful in determining renal size, major renal scars, and altered renal function. If RAD remains highly suspect, arteriography is indicated when adequate BP control has been achieved. Renal vein renin sampling may prove valuable just prior to the arterial study. Subtraction digital angiography has been disappointing, and is not used at CHLA.

Prepubertal Children

Guidelines for the *initial* investigation of prepubertal children suspected of having primary hypertension differ from those used for postpubertal children in the number of *first-ordered* tests. Experience at CHLA indicates that many children with secondary forms of hypertension (often renal) can be identified using a selective approach (Fig. 16.5). If the initial findings are normal, the evaluation should *sequentially* proceed to exclude all reasonable possibilities. The higher the BP and the more severe its manifestations, the more likely the hypertension has a secondary cause, most likely renal parenchymal disease (Table 16.7). Nevertheless, a significant proportion of prepubertal hypertensive children, perhaps 10% to 15%, will not have a recognizable secondary cause. In symptomatic prepubertal FH- children whose physical examination does not reveal diagnostic clues, the same laboratory studies advocated for adolescents, plus renal ultrasonography and renal scans, are recommended (Table 16.6). Even though subtle adrenal cortical abnormalities are extraordinarily rare in this age group, serum potassium and bicarbonate levels should be obtained to search for primary or secondary hyperaldosteronism. Measurement of plasma renin activity (PRA) has been advocated in children with primary hypertension (Gruskin et al., 1986), but the use of such profiles as the basis for therapy is untried in pediatrics. PRA levels are high in infancy and fall to adult levels by 16 years; they must be obtained under standardized conditions (Kotchen et al., 1972; Stark et al., 1975; Hiner et al., 1976).

Treatment

Treatment of primary hypertension is still empirical because long-term studies of dietary

Table 16.6. Recommendations for Initial Investigation of Sustained Hypertension

Test	Lieberman (CHLA), 1983	Task Force, 1987	Schärer et al., 1986	Dillon, 1987	Ogburn and Crocker, 1987	Feld and Springate, 1988
Urinalysis	X	X (+ culture)	X	X	X	X
Blood count	X	X	X			
BUN/creatinine	X	X	X	X	X	X
Uric acid		X				X
Electrolytes		X	X	X		X
PRA		X	X	X		
P-aldosterone			X	X		
P-catechol				X		
U-VMA/metabolites			X	X	X	
24-hr U-protein, creatinine					X	
P-magnesium, calcium, phosphorus, alkaline phosphatase					X	
Thyroid function					X	
P-cortisol					X	
Chest radiograph			X	X	X	X
Electrocardiogram			X	X	X	
Echocardiography	X	X	X			X
DMSA/DTPA	X		X	X	X	X
Renal ultrasound	X		X	X		X (or IVP)

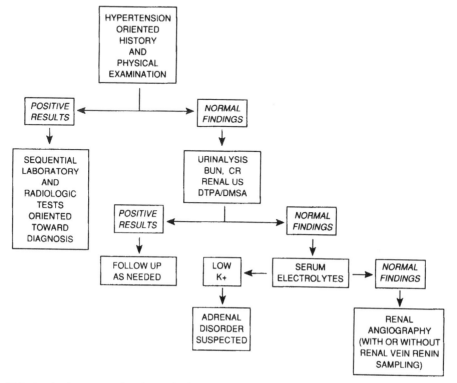

Figure. 16.5. A selective approach to the evaluation of sustained hypertension in a prepubertal child.

intervention with or without drug therapy do not exist. Short-term observations suggest that weight reduction in obese children and adolescents often leads to normalization of elevated pressures (Court et al., 1974; Rames et al., 1978; Rocchini et al., 1989). In the absence of adequate data on safety and effectiveness of drug therapy, the decision as to whether a specific child should receive medication must be individualized. The question has not been answered as to whether pharmacologic therapy in an asymptomatic, hypertensive, prepubertal child interferes with growth and development, but there are no data to suggest such adverse effects.

The first step in young children with persistently elevated levels of pressure is a dietary assessment of caloric and of salt intake. This evaluation should be undertaken in the context of the family's nutritional habits as well as their own cultural matrix. Food plays a central role in the nurturing of children. Primary hypertensives may be salt-sensitive, and this tendency may be greater in blacks than in other groups; therefore, attempts to reduce salt intake in black children may be more useful than is indicated in the current pediatric literature. It is not known whether salt reduction should be accompanied by potassium supplementation, but enough evidence is available to suggest that a potassium-rich diet might be useful. Supplementation with calcium has not been evaluated.

Older children and adolescents often eat in places other than their own homes. The ubiquitous presence of sodium creates difficulties for patients on a sodium-restricted intake to find easy ways of eating foods with their friends. Many fast food chains now offer salad bars, but peer pressure may result in the selection of high-sodium foods. An order of one superburger, french fries, and a chocolate shake contains about 1100 calories and at least 1 g of sodium before addition of salt at the table. The adolescent and his or her physician must agree on a therapeutic approach and must determine whether altering sodium intake will pose a significant burden. If they decide to lower salt intake, dietary counseling coupled with self-monitoring of urinary sodium may prove effective (Tochikubo et al., 1986).

Drug Therapy

Treatment of asymptomatic, mildly hypertensive individuals requires confronting young people with the threat of illness, even though they do not feel sick. In particular, affected adolescents must cope with the notion of a long-term, unremitting illness that may shorten their life span if they do not comply with treatment. Treatment requires sensitivity to their special problems, including their need to participate in decisions. In hypertensive children and adolescents who cannot or will not reduce their salt and caloric intake or in children whose BP remains abnormal despite dietary intervention, pharmacologic therapy is recommended with the usual choice of diuretic or beta blocker. The 1987 Second Task Force recommends beginning with less than a full dose of thiazide-type diuretics or less than a full dose of adrenergic inhibitor. In children with mild elevations of BP, thiazide therapy is often successful and has few side effects, although acute volume depletion is an immediate adverse effect. Long-term metabolic changes in children and adolescents treated with diuretics have not been reported; nevertheless, it is prudent to monitor young people for changes in lipids, glucose, and uric acid (Perez-Stable and Carolis, 1983). If the child does not respond to thiazide diuretics, the addition of a beta blocker is recommended for those without asthma. All children and adolescents receiving a beta blocker should have their pulse rate recorded and should exercise for 1 to 2 minutes to ensure that they can raise their pulse adequately when they are stressed (i.e., 20 beats/ minute or more). Children and parents should be cautioned about rebound hypertension if vomiting occurs or if the drug is abruptly stopped. Gill et al. (1976) noted that propranolol induced excessive bradycardia in several children and cardiac failure in two; Kallen et al. (1980) reported life-threatening hypoglycemia in children receiving propranolol.

Unlike the situation among adults, concern about long-term adverse cardiovascular effects has not yet changed pediatric recommendations to consider starting with angiotensin-converting enzyme (ACE) inhibitors or calcium channel blockers that do not alter cholesterol and triglycerides. If either diuretics or beta blockers in sufficient dosage do not provide BP control, an ACE inhibitor or calcium channel blocker may be warranted. These agents have been used in children with renal hypertension but not in children with primary hypertension. If adequate control is still not achieved, the drug may not have been taken or the diagnosis may be incorrect. Accordingly, if a response is not achieved, reevaluation with or without consultation is required.

Sometimes drug therapy can be stopped to determine whether it is still needed. Although there are few data about discontinuation of therapy, experience at CHLA suggests that the greatest success, although uncommon, occurs with concomitant salt and/or weight reduction. Periodic BP measurements should be continued to document the course of the child's BP, because many children still require treatment.

Further discussion of treatment of hypertension appears in the section on secondary causes.

Recommendations About Athletics

In the absence of definitive data, asymptomatic children and adolescents with mildly elevated BPs should be encouraged to participate in dynamic exercises. If they become symptomatic, they should be evaluated. Some sports, especially football, require participation in weightlifting programs. Youngsters who are asymptomatic before, during, and after these exercises should be allowed to play. However, the Second Task Force (1987) cautions that weight-lifting may lead to an increase in BP. The Task Force (1987) recommends aerobic exercises; in the absence of data on long-term effects of weightlifting on heart disease, isometric exercise should be avoided. In all symptomatic individuals, in all youngsters on treatment, and in those with electrocardiographic or echocardiographic changes of left ventricular hypertrophy, isometric exercises are potentially hazardous, and aerobic exercises should be substituted.

SECONDARY HYPERTENSION (TABLE 16.7)

The cause of most *prepubertal* hypertension is renal. The results of several published series differ in the distribution of causes and in the percentage of primary hypertension because of the sources of the data. Those publications describing severely ill children (Gill et al., 1976; Still and Cottom, 1967) are skewed toward renal causes, whereas Lieberman (1983) surveyed five Los Angeles hospitals for both inpatients and outpatients identified as hypertensive. Ogborn and Crocker (1987) studied children with sustained hypertension. In these five series, neither primary aldosteronism nor thyroid disease was reported. The need to include tests to diagnose primary aldosteronism and dexamethasone-suppressible hypertension during the *initial* evaluation phase is unclear, although PRA and electrolytes are recommended by some (Schärer et al., 1986; Dillon, 1987; Ogborn and Crocker, 1987).

The number of *postpubertal* children with renal hypertension also varies with the setting. Adolescents with severe hypertension sent to a referral service for evaluation and treatment are most likely to have a renal etiology, whereas those with mild hypertension are more likely to have primary hypertension. The number of pediatric patients with obscure etiologies for underlying hypertension is quite small. That fact should be kept in perspective so that expensive and invasive tests are reserved for individuals with significant symptomatic hypertension of unclear cause.

Neonatal Hypertension

Neonatal hypertension is a special situation. Recent detailed reviews are available (Rasoulpour and Martinelli, 1992; Singh et al., 1992). Data are now available for determining whether given levels of BP represent significant abnormalities for term infants (Table 16.8). With the advent of highly organized and well-equipped Neonatal Intensive Care Units, neonatal hypertension has been increasingly recognized since the 1970s.

Etiology

Major causes of neonatal hypertension are presented in Table 16.9. Singh et al. (1992) reported that 26 of 3179 infants admitted to a Neonatal Intensive Care Unit had hypertension (incidence 0.81%). They identified bronchopulmonary dysplasia (BPD), patent ductus arteriosus (PDA), intraventricular hemorrhage (IVH), and umbilical artery catheterization (UAC) as significant risk factors. Buchi and Siegler (1986) reported 53 infants admitted with hypertension representing 0.7% of all neonatal tertiary care admissions. These workers found that urinalysis, BUN, serum creatinine, and PRA (screening tests) were predictive of both etiology and outcome. Of the 53 infants studied, 23 had an identifiable etiology: 21 renal and 2 coarctation. Among the 53, 81% were normotensive without therapy by 1 year of age (Buchi and Siegler, 1986); 4 of 53 died, 2 of causes unrelated to hypertension, 1 of hypertension-related heart failure, and 1 of hypertensive encephalopathy.

If screening tests are abnormal, renal ultrasonography is advised. Pyelography has virtually been abandoned. Nuclear scans are not mentioned, although Adelman (1987) recommends them. If the response to treatment is unsatisfactory, additional diagnostic tests may be required,

Table 16.7. Causes of Hypertension in Children and Adolescents

Cause	Comments
Renal	
Bilateral involvement	
Glomerulonephritis, acute or chronic	Children and adolescents with these renal disorders have a characteristic constellation of symptoms, signs, and laboratory findings; diagnostic studies should be expedited and intervention should be prompt.
Previous infection (e.g., streptococcal)	
Henoch-Schönlein purpura	
Hemolytic-uremic syndrome	
Acute renal failure (acute interstitial nephritis, acute shutdown, acute tubular necrosis)	Hypertension is most often due to volume overload.
End-stage renal disease (ESRD)	Severe, chronic, resistant hypertension often is present when glomerular filtration rate (GFR) is < 5 ml/min/ 1.73 m^2
Bilateral or unilateral involvement	
Asymmetric renal disease (unilateral small kidney)	A significant cause of *malignant* and life-threatening hypertension in pediatrics. This diagnosis has generally been underemphasized in the literature.
Malformations including bilateral polycystic kidneys, hypoplasia, ureteropelvic junction obstruction	These anomalies are readily documented by renal ultrasonography ± nuclear scans in patients older than 1 month and with normal renal function. Patients with autosomal recessive polycystic renal disease often have life-threatening hypertension and congestive heart failure in the first months of life.
Pyelonephritis with or without hydronephrosis	*Reflux nephropathy* with scarred, small kidneys is a prominent cause of *malignant* hypertension, especially in girls ages 7 to 18 years.
Renal arterial disorders	
Renal artery stenosis (unilateral, bilateral or segmental), Takayasu's disease (affecting renal arteries), neurofibromatosis	Usually associated with moderate to *malignant* hypertension in pediatric patients from < 16 months to 18 years. Evaluation may be indicated in those with milder hypertension.
Thrombosis, embolus	*Especially important in neonates* and young infants. Hypertension may resolve after 6 months or more of medical therapy.
Tumors (renal): Wilms' juxtaglomerular tumors	Wilms' tumor has characteristic features and usually minimal if any hypertension; rarely associated with hyperreninemia and severe hypertension.
Trauma	Renal trauma acutely usually does not cause severe hypertension; long-term follow-up of severe trauma may uncover moderate to severe hypertension, however.
Cardiovascular	
Coarctation of the aorta	May be difficult to diagnose in neonate, readily diagnosed in older pediatric patients. The second most common cause of secondary hypertension after renal disorders.

Table 16.7. Causes of Hypertension in Children and Adolescents, *continued*

Cause	Comments
Hypoplasia of abdominal aorta (coarctation of the abdominal aorta; mid-aortic arch syndrome)	May be associated with markedly stunted growth. The severity of hypertension is correlated with the magnitude of renal artery involvement.
Endocrine Adrenal	
Congenital adrenal hyperplasia	Rare forms of hypertension in infancy and childhood.
Pheochromocytoma	Patients have wide variety of complaints, including *malignant hypertension.*
Central nervous system	
Infections, space-occupying lesions	Hypertension is component of altered central nervous system function. Usually not severe.
Dysautonomia (Riley Day syndrome)	Hypertension and hypotension often noted.
Burns	*Severe,* typically transient hypertension may accompany extensive third-degree burns, likely secondary to catecholamine discharge.
Orthopedic injuries and procedures	Hypertension frequently accompanies transient trauma to long bones, leg lengthening, and placement of Harrington rods for scoliosis.
Drug ingestion and abuse	
Sympathomimetics including amphetamines, ephedrine, phenylephrine eye drops	Patients may present with severe hypertension that readily resolves with drug withdrawal unless renal damage has occurred.
Glucocorticoids and mineralocorticoids	Mild hypertension unless agents are being used as part of regimen for significant underlying renal disease.
Rebound hypertension with withdrawal of antihypertensive agents	Important in young children who develop acute gastroenteritis and vomit maintenance oral antihypertensive agents.
Poisonings (lead, mercury)	

Table 16.8. Definition of Hypertension in Term Infants

Age Group	95th Percentile Value (mm Hg)		
	Systolic	Diastolic	Mean
Birth	90	60	70
7 days	92	69	77
8 days to 1 month	106	74	85

From Feld LG, Springate JE. Hypertension in children. *Curr Prob Pediatr* 1988;18(6):317.

but the risk/benefit ratio of invasive tests must be continuously borne in mind.

Renal Artery Disease. Before UAC became routine in neonatal centers, acquired renal arterial abnormalities were usually associated with extension of neonatal renal vein thrombosis or with embolization from patent ductus arteriosus (Durante et al., 1976). Now UAC has become commonplace, as has extracorporeal membrane oxygenation (ECMO). Complications of their use include renal artery thrombosis and stenosis with associated hypertension (Adelman, 1987). Initial experience with early nephrectomy for renal artery thrombosis was associated with a high death rate (Plumer et al., 1976). Subsequent use of aggressive medical therapy resulted in improved survival and decreased the need for surgery (Adelman, 1978).

Evaluation

The major difference in the approach advocated by Adelman (1984), by Vailas et al. (1986), and by myself is the need for diagnostic studies during the neonatal period. If the diagnosis of neonatal renovascular hypertension is suspected, renal scans and pyelograms are not

has permitted in utero detection of fetal abnormalities, especially renal ones (Elder, 1992). High-grade hydronephrosis in neonates has been attributed to high-grade reflux, which has been reported more often in boys than in girls (Elder, 1992). These infants are at some risk for serious long-term sequelae, which include proteinuria, hypertension, and ultimately renal failure (Bailey et al., 1983). Reports of long-term follow-up of large series of severely affected infants is not available, but all experts concur that heightened surveillance is required.

Although the incidence and prevalence of RN are unknown, it is more common in girls. The diagnosis should be considered in any child with urinary tract infection, especially if there is a family history of reflux nephropathy (Bailey et al., 1983). Children with uncomplicated infections have urinalyses that are protein-free unless they have high fever. If proteinuria is detected in a hypertensive child with a history of urinary tract infections and in the absence of fever, the child should be evaluated for reflux nephropathy. If reflux is detected, siblings also should be screened for reflux because of the known familial incidence of reflux and reflux nephropathy (Noe, 1992). Noninvasive screening for upper tract abnormalities can now easily be accomplished with renal ultrasonography. If any suspicious findings are encountered, voiding cystourethrography (VCUG) under standardized conditions should be done when the child is not infected.

The decision as to the optimal management plan rests on the severity of reflux, analysis of renal function, assessment of the family's ability to carry out long-term medical therapy, and cost considerations. The International Reflux Study in children was designed to study the impact of reflux on renal scarring, renal growth, renal function, urinary tract infections, and hypertension (International Reflux Study Committee, 1981). The long-term follow-up was designed to compare results of surgical versus nonsurgical intervention in children randomized according to degrees of reflux (Weiss et al., 1992). In summary, early and severe scarring associated with high-grade reflux (Grade IV) puts young children at significant risk whether they are treated conservatively (medically) or surgically with reimplantation.

Management of Sustained Hypertension (Table 16.11)

Clinicians responsible for the management of children with disorders not amenable to surgery are handicapped by the absence of long-term studies of treatment, including the follow-up of children and adolescents through periods of normal growth. Moreover, in the past, articles describing therapy could not separate the impact of each drug from that of polypharmacy (Potter et al., 1977; Sinaiko et al., 1980; Green et al., 1981).

Captopril, the most frequently used ACE inhibitor in pediatrics, is effective (Callis et al., 1986; O'Dea et al., 1988). Hyperkalemia as an acute event and proteinuria associated with immune complex nephropathy as a long-term problem have been reported (Mirkin and Newman, 1985). Other problems include cough, ageusia, and renal failure, especially in children with renal arterial disease. Bouissou et al. (1986) described 25 children (ages 1.5 to 18 years) with renal hypertension who received 29 courses of captopril therapy during a mean period of 14.8 months. Effective BP control occurred in all but 13%; the latter improved with addition of a beta blocker. Miller et al. (1986) studied 14 children with renal hypertension treated with enalapril, a longer-acting ACE inhibitor, for 3½ months to 1 year. The drug was well tolerated; however, two children had an increase in proteinuria. The major advantage of ACE inhibitors is their beneficial effect on renal hemodynamics in children with altered renal function. Studies with longer-acting ACE inhibitors have not been reported in young people.

The beneficial effects of sublingual nifedipine as a first-line drug for hypertensive emergencies in children are well recognized. Long-acting nifedipine has been used to treat chronic hypertension, but neither controlled studies nor specific guidelines for dosing schedules are available.

Children with chronic renal hypertension may require one or more agents shown in Table 16.11. Titration of dosages up to desired levels with avoidance of unpleasant reactions is a formidable task. Affected children, their families, and responsible caregivers all face a time-consuming, often tedious process of controlling BP without precipitating renal dysfunction.

Despite limitations concerning treatment of children with chronic renal hypertension, therapeutic goals can be set and reached. BP levels should be reduced over weeks to months to safe, tolerable levels. Although lowering of BP levels more quickly may alleviate both physician and patient anxiety, the short time spans do not permit the child adequate time for equilibration. In

Table 16.11. Treatment of Chronic Hypertension

Name of Drug	Oral Dose[a]	Comment
Diuretics		
Chlorothiazide	10 mg/kg/q 12 hours	Not effective in patients with decreased glomerular filtration rate (GFR). Observe for *acute volume depletion*, decreased K_s, decreased Na_s; long-term effects for children unknown.
or		
Hydrochlorothiazide	1 mg/kg/q 12 hours	
Furosemide	1 mg/kg/dose q 6 hours	Especially valuable in patients with decreased GFR. Causes hypercalciuria, *nephrocalcinosis,* and bone demineralization.
Vasodilators		
Hydralazine	0.5–1 mg/kg/dose q 8 hours	Frequently causes reflex tachycardia, abdominal discomfort, headache, especially IV; *lupus-like syndrome is rare in pediatrics.*
Minoxidil	0.025–0.05 mg/kg/q 12 hours	Salt and water retention can be modulated or prevented by concomitant diuretics. *Hypertrichosis* is important problem in pediatrics; resolves with discontinuation of drug. *Rebound hypertension* occurs with abrupt discontinuation. (Dose lower than that used by Second Task Force, 1987.)
Prazosin	20–25 µg/kg/dose q 8 hours	No studies of drug in pediatrics; clinical experience indicates that drug is well tolerated. First-dose effect dictates that patient receives initial dose supine; some children have *hair loss* with chronic use.
Nifedipine	0.25–0.5 mg/kg/dose 10 mg—adolescents	Evidence suggests useful drug for severe, symptomatic hypertension. Well tolerated except for tachycardia. Headache, flushing, dizziness occur.
Beta-adrenergic antagonists		
Propranolol	0.5–2.0 mg/kg/q 12 hours	Avoid in asthma and heart failure; may have problem with bradycardia, bronchospasm; hypoglycemia reported, especially in patients with inadequate oral intake; *rebound hypertension* with drug interruption. May impair mental performance and adversely affect lipids.
Atenolol	1–2 mg/kg/q 24 hours	No published experience in pediatrics; may be associated with some bronchospasm or mild bradycardia. Advantage over other adrenergic agents is lack of central nervous system effects, once-only daily dosage, fewer side effects than other adrenergic blockers.
Labetalol	100 mg BID—adolescents	Has alpha- and beta-adrenergic actions; does not affect exercise or alter lipids.
Central nervous system alpha-adrenergic agonists		
Methyldopa	10 mg/kg/q 6 hours	Dose adjustment required with decreased GFR. Interferes with mental concentration; sedation is common. May cause Coombs-positive test. *Rebound hypertension* reported on interrupting drug.

Table 16.11. Treatment of Chronic Hypertension, *continued*

Name of Drug	Oral Dose[a]	Comment
Clonidine	0.1–0.2 mg/24 hours	May be effective once daily; initial drowsiness; *rebound hypertension* occurs with abrupt discontinuation. Experience with use of weekly patch in children/adolescents is not published.
Clonidine patch	Dose not established	Some have trouble with the tape.
Angiotensin-converting (ACE) inhibitors		

Captopril
  Infants:
  Older:
	
	0.01–0.25 mg/kg q 12 hours
	0.25–0.5 mg/kg/q 8 hours
		Modification of dose needed in neonates, decreased GFR and renal artery stenosis. In these three, monitor blood pressure and creatinine carefully. May cause increased K_s, thrombocytopenia, neutropenia, nephropathy with secondary proteinuria, ageusia, cough, immune complex.

Enalapril	mg/kg/dose not established; start at 2.5 mg/kg/day and monitor need to increase to BID, and then to larger dose.	Currently being studied in pediatrics. Initial experience suggest agent is superior to captopril in terms of side effects, tolerance, and effectiveness. Monitor for neutropenia in lupus and other connective diseases. No adverse lipid effects.
Lisinopril and others	Dose not established	

[a]Lowest starting dose is given.

general, unless the child has significant symptomatic hypertension, there is no urgency to lower levels rapidly. The child's vasculature is less vulnerable to the ravages of hypertension, so that the known complications of stroke, myocardial infarction, and progressive kidney failure seen in the adult are unlikely.

Hypertensive Emergencies

An emergency exists when the BP becomes markedly elevated and symptoms or signs directly attributable to uncontrolled high BP develop, including CNS and visual disturbances.

The major causes of hypertensive emergencies in pediatrics usually are diagnosed easily (Table 16.12).

Treatment of hypertensive emergencies in young individuals has been made safer, easier, and more effective with the availability of agents listed in Table 16.13. The goal of treatment is a safe reduction of elevated pressure by decreasing both the systolic and the diastolic levels by approximately 33% of the elevation within the first 6 hours. The remainder of BP reduction to a preset goal, but not normalization, should take place within 36 to 72 hours. Sublingual nifedipine has been successfully used in infants and

Table 16.12. Causes of Hypertensive Emergencies in Pediatrics

Renal
  Acute glomerulonephritis
  Chronic renal failure and end-stage renal
    disease
  Hemolytic uremic syndrome
  Reflux nephropathy
  Renal artery stenosis
  Systemic lupus erythematosus
  Transplant rejection

Nonrenal
  Coarctation of the aorta
  Drug ingestion
  Pheochromocytoma
  Volume overload

children (Siegler and Brewer, 1988; Evans et al., 1988); the majority of patients respond without serious side effects. The duration of response, however, is highly variable. Intravenous labetolol (Houtman and Dillon, 1992) has been advocated, but it is less popular in the United States than in Europe. Once the BP is lowered to a level at which the patient becomes asymptomatic, oral agents can be introduced.

Table 16.13. Treatment of Hypertensive Emergencies

Drug	Onset of Action	Dose and Route	Comments
Nifedipine	Minutes	0.25–0.5 mg/kg/dose sublingual	Excellent first-line drug Avoids acute drops in BP
Captopril	Minutes	*Infants:* 0.01–0.25 mg/kg/dose *Children:* 0.1–0.2 mg/kg/dose PO	May acutely drop BP and cause acute renal failure
Hydralazine	Minutes	0.1–0.2 mg/kg IV	Tachycardia, headache
Diazoxide	Minutes	3–5 mg IV bolus	Usually requires furosemide because of salt and H_2O retention. Do not repeat within 1 hour.
Labetolol	Minutes	1–3 mg/kg IV	May drop BP acutely
Nitroprusside	Seconds	1–8 μm/kg/min IV	Drug of choice, requires admission to intensive care unit
Phentolamine	Seconds	0.1–0.2 mg/kg IV	Alpha blocker, for treatment of pheochromocytoma.

CONCLUSIONS

Hypertension in children and adolescents is now recognized as an important pediatric problem. Guidelines for the evaluation of single measurements of the blood pressure as well as multiple recordings are available. The factors associated with elevated levels are better understood. The approach to diagnosis, evaluation, and therapy can be systematized in a sequential, cost-effective, and psyche-protective fashion. The recommendations in this chapter should guide the clinician in the management of most children and adolescents with hypertension.

The author wishes to acknowledge the excellent secretarial help of Cari Adams.

References

Adelman RD. Neonatal hypertension. *Pediatr Clin North Am* 1978;25:99–109.

Adelman RD. Neonatal hypertension. In: Loggie JMH, Horan MJ, Gruskin AB, Hohn AR, Dunbar JB, Havlik RJ, eds. *NHLBI Workshop on Juvenile Hypertension.* New York: Biomedical Information Corporation, 1984:267–282.

Adelman RD. Long-term followup of neonatal renovascular hypertension. *Pediatr Nephrol* 1987;1:35–41.

Alpert BS, Fox ME. Racial aspects of blood pressure in children and adolescents. *Ped Clin North Am* 1993;40:13–22.

Anderson EA, Mahoney LT, Lauer RM, Clarke WR. Enhanced forearm blood flow during mental stress in children of hypertensive parents. *Hypertension* 1987;10:544–549.

Anderson NB. Racial differences in stress-induced cardiovascular reactivity and hypertension: current status and substantive issues. *Psychol Bull* 1989;105:89–105.

Aristimuno GG, Foster TA, Voors AW, Srinivasan SR, Berenson GS. Influence of persistent obesity in children on cardiovascular risk factors: the Bogalusa Study. *Circulation* 1984;69:895–904.

Aschinberg LC, Zeis PM, Miller RA, John EG, Chan LL. Essential hypertension in childhood. *JAMA* 238:322–324, 1977.

Bailey RR, Janus E, McLoughlin K, Lynn KL, Abbott GD. Familial and genetic data in reflux nephropathy. In: Hodson CJ, Heptinstall RH, Winberg J, eds. *Reflux Nephropathy Update: 1983.* Basel: Karger, 1984:40–51.

Bailey RR, Lynn KL. End-stage reflux nephropathy, In: Hodson CJ, Heptinstall RH, Winberg J, eds. *Reflux Nephropathy Update: 1983.* Basel: Karger, 1984:102–110.

Becque MD, Katch VL, Rocchini AP, Marks CR, Moorehead C. Coronary risk incidence of obese adolescents: reduction by exercise plus diet intervention. *Pediatrics* 1988;81:605–612.

Berenson GS, Lawrence M, Soto L. The heart and hypertension in childhood. *Semin Nephrol* 1989;9:236–246.

Bifano E, Post EM, Springer J, Williams ML, Streeten DHP. Treatment of neonatal hypertension with captopril. *J Pediatr* 1982;100:143–146.

Bouissou F, Meguira B, Rostin M, Fontaine C, Charlet JP, Barthe P. Long term therapy by captopril in children with renal hypertension. *Clin Exp Hypertens [A]* 1986;8:841–845.

Buchi KF and Siegler RL. Hypertension in the first month of life. *J Hypertens* 1986;4:525–528.

Calabrese EJ, Tuthill RW. The influence of elevated levels of sodium in drinking water on elementary and high school children in Massachusetts. In: Fregly MJ, Karl ML, eds. *The Role of Salt in Cardiovascular Hypertension.* New York: Academic Press, 1982:33–48.

Callis L, Vila A, Catalá J, Gras X. Long term treatment with captopril in pediatric patients with severe hypertension and chronic renal failure. *Clin Exp Hypertens [A]* 1986;8:847–851.

Canessa M, Adragna N, Solomon HS, Connolly TM, Tosteson DC. Increased sodium-lithium countertransport in red cells of patients with essential hypertension. *N Engl J Med* 1980;302:772–776.

Clarke WR, Woolson RF, Lever RM. Changes in ponderosity and blood pressure in childhood: the Muscatine Study. *Am J Epidemiol* 1986;124:195–206.

Cooper R, Liu K, Trevisan M, Miller W, Stamler J. Urinary sodium excretion and blood pressure in children: absence of a reproducible association. *Hypertension* 1983;5:135–139.

Cooper R, Van Horn L, Liu K, Trevisan M, Nans, S, Veshima H, Larbi E, Yu C, Sempos C, LeGrady D, Stamler J. A randomized trial on the effect of decreased dietary sodium intake on blood pressure in adolescents. *J Hypertens* 1984;2:361–366.

Court JM, Hill GJ, Dunlop M, Boulton TJC. Hypertension in childhood obesity. *Aust Paediatr J* 1974;10:296–300.

Daniels SR, Loggie JMH, Burton T, Kaplan S. Difficulties with ambulatory blood pressure monitoring in children. *J Pediatr* 1987;111:397–400.

Daniels SR, Meyer RA, Loggie JMH. Determinants of cardiac involvement in children and adolescents with essential hypertension. *Circulation* 1990;82:1243–1248.

deLeonardis V, DeScalzi M, Falchetti A, Cinelli P, Croppi E, Livi R, Scarpelli L, Scarpelli PT. Echocardiographic evaluation of children with and without family history of hypertension. *Am J Hypertens* 1988;1:305–308.

deSwiet M. The epidemiology of hypertension in children. *Br Med Bull* 1986;42: 172–175.

deSwiet M, Fayers PM, Shinebourne EA. Systolic blood pressure in a population of infants in the first year of life: the Brompton Study. *Pediatrics* 1980;65:1028–1035.

deSwiet M, Fayers PM, Shinebourne EA. Value of repeated blood pressure measurements in children—the Brompton Study. *Br Med J* 1980;1:567–569.

Dillon MJ. Investigation and management of hypertension in children. A personal perspective. *Pediatr Nephrol* 1987;1:59–68.

Dillon MJ. Blood pressure. *Arch Dis Child* 1988;63:347–349.

Durante D, Jones D, Spitzer R. Neonatal renal arterial embolism syndrome. J Pediatr 1976;89:978–979.

Dweck HS, Reynolds DW, Cassady G. Indirect blood pressure measurement in newborns. *Am J Dis Child* 1974;127:492–494.

Elder JS. Commentary: importance of antenatal diagnosis of vesicoureteral reflux. *J Urol* 1992;148:1750–1754.

Evans JHC, Shaw NJ, Brocklebank. Sublingual nifedipine in acute severe hypertension. *Arch Dis Child* 1988;63:975–977.

Falkner B. Vascular reactivity and hypertension in childhood. *Semin Nephrol* 1989;9: 247–252.

Falkner B, Kushner H, Khalsa DK, Canessa M, Katz S. Sodium sensitivity, growth and family history of hypertension in young blacks. *J Hypertens* 1986;4(Suppl):381–383.

Falkner B, Kushner H, Onesti G, Angelakos ET. Cardiovascular characteristics in adolescents who develop essential hypertension. *Hypertension* 1981;3:521–527.

Falkner B, Onesti G, Angelakos ET, Fernandes M, Langman C. Cardiovascular response to mental stress in normal adolescents with hypertensive patients. *Hypertension* 1979;1:23–30.

Falkner B, Onesti G, Angelakos ET. Effect of salt loading on the cardiovascular response to stress in adolescents. *Hypertension* 1981;3(Suppl 2):195–199.

Feld LG and Springate JF. Hypertension in children. *Curr Prob Pediatr* 1988;18: 317–373.

Ferrara LA, Moscato TS, Pisanti N, Marotta T, Krogh V, Capone D, Mancini M. Is the sympathetic nervous system altered in children with familial history of arterial hypertension? *Cardiology* 1988;75:200–205.

Filer LJ, Clarke WR, Lauer R, Burke GL. Blood pressure and sodium-lithium countertransport. In: Loggie JMH, Horan MJ, Gruskin AB, Hohn AR, Dunbar JB, Havlik RJ, eds. *NHLBI Workshop on Juvenile Hypertension*. New York: Biomedical Information Corporation, 1984:173–179.

Fixler DE, Laird WP, Fitzgerald V, Stead S, Adams R. Hypertension screening in schools: results of the Dallas study. *Pediatrics* 1979;63:32–36.

Garay RP, Elghozi J-L, Dagher G, Meyer P. Laboratory distinction between essential and secondary hypertension by measurement of erythrocyte cation fluxes. *N Engl J Med* 1980;302:769–771.

Gelenijnse JM, Grobbee DE, Hofman A. Sodium and potassium intake and blood pressure change in childhood. *Br Med J* 1990;300:899–902.

Gill DG, Mendes da Costa B, Cameron JS, Joseph MC, Chantler C. Analysis of 100 children with severe and persistent hypertension. *Arch Dis Child* 1976;51:951–956.

Gillman MW, Rosner B, Evans DA, Keough ME, Smith LA, Taylor JO, Hennekens CH. Use of multiple visits to increase blood pressure tracking correlations in childhood. *Pediatrics* 1991;87:708–711.

Gillum RF, Elmer PJ, Prineas RJ, Surbey D. Changing sodium intake in children. The Minneapolis children's blood pressure study. *Hypertension* 1981;3:698–703.

Gillum RF, Prineas RJ, Gomez-Marin O, Finn S, Chang P-N. Personality, behavior, family environment, family social status and hypertension risk factors in children. The Minneapolis Children's Blood Pressure Study. *J Chron Dis* 1985;38:187–194.

Goldring D, Londe S, Sivahoff M, Hernandez A, Britton C. Blood pressure in a high school population. *J Pediatr* 1977;91: 884–889.

Gomez-Marin O, Prineas RJ, Ristam L. Cuff bladder width and blood pressure measurement in children and adolescents. *J Hypertens* 1992;10:1235–1241.

Green TP, Nevins TE, Houser MT, Sibley R, Fish AJ, Sinaiko AR. Renal failure as a complication of acute antihypertensive therapy. *Pediatrics* 1981;67:850–854.

Grobbee DE. Predicting hypertension in childhood: Value of blood pressure measurement and family history. *J Am Coll Nutr* 1992;11:55S–59S.

Grobbee DE, Bak AAA. Electrolyte intake and hypertension in children, In: Rettig R, Ganten D, Luft F, eds. *Salt and Hypertension*. Heidelberg: Springer, 1989:283.

Grobbee DE, Hofman A. Results of intervention studies of blood pressure in childhood and adolescence. *Scand J Lab Clin Invest* 1989;192(Suppl):19–31.

Gruskin AB, Perlman SA, Baluarte JH, Morgenstern BZ, Polinsky MS, Kaiser BA. Primary hypertension in the adolescent: facts and unresolved issues. In: Loggie JMH, Horan MJ, Gruskin AB, Hohn AR, Dunbar JB, Havlik RJ, eds. *NHLBI Workshop on Juvenile Hypertension*. New York: Biomedical Information Corporation, 1983:305–333.

Gruskin AB, Perlman SA, Baluarte JH, Polinsky MS, Kaiser BA, Morgenstern BZ: The utility of renin profiling in childhood hypertension. *Clin Exp Hypertens [A]* 1986; 8:741–745.

Gutgesell M, Terrell G, Labarthe D. Pediatric blood pressure: ethnic comparisons in a primary care center. *Hypertension* 1981; 3:39–47.

Hansen HS, Nielsen JR, Hyldebrandt N, Froberg K. Blood pressure and cardiac structure in children with a parental history of hypertension: the Odense School Child Study. *J Hypertens* 1992;10:677–682.

Havlik RJ, Garrison RJ, Katz SH, Ellison RC, Feinleib M, Myrianthopoulos NC. Detection of genetic variance in blood pressure of seven-year-old twins. *Am J Epidemiol* 1979;109:512–516.

Hediger ML, Schall JI, Katz SH, Gruskin AB, Eveleth PB. Resting blood pressure and pulse rate distributions in black adolescents: the Philadelphia Blood Pressure Project. *Pediatrics* 1984;74:1016–1021.

Henningsen NC, Mattsson S, Nosslin B, Nelson D, Ohlsson O. Abnormal whole-body and cellular (erythrocytes) turnover of $^{22}Na^+$ in normotensive relatives of probands with established essential hypertension. *Clin Sci* 1979;57(Suppl 5):321–324.

Higgins M, Keller JB, Metzner HL, Moore FE, Ostrander LD Jr. Studies of blood pressure in Tecumseh, Michigan: II. Antecedents in children of high blood pressure in young adults. *Hypertension* 1980;2(Suppl 1):117–123.

Hiner LB, Gruskin AB, Baluarte HJ, Cote ML. Plasma renin activity in normal children. *J Pediatr* 1976;89:258–261.

Hofman A, Hazebroek A, Valkenburg HA. A randomized trial of sodium intake and blood pressure in newborn infants. *JAMA* 1983;250:370–373.

Horn PT. Persistent hypertension after prenatal cocaine exposure. *J Pediatr* 1992;121: 288–291.

Houtman PN, Dillon MJ. Medical management of hypertension in childhood. *Child Nephrol Urol* 1992;12:154–161.

Huai-yong C, Li-sheng L, De-yu Z. Comparison of erythrocyte membrane Ca^{2+}-Mg^{2+}-ATPase activity in children with and without family history of essential hypertension. *J Hum Hypertens* 1990;4:147–148.

International Reflux Study Committee. Medical versus surgical treatment of vesicoureteral reflux: a prospective international reflux study in children. *J Urol* 1981; 125:277–283.

Johnson EH, Spielbarger CD, Worden TJ, Jacobs GA. Emotional and familial determinants of elevated blood pressure in black and white adolescent males. *J Psychosom Res* 1987;31:287–300.

Johnson GL, Kotchen JM, McKean HE, Cottrill CM, Kotchen TA. Blood pressure related echocardiographic changes in adolescents and young adults. *Am Heart J* 1983;105:113–118.

Kallen RJ, Mohler JH, Lin HL. Hypoglycemia: a complication of treatment of hypertension with propranolol. *Clin Pediatr* 1980;19:567–568.

Kanai H, Matsuzawa Y, Tokunaga K, Keno Y, Kobatake T, Fujioka S, Nakajima T, Tarui S. Hypertension in obese children: fasting serum insulin levels are closely correlated with blood pressure. *Int J Obesity* 1990;14:1047–1056.

Kilcoyne MM. Adolescent hypertension II. Characteristics and response to treatment. *Circulation* 1974;50:1014–1019.

Kilcoyne MM, Richter RW, Alsup PA. Adolescent hypertension I. Detection and prevalence. *Circulation* 1974;50:758–764.

Kirkendall WM, Feinleib M, Freis ED, Mark AL. Recommendations for human blood pressure determinations by sphygmomanometers. Subcommittee of the AHA Postgraduate Education Committee. *Hypertension* 1981;3:510A–519A.

Kirkland RT, Kirkland JL. Systolic blood pressure measurements in the newborn infant with the transcutaneous Doppler method. *J Pediatr* 1972;80:52–56.

Korobkin M, Perloff DL, Palubinskas AJ. Renal arteriography in the evaluation of unexplained hypertension in children and adolescents. *J Pediatr* 1976;88:388–393.

Kotchen JM, Kotchen TA. Geographic effect on racial blood pressure differences in adolescents. *J Chron Dis* 1978;31:581–586.

Kotchen JM, Kotchen TA, Cottrill CM, Guthrie GP, Somes G. Blood pressures of young mothers and their first children 3–6 years following hypertension during pregnancy. *J Chron Dis* 1979;32:653–659.

Kotchen TA, Strickland AL, Rice TW, Walters DR. A study of the renin-angiotensin system in newborn infants. *J Pediatr* 1972;80:938–946.

Laird WB, Fixler DE. Left ventricular hypertrophy in adolescents with elevated blood pressure: assessment by chest roentgenography, electrocardiography, and echocardiography. *Pediatrics* 1981;67:255–259.

Lauer RM, Clarke WR, Beaglehoe R. Level, trend and variability of blood pressure during childhood: the Muscatine Study. *Circulation* 1984;69:242–249.

Lauer RM, Clarke WR, Mahoney LT, Witt J. Childhood predictors for high adult blood pressure. The Muscatine Study. *Pediatr Clin North Am* 1993;40:23–40.

Lever AF, Harrap SB. Essential hypertension: a disorder of growth with origins in childhood. *J Hypertens* 1992;10:101–120.

Levine LS, Lewy JE, New MI. Hypertension in high school students: screening results. *N Y State J Med* 1976;76:40–44.

Levinson S, Liu K, Stamler J, Stamler R, Whipple I, Ausbrook D, Berkson D. Ethnic differences in blood pressure in a biracial adolescent female population. *Am J Epidemiol* 1985;122:366–377.

Lieberman E. Clinical assessment of the hypertensive patient, In: Kotchen TA, Kotchen JM, eds. *Clinical Approaches to High Blood Pressure in the Young*. Boston: John Wright, 1983:237–248.

Loggie JMH. Essential hypertension in adolescents. *Postgrad Med* 1974;56:133–140.

Loggie JMH. Hypertension in children and adolescents. *Hosp Pract* 1975;10:81–92.

Loirat C, Pillion G, Blum C. Hypertension in children: present data and problems. *Adv Nephrol* 1982;11:65–98.

Londe S, Bourgoignie JJ, Robson AM, Goldring D. Hypertension in apparently normal children. *J Pediatr* 1971;78:569–577.

Luft FC, Miller JZ, Cohen SJ, Fineberg NS, Weinberger MH. Heritable aspects of salt sensitivity. *Am J Cardiol* 1988;61:1H–6H.

Macintyre S, Watt G, West P, Ecob R. Correlates of blood pressure in 15 year olds in the west of Scotland. *J Epid And Comm Health* 1991;45:143–147.

Mason T, Polak MJ, Pyles L, Mullet M, Swanke C. Treatment of neonatal renovascular hypertension with intravenous enalapril. *Am J Perinat* 1992;9:254–257.

McDonald A, Trevisan M, Cooper R, Stamler R, Gosch F, Ostrow D, Stamler J. Epidemiological studies of sodium transport and hypertension. *Hypertension* 1987;10(Suppl 1):42–47.

McGonigle LF, Beaudry MA, Coe JY. Recovery from neonatal myocardial dysfunction after treatment of acute hypertension. *Arch Dis Childh* 1987;62:614.

Michel MC, Galal O, Stroermer J, Bock KD, Brodde OE. Alpha and beta adrenoreceptors in hypertension. II. Platelet alpha$_2$ and lymphocyte beta$_2$-adrenoreceptors in children of parents with essential hypertension. A model for the pathogenesis of hypertension. *J Cardiovasc Pharm* 1989;13:432–439.

Michels VV, Bergstrath EJ, Hoverman VR, O'Fallon WM, Weidman WH. Tracking and prediction of blood pressure in children. *Mayo Clin Proc* 1987;62:875–881.

Miller K, Atkin B, Rodel PV, Walker JF. Enalapril: a well-tolerated and efficacious agent for the paediatric hypertensive patient. *J Hypertens* 1986;4(Suppl 5):413–416.

Mirkin BL, Newman TJ. Efficacy and safety of captopril in the treatment of severe childhood hypertension: report of the International Study Group. *Pediatrics* 1985;75:1091–1100.

Molineux, Steptoe A. Exaggerated blood pressure responses to submaximal exercise in normotensive adolescents with a family history of hypertension. *J Hypertens* 1988;6:361–365.

Mongeau JG. Erythrocyte cation fluxes in essential hypertension of children and adolescents. *Int J Pediatr Nephrol* 1985;6:41–46.

Mongeau JG. Heredity and blood pressure in humans: an overview. *Pediatr Nephrol* 1987;1:69–75.

Moss AJ: Blood pressure in infants, children and adolescents. *West J Med* 1981;134:296–314.

Munger RG, Prineas RJ, Gomez-Marin O. Persistent elevation of blood pressure among children with a family history of hypertension: the Minneapolis Children's Blood Pressure Study. *J Hypertens* 1988;6:647.

Murphy JK, Alpert BS, Walker SS. Ethnicity, pressor reactivity and children's blood pressure. *Hypertension* 1992;20:327–332.

Newman WP III, Freedman DS, Voors AW, Gard PD, Srinivasan SR, Cresanta JL, Williamson GD, Webber LS, Berenson GS. Relation of serum lipoprotein levels and systolic blood pressure to early atherosclerosis. The Bogalusa Heart Study. *N Engl J Med* 1986;314:138–144.

Noe HN. The long-term results of prospective sibling reflux screening. *J Urol* 1992;148:1739–1742.

O'Dea RF, Mirkin BL. Metabolic disposition of methyldopa in hypertensive and renal-insufficient children. *Clin Pharmacol Ther* 1980;27:37–43.

O'Dea RF, Mirkin BL, Alward CT, Sinaiko AR. Treatment of neonatal hypertension with captopril. *J Pediatr* 1988;113:403–406.

Ogborn MR, Crocker JFS. Investigation of pediatric hypertension. *Am J Dis Child* 1987;141:1205–1209.

Parker FC, Croft JB, Cresanta JL, Freedman DS, Burke GL, Webber LS, Berenson GS. The association between cardiovascular response tasks and future blood pressure levels in children: Bogalusa Heart Study. *Am Heart J* 1987;113:1174–1179.

Pennisi AJ, Takahashi M, Bernstein BH, Singsen BH, Uittenbogaart C, Ettenger RB, Malekzadeh MH, Hanson V, Fine RN. Minoxidil therapy in children with severe hypertension. *J Pediatr* 1977;90:813–819.

Perez-Stable E, Carolis PV. Thiazide-induced disturbance in carbohydrate, lipid and potassium metabolism. *Am Heart J* 1983;106:245–251.

Perlman JM, Volpe JJ. Neurologic complications of captopril treatment of neonatal hypertension. *Pediatrics* 1989;83:47–52.

Perlman SA, Prebis JW, Gruskin AB, Polinsky MS, Kaiser BA, Baluarte HJ, Morgenstern BZ. Calcium homeostasis in adolescents with essential hypertension. *Semin Nephrol* 1983;3:149–158.

Plumer LB, Kaplan GW, Mendoza SA. Hypertension in infants: a complication of umbilical arterial catheterization. *J Pediatr* 1976;89:802–805.

Potter DE, Schambelan M, Salvatierra O Jr, Orloff S, Holliday MA. Treatment of high-renin hypertension with propranolol in children after renal transplantation. *J Pediatr* 1977;90:307–311.

Prineas RJ, Gillum RF, Gomez-Marin O. The determinants of blood pressure levels in children: the Minneapolis children's blood pressure study. In: Loggie JMH, Horan MJ, Gruskin AB, Hohn AR, Dunbar JB, Havlik RJ, eds. *NHLBI Workshop on Juvenile Hypertension*. New York: Biomedical Information Corporation, 1984:21–35.

Prineas RJ, Gomez-Marin O, Gillum RF. Children's blood pressure. Dietary control of blood pressure by weight loss. In: *Report of the 85th Ross Conference on Pediatric Research*, 1985:120.

Rames LK, Clarke WR, Connor WE, Reiter MA, Lauer RM. Normal blood pressures and the evaluation of sustained blood pressure elevation in childhood: the Muscatine study. *Pediatrics* 1978;61:245–251.

Rasoulpour M, Martinelli K. Systemic hypertension. *Clin Perinatol* 1992;19:121–137.

Report of the Second Task Force on Blood Pressure Control in Children—1987. *Pediatrics* 1987;79:1–25.

Rocchini AP. Adolescent obesity and hypertension. *Pediatr Clin North Am* 1993;40:81–92.

Rocchini AP, Katch V, Anderson J, Hinderliter J, Becque D, Martin M, Marks C: Blood pressure and obese adolescents: effect of weight loss. *Pediatrics* 1988;82:16–23.

Rocchini AP, Key J, Bondie D, Chico R, Moorehead C, Katch V, Martin M. The effect of weight loss on the sensitivity of blood pressure to sodium in obese adolescents. *N Eng J Med* 1989;321:580–585.

Rose RJ, Miller JZ, Grim CE, Christian JC. Aggregation of blood pressure in the families of identical twins. *Am J Epidemiol* 1979;109:503–511.

Rosner B, Hennekens CH, Kass EH, Miall WE. Age-specific correlation analysis of longitudinal blood pressure data. *Am J Epidemiol* 1977;106:306–313.

Schärer K, Rascher W, Ganten D, et al, eds. Proceedings of the Second International Symposium on Hypertension in Children and Adolescents, Heidelberg (FRG): Recommendations for the diagnosis of hypertension in children and adolescents. *Clin Exp Hypertens [A]* 1986;8:913–914.

Schieken RM. Exercise study of blood pressure. a predictor of future hypertension? In: Loggie JMH, Horan MJ, Gruskin AB, Hohn AR, Dunbar JB, Havlik RJ, eds. *NHLBI Workshop on Juvenile Hypertension.* New York: Biomedical Information Corporation, 1984:145–159.

Schieken RM, Clarke WR, Lauer RM. Left ventricular hypertrophy in children with blood pressures in the upper quintile of the distribution: the Muscatine Study. *Hypertension* 1981;3:669–675.

Schieken RM, Clarke WR, Prineas R, Klein V, Lauer RM. Electrocardiographic measures of the left ventricular hypertrophy across the distribution of blood pressure: the Muscatine Study. *Circulation* 1982;66: 428–432.

Sfakianakis GN, Sfakianakis E, Paredes A, Abitbol C, Zilleruelo G, Goldberg RN, Strauss J. Single-dose captopril scintigraphy in the neonate with renovascular hypertension: reduction of renal failure, a side effect of captopril therapy. *Biol Neonate* 1988;54:246–253.

Shear CL, Burke GL, Freedman DS, Berenson GS. Value of childhood blood pressure measurements and family history in predicting future blood pressure status: results from 8 years of followup in the Bogalusa Heart Study. *Pediatrics* 1986;77:862–869.

Shibutani Y, Sakamoto K, Katsuno S, Yoshimoto S, Matsuura T. An epidemiological study of plasma renin activity in schoolchildren in Japan: distribution and its relation with family history of hypertension. *J Hypertens* 1989;6:489–493.

Siegler RL, Brewer ED. Effect of sublingual or oral nifedipine in the treatment of hypertension. *J Pediatr* 1988;112:811–813.

Siegler RL, Brewer ED, Corneli HH, Thompson JA. Hypertension first seen as facial paralysis: case reports and review of the literature. *Pediatrics* 1991;87:387–389.

Silverberg DS, Van Nostrand C, Juchli B, Smith ESO, Van Dorsser E. Screening for hypertension in a high school population. *Can Med Assoc J* 1975;113:103–113.

Sinaiko AR. Pharmacologic management of childhood hypertension. *Pediatr Clin North Am* 1993;40:195–212.

Sinaiko AR, Gomez-Marin O, Prineas RJ. Prevalence of significant hypertension in junior high school-aged children. The Children and Adolescent Blood Pressure Program. *J Pediatr* 1989;114:664–669.

Sinaiko AR, Kashtan CE, Mirkin BL. Antihypertensive drug therapy with captopril in children and adolescents. *Clin Exp Hypertens [A]* 1986;8:829–839.

Sinaiko AR, O'Dea RF, Mirkin BL. Clinical response of hypertensive children to long-term minoxidil therapy. *J Cardiovasc Pharmacol* 1980;2(Suppl 2):181–188.

Singh HP, Hurley M, Myers TG. Neonatal hypertension: incidence and risk factors. *Am J Hypertens* 1992;5:51–55.

Stark P, Beckerhoff R, Leumann EP, Vetter W. Siegenthaler W. Control of plasma aldosterone in infancy and childhood. A study of plasma renin activity, plasma cortisol and plasma aldosterone. *Helv Paediatr Acta* 1975;30:349–356.

Steinberger J, Rocchini AP. Is insulin resistance responsible for the lipid abnormalities seen in obesity? *Circulation* 1991; 84(Suppl 2):5.

Still JL, Cottom D. Severe hypertension in childhood. *Arch Dis Child* 1967;42:34–39.

Subcommittee on Atherosclerosis and Hypertension in Childhood of the Council on Cardiovascular Disease in the Young, American Heart Association. integrated cardiovascular health promotion in childhood. *Circulation* 85:1638, 1992.

Tochikubo O, Sasaki O, Umemura S, Kaneko Y. Management of hypertension in high school students by using new salt titrator tape. *Hypertension* 1986;8:1164–1171.

Trevisan M, Strazzullo P, Cappuccio FP, DiMuro MR, DeColle S, Franzese A, Iacone R, Krogh V. Red blood cell Na content, Na, Li-countertransport, family history of hypertension and blood pressure in school children. *J Hypertens* 1988;6: 227–230.

Uhari M, Koskimies O. A survey of 164 Finnish children and adolescents with hypertension. *Acta Paediatr Scand* 1979;68: 193–198.

Vailas GN, Brouillette RT, Scott JP, Shkolnik A, Conway J, Wiringa K. Neonatal aortic thrombosis: recent experience. *J Pediatr* 1986;109:101–108.

Voors AW, Webber LS, Frerichs RR, Berenson GS. Body height and body mass: a determinant of basal blood pressure in children: the Bogalusa Heart Study. *Am J Epidemiol* 1977;106:101–115.

Voors AW, Webber LS, Berenson GL. Racial contrasts in cardiovascular response tests for children from a total community. *Hypertension* 1980;2:686.

Weinberger MH, Miller JZ, Fineberg NS, Luft FC, Grim CE, Christian JC. Association of haptoglobin with sodium sensitivity and resistance of blood pressure. *Hypertension* 1987;10:443–446.

Weismann DN. Systolic or diastolic blood pressure significance. *Pediatrics* 1988;82:112.

Weiss R, Duckett J, Spitzer A. Results of a randomized clinical trial of medical versus surgical management of infants and children with grades III and IV primary vesicoureteral reflux (United States). *J Urol* 1992;148:1667–1673.

Wells TG, Bunchman TE, Kearns GL. Treatment of neonatal hypertension with enalaprilat. *J Pediatr* 1990;117:664–667.

Williams S, St George IM, Silva PA. Intrauterine growth retardation and blood pressure at age seven and eighteen. *J Clin Epidiol* 1992;45:1257–1263.

Wilson PD, Ferencz C, Dischinger PC, Brennar JI, Zeger SL. Twenty-four-hour ambulatory blood pressure in normotensive adolescent children of hypertensive and normotensive parents. *Am J Epidemiol* 1988;127:946–954.

Wilson SL, Gaffney FA, Laird WP, Fixler DE. Body size, composition and fitness in adolescents with elevated blood pressure. *Hypertension* 1985;7:417–422.

Zinner SH, Levy PS, Kass EH. Familial aggregation of blood pressure in childhood. *N Engl J Med* 1971;284:401–404.

Zinner SH, Margolius HS, Rosner B, Keiser HR, Kass WH. Familial aggregation of urinary kallikrein excretion in childhood: relation to blood pressure, race and urinary electrolytes. *Am J Epidemiol* 1976;104:124–132.

Zinner SH, Margolius HS, Rosner B, Kass EH. Stability of blood pressure rank and urinary kallikrein concentration in childhood: an eight-year followup. *Circulation* 1978;58:908–915.

Index

Page numbers in *italics* denote figures; those followed by "t" denote tables.